Neonatology Questions and Controversies

Infectious Disease, Immunology, and Pharmacology

Neonatology Questions and Controversies

Infectious Disease, Immunology, and Pharmacology

Second Edition

Series Editor

Richard A. Polin, MD
William T Speck Professor of Pediatrics
Executive Vice Chair Department of Pediatrics
Vagelos College of Physicians and Surgeons
Columbia University

Other Volumes in the Neonatology Questions and Controversies Series

GASTROENTEROLOGY AND NUTRITION

HEMATOLOGY AND TRANSFUSION MEDICINE

NEONATAL HEMODYNAMICS

NEUROLOGY

RENAL, FLUID AND ELECTROLYTE DISORDERS

THE NEWBORN LUNG

2nd Edition

Neonatology Questions and Controversies

Infectious Disease, Immunology, and Pharmacology

William E. Benitz, MD
Philip Sunshine Professor in Neonatology
Emeritus
Pediatrics/Neonatal & Developmental
Medicine
Stanford University
Stanford, California
United States

James L. Wynn, MD
Professor of Pediatrics,
University of Florida
Gainesville, Florida
United States

P. Brian Smith, MD MPH MHS
Samuel L. Katz Professor
Pediatrics
Duke University Medical Center
Durham, North Carolina
United States

Consulting Editor

Richard A. Polin, MD
William T Speck Professor of Pediatrics
Executive Vice Chair Department of Pediatrics
Vagelos College of Physicians and Surgeons
Columbia University
New York City, New York
United States

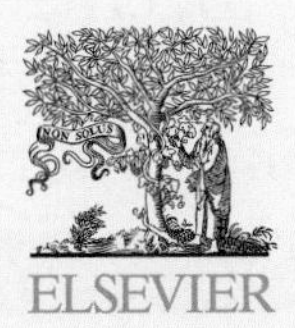

ELSEVIER

Elsevier
1600 John F. Kennedy Blvd.
Ste 1800
Philadelphia, PA 19103-2899

NEONATOLOGY QUESTIONS AND CONTROVERSIES:
INFECTIOUS DISEASE, IMMUNOLOGY, AND PHARMACOLOGY
ISBN: 978-0-323-87906-4

Content Strategist: Sarah Barth
Senior Content Development Specialist: Vasowati Shome
Content Development Manager: Ranjana Sharma
Publishing Services Manager: Shereen Jameel
Project Manager: Haritha Dharmarajan
Design Direction: Margaret Reid

Printed in India

Last digit is the print number: 9 8 7 6 5 4 3 2 1

Contributors

Julie Autmizguine, MD, MHS
Associate Professor
Pharmacology and Physiology
Université de Montréal
Associate Professor
Pediatrics
Université de Montréal
Infectious Disease Pediatrician
Pediatrics
CHU Sainte-Justine
Montréal, Québec
Canada
Antibiotic Considerations for Necrotizing Enterocolitis

Alejandra Barrero-Castillero, MD, MPH
Attending Neonatologist
Department of Neonatology
Beth Israel Deaconess Medical Center
Neonatologist
Department of Newborn Medicine
Boston Children's Hospital;
Instructor
Department of Pediatrics
Harvard Medical School
Boston, Massachusetts
United States
Perinatal and Neonatal Considerations in COVID-19

Sonia Lomeli Bonifacio, MD
Clinical Professor of Pediatrics
Division of Neonatal & Developmental Medicine
Stanford University
Palo Alto, California
United States
Neuroprotective Therapies in Newborns

C. Michael Cotten, MD, MHS
Professor
Department of Pediatrics
Duke University
Durham, North Carolina
United States
Antibiotic Stewardship

Jessica E. Ericson, MD, MPH
Associate Professor
Department of Pediatrics
Pennsylvania State College of Medicine
Hershey, Pennsylvania
United States
Empiric Therapy for Neonatal Sepsis

Laura Fillistorf, MS
Department Mother-Woman-Child
Clinic of Neonatology
Lausanne University Hospital and University of Lausanne
Switzerland
Clinical and Molecular Markers to Assist Decision-Making in Neonatal Sepsis

Susannah Franco, PharmD
Neonatal and Pediatric Clinical Pharmacist
Department of Pharmacy
SUNY Downstate Health Sciences University
University Hospital at Downstate
Brooklyn, New York
United States
Gonococcal Eye Prophylaxis—Are Mandates Still Justified?

Eric Giannoni, MD
Department Mother-Woman-Child
Lausanne University Hospital and University of Lausanne
Switzerland
Clinical and Molecular Markers to Assist Decision-Making in Neonatal Sepsis

Rachel G. Greenberg, MD, MB, MHS
Associate Professor
Department of Pediatrics
Duke Clinical Research Institute
Durham, North Carolina
United States
When to Perform Lumbar Puncture in Infants at Risk for Meningitis in the Neonatal Intensive Care Unit

Margaret R. Hammerschlag, MD
Professor
Department of Pediatrics
Division of Pediatric Infectious Diseases
SUNY Downstate Health Sciences University
Professor
Department of Medicine
SUNY Downstate Health Sciences University
Brooklyn, New York
United States
Gonococcal Eye Prophylaxis—Are Mandates Still Justified?

Mina Hanna, MD
Associate Professor of Pediatrics
Department of Pediatrics
University of Kentucky
Lexington, Kentucky
United States
Drug-Associated Acute Kidney Injury in Neonates

Rachel K. Hopper, MD
Clinical Associate Professor
Department of Pediatrics (Cardiology)
Stanford University School of Medicine
Palo Alto, California
United States
Vasodilator Drugs for Pulmonary Hypertension in Bronchopulmonary Dysplasia

Nazia Kabani, MD, MSPH
Assistant Professor
Department of Pediatrics
University of Alabama at Birmingham
Divisions of Neonatology and Pediatric Infectious Diseases
University of Alabama at Birmingham
Birmingham, Alabama
United States
Neonatal Herpes Simplex Virus Infection

David Alan Kaufman, MD
Professor
Department of Pediatrics
University of Virginia School of Medicine
Charlottesville, Virginia
United States
Neonatal Fungal Infections

Julie J. Kim-Chang, MD
Assistant Professor
Department of Pediatrics
Duke University School of Medicine
Durham, North Carolina
United States
Recent Advances and Controversies in Inborn Errors of Immunity Presenting in the Newborn Period

David W. Kimberlin, MD
Professor
Department of Pediatrics
University of Alabama at Birmingham;
Sergio Stagno Endowed Chair in Pediatric Infectious Diseases
University of Alabama at Birmingham;
Co-Director, Division of Pediatric Infectious Diseases
University of Alabama at Birmingham
Birmingham, Alabama
United States
Neonatal Herpes Simplex Virus Infection

Prabhakar Kocherlakota, MD, FAAP
Director
Elaine Kaplan Neonatal Intensive Care Unit
Montefiore St. Luke's Cornwall Hospital
Newburgh
Associate Professor of Pediatrics
New York Medical College
Valhalla, New York
United States
Pharmacological Therapy of Neonatal Abstinence Syndrome

Edmund F. La Gamma, MD, FAAP
Chief
Division of Newborn Medicine
Director
Neonatal-Perinatal Fellowship Program
Professor of Pediatrics
Biochemistry & Molecular Biology
The Regional Neonatal Center
Maria Fareri Children's Hospital
Westchester Medical Center
New York Medical College
Valhalla, New York
United States
Pharmacological Therapy of Neonatal Abstinence Syndrome

Shelley M. Lawrence, MD, MS
Associate Professor
Department of Pediatrics
Division of Neonatology
University of Utah
Salt Lake City, Utah
United States
Congenital Syphilis

Hillary Liken, MD
Pediatric Cardiology Fellowship Program
University of Michigan
Ann Arbor, Michigan
United States
Neonatal Fungal Infections

Ahmed Moussa, MD, MEd
Neonatologist
Department of Pediatrics
CHU Sainte-Justine;
Associate Professor
Department of Pediatrics
University of Montreal
Montreal, Quebec
Canada
Antibiotic Considerations for Necrotizing Enterocolitis

Sagori Mukhopadhyay, MD, MMSc
Assistant Professor
Department of Pediatric Medicine
University of Pennsylvania
Children's Hospital of Philadelphia
Philadelphia, Pennsylvania
United States
Management of the Asymptomatic Newborn at Risk for Sepsis

Namrita J. Odackal, DO
Assistant Professor
Department of Pediatrics
Nationwide Children's Hospital
The Ohio State University
Columbus, Ohio
United States
Neonatal Fungal Infections

Sallie R. Permar, MD, PhD
Nancy C. Paduano and Chair
Department of Pediatrics
Weill Cornell Medical Center
New York
United States
When and How to Treat Neonatal CMV Infection

Karen Marie Puopolo, MD, PhD
Professor
Department of Pediatric Medicine
University of Pennsylvania, Children's Hospital of Philadelphia
New York, Pennsylvania
United States
Management of the Asymptomatic Newborn at Risk for Sepsis

Christine M. Salvatore, MD
Associate Professor and Chief
Division of Pediatric Infectious Diseases
Weill Cornell Medicine
New York, New York
United States
When and How to Treat Neonatal CMV Infection

Amanda G. Sandoval Karamian, MD
Assistant Professor
Division of Pediatric Neurology
University of Utah
Salt Lake City, Utah
United States
Antiseizure Medications and Treatments in Neonates

John William Sleasman, MD
Dr. Glenn A. Kiser and Eltha Muriel Kiser Professor of Pediatrics
Department of Pediatrics
Duke University School of Medicine
Durham, North Carolina
United States
Recent Advances and Controversies in Inborn Errors of Immunity Presenting in the Newborn Period

Ashley Stark, MD, MS
Physician
Department of Neonatology
Duke University
Durham, North Carolina
United States
When to Perform Lumbar Puncture in Infants at Risk for Meningitis in the Neonatal Intensive Care Unit

Martin Stocker, MD, MME
Clinic of Neonatology and Paediatric Intensive Care
Children's Hospital
Lucerne
Switzerland
Clinical and Molecular Markers to Assist Decision-Making in Neonatal Sepsis

Brynne Archer Sullivan, MD, MSCR
Assistant Professor
Department of Pediatrics
University of Virginia
Charlottesville, Virginia
United States
Organ Dysfunction in Sepsis and Necrotizing Enterocolitis

Rachel T. Sullivan, MD
Assistant Professor
Department of Pediatric (Cardiology)
Vanderbilt University
Nashville, Tennessee
United States
Vasodilator Drugs for Pulmonary Hypertension in Bronchopulmonary Dysplasia

Joseph Y. Ting, MBBS, MPH
Associate Professor
Division of Neonatal-Perinatal Care, Department of Pediatrics,
University of Alberta,
Edmonton, Alberta
Canada
Antibiotic Considerations for Necrotizing Enterocolitis

Krisa P. Van Meurs, MD
Rosemarie Hess Professor of Neonatal and Developmental Medicine
Department of Pediatrics
Stanford University School of Medicine
Palo Alto, California
Medical Director
NeuroNICU
Lucile Packard Children's Hospital Stanford
Palo Alto, California
United States
Neuroprotective Therapies in Newborns

Zachary Andrew Vesoulis, MD, MSCI
Assistant Professor
Department of Pediatrics
Washington University
St. Louis, Missouri
United States
Organ Dysfunction in Sepsis and Necrotizing Enterocolitis

Courtney J. Wusthoff, MD, MS
Associate Professor
Division of Child Neurology
Stanford University
Neurology Director
NeuroNICU
Lucile Packard Children's Hospital Stanford
Palo Alto, California
United States
Antiseizure Medications and Treatments in Neonates

Series Foreword

"To study the phenomena of disease without books is to sail an uncharted sea, while to study books without patients is not to go to sea at all."

"Medicine is learned by the bedside and not in the classroom. Let not your conceptions of disease come from the words heard in the lecture room or read from the book. See and then reason and compare and control. But see first."

Sir William Osler

Before the invention of movable type by Johannes Gutenberg in the 15th century, physicians learned medicine through apprenticeships with individuals considered experienced. There were no printed textbooks, and medical journals were not published until the beginning of the 19th century. By serving as an apprentice to a physician over a period of years, one could learn how to be a competent practitioner. Internships in the United States evolved from those early apprenticeships in the 18th century. The term "residency" came into use because a physician in training had a residence at the hospital. Modern-day internships began in 1904 at The Johns Hopkins Hospital, which was founded by Sir Williams Osler, William S. Halstead, William H. Welch, and Howard A. Kelly. Halstead is credited with creating the first surgical residency, and he coined the phrase "see one, do one, teach one" (SODOTO). That educational philosophy has been adopted by nearly every specialty in medicine including neonatology.

Modern-day trainees in neonatology still learn how to care for critically ill infants and how to perform procedures by watching, assisting, and listening to more experienced individuals at the bedside. The SODOTO approach is considered a fundamental educational tool. However, over a 3-year period, much of education occurs remote from the bedside during teaching rounds and conferences. The teaching is often more theoretical, and, by design, rounds in the nursery and conferences are passive learning exercises. In those settings, trainees listen but do not take an active role in the educational process. Learning is always more effective when recipients take an active role in their own education. Ideally, they should be questioning what they hear, reading pertinent literature, and, when the opportunity arises, teaching others. Unfortunately, the transmission of information in such settings is not usually followed by an active phase of questioning and reading by the trainees.

Most graduates of fellowship programs turn out to be excellent practitioners, but when they leave the fellowship program new information is acquired only intermittently, either at conferences or from journals and textbooks. As a source of new information, journals provide access to the most up-to-date information. However, that information can be unfiltered, and the conclusions of a study may not be appropriate (or perhaps risky) for a critically ill infant. Textbooks such as those in the Neonatology Questions and Controversies Series offer an opportunity to hear from experts in neonatal–perinatal medicine who have synthesized (and filtered) the existing literature and can provide up-to-date recommendations.

The fourth edition of the Neonatology Questions and Controversies Series also has seven volumes. Each of them has been extensively revised, and we have added several new editors: Terri Inder has joined Jeffrey Perlman for the *Neurology* volume; James Wynn joined William Benitz and P. Brian Smith as a coeditor for the *Infectious Disease and Pharmacology* volume; and Patrick McNamara is now a coeditor with Martin Kluckow for the *Hemodynamics and Cardiology* volume. The reader will find many completely new chapters; however, just as in the previous edition, each of them is focused on day-to day clinical decisions encountered by neonatologists. Nothing will replace the teaching that occurs at the bedside when confronted with a critically ill neonate, and the SODOTO educational approach still plays an important role in education. Procedures are best learned by simulations and the guidance of experienced practitioners at the bedside. However, expertise as a practitioner can only be enhanced by reading and incorporating new information into daily practice, when that information has been proven safe and effective. Perhaps SODOTO should be changed to LQRT (listen, question, read, teach). The Neonatology Questions and Controversies Series is a unique resource for learning from experts in the field who have been through the LQRT process many times. The quotes by Sir Osler at the top of this Foreword suggest that both bedside teaching and journals and textbooks have synergistic roles in physician education, and neither alone is sufficient.

As with all prior editions, I am indebted to an exceptional group of volume editors who chose the content and authors and edited the manuscripts. I also want to thank Sarah Barth (Publisher), as well as Vasowati Shome and Vaishali Singh (Senior Content Development Specialists), at Elsevier who have guided the development of this series.

Richard A. Polin, MD

Preface

Infants have distinct immune system function that renders them susceptible to a broad array of infections. Many of these infections carry lifelong consequences. Infants also have rapidly changing hepatic and renal systems, leading to marked differences in how they metabolize and eliminate drugs. In this second edition of the *Infectious Disease and Pharmacology* volume of the Neonatology Questions and Controversies Series, we present three sections to address the unique pathophysiology of the infant. Section 1, Infectious Disease, includes a number of chapters on infectious diseases, among them new chapters on COVID-19, congenital syphilis, gonococcal eye prophylaxis, and organ dysfunction in sepsis and necrotizing enterocolitis. Section 2, Pharmacology, includes a new chapter on drug-associated acute kidney injury. Finally, we added a third section specifically focused on immunology which includes two chapters: one on inborn errors of immunity presenting in the newborn period and one on clinical and molecular markers for the diagnosis of neonatal sepsis. Contributors to this edition include pediatricians, neonatologists, and experts in pediatric infectious disease, neurology, and pharmacology, representing a wide variety of research interests. We hope that these updates will prove valuable to our colleagues who are responsible for the management of newborn babies as they navigate the often hazardous transition to extrauterine life.

William E. Benitz, MD
James L. Wynn, MD
P. Brian Smith, MD, MPH, MHS

Contents

Neonatology Questions and Controversies

Infectious Disease, Immunology, and Pharmacology

SECTION 1

Infectious Disease

Chapter 1

Management of the Asymptomatic Newborn at Risk for Sepsis

Sagori Mukhopadhyay, MD, MMSc; Karen Marie Puopolo, MD, PhD

Key Points

- The current incidence of neonatal early-onset sepsis (EOS) among infants born ≥37 weeks is relatively low (≈1/2000) and as much as 20-fold lower among well-appearing term infants.
- There are three major approaches to EOS risk assessment among term infants: categorical consideration of risk factors, multivariate consideration of risk factors in combination with clinical condition, and consideration of the clinical condition alone as it evolves in the first 48 hours after birth.
- Currently available laboratory tests lack sensitivity for predicting culture-confirmed EOS among term infants.
- EOS-associated clinical activities may have a significant impact on early mother–newborn interactions and initiation of breastfeeding.
- Depending on the local structure of care, EOS risk assessment activities are costly in terms of caregiver time, resource allocation, and monetary expenditures.
- Preclinical animal and clinical human studies demonstrate an impact of perinatally administered antibiotics on the initial composition of the newborn gut microbiome.
- Retrospective human epidemiologic studies associate perinatal and early infancy antibiotics with multiple morbidities in early childhood.

Introduction

Management of newborns at risk of early-onset bacterial sepsis (EOS) is one of the most common clinical tasks conducted by perinatal clinicians. Depending on the local structure of care, decisions are made by midwives, community pediatricians, resident house staff, newborn hospitalists, or neonatal intensive care specialists. EOS risk management begins with an assessment of whether the newborn is at a higher-than-average risk for EOS, continues to deciding whether or not to administer empiric antibiotic therapy, and ends with the decision to stop or extend empiric therapies, if given. Caregivers engage in this management to protect newborns from what may be a serious and even life-threatening infection. However, as the incidence of EOS has declined in the United States and the potential effects of early antibiotic exposures are considered, risk management has become increasingly controversial, especially among initially well-appearing infants born at term.[1,2] The incidence of EOS among all infants born ≥37 weeks' gestation is now approximately 1 case per 2000 live births[3,4]; among well-appearing term infants born by vaginal delivery to mothers without concern for intrapartum infection, the incidence may be as low as 1 case in 25,000 births.[5] Among term infants born by elective cesarean section before the onset of labor and before rupture of membranes, the incidence is close to zero.[6] Faced with a low-incidence, high-consequence condition, neonatal caregivers are challenged to determine the best approach to ensure newborn health. The difficulty of this task has been brought forward in a national surveys of EOS practices among American newborn nurseries. Wide variation was identified in most aspects of EOS risk management, with a significant impact on the newborn and on the maternal–infant dyad.[7,8]

Two newborn characteristics can be used to identify categories of infants at markedly higher risk of EOS compared with infants without such characteristics. The first is gestational age (or birth weight used as a surrogate for gestational age). Centers for Disease Control and Prevention (CDC) multistate surveillance data in the United States demonstrate that the incidence among infants born at <37 weeks' gestation is five to six times higher compared with the incidence among infants born at ≥37 weeks' gestation. The incidence of EOS among those born with birth weight <1500g is approximately 20 times higher than among those born at term.[3,4,9] The microbiology of EOS also differs among premature infants: despite widespread application of intrapartum antibiotic prophylaxis (IAP) to prevent group B *Streptococcus* (GBS)-specific EOS,[10] GBS remains the most common organism isolated in term infants with EOS.[3,4] In contrast, *Escherichia coli* is the most common isolate among premature infants.[3,4,9]

The second characteristic predictive of EOS is infant clinical presentation. Escobar and colleagues[11] evaluated the outcomes of EOS evaluation among 2875 newborns evaluated for EOS. Roughly half of the infants were evaluated due to clinical symptoms, and the other half were evaluated based on the presence of specific risk factors (e.g., maternal chorioamnionitis, rupture of membranes >18 hours). The unadjusted incidence of EOS was 10-fold higher among infants who were critically ill compared with those who were initially asymptomatic; on multivariate analysis, initial asymptomatic status predicted an approximately 60% lower risk of EOS compared with presentation with any degree of instability.[11] In subsequent multivariate analyses, Escobar and colleagues[12] observed similar magnitudes of risk associated with good and poor clinical status.

Despite a high relative risk of infection, not all premature infants are infected, and not all symptomatic term infants are infected. The challenge among such infants is to determine which infants may not require EOS evaluation and empiric antibiotics. Among term, well-appearing infants, in contrast, the primary challenge is to determine who, despite initial reassuring clinical condition, is at highest risk to develop symptomatic EOS. For these infants, the task is to determine which infants may require EOS evaluation and empiric antibiotics. In this chapter, we will evaluate the merits and limitations of different approaches to assessing the risk of EOS among term, well-appearing newborns.

Approaches to EOS Risk Assessment Among Well-Appearing Term Infants

The first national consensus guidelines addressing EOS were issued by the American Academy of Pediatrics (AAP) in 1992,[13] by the CDC in 1996,[14] and by the American College of Obstetricians and Gynecologists (ACOG) in 1996.[15] These guidelines were directed at reducing GBS-specific EOS incidence by interrupting mother-to-infant GBS transmission during labor. The evidence for specific chemoprophylaxis approaches to mediate such interruption and effectiveness of the various approaches was reviewed in each subsequent revision.[16,17] Universal GBS screening and intrapartum chemoprophylaxis were recommended in the revised CDC guidelines in 2002[16] and 2010.[17] Responsibility for ongoing updates to perinatal GBS guidance was assumed by the individual professional societies in 2019. Recommended practices are addressed in separate guidance documents collaboratively authored by the AAP and ACOG.[18,19] The American Society of Microbiology provides guidance for GBS laboratory practice.[20]

Current AAP guidance also contains recommendations for the management of newborns after delivery with the goal of early identification of EOS cases and early initiation of antibiotics to halt the progression of disease. Separate risk assessment recommendations for term and late preterm infants born at ≥35 weeks' gestation and preterm infants born at ≤34 weeks' gestation are available.[21,22] There are three recommended practice approaches for the evaluation of term and late preterm infants.[21] The context, advantages, and limitations of each are summarized in Table 1.1.

Categorical approaches to EOS risk assessment: This approach utilizes decision trees to direct management with a series of categorical consideration of risk factors, using these factors in dichotomous fashion with clear cutoff values. Decision trees ensure ease of clinical use and direct immediate decision-making, and they are often used when time is a critical factor in determining the success of the outcome.[37] This approach does not require computation or longitudinal monitoring. The aim of the categorical approach is to maximize sensitivity at the expense of specificity. With the goal to "not miss" EOS cases (defining this goal as

TABLE 1.1 EOS Risk Assessment Options for Newborns At ≥35 0/7 Weeks' Gestation[21]

	Categorical Approach	Neonatal Early-Onset Sepsis Calculator[a]	Observation Approach
Risk factors considered	• Signs of newborn clinical illness • Maternal intrapartum temperature ≥100.4°F (≥38°C) • Inadequate IAP in a GBS-colonized mother	• Gestational age at birth • Highest maternal intrapartum temperature • Duration of rupture of membranes • Maternal GBS status • Type and duration of intrapartum antibiotic • Infant clinical status over the first 6–12 hr of age	• Signs of newborn clinical illness • Maternal intrapartum temperature ≥ 100.4°F (≥ 38°C) • Inadequate IAP in a GBS-colonized mother
Infant clinical status	Local center determines what constitutes "signs of newborn clinical illness."	Guidance on content and duration of vital signs and specifics of clinical status provided to determine one of three clinical states: • Clinical illness • Equivocal • Well-appearing	Local center determines what constitutes "signs of newborn clinical illness."

Recommended clinical actions	• Blood culture and empiric antibiotics are recommended for infants:
	  • With clinical illness
	  • Born to mother with intrapartum temperature ≥38°C/100.4°F
	• Clinical observation for 24–36 hr in the birth hospital for infants born to mothers with inadequate GBS IAP
		Recommended actions are provided based on final risk estimates at birth, as well as risk estimates adjusted for clinical condition.	• Blood culture and empiric antibiotics are recommended for infants with clinical illness
			• At-risk infants who appear well at birth undergo serial, structured clinical assessments from birth through 36-48 hr of age and undergo EOS evaluation if signs of illness develop

Advantages	• Familiar • Multiple retrospective studies	• Prospectively validated in large cohorts and multiple smaller centers • Individualized management • Overall lower use of empiric antibiotics compared with categorical approach	Overall lower use of empiric antibiotics compared with categorical and (possibly) multivariate approach
Limitations	• Poor discrimination within risk categories • Higher use of empiric antibiotics compared with multivariate and observation-based approaches	• Requires structures for risk calculation • Requires process for enhanced newborn observation at some levels of estimated risk	• Validation in small cohorts where risk was primarily determined by obstetric diagnosis of chorioamnionitis • Requires structures for serial newborn observation and development of rules for evaluation and empiric treatment
References	16, 17, 23, 28–32	5, 12, 23–27	32–36

[a] The Neonatal Early-Onset Sepsis Calculator can be found at https://neonatalsepsiscalculator.kaiserpermanente.org/.

the identification of invasive infection before the newborn is clinically ill), a wide margin for categorizing infants as "at risk" is seen as beneficial, and the likelihood of overtreatment is judged to be acceptable. Originally designed to provide a secondary means of identifying infants at risk for GBS-specific EOS, the categorical approach has evolved to provide more holistic guidance for all bacterial causes of EOS. This approach is familiar and has been used widely in recent years, with multiple publications detailing the proportion of term and late preterm infants subject to laboratory testing and empiric antibiotic treatment.[23,28–32] An important component of this approach is that all infants born to women with intrapartum fever are considered at equal risk of EOS and are administered empiric antibiotics—regardless of clinical appearance.

Multivariate risk assessment: This approach utilizes established risk factors and newborn clinical condition to estimate the individual infant's risk of EOS. In their study of infants being evaluated for EOS using a CDC-recommended categorical approach, Escobar and colleagues[11] demonstrated that a limited number of risk factors could be used to predict infection. Subsequently, these investigators used a cohort of 608,000 infants born at ≥34 weeks' gestation to develop predictive models for culture-confirmed EOS based on objective data known at the moment of birth[24] and the evolving newborn condition in the first 6 to 12 hours after birth.[12] The objective data used include gestational age, highest intrapartum maternal temperature, maternal GBS status, duration of rupture of membranes, and type and duration of intrapartum antibiotics. The models were used to develop the web-based Neonatal Early-Onset Sepsis Calculator with recommended clinical algorithms based on the final risk estimate.[5,23,25]

Blood culture and enhanced clinical observation are recommended for infants with EOS risk estimated at ≥1/1000, and blood culture and empiric antibiotics are recommended for infants with EOS risk estimated at ≥3/1000. The primary advantage of the multivariate approach is that it accounts for interactions among risk factors, providing differential information on an individual infant's risk rather than placing infants in categories with a wide range of risk. A further advantage is that it uses only objective data, including maternal fever, without requiring obstetric clinical judgment with respect to clinical chorioamnionitis. If needed, the risk estimated can be recalculated during the first 6 to 12 hours as the newborn clinical condition evolves. Care pathways must be established to ensure that the risk estimate is accurately calculated and recorded at birth. The clinical care algorithms rely on enhanced clinical surveillance for infants, with estimates of 1/1000 requiring birth hospitalization for a minimum of 24 to 36 hours, as well as frequent vital signs and clinical nursing assessments. Institutions opting for this approach may set different risk thresholds for specific actions if local resources mandate more conservative algorithms,[26] but the use of more liberal thresholds has not been validated. Multiple centers have reported use of the sepsis calculator; all prospective implementation studies and a meta-analysis document decreased use of empiric antibiotic treatments compared with the use of categorical approaches without safety concerns.[27]

Risk assessment based primarily on newborn clinical condition: A third strategy for evaluating risk among well-appearing term infants consists of reliance on clinical signs of illness to identify infants with EOS. Such an approach is based on the observation that, among term infants, an asymptomatic condition at birth is associated with an approximately 60% to 70% reduction in risk for EOS.[11,12] EOS in persistently asymptomatic infants is uncommon. In a prospective neonatal early-onset sepsis calculator validation report, only 1/56,261 infants managed using the sepsis risk calculator had bacteremia, despite never manifesting signs of illness.[23] Other centers report the convergence of EOS with symptoms, demonstrating that term infants with EOS generally have signs of illness at birth or develop signs with 48 hours of birth.[28,38] CDC investigators reported on national surveillance for early-onset GBS infection in the United States from 2006 to 2015, including over 4 million live births. This study found that 94.7% of cases of GBS-specific EOS occurred within 48 hours of birth, with only 14 cases identified after a newborn was discharged from the birth hospital.[39] Centers in Italy have reported their experiences with strategies based on identification of at-risk newborns using categorical approaches to risk, accompanied by laboratory tests and serial examinations of at-risk newborns.[33,34] One U.S. center has reported on a stepwise adoption of an approach based on clinical monitoring for infants born to mothers with an obstetric clinical diagnosis of chorioamnionitis.[32,35,36] Utilizing a quality-improvement framework, this center made serial changes in management, initially focused on the care of infants born at ≥34 to 35 weeks' gestation. Prior to the quality-improvement initiative, blood cultures, complete blood count (CBC), and serial C-reactive protein (CRP) were obtained for all newborns of women with an obstetric diagnosis of intraamniotic infection (chorioamnionitis), and all were administered empiric antibiotics. In the first iteration, such infants were only cared for in this manner if clinically ill at birth. Otherwise, newborns were admitted to a neonatal intensive care unit (NICU) and monitored for a minimum of 24 hours, and they were administered antibiotics if the care team identified signs of instability. With this approach, the rate of empiric antibiotic administration declined from 100% to 21% among 310 infants born at ≥34 to 35 weeks' gestation.[32] In the second iteration, at-risk infants born at ≥35 weeks' gestation were cared for in maternal/newborn couplet care with enhanced clinical monitoring performed by NICU and well-baby nurses. During this period, 25 out of 339 infants (7.4%) had laboratory studies and were administered empiric antibiotics.[35] After 5 years of utilizing this approach, the center reported an overall decline in the use of empiric antibiotic therapy among all infants born at ≥35 weeks' gestation from 11.1% to 4.1%, as well as a decline in the use of CRP from 15.3% to 6.3%.[36]

Areas of Controversy

EOS risk assessment for initially well-appearing term infants is a matter of considerable controversy among newborn caregivers, with debate centered on four main issues: (1) how many newborns is it acceptable to evaluate and empirically treat to identify one case of EOS; (2) what is the best way to use available laboratory tests to assess risk; (3) what are the economic and social costs of EOS risk assessment; and (4) what unintended consequences result from perinatal antibiotic administration?

How many infants should be empirically evaluated and empirically treated for risk of EOS? This judgment is perhaps the most controversial aspect of the categorical risk approach. AAP guidance endorses the use of one of the three general approaches to EOS risk assessment, allowing centers to determine what is best suited to their local structure of care and local acceptance of risk.[21] The impact of the categorical approach recommended in the earliest GBS prevention guidance has been described in a variety of reports (Table 1.1).[23,28–32] Depending on which categorical approach is taken, 5% to 20% of term and late preterm infants are evaluated with laboratory tests, and 5% to 11% are administered neonatal antibiotics for risk of EOS.

Multiple reports have documented that the multivariate risk approach results in fewer newborns evaluated and empirically treated with antibiotics (Table 1.1).[27] A prospective validation report including 204,685 infants born at ≥35 weeks' gestation cared for in the Kaiser Permanente Northern California integrated healthcare system demonstrated that blood culture testing declined by 66% and empiric antibiotic administration declined by 48% (to 2.6% overall) with use of the multivariate risk approach, compared with the use of a risk algorithm based on CDC 2010 recommendations.[23] No adverse impacts of the multivariate risk approach were noted during the birth hospitalization or after-birth hospital discharge. Hospital readmissions within 7 days of birth for culture-confirmed EOS were rare, occurring at a rate of approximately 5/100,000 births, regardless of the approach taken for risk assessment at birth. Strategies based on clinical observation are predicted to result in very low rates of empiric antibiotic administration. In the reports published by Stanford University investigators, the overall rate of antibiotic administration after adoption of an observation-based approach declined by 2/3 (11.1% using the categorical approach dropped to 3.7% in the final phase of observation implementation)[36] but still remained higher than that reported by the Kaiser Permanente investigators. Both the multivariate model and observation-based approach provide significant practical challenges compared with the categorical decision-tree approach.

The neonatal early-onset sepsis calculator was designed for use with all live births ≥34 weeks; it has not been validated for secondary assessment of infants flagged at risk by categorical approaches, as has been done in some retrospective studies.[40,41] It does not rely on categorical risk flags but uses objective risk data to provide an estimated risk of EOS at the moment of birth. This estimate is subsequently adjusted based on the evolving newborn clinical condition. Centers adopting this approach must develop processes for ensuring that the data required for the multivariate risk estimate are available and that the risk output is properly calculated, recorded, and communicated to caregivers. One center reported success with integration of the calculator models into their local electronic medical record.[42]

Observation-based approaches require centers to decide who is eligible for observation versus intervention, how to screen for risk (using a categorical or multivariate approach, with or without laboratory testing), and how serial clinical examinations will be conducted, recorded, and communicated. Furthermore, centers need to develop explicit guidance for intervention based on specific changes in the newborn clinical condition. Theoretically, a center could dispense with all EOS risk assessment and implement serial clinical observation for all well-appearing term newborns, intervening with laboratory testing and/or empiric antibiotics only when signs of illness became apparent. Such an approach would significantly affect the structure of well-nursery care. The need for frequent clinical assessments and vital sign measurements would affect mother–infant couplet care and could result in increased labor costs resulting from increased demands on both nursing and pediatric providers. The Stanford University investigators reported 24/7 physician assessment followed by the use of NICU-skilled nurses for direct observation of infants at risk of EOS for at least 2 hours after birth.[36] This center maintains a relatively low (1:3) nurse/dyad ratio for all mothers and newborns in their postpartum setting and frequent vital sign assessment to facilitate their observation-based approach—staff utilization decisions that have significant associated costs. Most importantly, clinicians using an observation-based approach to EOS risk assessment will need to view a newborn transition from well appearing to symptomatic as an expected outcome and not a failure of care.

Are there infants at no risk of EOS? Consideration of the newborn evolving clinical status is a key component of multivariate risk assessment and observation-based strategies. However, both strategies assume that the newborn is at some baseline risk of EOS. Such risk is primarily driven by exposure to normal maternal genitourinary and gastrointestinal flora during the process of labor and delivery. Rarely, transplacental bacterial infection may occur with select organisms, notably *Listeria monocytogenes*; also, cases of in utero–onset GBS EOS have been reported.[43,44] Such cases generally present with nonreassuring fetal status or even in utero fetal demise. Scheduled cesarean section delivery prior to the onset of labor, attempts to induce labor, or rupture of membranes prior to delivery have been identified as scenarios that result in very low risk of EOS even among extremely preterm infants.[45]

A recent study addressed the risk of EOS among infants of all gestational ages based on delivery characteristics.[6] Among a cohort of 53,575 births of all gestational ages, 7549 infants were evaluated for EOS and 41 cases were detected. No EOS cases occurred among infants born by cesarean delivery, without labor or membrane rupture before delivery, and without any antepartum obstetric concern for intraamniotic infection or nonreassuring fetal status. Because infants born under such strictly defined circumstances may have signs of clinical instability due to physiologic transition, retained fetal lung fluid, or pulmonary immaturity, recognition of the extremely low a priori risk of EOS is critical to determining if such infants ever warrant empiric antibiotic treatments.

What is the best way to use available laboratory tests to assess EOS risk? Clinicians seek to use laboratory tests to both predict and diagnose EOS. Bacterial culture; white blood cell (WBC) count and differential, including absolute neutrophil count (ANC) and the ratio of immature to total neutrophil forms (I/T); proinflammatory cytokines such as interleukins IL-1β, IL-6, IL-8, and IL-10 and tumor necrosis factor alpha; acute-phase reactants, such as procalcitonin and CRP; and cell surface markers such as CD64 have been variably correlated with culture-proven, clinical, and viral sepsis. Most recently, molecular methods such as microarray and proteome analysis have sought to characterize molecular signatures that correlate with culture-confirmed infection.

Bacterial culture and the definition of EOS: Epidemiologic studies of EOS are based on culture-confirmed isolation of pathogenic bacterial species from normally sterile compartments, most commonly blood and cerebrospinal fluid, and rarely, in some circumstances, pleural or peritoneal fluid. Neonatal surface cultures taken at birth are generally considered to represent colonization. Although they are used to test the efficacy of GBS IAP, cultures of the nares, inner ear, periumbilical, and perianal regions or swallowed amniotic fluid do not reflect invasive infection. Among symptomatic infants, evidence of surface colonization has been used to justify the diagnosis of "culture-negative sepsis" by arguing that blood cultures are sterile due to the use of maternally administered intrapartum antibiotic administration. Currently available blood culture systems use optimized enriched culture media with antimicrobial-inactivating elements that efficiently neutralize commonly used beta-lactam antibiotics, as well as gentamicin. These culture systems detect bacteremia at a level of 1 to 10 colony-forming units if a minimum of 1mL of blood is inoculated.[46–48] A quality-improvement initiation based on both the clinical report of blood culture bottle inoculate and bottle weights to verify the clinical report demonstrated the feasibility of obtaining 1 to 2mL of blood for culture among infants of all gestational ages.[49] Studies report no impact of intrapartum antibiotics on blood culture time to positivity among bacteremic infants.[50,51] Nonetheless, concern for culture-negative EOS persists and drives prolonged empiric antibiotic use. Some authors have advocated for a neonatal consensus diagnosis of EOS, based on the presence of symptoms and elevations of specific inflammatory markers.[52] Given the lack of sensitivity for detecting true infection associated with currently available laboratory tests (see below), adoption of such a definition in high-income countries will inevitably lead to increases in empiric antibiotic administration. However, epidemiologic studies and clinical intervention trials may benefit from a neonatal consensus definition of EOS that extends beyond culture-confirmed disease, particularly in low-resource settings where culture-based diagnostics are not widely available. Among adult patients, early recognition of sepsis syndrome and prompt initiation of volume resuscitation, as well as antibiotics, are critical to intact survival. There is no equivalent clinical imperative among well-appearing term newborns. The most straightforward approach to evaluating the predictive performance of laboratory tests is to use the outcome of culture-confirmed infection.

Complete blood count: The most commonly used laboratory test to evaluate the risk of EOS among newborns is the CBC and its components.[7] Recent studies suggest this practice should be reconsidered. Multiple single centers have reported the poor sensitivity of total WBC and differential for identifying culture-confirmed EOS among initially well-appearing infants. The rates at which newborns are flagged with "abnormal" WBC vary widely, influenced by the metric chosen, the definition of abnormal, and the time at which the test is obtained (see Table 1.2). A multicenter study addressed these issues with a cohort that included 67,623 CBC/differential tests obtained within 1 hour of a blood culture, finding 245 cases of culture-confirmed infection (incidence of EOS was 0.4% among the tested infants).[53] Test performance was analyzed using multiple approaches, including determining the mean values and distribution of values comparing infected and uninfected infants and sensitivity, specificity, and likelihood ratios for infection at different thresholds of "abnormal." In addition, multiple models were built to determine if adjusting for age, birth weight, birth facility, year of birth, maternal diagnosis of preeclampsia, mode of delivery, and 5-minute Apgar score would improve test performance. The best test performance was obtained by accounting for age in hours after birth. The poorest test performance associated with values obtained immediately after birth was particularly notable: the receiver–operator curve for total WBC was 0.52 at <1 hour of age. Platelet count was also nonpredictive, even for values obtained at >4 hours of age. The best test performance was obtained for extremely low WBC and ANC values obtained after 4 hours of age; the I/T^2 (essentially the I/T divided by the ANC) was the only test characteristic with good performance independent of newborn age.[53,54] A larger multicenter study including 293 centers in the Pediatrix Medical Group performed similar analyses: 168,604 blood cultures from infants admitted to NICUs were matched to CBC obtained within 24 hours of the blood culture, including 2001 cases of culture-confirmed EOS.[55] This study included infants of all gestational ages, with results provided in gestational age categories. Poor sensitivity was again found

TABLE 1.2 WBC Testing Among Well-Appearing Newborns at Risk for EOS

References	Years	Infants With CBC	CBC Timing (Hours of Age)	Abnormal CBC Definition	Abnormal CBC, *n*	EOS Among Tested Infants, *n* (%)
28	1996–1999	≥35 wk All EOS risk (*n* = 1665)	<4	WBC ≤ 5000 or ≥ 30,000 ANC < 1500 I/T > 0.2	454/1665	0 (0.0)
30	2008–2009	≥35 wk All EOS risk (*n* = 1062)	0–2	WBC ≤ 5000 I/T > 0.2	32/1062	3 (0.3)[a]
29	2011–2012	≥35 wk Exposed to CAM (*n* = 692)	0, 12, and 24	At least one abnormal value of ANC, ATI, or I/T	686/692	3 (0.4)
56	2006–2012	≥35 wk Exposed to CAM (*n* = 535)	0 and 12	I/T > 0.2[b]	185/535	3 (0.6)[c]
34	2004–2005	≥35 wk All EOS risk (*n* = 477)	0–48	WBC ≤ 5000 or ≥ 15,000[b]	327/477	3 (0.6)

For each study, the number of infants includes only those for whom the whole CBC was obtained. *ATI*, absolute immature neutrophil count; *CAM*, chorioamnionitis.
[a]None of the three cases of EOS was among the 32 infants with abnormal CBC.
[b]Clinicians also variably obtained CRP levels.
[c]Although three cases of EOS were well appearing by 6 to 8 hours of age, all were depressed at birth, requiring positive pressure ventilation, continuous positive airway pressure (CPAP), or bag/mask ventilation.

for WBC, the differential components, and the platelet count. Among infants born at ≥37 weeks' gestation, the highest likelihood ratios were associated with WBC < 5000, ANC < 1500, and I/T > 0.5, and platelet counts were nonpredictive. Current AAP guidance does not recommend use of the WBC and differential in EOS risk assessment.[21]

CRP and other markers of inflammation: Most studies of inflammatory molecules and biomarkers have been performed on infants who are symptomatic and being evaluated for sepsis. None of these has yet proven useful in predicting infection in initially well-appearing infants. Nonetheless, CRP was the second most common laboratory test used to identify infants at risk for EOS in a national survey of neonatal providers.[7] CRP is one of several acute-phase reactant proteins synthesized in the liver in response to proinflammatory cytokines. CRP is documented to rise and fall over the course of neonatal GBS infection with a variable course.[57] A single measurement of CRP sent at the same time as blood culture lacks sensitivity for EOS, although serial measurements have a likelihood ratio of approximately 3 for predicting culture-confirmed infection.[58] CRP is particularly problematic for use in the immediate neonatal period, as it rises in response to other common neonatal conditions such as bruising and cephalohematoma and in generalized conditions of fetal distress that lead to meconium-stained amniotic fluid.[59] Similarly, procalcitonin is an acute-phase reactant that increases earlier than CRP in the course of infection, but it also rises in response to asphyxia, respiratory distress syndrome, and pneumothorax; procalcitonin also appears to naturally rise and decline in the first 48 hours after birth.[60] A review of 18 neonatal procalcitonin studies demonstrated a wide range of cutoff values, definitions for outcomes, and ultimately variable test performance.[61] Molecular methods that simultaneously measure multiple mediators of host response may be used to identify a "molecular signature" of EOS. Sweeney and colleagues[62] employed an 11-gene microarray to identify culture-confirmed early- and late-onset infection in a retrospective analysis of three different study cohorts including a wide range of gestational ages. The study found high diagnostic accuracy in distinguishing culture-confirmed infection. Development of rapid, point-of-care assays that rely on small volumes of cord or peripheral blood and use of alternative biospecimens such as saliva and breath may provide novel means of sepsis diagnosis.[63] Currently, however, AAP guidance does not recommend the use of inflammatory markers such as CRP to assess well-appearing term newborn infants for risk of EOS, nor to determine whether to extend empiric antibiotics in the absence of culture-confirmed infection.[21]

What are the economic and social costs of EOS risk assessment? Many reports have focused on the economic impact of maternal GBS screening and IAP, but few have addressed the costs of neonatal assessment and treatment. Economic analysis of EOS risk activities is complicated by variation across centers in the both diagnostic and therapeutic approach and, importantly, whether newborns are admitted to higher-cost intensive care units or primarily cared for in well-nursery settings. We performed an economic analysis addressing the costs associated with EOS risk assessment among well-appearing infants born at ≥36 weeks' gestation who were ultimately found to be uninfected. We estimated that a local algorithm aligned with the categorical approach recommended in the 2010 CDC GBS guidelines results in $110,000 to $150,000 in costs per 1000 live births.[31] Extrapolated to approximately 3.6 million term births per year in the United States, approximately $400 to $500 million is spent annually on EOS-associated procedures. A simulated decision-tree analysis based on perinatal care in Australia for infants born at ≥35 weeks' gestation estimated that use of the neonatal sepsis risk calculator in place of a categorical approach to EOS risk assessment would result in savings of approximately $25,000 to $50,000 per 1000 live births.[64] The social costs are also considerable. In most perinatal centers, blood tests, intravenous line placement, and antibiotic administration are performed in neonatal care settings separate from maternal care settings, resulting in mother–infant separation after birth. In a survey of national EOS, 95% of respondents reported separating the mother and infant to perform laboratory testing, and approximately 40% of newborns receiving antibiotics for EOS are separated from the mother for the duration of care.[7] Such separation has a significantly negative effect on the establishment of breastfeeding, an unintended consequence of EOS evaluation that may have long-term child health implications. In a study of 692 asymptomatic term infants separated from the mother for the evaluation of EOS, separation during the first 2 hours after birth resulted in significantly lower incidence of exclusive breastfeeding and increased use of formula in the absence of a medical indication.[65] Centers have reported increased rates of breast milk feeding among newborns at risk for EOS after transition from a categorical approach for risk assessment to an approach based on use of the neonatal early-onset sepsis calculator.[66,67]

Are there long-term consequences that result from perinatal antibiotic administration? Microbial exposure has been shown to play a role in determining host immune behavior as early as prenatal life, via the maternal microflora.[68] This is followed by a postnatal period when the increase in microbial exposure at birth overlaps with the critical developmental window of immune cell programming.[69–72] The roles of commensal microflora exposure in innate and adaptive immune pathways, including induction of toll-like receptor tolerance to exogenous endotoxin and production of short-chain fatty acids that stimulate the regulatory T-cell population, have been demonstrated.[73,74] In preclinical studies, disruption of the early host microflora—either absolutely (as in germ-free mice) or partially by antibiotic exposure—results in an increased proinflammatory response in the host gut to environmental irritants and an increased mortality when fighting invasive pathogens.[75,76] Mice given subtherapeutic levels of antibiotics after weaning exhibit increased adiposity and increased bacterial SFCA metabolism and energy extraction.[77,78] Early low-dose antibiotics combined with a high-fat diet cause even greater increases in adiposity.[79,80] Many of these effects occur only during the newborn period, highlighting the importance of early-life microbiota and the potential for disruption to cause lasting adverse health outcomes. Intrapartum antibiotics are administered with the intent of altering colonization of the newborn with pathogenic bacterial species.

TABLE 1.3 Studies Addessing Perinatal Antibiotics and Neonatal Microbiome

References	Infant Population (*n*)	Exposure (*n*)	Microbiota Source and Timing	Impact on Exposed Compared With Unexposed
81, 82	Term (52)	IAP (ampicillin)	Infant stool at 7 and 30 days	↑ Enterobacteriaceae and ↓ *Bifidobacterium* at both 7 and 30 days
83	Term (198)	IAP/VD (96) No IAP/VD (40) IAP/CS/P (17) IAP/CS/E (23)	Infant stool at 3 months and 1 year	↑ *Proteobacterium* and *Clostridia* (especially CS) ↓ Bacteroidetes BF impact
84	Term dyads (262)	GBS status IAP	Infant stool at 1 and 6 months	↑ Clostridiaceae, Ruminococcoceae, and Enterococcaceae in infants born to GBS+ mothers when adjusting for IAP
85	Women at <32 weeks' gestation (27)	IAP for GBS+ and GBS unknown	Maternal vaginal microbiota	Most *Lactobacillus* in GBS+/no IAP Most *Pseudomonas* in GBS–/+IAP
86	Term dyads (36) Mothers with elevated BMI	IAP (cefazolin or penicillin G)	Placenta Oral (mother and infant) Gut (mother)	↑ Proteobacteria ↓ Streptococcaceae, Gemellaceae, and lactobacilli ↓ Maternal–infant similarity
87	Term dyads (45)	Observational	Vertical transmission of *Lactobacillus*	Both IAP and PROM ↓ *Lactobacillus* in infant
88	Term (50)	IAP for GBS	Infant stool culture at day 3	↓ *Clostridia*
89, 90	Preterm (27) Term (13)	Prematurity	Infant stool over 3 months	↑ Enterobacteriaceae even when adjusting for prematurity
91	Preterm (41) Term (17)	Postnatal antibiotics	Infant stool at 110 days	↓ Shannon diversity
92	Very preterm (23)	Total days of postnatal antibiotics	Stool at days 15, 30, and 90	↑ *Clostridia* days 15 and 30 ↓ *Bacteroides fragilis* at day 30
93	Term (105)	Maternal prenatal and intrapartum antibiotics	First meconium < 48 hr	↑ Shannon diversity Beta diversity associated with antibiotic exposure

BF, breastfeeding; *BMI*, body mass index; *CS/P*, planned cesarean section delivery; *CS/E*, emergent cesarean section delivery; *PROM*, premature rupture of membranes; *VD*, vaginal delivery.

An unintended consequence may be more global alteration of the early microbiota in both diversity and composition. Recently, multiple studies have documented the impact of perinatal antibiotics, with effects extending days to months (Table 1.3).[81–93] Neonatal antibiotics administered for risk of EOS have not been as well studied to date but are anticipated to have some impact on the developing microbiota, as well. Epidemiologic studies have reported an association of early-life antibiotics with increased risk of multiple adverse outcomes, including obesity, diabetes, asthma, eczema, and food allergies and altered response to subsequent infections.[94–99] The effects on antibiotics administered specifically for GBS prophylaxis were evaluated in two large U.S. perinatal cohorts with different socioeconomic and race/ethnicity characteristics.[100,101] The administration of adequate GBS intrapartum antibiotic prophylaxis was associated with increased rates of infant and child weight gain and higher body mass index up to 5 years of age in both cohorts. Studies such as these that address whether intrapartum and neonatal antibiotics specifically have enduring health consequences for the infant will continue to fuel the debate surrounding the risk/benefit balance of EOS prevention and risk assessment practices.

REFERENCES

1. Taylor JA, Opel DJ. Choriophobia: a 1-act play. *Pediatrics*. 2012;130:342-346.
2. Benitz WE, Wynn JL, Polin RA. Reappraisal of guidelines for management of neonates with suspected early-onset sepsis. *J Pediatr*. 2015;166:1070-1074.
3. Schrag SJ, Farley MM, Petit S, et al. Epidemiology of invasive early-onset neonatal sepsis, 2005 to 2014. *Pediatrics*. 2016; 138:e20162013.
4. Stoll BJ, Puopolo KM, Hansen NI, et al. Early-onset neonatal sepsis 2015 to 2017, the rise of *Escherichia coli*, and the need for novel prevention strategies. *JAMA Pediatr*. 2020;174: e200593.
5. Kaiser Permanente Division of Research. *Neonatal Early-Onset Sepsis Calculator*. Available at: https://neonatalsepsiscalculator.kaiserpermanente.org. Accessed January 17, 2023.
6. Flannery DD, Mukhopadhyay S, Morales KH, et al. Delivery characteristics and the risk of early-onset neonatal sepsis. *Pediatrics*. 2022;149:e2021052900.
7. Mukhopadhyay S, Taylor JA, Von Kohorn I, et al. Variation in sepsis evaluation across a national network of nurseries. *Pediatrics*. 2017;139:e20162845.
8. Payton KSE, Wirtschafter D, Bennett MV, et al. Vignettes identify variation in antibiotic use for suspected early onset sepsis. *Hosp Pediatr*. 2021;11:770-774.
9. Flannery DD, Edwards EM, Puopolo KM, Horbar JD. Early-onset sepsis among very preterm infants. *Pediatrics*. 2021;148: e2021052456.
10. Van Dyke MK, Phares CR, Lynfield R, et al. Evaluation of universal antenatal screening for group B streptococcus. *N Engl J Med*. 2009;360:2626-2636.
11. Escobar GJ, Li DK, Armstrong MA, et al. Neonatal sepsis workups in infants ≥ 2000 grams at birth: a population-based study. *Pediatrics*. 2000;106:256-263.
12. Escobar GJ, Puopolo KM, Wi S, et al. Stratification of risk of early-onset sepsis in newborns ≥34 weeks' gestation. *Pediatrics*. 2014;133:30-36.
13. American Academy of Pediatrics. American Academy of Pediatrics Committee on Infectious Diseases and Committee on Fetus and Newborn: guidelines for prevention of group B streptococcal (GBS) infection by chemoprophylaxis. *Pediatrics*. 1992; 90:775-778.
14. Centers for Disease Control and Prevention. Prevention of perinatal group B streptococcal disease: a public health perspective. *MMWR Recomm Rep*. 1996;45:1-24.
15. American College of Obstetricians and Gynecologists. Prevention of early-onset group B streptococcal disease in newborns. *Int J Gynaecol Obstet*. 2003;81:115-122.
16. Schrag S, Gorwitz R, Fultz-Butts K, et al. Prevention of perinatal group B streptococcal disease. Revised guidelines from CDC. *MMWR Recomm Rep*. 2002;51:1-22.
17. Verani JR, McGee L, Schrag SJ. Prevention of perinatal group B streptococcal disease—revised guidelines from CDC, 2010. *MMWR Recomm Rep*. 2010;59:1-36.
18. Puopolo KM, Lynfield R, Cummings JJ, American Academy of Pediatrics, Committee on Fetus and Newborn, Committee on Infectious Diseases. Management of infants at risk for group B streptococcal disease. *Pediatrics*. 2019;144:e20191881.
19. American College of Obstetricians and Gynecologists. Prevention of group B streptococcal early-onset disease in newborns: ACOG committee opinion, number 797. *Obstet Gynecol*. 2020;135:e51-e72.
20. American Society for Microbiology. *Guidelines for the Detection and Identification of Group B Streptococcus*. Available at: https://asm.org/Guideline/Guidelines-for-the-Detection-and-Identification-of. Accessed April 5, 2022.
21. Puopolo KM, Benitz WE, Zaoutis TE, Committee on Fetus and Newborn, Committee on Infectious Diseases. Management of neonates born at ≥35 0/7 weeks' gestation with suspected or proven early-onset bacterial sepsis. *Pediatrics*. 2018;142: e20182894.
22. Puopolo KM, Benitz WE, Zaoutis TE, Committee on Fetus and Newborn, Committee on Infectious Diseases. Management of neonates born at ≤34 6/7 weeks' gestation with suspected or proven early-onset bacterial sepsis. *Pediatrics*. 2018;142: e20182896.
23. Kuzniewicz MW, Puopolo KM, Fischer A, et al. A quantitative, risk-based approach to the management of neonatal early-onset sepsis. *JAMA Pediatr*. 2017;171:365-371.
24. Puopolo KM, Draper D, Wi S, et al. Estimating the probability of neonatal early-onset infection on the basis of maternal risk factors. *Pediatrics*. 2011;128:e1155-e1163.
25. Kuzniewicz MW, Walsh EM, Li S, Fischer A, Escobar GJ. Development and implementation of an early-onset sepsis calculator to guide antibiotic management in late preterm and term neonates. *Jt Comm J Qual Patient Saf*. 2016;42:232-239.
26. Dhudasia MB, Mukhopadhyay S, Puopolo KM. Implementation of the sepsis risk calculator at an academic birth hospital. *Hosp Pediatr*. 2018;8(5):243-250.
27. Achten NB, Klingenberg C, Benitz WE, et al. Association of use of the neonatal early-onset sepsis calculator with reduction in antibiotic therapy and safety: a systematic review and meta-analysis. *JAMA Pediatr*. 2019;173:1032-1040.
28. Ottolini MC, Lundgren K, Mirkinson LJ, et al. Utility of complete blood count and blood culture screening to diagnose neonatal sepsis in the asymptomatic at risk newborn. *Pediatr Infect Dis J*. 2003;22:430-434.
29. Jackson GL, Engle WD, Sendelbach DM, et al. Are complete blood cell counts useful in the evaluation of asymptomatic neonates exposed to suspected chorioamnionitis? *Pediatrics*. 2004; 113:1173-1180.
30. Mukhopadhyay S, Eichenwald EC, Puopolo KM. Neonatal early-onset sepsis evaluations among well-appearing infants: projected impact of changes in CDC GBS guidelines. *J Perinatol*. 2013;33:198-205.
31. Mukhopadhyay S, Dukhovny D, Mao W, et al. 2010 perinatal GBS prevention guideline and resource utilization. *Pediatrics*. 2014;133:196-203.
32. Joshi NS, Gupta A, Allan JM, et al. Clinical monitoring of well-appearing infants born to mothers with chorioamnionitis. *Pediatrics*. 2018;141:e20172056.
33. Berardi A, Fornaciari S, Rossi C, et al. Safety of physical examination alone for managing well-appearing neonates ≥ 35 weeks' gestation at risk for early-onset sepsis. *J Matern Fetal Neonatal Med*. 2015;28:1123-1127.
34. Cantoni L, Ronfani L, Da Riol R, et al. Physical examination instead of laboratory tests for most infants born to mothers colonized with group B streptococcus: support for the Centers for Disease Control and Prevention's 2010 recommendations. *J Pediatr*. 2013;163:568-573.
35. Joshi NS, Gupta A, Allan JM, et al. Management of chorioamnionitis-exposed infants in the newborn nursery using a clinical examination-based approach. *Hosp Pediatr*. 2019;9: 227-233.

36. Frymoyer A, Joshi NS, Allan JM, et al. Sustainability of a clinical examination-based approach for ascertainment of early-onset sepsis in late preterm and term neonates. *J Pediatr*. 2020;225:263-268.
37. Penaloza-Ramos MC, Sheppard JP, Jowett S, et al. Cost-effectiveness of optimizing acute stroke care services for thrombolysis. *Stroke*. 2014;45:553-562.
38. Hashavya S, Benenson S, Ergaz-Shaltiel Z, et al. The use of blood counts and blood cultures to screen neonates born to partially treated group B streptococcus-carrier mothers for early-onset sepsis: is it justified? *Pediatr Infect Dis J*. 2011; 30:840-843.
39. Nanduri SA, Petit S, Smelser C, et al. Epidemiology of invasive early-onset and late-onset group B streptococcal disease in the United States, 2006 to 2015: multistate laboratory and population-based surveillance. *JAMA Pediatr*. 2019;173:224-233.
40. Shakib J, Buchi K, Smith E, et al. Management of newborns born to mothers with chorioamnionitis: is it time for a kinder, gentler approach? *Acad Pediatr*. 2015;15:340-344.
41. Warren S, Garcia M, Hankins C. Impact of neonatal early-onset sepsis calculator on antibiotic use within two tertiary healthcare centers. *J Perinatol*. 2017;37:394-397.
42. Fowler NT, Garcia M, Hankins C. Impact of integrating a neonatal early-onset sepsis risk calculator into the electronic health record. *Pediatr Qual Saf*. 2019;4:e235.
43. Gibbs RS, Roberts DJ. Case records of the Massachusetts General Hospital. Case 27-2007. A 30-year-old pregnant woman with intrauterine fetal death. *N Engl J Med*. 2007;357:918-925.
44. Lamont RF, Sobel J, Mazaki-Tovi S, et al. Listeriosis in human pregnancy: a systematic review. *J Perinat Med*. 2011;39:227-236.
45. Puopolo KM, Mukhopadhyay S, Hansen NI, et al. Identification of extremely premature infants at low risk for early-onset sepsis. *Pediatrics*. 2017;140:e20170925.
46. Jorgensen JH, Mirrett S, McDonald LC, et al. Controlled clinical laboratory comparison of BACTEC plus aerobic/F resin medium with BacT/Alert aerobic FAN medium for detection of bacteremia and fungemia. *J Clin Microbiol*. 1997;35:53-58.
47. Flayhart D, Borek AP, Wakefield T, et al. Comparison of BACTEC PLUS blood culture media to BacT/Alert FA blood culture media for detection of bacterial pathogens in samples containing therapeutic levels of antibiotics. *J Clin Microbiol*. 2007;45:816-821.
48. Dunne Jr WM, Case LK, Isgriggs L, et al. In-house validation of the BACTEC 9240 blood culture system for detection of bacterial contamination in platelet concentrates. *Transfusion*. 2005;45: 1138-1142.
49. Woodford EC, Dhudasia MB, Puopolo KM, et al. Neonatal blood culture inoculant volume: feasibility and challenges. *Pediatr Res*. 2021;90:1086-1092.
50. Sarkar SS, Bhagat I, Bhatt-Mehta V, et al. Does maternal intrapartum antibiotic treatment prolong the incubation time required for blood cultures to become positive for infants with early-onset sepsis? *Am J Perinatol*. 2015;32:357-362.
51. Kuzniewicz MW, Mukhopadhyay S, Li S, Walsh EM, Puopolo KM. Time to positivity of neonatal blood cultures for early-onset sepsis. *Pediatr Infect Dis J*. 2020;39:634-640.
52. Wynn JL, Wong HR, Shanley TP, et al. Time for a neonatal-specific consensus definition for sepsis. *Pediatr Crit Care Med*. 2014;15:523-528.
53. Newman TB, Puopolo KM, Wi S, et al. Interpreting complete blood counts soon after birth in newborns at risk for sepsis. *Pediatrics*. 2010;126:903-909.
54. Newman TB, Draper D, Puopolo KM, et al. Combining immature and total neutrophil counts to predict early onset sepsis in term and late preterm newborns: use of the I/T2. *Pediatr Infect Dis J*. 2014;33:798-802.
55. Hornik CP, Benjamin DK, Becker KC, et al. Use of the complete blood cell count in early-onset neonatal sepsis. *Pediatr Infect Dis J*. 2012;31:799-802.
56. Kiser C, Nawab U, McKenna K, et al. Role of guidelines on length of therapy in chorioamnionitis and neonatal sepsis. *Pediatrics*. 2014;133:992-998.
57. Philip AG. Response of C-reactive protein in neonatal Group B streptococcal infection. *Pediatr Infect Dis*. 1985;4:145-148.
58. Benitz WE, Han MY, Madan A, et al. Serial serum C-reactive protein levels in the diagnosis of neonatal infection. *Pediatrics*. 1998;102:E41.
59. Pourcyrous M, Bada HS, Korones SB, et al. Significance of serial C-reactive protein responses in neonatal infection and other disorders. *Pediatrics*. 1993;92:431-435.
60. Benitz WE. Adjunct laboratory tests in the diagnosis of early-onset neonatal sepsis. *Clin Perinatol*. 2010;37:421-438.
61. Chiesa C, Pacifico L, Osborn JF, et al. Early-onset neonatal sepsis: still room for improvement in procalcitonin diagnostic accuracy studies. *Medicine (Baltimore)*. 2015;94:e1230.
62. Sweeney TE, Wynn JL, Cernada M, et al. Validation of the Sepsis MetaScore for diagnosis of neonatal sepsis. *J Pediatric Infect Dis Soc*. 2018;7:129-135.
63. Celik IH, Hanna M, Canpolat FE, Pammi M. Diagnosis of neonatal sepsis: the past, present and future. *Pediatr Res*. 2022;91: 337-350.
64. Cussen A, Guinness L. Cost savings from use of a neonatal sepsis calculator in Australia: a modelled economic analysis. *J Paediatr Child Health*. 2021;57:1037-1043.
65. Mukhopadhyay S, Lieberman ES, Puopolo KM, et al. Effect of early-onset sepsis evaluations on in-hospital breastfeeding practices among asymptomatic term neonates. *Hosp Pediatr*. 2015;5:203-210.
66. Leonardi BM, Binder M, Griswold KJ, Yalcinkaya GF, Walsh MC. Utilization of a neonatal early-onset sepsis calculator to guide initial newborn management. *Pediatr Qual Saf*. 2019; 4:e214.
67. Kasat K, Ahn S, Smith S, Zoullas S, Ellington M. Impact of early-onset sepsis guidelines on breastfeeding. *J Perinatol*. 2021;41:2499-2504.
68. Gomez de Aguero M, Ganal-Vonarburg SC, Fuhrer T, et al. The maternal microbiota drives early postnatal innate immune development. *Science*. 2016;351:1296-1302.
69. Vangay P, Ward T, Gerber JS, et al. Antibiotics, pediatric dysbiosis, and disease. *Cell Host Microbe*. 2015;17:553-564.
70. Dominguez-Bello MG, Costello EK, Contreras M, et al. Delivery mode shapes the acquisition and structure of the initial microbiota across multiple body habitats in newborns. *Proc Natl Acad Sci U S A*. 2010;107:11971-11975.
71. Chu DM, Ma J, Prince AL, et al. Maturation of the infant microbiome community structure and function across multiple body sites and in relation to mode of delivery. *Nat Med*. 2017;23: 314-326.
72. Renz H, Brandtzaeg P, Hornef M. The impact of perinatal immune development on mucosal homeostasis and chronic inflammation. *Nat Rev Immunol*. 2011;12:9-23.
73. Lotz M, Gutle D, Walther S, et al. Postnatal acquisition of endotoxin tolerance in intestinal epithelial cells. *J Exp Med*. 2006;203:973-984.

74. Smith PM, Howitt MR, Panikov N, et al. The microbial metabolites, short-chain fatty acids, regulate colonic Treg cell homeostasis. *Science*. 2013;341:569-573.
75. Deshmukh HS, Liu Y, Menkiti OR, et al. The microbiota regulates neutrophil homeostasis and host resistance to Escherichia coli K1 sepsis in neonatal mice. *Nat Med*. 2014;20:524-530.
76. Olszak T, An D, Zeissig S, et al. Microbial exposure during early life has persistent effects on natural killer T cell function. *Science*. 2012;336:489-493.
77. Cho I, Yamanishi S, Cox L, et al. Antibiotics in early life alter the murine colonic microbiome and adiposity. *Nature*. 2012; 488:621-626.
78. Samuel BS, Shaito A, Motoike T, et al. Effects of the gut microbiota on host adiposity are modulated by the short-chain fatty-acid binding G protein-coupled receptor, Gpr41. *Proc Natl Acad Sci U S A*. 2008;105:16767-16772.
79. Cox LM, Yamanishi S, Sohn J, et al. Altering the intestinal microbiota during a critical developmental window has lasting metabolic consequences. *Cell*. 2014;158:705-721.
80. Ridaura VK, Faith JJ, Rey FE, et al. Gut microbiota from twins discordant for obesity modulate metabolism in mice. *Science*. 2013;341:1241214.
81. Corvaglia L, Tonti G, Martini S, et al. Influence of intrapartum antibiotic prophylaxis for group B streptococcus on gut microbiota in the first month of life. *J Pediatr Gastroenterol Nutr*. 2016;62:304-308.
82. Mazzola G, Murphy K, Ross RP, et al. Early gut microbiota perturbations following intrapartum antibiotic prophylaxis to prevent group B streptococcal disease. *PLoS ONE*. 2016;11: e0157527.
83. Azad MB, Konya T, Persaud RR, et al. Impact of maternal intrapartum antibiotics, method of birth and breastfeeding on gut microbiota during the first year of life: a prospective cohort study. *BJOG*. 2016;123:983-993.
84. Cassidy-Bushrow AE, Sitarik A, Levin AM, et al. Maternal group B streptococcus and the infant gut microbiota. *J Dev Orig Health Dis*. 2016;7:45-53.
85. Roesch LF, Silveira RC, Corso AL, et al. Diversity and composition of vaginal microbiota of pregnant women at risk for transmitting Group B streptococcus treated with intrapartum penicillin. *PLoS ONE*. 2017;12:e0169916.
86. Gomez-Arango LF, Barrett HL, McIntyre HD, et al. Antibiotic treatment at delivery shapes the initial oral microbiome in neonates. *Sci Rep*. 2017;7:43481.
87. Keski-Nisula L, Kyynarainen HR, Karkkainen U, et al. Maternal intrapartum antibiotics and decreased vertical transmission of lactobacillus to neonates during birth. *Acta Paediatr*. 2013; 102:480-485.
88. Jaureguy F, Carton M, Panel P, et al. Effects of intrapartum penicillin prophylaxis on intestinal bacterial colonization in infants. *J Clin Microbiol*. 2004;42:5184-5188.
89. Arboleya S, Sanchez B, Solis G, et al. Impact of prematurity and perinatal antibiotics on the developing intestinal microbiota: a functional inference study. *Int J Mol Sci*. 2016;17:e649.
90. Arboleya S, Sanchez B, Milani C, et al. Intestinal microbiota development in preterm neonates and effect of perinatal antibiotics. *J Pediatr*. 2015;166:538-544.
91. Gasparrini AJ, Wang B, Sun X, et al. Persistent metagenomic signatures of early-life hospitalization and antibiotic treatment in the infant gut microbiota and resistome. *Nat Microbiol*. 2019;4:2285-2297.
92. Bozzi Cionci N, Lucaccioni L, Pietrella E, et al. Antibiotic exposure, common morbidities and main intestinal microbial groups in very preterm neonates: a pilot study. *Antibiotics (Basel)*. 2022;11:237.
93. Wong WSW, Sabu P, Deopujari V, et al. Prenatal and peripartum exposure to antibiotics and cesarean section delivery are associated with differences in diversity and composition of the infant meconium microbiome. *Microorganisms*. 2020; 8:179.
94. Metsala J, Lundqvist A, Virta LJ, et al. Mother's and offspring's use of antibiotics and infant allergy to cow's milk. *Epidemiology*. 2013;24:303-309.
95. Marrs T, Bruce KD, Logan K, et al. Is there an association between microbial exposure and food allergy? A systematic review. *Pediatr Allergy Immunol*. 2013;24:311-320.e8.
96. Tsakok T, McKeever TM, Yeo L, et al. Does early life exposure to antibiotics increase the risk of eczema? A systematic review. *Br J Dermatol*. 2013;169:983-991.
97. Murk W, Risnes KR, Bracken MB. Prenatal or early-life exposure to antibiotics and risk of childhood asthma: a systematic review. *Pediatrics*. 2011;127:1125-1138.
98. Kummeling I, Stelma FF, Dagnelie PC, et al. Early life exposure to antibiotics and the subsequent development of eczema, wheeze, and allergic sensitization in the first 2 years of life: the KOALA Birth Cohort Study. *Pediatrics*. 2007; 119:e225-e231.
99. Penders J, Kummeling I, Thijs Ç. Infant antibiotic use and wheeze and asthma risk: a systematic review and meta-analysis. *Eur Respir J*. 2011;38:295-302.
100. Mukhopadhyay S, Bryan M, Dhudasia MB, et al. Intrapartum group B streptococcal prophylaxis and childhood weight gain. *Arch Dis Child Fetal Neonatal Ed*. 2021;106:649-656.
101. Koebnick C, Sidell MA, Getahun D, et al. Intrapartum antibiotic exposure and body mass index in children. *Clin Infect Dis*. 2021;73:e938-e946.

Chapter 2

Empiric Therapy for Neonatal Sepsis

Jessica E. Ericson, MD, MPH

Key Points

- Most early-onset infections in high-resource settings are caused by group B *Streptococcus* and *Escherichia coli.*
- Ampicillin + gentamicin is an appropriate empirical antibiotic regimen for early-onset sepsis in most settings.
- Most late-onset infections are caused by Gram-positive organisms.
- Nafcillin + gentamicin balances the need for a narrow spectrum with the risks of potentially providing inadequate empirical treatment in most cases.
- Empirical antimicrobials targeting methicillin-resistant *Staphylococcus aureus*, *Pseudomonas*, yeast, and viruses should be considered if risk factors are present but are unnecessary in most cases.

Neonatal sepsis refers to the onset of systemic symptoms triggered by a pathogen during the first month of age and is associated with significant morbidity and mortality.[1] Although neonatal sepsis can be due to bacteria, viruses,[2] fungi,[3] and parasites,[4] bacterial infections account for the vast majority of cases, and the term "neonatal sepsis" is often used to refer to bacterial infections specifically.[1] There is not currently a consensus definition for neonatal sepsis.[5] Neonatal infections are differentiated into early onset and late onset based on the age of the infant when symptoms develop.[1]

Clinical signs of neonatal sepsis are often nonspecific and can include lethargy, poor feeding, irritability, and temperature instability.[6] Blood culture and antibiotic susceptibility testing results are often not available for 48 to 72 hours after collection, prolonging the amount of time before an infection can be proven and targeted treatment initiated. Delaying treatment for infants with bacterial infections may increase their risk of morbidity and mortality.[7] For this reason, empiric treatment is often started while awaiting culture results. Changes in the epidemiology of neonatal sepsis, as well as the growing number of cases due to antibiotic-resistant pathogens, have made the optimal antibiotic combination for empiric treatment in the modern era uncertain.[8,9] Pathogens causing neonatal sepsis in low- and middle-income countries are often quite different from those seen in higher-income settings.[10] Local and regional pathogen distributions and antibiotic susceptibility patterns should be used to inform empirical antibiotic selection. This review will discuss the relative risks and benefits of antibiotics currently used for the empiric treatment of neonatal sepsis in higher-income settings.

Early-Onset Sepsis

Pathogens responsible for early-onset infections are typically acquired from the mother's genital tract during delivery and cause symptoms within the first 3 days of life.[11] Prolonged membrane rupture, chorioamnionitis, and prematurity increase the risk of early-onset sepsis (EOS).[12] Approximately 65% of EOS cases are due to *Streptococcus agalactiae* (group B *Streptococcus* [GBS]) or *Escherichia coli* (Table 2.1).[11] Other bacteria that cause EOS include viridans group streptococci, *Enterococcus* species, enteric Gram-negative bacilli, and *Listeria monocytogenes*.[11] Mortality due to EOS varies by gestational age but can be as high as 29%.[11] For this reason, antibiotics are started empirically while awaiting culture results.

AMPICILLIN AND GENTAMICIN

The American Academy of Pediatrics and the World Health Organization recommend empiric treatment

TABLE 2.1 Organisms Causing ≥5% of Neonatal EOS Cases[11]

Organism	% of Cases
≥37 weeks' gestational age	
Streptococcus agalactiae	51
Escherichia coli	15
Enterococcus spp.	9
Streptococcus pyogenes	6
<37 weeks' gestational age	
Escherichia coli	51
Streptococcus agalactiae	13
Haemophilus spp.	5
Klebsiella spp.	5

with ampicillin or penicillin in combination with gentamicin for infants with suspected EOS.[8,13,14] Ampicillin provides coverage against many Gram-positive infections, including GBS, *Enterococcus* species, and *L. monocytogenes*, as well as some Gram-negative pathogens.[15] The addition of gentamicin allows for coverage of a greater number of Gram-negative bacteria, including ampicillin-resistant *E. coli*.[15] Other advantages include relatively low cost and extensive experience with this specific combination.[16]

Ampicillin

Penicillins, such as ampicillin, are relatively safe and inexpensive to use in infants.[16] Rare side effects include allergic reactions, neutropenia, and, with high exposures, seizures.[17] Furthermore, GBS remains a leading cause of EOS, despite widespread implementation of intrapartum antibiotic prophylaxis (IAP) for pregnant women colonized with GBS.[11] Multiple studies conducted over the past 2 decades confirm that GBS isolates remain fully susceptible to beta-lactams, including penicillin and ampicillin.[11,18,19]

Ampicillin is additionally the drug of choice for susceptible infections due to *Enterococcus* species and *L. monocytogenes*.[20] *L. monocytogenes* is a well-known but uncommon cause of maternal and neonatal infection.[11,21] EOS develops in the infant when transplacental transmission of listeriosis occurs following maternal infection or through acquisition of maternal gastrointestinal and vaginal flora during the birth process.[22] Despite its rarity, EOS due to *L. monocytogenes* is associated with a high mortality and significant sequelae in survivors.[23,24] Although no study has demonstrated the benefits of early effective therapy for this particular condition, given the available evidence it seems prudent to provide optimal empiric therapy for this organism until it has been ruled out.

Gentamicin

Aminoglycosides, such as gentamicin, provide excellent activity against Gram-negative bacilli and also provide synergy with penicillins to increase activity against GBS, *S. aureus*, enterococci, and *L. monocytogenes*.[25,26] Additional advantages of gentamicin treatment include infrequent resistance and low cost compared to many newer antibiotics.[11] Although infections due to ampicillin-resistant *E. coli* have increased, gentamicin-resistant *E. coli* infections are rare.[11] Recent studies in the United States, England, and Germany have found that, although ampicillin resistance in *E. coli* is common, >90% remain susceptible to gentamicin.[11,27,28] These studies suggest that the specific combination of ampicillin and gentamicin remains an appropriate empiric therapy for EOS in most centers.

LIMITATIONS OF AMPICILLIN AND GENTAMICIN

Although ampicillin plus gentamicin is the most common antibiotic combination used for EOS, the continued appropriateness of this antibiotic strategy has been questioned by several investigators who argue that other agents may be more advantageous.

Ampicillin Concerns

A commonly noted problem with using ampicillin as empirical treatment for EOS is the trend of increasing ampicillin resistance among EOS cases due to *E. coli*.[9,11,29] Since widespread IAP with ampicillin was recommended in 1996, the proportion of EOS *E. coli* infections resistant to ampicillin has increased, especially among premature and very-low-birth-weight infants.[29,30] As many as 78% to 85% of early-onset *E. coli* infections are due to ampicillin-resistant strains.[31]

Gentamicin Concerns

The greatest concerns with gentamicin, as with all aminoglycosides, are the risks of ototoxicity and nephrotoxicity.[32] High doses of aminoglycosides can damage the sensory hair cells, leading to irreversible hearing loss.[32] Nephrotoxicity typically presents as a reversible inability to concentrate urine along with proteinuria. These risks can be reduced with careful therapeutic drug monitoring of blood levels but toxicity sometimes occurs even at low concentrations and short durations.[32] In particular, it has been estimated that 1 in 500 individuals has a mitochondrial DNA mutation that increases the risk of hearing loss with aminoglycoside therapy, even when blood concentrations are within the target range.[33] Additionally, aminoglycosides may potentiate the effect of environmental noise on the developing cochlea such that low concentrations of gentamicin may lead to ototoxicity if administered in a noisy environment, such as a neonatal intensive care unit.[34] Unfortunately, it has been difficult to determine the true risk of these toxicities for infants exposed to aminoglycosides because there are many potential confounding factors, including concomitant medications and sepsis.[33,35]

For infants who have meningitis as a component of their sepsis syndrome, gentamicin may not provide adequate penetration into the central nervous system to effectively treat ampicillin-resistant organisms.[36] Newer antibiotics with superior penetration across the blood–brain barrier may improve outcomes for Gram-negative meningitis resistant to ampicillin, but no clear best alternative to gentamicin has yet been established.[37,38]

Although uncommon, cases of ampicillin- and gentamicin-resistant *E. coli* have been reported; therefore, although the combination of ampicillin and gentamicin appears to currently be the most rational empiric regimen for EOS, the incidence of resistant infections should be closely monitored.[28,39]

TIMING OF ANTIBIOTIC INITIATION

For symptomatic infants, prompt initiation of empirical antibiotics is warranted[13]; however, for asymptomatic infants at risk for EOS, the optimal timing of antibiotic initiation is less clear. Treating all infants at risk of EOS with antibiotics unnecessarily exposes many infants to antibiotic therapy, increasing the risks of adverse events without providing benefit. Waiting until the infant develops signs of sepsis increases the risks of sequelae and, in some cases, death. Measures to improve prompt identification of infants who are truly infected are under investigation. Use of a calculator (https://neonatalsepsiscalculator.kaiserpermanente.org) to quantify the risk of EOS based on maternal and neonatal characteristics is a promising strategy to safely reduce the number of infants unnecessarily exposed to antibiotics.[40,41]

Late-Onset Sepsis

In contrast to EOS, most late-onset sepsis (LOS) pathogens are acquired from the environment following parturition, resulting in the development of symptoms between days 4 and 120 of life.[42] Gram-positive organisms predominate LOS cases (Table 2.2).[42,43] For hospitalized infants, invasive procedures such as the placement of intravascular catheters, chest tubes and other drains, mechanical ventilation, parenteral nutrition, and surgical procedures interfere with the infant's immune barriers, making them more susceptible to infection.[43] Coagulase-negative staphylococci (CoNS) are the most common cause of LOS (45%–53%), followed by *S. aureus* (11%–13%), *E. coli* (5%–7%), and GBS (2%–7%).[43,44]

As with EOS infections, cases of suspected LOS should be treated empirically in most cases. Because the pathogen distribution is different for LOS compared to EOS, there is greater variability among centers and clinicians in the preferred antibiotic regimen.[45–47] A common strategy is to use one antibiotic with predominantly Gram-positive activity (i.e., ampicillin, nafcillin, or vancomycin) and another with

TABLE 2.2 Organisms Frequently Causing Late-Onset Sepsis in Infants[42,43]

Organism	% of Cases
≥37 weeks' gestational age	
Escherichia coli	20
Coagulase-negative staphylococci	19
Staphylococcus aureus	18
Streptococcus agalactiae	8
Pseudomonas aeruginosa	2
<37 weeks' gestational age	
Coagulase-negative staphylococci	53
Staphylococcus aureus	11
Escherichia coli	5
Streptococcus agalactiae	2
Pseudomonas aeruginosa	2

predominantly Gram-negative activity (gentamicin or ceftazidime). Given that a substantial percentage of LOS infections are nosocomial, it is crucial to consider local and institutional epidemiology when determining the most appropriate empiric treatment.[15,48]

AMPICILLIN

Ampicillin is often used as an empirical treatment for LOS for the same reasons that it is used for EOS: good coverage of GBS, *Enterococcus* species, and *L. monocytogenes*, along with some coverage of *E. coli* and other Gram-negative bacteria. However, LOS is more likely to be due to CoNS or *S. aureus*, and ampicillin is only very rarely effective against CoNS and *S. aureus*. GBS causes disease, but is much less common than during the first 3 days of life, accounting for <10% of LOS cases.[42,43] For these reasons, many clinicians limit empirical ampicillin use to the first 3 days of life and use broader-spectrum agents thereafter.

VANCOMYCIN

Vancomycin is commonly used as the Gram-positive antibiotic of choice for empirical treatment of LOS because of its broad spectrum. CoNS and *S. aureus* are the most common causes of LOS in infants born at term, and approximately 50% of CoNS and 28% of *S. aureus* are resistant to beta-lactams.[49,50] Vancomycin is also effective against GBS, *Enterococcus*, and *L. monocytogenes*, less common causes of LOS.[51,52] However, empirical treatment is not beneficial in most cases of bacteremia with these organisms. A retrospective study of 4364 infants with CoNS bacteremia found that the 2848 infants who received empiric vancomycin had similar mortality when compared to 1516 infants who received vancomycin 1 to 3 days after the first positive blood culture was collected (9% vs. 8%; adjusted odds ratio = 1.06; 95% confidence interval [CI], 0.81–1.39).[53] The duration of bacteremia and duration of hospital stay were also similar.[53] Although this study did not compare other important sequelae of CoNS bacteremia, including neurodevelopmental impairment, it did suggest that, for infants with beta-lactam–resistant CoNS infections, definitive therapy with vancomycin could likely be delayed until susceptibility results are available without substantial increases in risk.[54] A single-center study reported no change in the frequency of fulminant sepsis or the duration of the sepsis episodes for 2 years with oxacillin compared with 7 years with vancomycin as the standard empiric Gram-positive antibiotic.[55]

In addition to limited data supporting its effectiveness compared to antibiotics with narrower spectrums, the Centers for Disease Control and Prevention has specifically targeted reducing excessive vancomycin use as a healthcare improvement goal.[56] In addition to the short-term consequences of vancomycin exposure, nephrotoxicity, and ototoxicity,[57,58] vancomycin use increases the risk of future sepsis in general, as well as infections with vancomycin-resistant enterococci,[59] multidrug-resistant Gram-negative bacilli,[60] vancomycin-intermediate and -resistant *S. aureus*, and invasive candidiasis for both the individual and the patient care unit.[61]

However, in centers where LOS due to methicillin-resistant *S. aureus* (MRSA) is common, empirical vancomycin may be appropriate. A large retrospective study found that, for infants with MRSA bacteremia, empirical vancomycin therapy was associated with improved survival at 30 days.[7] Of the infants with MRSA who received adequate empirical antibiotics, 8% died (39/493) compared to 9% of those given inadequate empirical antibiotics (24/255).[7] When the odds of 30-day survival were adjusted for confounding factors, adequate empirical antibiotic therapy with vancomycin doubled the odds of survival (odds ratio = 2.06; 95% CI, 1.08–3.82).[7]

NAFCILLIN AND OXACILLIN

The anti-staphylococcal penicillins, nafcillin and oxacillin, are frequently used as empirical therapy for LOS.[54] These antibiotics provide good activity against methicillin-susceptible *S. aureus* (MSSA), susceptible CoNS isolates, GBS, and other *Streptococcus* species but have a narrower spectrum and lower toxicity than vancomycin.

Recently, empiric use of oxacillin for LOS has been associated with an unexpected decrease in the incidence of LOS due to *S. aureus*.[62] This may be related to the corresponding increase in CoNS infections. Because CoNS are less pathogenic than *S. aureus*, this change resulted in three fewer deaths during the 2-year oxacillin period compared to the 2-year vancomycin period.[62] Several other centers found that they were able to reduce vancomycin use dramatically without increases in mortality or measured morbidities. One center decreased their vancomycin use from 81% of antibiotic courses to 23% of antibiotic courses with no changes in mortality.[63] A multicenter study of medication use in 220 neonatal intensive care units found that nafcillin use increased by 158% over the 5 years of the study period.[64] Over that same time period, mortality among the infants born weighing ≤1500g did not change.[65]

The major therapeutic hole for these penicillins is MRSA; however, invasive MSSA infections are more common than MRSA infections in infants, and beta-lactam antibiotics are superior to vancomycin for the treatment of invasive MSSA.[49,66] Unless the MRSA rate is particularly high or there are very clear risk factors for MRSA, it seems appropriate to use the class of antibiotics that will be the most effective for the common organisms rather than using an antibiotic that, although it provides a more complete Gram-positive spectrum of activity, is a less effective drug for most non-MRSA organisms. Although infants colonized with MRSA can have LOS caused by other types of organisms, due to the increased risk of invasive MRSA infection infants known to be colonized with MRSA should probably be treated empirically with vancomycin should signs of LOS develop.[67]

Nafcillin and oxacillin likely have some activity against *Enterococcus* species and *L. monocytogenes* but there are no approved criteria for testing for the susceptibility of these antibiotic/organism combinations. Ampicillin or vancomycin should be used if these organisms are suspected; however, concern for these two organisms should not have a significant impact on antibiotic selection for LOS. Infections due to *L. monocytogenes* are exceeding rare after the first month of life.[68]

CEFAZOLIN

Cefazolin, a first-generation cephalosporin, has advantages and disadvantages similar to those for nafcillin/oxacillin with regard to a narrower spectrum of activity and lower toxicity than vancomycin. There is less experience with the use of cefazolin for LOS than with the anti-staphylococcal penicillins, but it appears to have similar efficacy for the treatment of invasive Gram-positive infections.[69-71] Cefazolin has the additional theoretical benefit as an empirical agent for neonatal LOS of a spectrum that includes some *E. coli* and *Klebsiella* species in addition to Gram-positive organisms.[72] Like all cephalosporins, cefazolin is not sufficiently effective to use as monotherapy for treatment of infections due to *Enterococcus* species or *L. monocytogenes*. Cefazolin does not provide adequate treatment of the central nervous system and should not be used until meningitis has been excluded.[36] Additional studies in infants should be conducted prior to widespread use of empirical cefazolin.

THIRD-GENERATION CEPHALOSPORINS

Cefotaxime and ceftriaxone are third-generation cephalosporins that provide increased coverage against Gram-negative bacteria compared with ampicillin or nafcillin/oxacillin while maintaining fair Gram-positive activity.[25] Cefotaxime is the preferred treatment for cases of suspected or proven neonatal meningitis due to its superior central nervous system penetration and tolerability.[15,73] Unfortunately, cefotaxime is no longer being produced in the United States, so an alternative third-generation cephalosporin is often necessary.[74] Ceftriaxone has the most similar spectrum of activity but must be carefully used early in life due to its ability to displace bilirubin and increase risk of bilirubin-associated encephalopathy. This risk is unlikely to be clinically significant after the first 2 weeks of age and can be closely monitored during the antibiotic course.[75]

In contrast to ampicillin, most *E. coli* infections are susceptible to third-generation cephalosporins. In one study, 3% to 9% of early-onset *E. coli* infections were due to cephalosporin-resistant strains.[76] Similarly, a national surveillance study conducted in Germany found that 4% of 158 neonatal *E. coli* infections were resistant to cefotaxime.[28] Another surveillance study that included 5 years of neonatal bloodstream infections in England and Wales found that ~3% of *E. coli* infections were resistant to cefotaxime.[77] Because of the broader spectrum of cefotaxime and ceftriaxone compared to ampicillin, this antibiotic is often used as a single agent that has the advantage of reduced line entries and, potentially, lower toxicity. Ceftazidime is also a third-generation cephalosporin but has inferior Gram-positive activity and should not be used as monotherapy empirically.

Cephalosporins are not effective as monotherapy against *Enterococcus* or *L. monocytogenes*, so ampicillin should be used in addition to cefotaxime if these organisms are suspected.[21] Additionally, third-generation cephalosporins are thought to be less effective than first-generation cephalosporins or anti-staphylococcal penicillins against *S. aureus*.[78] Cefotaxime also does not exhibit synergy when combined with gentamicin such that the addition of gentamicin to cefotaxime is less useful than when it is used alongside ampicillin or nafcillin.[25]

An additional concern with widespread cephalosporin use is the associated increase in resistant isolates such that caution must be exercised prior to using cefotaxime as part of the standard empirical antibiotic strategy for infants. In settings where broad-spectrum antibiotic use is common, cephalosporin resistance among Gram-negative bacteria causing LOS can reach 50%.[79] Studies in adults have linked cephalosporin use to the selection of highly resistant Gram-negative isolates and increased rates of infections due to *Pseudomonas aeruginosa* and extended-spectrum penicillinase producing enterobactericeae.[80] Additionally, cephalosporin use in infants increases the risk of invasive candidiasis, which has significant associated morbidity and mortality and may be associated with an increased risk of all-cause mortality in hospitalized infants.[38,52] A multicenter study of 3702 infants with birth weights $<$1000g found that candidiasis was significantly correlated with the average number of cephalosporin days (correlation coefficient = 0.67; $P = 0.017$).[38] Due to these concerns with efficacy and safety, many experts recommend the use of cefotaxime only with suspected or proven neonatal meningitis or as an alternative to gentamicin in instances of neonatal renal or auditory problems.[15]

GENTAMICIN

Similar to its role in EOS, gentamicin provides broad-spectrum Gram-negative coverage with the additional potential benefit of synergy with other antibiotics for the treatment of some Gram-positive infections.[25,26] Because Gram-positive infections predominate after 3 days of age, the combinations of ampicillin/gentamicin or nafcillin or oxacillin/gentamicin would be expected to provide a good balance of a relatively narrow spectrum that still provides effective coverage for the majority of expected pathogens.[63] Gentamicin is not typically used in combination with cefotaxime because cefotaxime has good Gram-negative coverage by itself.

PSEUDOMONAS COVERAGE

Approximately 2% to 5% of LOS cases are due to *P. aeruginosa*.[27,43] Because of this low incidence, empiric coverage of *P. aeruginosa* is not usually warranted. However, compared to other pathogens, *P. aeruginosa* is more likely to cause fulminant disease and has a higher mortality than other pathogens.[81,82] An Australian surveillance study with an unusually high incidence of *Pseudomonas* LOS found that 52% of infants with *Pseudomonas* infection died, resulting in a significantly increased odds of mortality compared to other Gram-negative bacilli (odds ratio = 5.91; 95% CI, 3.69–9.47).[83] Consideration should be given to including empiric antibiotics that are effective against *P. aeruginosa* for infants with rapidly progressive clinical decompensation.

Although most cases are sporadic, *P. aeruginosa* has caused outbreaks of disease in neonatal units in the past.[84] Compared to other organisms, the risk of infant-to-infant spread is much greater for *P. aeruginosa*. For this reason, empiric coverage of *P. aeruginosa* is warranted for neighbors of *Pseudomonas*-infected infants who develop signs of infection.[85] Ceftazidime, cefepime, piperacillin–tazobactam, and meropenem are the antibiotics most often used for empiric and definitive treatment of *P. aeruginosa*. Piperacillin–tazobactam and meropenem are also effective against anaerobic bacteria, so they may have greater detrimental effects on intestinal flora and risks of candidiasis and infections with resistant organisms in the future.[86] When meningitis is a possibility, piperacillin–tazobactam may not be as effective as other anti-pseudomonal antibiotics due to the need to achieve a proper ratio of both piperacillin and tazobactam across the blood–brain barrier.[87] Fluoroquinolones are used in adults for treatment of *P. aeruginosa* but should not generally be used in infants due to the lack of safety data. The U.S. Food and Drug Administration recently upgraded the "black-box" warning for fluoroquinolones due to findings that the risks of mitochondrial toxicity and other adverse events were more common than previously appreciated.[88] For highly resistant Gram-negative infections, ciprofloxacin may be necessary, but empirical use should be extremely rare.[89]

ANTIFUNGALS

Invasive candidiasis is a relatively uncommon cause of sepsis among infants but has a high mortality and leads to long-term neurodevelopmental impairment among survivors.[90] Empiric antifungal therapy should be considered for infants who do not show rapid improvement following initiation of empiric antibacterials. The risk of candidiasis is inversely related to gestational age and birth weight and is further increased by exposure to third-generation cephalosporins and other broad-spectrum antibiotics and the presence of central venous catheters.[91] Fluconazole is a reasonable first-line antifungal if it has not been used for prophylaxis, in which case, micafungin or amphotericin B deoxycholate should be considered.[92]

Early antifungal use reduces mortality due to *Candida* LOS. A study that included 136 infants found that empiric antifungal treatment improved neurodevelopmental impairment-free survival for infants with candidiasis compared to those who received only definitive therapy.[93] Fifty percent (19/38) of infants with invasive candidiasis who received empiric antifungal therapy had death or neurodevelopmental impairment compared to 64% (55/86) of those with delayed therapy (odds ratio = 0.27; 95% CI, 0.08–0.86).[93]

ANTIVIRALS

Neonatal herpes simplex virus (HSV) infections may lead to subtle or fulminant signs of sepsis in infants. Signs usually develop from days 5 to 14 of age depending on the manifestation of disease. Disseminated disease usually presents around day 7 of age; skin, eye, and mucous membrane disease around day 10 of age; central nervous system disease can occur as late as day 21 of age.[94] Delayed initiation of acyclovir to infants with HSV disease has been associated with increased mortality.[95] For infants who are ultimately diagnosed with HSV infection, empiric acyclovir therapy has been associated with improved survival compared to infants for whom acyclovir therapy is delayed until a definitive diagnosis is made (odds ratio = 2.63; 95% CI, 1.36–5.08).[95] Infants at high risk of neonatal HSV infection should be treated promptly with acyclovir.[96]

Low-Resource Settings

The epidemiology of neonatal sepsis varies significantly throughout the world. For example, GBS is an uncommon cause of neonatal sepsis in Sub-Saharan Africa.[10] Multidrug-resistant Gram-negative infections predominate in some settings.[97] The World Health Organization currently recommends that neonatal sepsis be treated with penicillin or ampicillin and gentamicin in all settings.[98] These recommendations fail to acknowledge that this regimen is unlikely to have similar efficacy in all communities. Regional surveillance of the organisms causing neonatal sepsis and their antibiotic susceptibility patterns is critical to optimize outcomes of affected neonates globally.[99]

Conclusion

Most infants that receive empiric antibiotic treatment do not have culture-proven sepsis. Uninfected infants receiving empiric treatment are exposed to the negative consequences of antimicrobial use without corresponding benefit.[16,100] Recent studies have demonstrated that even short courses of empirical antibiotics lead to reductions in the biodiversity of intestinal microbes with a shift toward more pathogenic species, such as *Enterobacter* species. These alterations in biodiversity have been linked to increased risks of necrotizing enterocolitis, bacterial sepsis, invasive candidiasis, and death during infancy, as well as longer-term consequences that are still under study.[101] As we seek to improve care to achieve better short- and long-term outcomes, we must develop (1) better methods for identifying which infants truly have infections, and (2) techniques that allow for accurate identification of the infecting organism rapidly enough that empiric therapy can promptly be replaced by definitive targeted therapy. While we await these capabilities, narrow-spectrum therapy with ampicillin and gentamicin or an anti-staphylococcal penicillin and gentamicin is probably the best approach in most cases. Special risk factors may warrant broader empiric therapy that should be narrowed as soon as culture results are available.

REFERENCES

1. Shane AL, Stoll BJ. Recent developments and current issues in the epidemiology, diagnosis, and management of bacterial and fungal neonatal sepsis. *Am J Perinatol*. 2013;30(2):131-141.
2. Davis KL, Shah SS, Frank G, Eppes SC. Why are young infants tested for herpes simplex virus? *Pediatr Emerg Care*. 2008; 24(10):673-678.
3. Rattani S, Farooqi J, Hussain AS, Jabeen K. Spectrum and antifungal resistance of candidemia in neonates with early- and late-onset sepsis in Pakistan. *Pediatr Infect Dis J*. 2021;40(9): 814-820.
4. Ekanem AD, Anah MU, Udo JJ. The prevalence of congenital malaria among neonates with suspected sepsis in Calabar, Nigeria. *Trop Doct*. 2008;38(2):73-76.
5. Wynn JL, Wong HR, Shanley TP, Bizzarro MJ, Saiman L, Polin RA. Time for a neonatal-specific consensus definition for sepsis. *Pediatr Crit Care Med*. 2014;15(6):523-528.
6. Berardi A, Buffagni AM, Rossi C, et al. Serial physical examinations, a simple and reliable tool for managing neonates at risk for early-onset sepsis. *World J Clin Pediatr*. 2016;5(4):358-364.
7. Thaden JT, Ericson JE, Cross H, et al. Survival benefit of empirical therapy for *Staphylococcus aureus* bloodstream infections in infants. *Pediatr Infect Dis J*. 2015;34(11):1175-1179.
8. Downie L, Armiento R, Subhi R, Kelly J, Clifford V, Duke T. Community-acquired neonatal and infant sepsis in developing countries: efficacy of WHO's currently recommended antibiotics—systematic review and meta-analysis. *Arch Dis Child*. 2013;98(2): 146-154.
9. Bergin SP, Thaden J, Ericson JE, et al. Neonatal Escherichia coli bloodstream infections: clinical outcomes and impact of initial antibiotic therapy. *Pediatr Infect Dis J*. 2015;34(9):933-936.
10. Mduma E, Halidou T, Kaboré B, et al. Etiology of severe invasive infections in young infants in rural settings in sub-Saharan Africa. *PLoS ONE*. 2022;17(2):e0264322.
11. Stoll BJ, Puopolo KM, Hansen NI, et al. Early-onset neonatal sepsis 2015 to 2017, the rise of Escherichia coli, and the need for novel prevention strategies. *JAMA Pediatr*. 2020;174(7):e200593.
12. Wortham JM, Hansen NI, Schrag SJ, et al. Chorioamnionitis and culture-confirmed, early-onset neonatal infections. *Pediatrics*. 2016;137(1):e20152323.
13. Puopolo KM, Benitz WE, Zaoutis TE, American Academy of Pediatrics Committee on Fetus and Newborn, Committee on Infectious Diseases. Management of neonates born at ≥35 0/7 weeks' gestation with suspected or proven early-onset bacterial sepsis. *Pediatrics*. 2018;142(6):e20182894.
14. Puopolo KM, Benitz WE, Zaoutis TE, American Academy of Pediatrics Committee on Fetus and Newborn, Committee on Infectious Diseases. Management of neonates born at ≤34 6/7 weeks' gestation with suspected or proven early-onset bacterial sepsis. *Pediatrics*. 2018;142(6):e20182896.
15. Stockmann C, Spigarelli MG, Campbell SC, et al. Considerations in the pharmacologic treatment and prevention of neonatal sepsis. *Paediatr Drugs*. 2014;16(1):67-81.
16. Baltimore RS. Neonatal sepsis: epidemiology and management. *Paediatr Drugs*. 2003;5(11):723-740.
17. Hornik CP, Benjamin DK, Smith PB, et al. Electronic health records and pharmacokinetic modeling to assess the relationship between ampicillin exposure and seizure risk in neonates. *J Pediatr*. 2016;178:125-129.e1.
18. Andrews JI, Diekema DJ, Hunter SK, et al. Group B streptococci causing neonatal bloodstream infection: antimicrobial susceptibility and serotyping results from SENTRY centers in the Western Hemisphere. *Am J Obstet Gynecol*. 2000;183(4): 859-862.
19. Fluegge K, Supper S, Siedler A, Berner R. Antibiotic susceptibility in neonatal invasive isolates of Streptococcus agalactiae in a 2-year nationwide surveillance study in Germany. *Antimicrob Agents Chemother*. 2004;48(11):4444-4446.
20. Mariani M, Parodi A, Minghetti D, et al. Early and late onset neonatal sepsis: epidemiology and effectiveness of empirical antibacterial therapy in a III level neonatal intensive care unit. *Antibiotics (Basel)*. 2022;11(2):284.
21. Leazer R, Perkins AM, Shomaker K, Fine B. A meta-analysis of the rates of Listeria monocytogenes and Enterococcus in febrile infants. *Hosp Pediatr*. 2016;6(4):187-195.
22. Mylonakis E, Paliou M, Hohmann EL, Calderwood SB, Wing EJ. Listeriosis during pregnancy: a case series and review of 222 cases. *Medicine (Baltimore)*. 2002;81(4):260-269.
23. Jiao Y, Zhang W, Ma J, et al. Early onset of neonatal listeriosis. *Pediatr Int*. 2011;53(6):1034-1037.
24. Charlier C, Kermorvant-Duchemin E, Perrodeau E, et al. Neonatal listeriosis presentation and outcome: a prospective study of 189 cases. *Clin Infect Dis*. 2022;74(1):8-16.
25. Darmstadt GL, Batra M, Zaidi AK. Parenteral antibiotics for the treatment of serious neonatal bacterial infections in developing country settings. *Pediatr Infect Dis J*. 2009;28(suppl 1): S37-S42.
26. Espaze EP, Reynaud AE. Antibiotic susceptibilities of Listeria: In vitro studies. *Infection*. 1988;16(suppl 2):S160-S164.
27. Vergnano S, Menson E, Kennea N, et al. Neonatal infections in England: the NeonIN surveillance network. *Arch Dis Child Fetal Neonatal Ed*. 2011;96(1):F9-F14.
28. Heideking M, Lander F, Hufnagel M, et al. Antibiotic susceptibility profiles of neonatal invasive isolates of Escherichia coli from a 2-year nationwide surveillance study in Germany, 2009–2010. *Eur J Clin Microbiol Infect Dis*. 2013;32(9): 1221-1223.
29. Bizzarro MJ, Dembry LM, Baltimore RS, Gallagher PG. Changing patterns in neonatal Escherichia coli sepsis and ampicillin resistance in the era of intrapartum antibiotic prophylaxis. *Pediatrics*. 2008;121(4):689-696.
30. Alarcon A, Peña P, Salas S, Sancha M, Omeñaca F. Neonatal early onset Escherichia coli sepsis: trends in incidence and antimicrobial resistance in the era of intrapartum antimicrobial prophylaxis. *Pediatr Infect Dis J*. 2004;23(4):295-299.
31. Weissman SJ, Hansen NI, Zaterka-Baxter K, Higgins RD, Stoll BJ. Emergence of antibiotic resistance-associated clones among Escherichia coli recovered from newborns with early-onset sepsis and meningitis in the United States, 2008–2009. *J Pediatric Infect Dis Soc*. 2016;5(3):269-276.
32. Touw DJ, Westerman EM, Sprij AJ. Therapeutic drug monitoring of aminoglycosides in neonates. *Clin Pharmacokinet*. 2009; 48(2):71-88.
33. Musiime GM, Seale AC, Moxon SG, Lawn JE. Risk of gentamicin toxicity in neonates treated for possible severe bacterial infection in low- and middle-income countries: systematic review. *Trop Med Int Health*. 2015;20(12):1593-1606.
34. Zimmerman E, Lahav A. Ototoxicity in preterm infants: effects of genetics, aminoglycosides, and loud environmental noise. *J Perinatol*. 2013;33(1):3-8.
35. Fuchs A, Zimmermann L, Bickle Graz M, et al. Gentamicin exposure and sensorineural hearing loss in preterm infants. *PLoS ONE*. 2016;11(7):e0158806.

36. Sullins AK, Abdel-Rahman SM. Pharmacokinetics of antibacterial agents in the CSF of children and adolescents. *Paediatr Drugs*. 2013;15(2):93-117.
37. Clark RH, Bloom BT, Spitzer AR, Gerstmann DR. Empiric use of ampicillin and cefotaxime, compared with ampicillin and gentamicin, for neonates at risk for sepsis is associated with an increased risk of neonatal death. *Pediatrics*. 2006;117(1):67-74.
38. Cotten CM, McDonald S, Stoll B, et al. The association of third-generation cephalosporin use and invasive candidiasis in extremely low birth-weight infants. *Pediatrics*. 2006;118(2):717-722.
39. Friedman S, Shah V, Ohlsson A, Matlow AG. Neonatal Escherichia coli infections: concerns regarding resistance to current therapy. *Acta Paediatr*. 2000;89(6):686-689.
40. Ellington M, Kasat K, Williams K, et al. Improving antibiotic stewardship among asymptomatic newborns using the early-onset sepsis risk calculator. *Pediatr Qual Saf*. 2021;6(5):e459.
41. Kuzniewicz MW, Puopolo KM, Fischer A, et al. A quantitative, risk-based approach to the management of neonatal early-onset sepsis. *JAMA Pediatr*. 2017;171(4):365-371.
42. Testoni D, Hayashi M, Cohen-Wolkowiez M, et al. Late-onset bloodstream infections in hospitalized term infants. *Pediatr Infect Dis J*. 2014;33(9):920-923.
43. Boghossian NS, Page GP, Bell EF, et al. Late-onset sepsis in very low birth weight infants from singleton and multiple-gestation births. *J Pediatr*. 2013;162(6):1120-1124.e1.
44. Song WS, Park HW, Oh MY, et al. Neonatal sepsis-causing bacterial pathogens and outcome of trends of their antimicrobial susceptibility a 20-year period at a neonatal intensive care unit. *Clin Exp Pediatr*. 2022;65(7):350-357.
45. Garrido F, Allegaert K, Arribas C, et al. Variations in antibiotic use and sepsis management in neonatal intensive care units: a European survey. *Antibiotics (Basel)*. 2021;10(9):1046.
46. Metsvaht T, Nellis G, Varendi H, et al. High variability in the dosing of commonly used antibiotics revealed by a Europe-wide point prevalence study: implications for research and dissemination. *BMC Pediatr*. 2015;15:41.
47. Arnold C, Clark R, Bosco J, Shoemaker C, Spitzer AR. Variability in vancomycin use in newborn intensive care units determined from data in an electronic medical record. *Infect Control Hosp Epidemiol*. 2008;29(7):667-670.
48. Muller-Pebody B, Johnson AP, Heath PT, et al. Empirical treatment of neonatal sepsis: are the current guidelines adequate? *Arch Dis Child Fetal Neonatal Ed*. 2011;96(1):F4-F8.
49. Ericson JE, Popoola VO, Smith PB, et al. Burden of invasive Staphylococcus aureus infections in hospitalized infants. *JAMA Pediatr*. 2015;169(12):1105-1111.
50. Mintz A, Mor M, Klinger G, et al. Changing epidemiology and resistance patterns of pathogens causing neonatal bacteremia. *Eur J Clin Microbiol Infect Dis*. 2020;39(10):1879-1884.
51. Korang SK, Safi S, Nava C, et al. Antibiotic regimens for late-onset neonatal sepsis. *Cochrane Database Syst Rev*. 2021;5:CD013836.
52. Wagstaff JS, Durrant RJ, Newman MG, et al. Antibiotic treatment of suspected and confirmed neonatal sepsis within 28 days of birth: a retrospective analysis. *Front Pharmacol*. 2019;10:1191.
53. Ericson JE, Thaden J, Cross HR, et al. No survival benefit with empirical vancomycin therapy for coagulase-negative staphylococcal bloodstream infections in infants. *Pediatr Infect Dis J*. 2015;34(4):371-375.
54. Chiu CH, Michelow IC, Cronin J, Ringer SA, Ferris TG, Puopolo KM. Effectiveness of a guideline to reduce vancomycin use in the neonatal intensive care unit. *Pediatr Infect Dis J*. 2011;30(4):273-278.
55. Blanchard AC, Quach C, Autmizguine J. Staphylococcal infections in infants: updates and current challenges. *Clin Perinatol*. 2015;42(1):119-132, ix.
56. Centers for Disease Control and Prevention. Recommendations for preventing the spread of vancomycin resistance. Recommendations of the Hospital Infection Control Practices Advisory Committee (HICPAC). *MMWR Recomm Rep*. 1995;44(RR-12):1-13.
57. Williams C, Hankinson C, McWilliam SJ, Oni L. Vancomycin-associated acute kidney injury epidemiology in children: a systematic review [published online ahead of print February 24, 2022]. *Arch Dis Child*. 2022. doi:10.1136/archdischild-2021-323429.
58. Marissen J, Fortmann I, Humberg A, et al. Vancomycin-induced ototoxicity in very-low-birthweight infants. *J Antimicrob Chemother*. 2020;75(8):2291-2298.
59. Iosifidis E, Evdoridou I, Agakidou E, et al. Vancomycin-resistant Enterococcus outbreak in a neonatal intensive care unit: epidemiology, molecular analysis and risk factors. *Am J Infect Control*. 2013;41(10):857-861.
60. Ofek-Shlomai N, Benenson S, Ergaz Z, Peleg O, Braunstein R, Bar-Oz B. Gastrointestinal colonization with ESBL-producing Klebsiella in preterm babies—is vancomycin to blame? *Eur J Clin Microbiol Infect Dis*. 2012;31(4):567-570.
61. Zaoutis TE, Prasad PA, Localio AR, et al. Risk factors and predictors for candidemia in pediatric intensive care unit patients: implications for prevention. *Clin Infect Dis*. 2010;51(5):e38-e45.
62. Romanelli RMC, Anchieta LM, Bueno E Silva AC, de Jesus LA, Rosado V, Clemente WT. Empirical antimicrobial therapy for late-onset sepsis in a neonatal unit with high prevalence of coagulase-negative Staphylococcus. *J Pediatr (Rio J)*. 2016;92(5):472-478.
63. Holzmann-Pazgal G, Khan AM, Northrup TF, Domonoske C, Eichenwald EC. Decreasing vancomycin utilization in a neonatal intensive care unit. *Am J Infect Control*. 2015;43(11):1255-1257.
64. Clark RH, Bloom BT, Spitzer AR, Gerstmann DR. Reported medication use in the neonatal intensive care unit: data from a large national data set. *Pediatrics*. 2006;117(6):1979-1987.
65. Stoll BJ, Hansen NI, Bell EF, et al. Trends in care practices, morbidity, and mortality of extremely preterm neonates, 1993–2012. *JAMA*. 2015;314(10):1039-1051.
66. Schweizer ML, Furuno JP, Harris AD, et al. Comparative effectiveness of nafcillin or cefazolin versus vancomycin in methicillin-susceptible Staphylococcus aureus bacteremia. *BMC Infect Dis*. 2011;11:279.
67. Popoola VO, Budd A, Wittig SM, et al. Methicillin-resistant Staphylococcus aureus transmission and infections in a neonatal intensive care unit despite active surveillance cultures and decolonization: challenges for infection prevention. *Infect Control Hosp Epidemiol*. 2014;35(4):412-418.
68. Okike IO, Awofisayo A, Adak B, Heath PT. Empirical antibiotic cover for Listeria monocytogenes infection beyond the neonatal period: a time for change? *Arch Dis Child*. 2015;100(5):423-425.
69. Ceriani Cernadas JM, Fernández Jonusas S, Márquez M, Garsd A, Mariani G. Clinical outcome of neonates with nosocomial suspected sepsis treated with cefazolin or vancomycin: a non-inferiority, randomized, controlled trial. *Arch Argent Pediatr*. 2014;112(4):308-314.

70. Pollett S, Baxi SM, Rutherford GW, Doernberg SB, Bacchetti P, Chambers HF. Cefazolin versus nafcillin for methicillin-sensitive Staphylococcus aureus bloodstream infection in a California tertiary medical center. *Antimicrob Agents Chemother*. 2016;60(8):4684-4689.
71. Rao SN, Rhodes NJ, Lee BJ, et al. Treatment outcomes with cefazolin versus oxacillin for deep-seated methicillin-susceptible Staphylococcus aureus bloodstream infections. *Antimicrob Agents Chemother*. 2015;59(9):5232-5238.
72. U.S. National Library of Medicine, National Institutes of Health. *CEFAZOLIN - (cefazolin sodium) Injection, Solution*. Available at: https://dailymed.nlm.nih.gov/dailymed/drugInfo.cfm?setid=13a33420-b1e1-4b7e-8e59-4d5badafe654. Accessed January 18, 2023.
73. Odio CM. Cefotaxime for treatment of neonatal sepsis and meningitis. *Diagn Microbiol Infect Dis*. 1995;22(1-2):111-117.
74. U.S. Food and Drug Administration. *Determination that CLAFORAN (cefotaxime sodium) for injection, 500 milligrams/vial, 1 gram/vial, 2 grams/vial and 10 grams/vial, was not withdrawn from sale for reasons of safety or effectiveness*. Available at: https://www.federalregister.gov/documents/2019/07/03/2019-14172/determination-that-claforan-cefotaxime-sodium-for-injection-500-milligramsvial-1-gramvial-2. Accessed January 18, 2023.
75. Hile GB, Musick KL, Dugan AJ, Bailey AM, Howington GT. Occurrence of hyperbilirubinemia in neonates given a short-term course of ceftriaxone versus cefotaxime for sepsis. *J Pediatr Pharmacol Ther*. 2021;26(1):99-103.
76. Flannery DD, Puopolo KM, Hansen NI, et al. Antimicrobial susceptibility profiles among neonatal early-onset sepsis pathogens. *Pediatr Infect Dis J*. 2022;41(3):263-271.
77. Blackburn RM, Verlander NQ, Heath PT, Muller-Pebody B. The changing antibiotic susceptibility of bloodstream infections in the first month of life: informing antibiotic policies for early- and late-onset neonatal sepsis. *Epidemiol Infect*. 2014;142(4):803-811.
78. Kang N, Housman ST, Nicolau DP. Assessing the surrogate susceptibility of oxacillin and cefoxitin for commonly utilized parenteral agents against methicillin-susceptible Staphylococcus aureus: focus on ceftriaxone discordance between predictive susceptibility and in vivo exposures. *Pathogens*. 2015;4(3):599-605.
79. Lona Reyes JC, Verdugo Robles M, Pérez Ramírez RO, Pérez Molina JJ, Ascencio Esparza EP, Benítez Vázquez EA. Etiology and antimicrobial resistance patterns in early and late neonatal sepsis in a neonatal intensive care unit. *Arch Argent Pediatr*. 2015;113(4):317-323.
80. Dancer SJ. The problem with cephalosporins. *J Antimicrob Chemother*. 2001;48(4):463-478.
81. Tsai MH, Hsu JF, Chu SM, et al. Incidence, clinical characteristics and risk factors for adverse outcome in neonates with late-onset sepsis. *Pediatr Infect Dis J*. 2014;33(1):e7-e13.
82. Hammoud MS, Al-Taiar A, Thalib L, Al-Sweih N, Pathan S, Isaacs D. Incidence, aetiology and resistance of late-onset neonatal sepsis: a five-year prospective study. *J Paediatr Child Health*. 2012;48(7):604-609.
83. Gordon A, Isaacs D. Late onset neonatal Gram-negative bacillary infection in Australia and New Zealand: 1992–2002. *Pediatr Infect Dis J*. 2006;25(1):25-29.
84. Jefferies JM, Cooper T, Yam T, Clarke SC. Pseudomonas aeruginosa outbreaks in the neonatal intensive care unit—a systematic review of risk factors and environmental sources. *J Med Microbiol*. 2012;61(Pt 8):1052-1061.
85. Reichert F, Piening B, Geffers C, Gastmeier P, Bührer C, Schwab F. Pathogen-specific clustering of nosocomial blood stream infections in very preterm infants. *Pediatrics*. 2016;137(4):e20152860.
86. Gibson MK, Wang B, Ahmadi S, et al. Developmental dynamics of the preterm infant gut microbiota and antibiotic resistome. *Nat Microbiol*. 2016;1:16024.
87. Leleu G, Kitzis MD, Vallois JM, Gutmann L, Decazes JM. Different ratios of the piperacillin–tazobactam combination for treatment of experimental meningitis due to Klebsiella pneumoniae producing the TEM-3 extended-spectrum beta-lactamase. *Antimicrob Agents Chemother*. 1994;38(2):195-199.
88. U.S. National Library of Medicine, National Institutes of Health. *CIPROFLOXACIN Injection, Solution*. Available at: https://dailymed.nlm.nih.gov/dailymed/drugInfo.cfm?setid=e82f52f2-ecf8-4c04-a206-f3253b265903. Accessed January 18, 2023.
89. Kaguelidou F, Turner MA, Choonara I, Jacqz-Aigrain E. Ciprofloxacin use in neonates: a systematic review of the literature. *Pediatr Infect Dis J*. 2011;30(2):e29-e37.
90. Adams-Chapman I, Bann CM, Das A, et al. Neurodevelopmental outcome of extremely low birth weight infants with Candida infection. *J Pediatr*. 2013;163(4):961-967.e3.
91. Kelly MS, Benjamin DK, Smith PB. The epidemiology and diagnosis of invasive candidiasis among premature infants. *Clin Perinatol*. 2015;42(1):105-117, viii-ix.
92. Botero-Calderon L, Benjamin DK, Cohen-Wolkowiez M. Advances in the treatment of invasive neonatal candidiasis. *Expert Opin Pharmacother*. 2015;16(7):1035-1048.
93. Greenberg RG, Benjamin DK, Gantz MG, et al. Empiric antifungal therapy and outcomes in extremely low birth weight infants with invasive candidiasis. *J Pediatr*. 2012;161(2):264-269.e2.
94. Curfman AL, Glissmeyer EW, Ahmad FA, et al. Initial presentation of neonatal herpes simplex virus infection. *J Pediatr*. 2016;172:121-126.e1.
95. Shah SS, Aronson PL, Mohamad Z, Lorch SA. Delayed acyclovir therapy and death among neonates with herpes simplex virus infection. *Pediatrics*. 2011;128(6):1153-1160.
96. Pittet LF, Curtis N. Postnatal exposure to herpes simplex virus: to treat or not to treat? *Pediatr Infect Dis J*. 2021;40(5S):S16-S21.
97. Panda SK, Nayak MK, Jena P, et al. Nonfermenting, Gram-negative bacilli causing neonatal sepsis in Odisha, India: four-year surveillance. *Cureus*. 2022;14(2):e22219.
98. Fuchs A, Bielicki J, Mathur S, Sharland M, Van Den Anker JN. Reviewing the WHO guidelines for antibiotic use for sepsis in neonates and children. *Paediatr Int Child Health*. 2018;38(suppl 1):S3-S15.
99. Sands K, Spiller OB, Thomson K, Portal EAR, Iregbu KC, Walsh TR. Early-onset neonatal sepsis in low- and middle-income countries: current challenges and future opportunities. *Infect Drug Resist*. 2022;15:933-946.
100. Tzialla C, Borghesi A, Serra G, Stronati M, Corsello G. Antimicrobial therapy in neonatal intensive care unit. *Ital J Pediatr*. 2015;41:27.
101. Greenwood C, Morrow AL, Lagomarcino AJ, et al. Early empiric antibiotic use in preterm infants is associated with lower bacterial diversity and higher relative abundance of Enterobacter. *J Pediatr*. 2014;165(1):23-29.

Chapter 3

When and How to Treat Neonatal CMV Infection

Sallie R. Permar, MD, PhD; Christine M. Salvatore, MD

Key Points

- Congenital cytomegalovirus (CMV) is the leading infectious cause of hearing loss and neurologic deficits, affecting up to 1% of live births worldwide.
- Symptomatic congenital CMV infection should be treated with ganciclovir or valganciclovir for 6 months to reduce or ameliorate long-term neurologic deficits, including hearing loss and developmental delay.
- Studies suggest that some infants with asymptomatic or mild congenital CMV infection at birth may benefit from treatment, but more studies are needed.
- In premature infants, postnatal CMV infection can cause severe sepsis-like disease and may contribute to long-term neurologic impairment and bronchopulmonary dysplasia.
- Premature infants with symptomatic postnatal CMV infection should be strongly considered for treatment.
- There is not enough evidence at this time to recommend routine treatment of asymptomatic premature infants with postnatal CMV infection.
- Universal screening of all newborns for CMV is warranted to identify congenitally infected infants who will benefit from enhanced neurodevelopmental monitoring and treatment.

Clinical Significance

Cytomegalovirus (CMV) is the most common infection in the newborn, affecting between 0.5% and 2.3% of live births worldwide.[1,2] The seroprevalence of CMV in adults ranges from 45% to 100%, depending on geographic location, socioeconomic status, and race.[3] Infants can acquire CMV infection in utero (congenital CMV), through maternal secretions at birth (perinatal), or after birth via breastfeeding (postnatal CMV). Historically, only congenital CMV was thought to cause clinically significant illness and lead to neurodevelopmental impairment in infants; however, new studies have shown that postnatal CMV infection in premature infants can cause severe disease and contribute to long-term sequelae. Although the infection types can be similar, the risk factors for transmission, severity of disease, long-term sequelae, and treatment recommendations differ based on route of infection (congenital vs. postnatal). We will therefore discuss these two modes of viral transmission separately.

CONGENITAL CMV TRANSMISSION AND OUTCOMES

The highest risk of acquiring congenital CMV occurs in fetuses whose mothers have no prior immunity to CMV (primary infection, ~40% transmission rate); however, transmission can occur with reactivation of a latent infection or with maternal infection with a new strain of CMV (1%–2% transmission rate).[4,5] In fact, because of the high global prevalence of CMV seropositivity among women of childbearing age, the majority of congenital CMV infections occur in infants of women with prior immunity to CMV.[6]

Only 10% to 15% of infants with congenital CMV are symptomatic at birth. Symptoms range from mild to life-threatening multiorgan dysfunction and can include intrauterine growth restriction (IUGR), petechiae, jaundice, hepatosplenomegaly, microcephaly, chorioretinitis, and sensorineural hearing loss (SNHL).[7,8] Long-term sequelae include intellectual disability, seizures, chorioretinitis, optic nerve atrophy, psychomotor and speech delays, learning disabilities, and dental defects.[9,10] Of those infants who are asymptomatic at birth, 10% to 20% will develop neurologic impairment by 2 years of age, most commonly SNHL.[10–13] SNHL associated with CMV has a fluctuating and progressive course, with some children not developing symptoms until 6 years of age.[14,15] Infants with congenital CMV from a primary maternal infection are more likely to have severe sequelae.[7,8,16] Mortality in infants secondary to congenital CMV is 100 to 200 cases in the United States annually.[12] Overall, congenital CMV is the leading cause of developmental impairment and the leading nongenetic cause of SNHL.[17,18]

POSTNATAL CMV TRANSMISSION AND OUTCOMES

Infants acquire postnatal CMV through virus shed in maternal breast milk.[19,20] In the past, CMV was frequently transmitted to hospitalized infants through blood transfusions, but the use of CMV-seronegative or leukoreduced blood has essentially eliminated this mode of transmission.[21] Although harmless in full-term infants, postnatal CMV infection in very-low-birth-weight (VLBW; <1500 g birth weight) infants can result in a severe sepsis-like illness characterized by pneumonitis, enteritis, hepatitis, and thrombocytopenia and may lead to long-term neurologic impairment.[22–24] In a meta-analysis of 17 studies, the risk of postnatal CMV infection in VLBW infants in the United States was approximately 6.5%, with 1.4% developing a sepsis-like syndrome.[23] In most neonatal intensive care units (NICUs), the true prevalence is likely underestimated because CMV is not routinely evaluated for during sepsis evaluations.

There is still debate regarding the outcomes of postnatally acquired CMV and if premature infants who survived a postnatal CMV infection, such as full-term infants after postnatal infection, have no long-term consequences. Gunkel et al.[25] followed 356 infants <32 weeks gestational age prospectively for 6 years, of whom 49 (14%) were CMV positive and 307 were CMV negative. The infants' neurodevelopment was assessed at 16 months, at 24 to 30 months, and at 6 years. The authors noticed no difference at 24 to 30 months, but at 6 years of age infected children scored slightly lower on formal neurodevelopmental testing. They did not observe significant differences in motor development, and none of the infected children developed sensorineural hearing loss. Another prospective study that followed infants with and without a diagnosis of postnatal CMV initially showed that there were no differences in neurodevelopmental outcome between the two groups.[26] Yet, again, when the same population was followed longer, significant differences in neurodevelopment could be found beginning at 6 years of age.[22] Further, a retrospective study on outcome data from over 300 NICUs found that VLBW infants with a diagnosis of postnatal CMV had an increased risk of bronchopulmonary dysplasia (BPD) at 36 weeks' corrected gestational age when compared with birth-weight–matched uninfected infants.[27] Other studies showed a variable association of postnatal CMV with BPD in premature infants.[28–33] A large, multicenter, prospective study is needed to fully determine the risk that postnatal CMV poses to premature infants and determine how best to prevent virus transmission or disease in this population.

Treatment of Congenital CMV

CONGENITAL CMV WITH CENTRAL NERVOUS SYSTEM INVOLVEMENT

Infants with congenital CMV infection and central nervous system (CNS) involvement represent the most well-studied and least controversial population (Figure 3.1). These infants have the highest risk for severe and permanent neurologic sequelae (up to 60%).[11,15,34,35] The National Institute of Allergy and Infectious Diseases Collaborative Antiviral Study Group (CASG) has led the majority of studies establishing a role for antiviral treatment of CMV in congenitally infected infants with CNS involvement. Ganciclovir, a nucleoside analog, was first found to inhibit CMV replication in vitro and in animal models in the 1980s.[36] Subsequent phase I and II trials in the 1990s established safe dosing in infants and demonstrated some stabilization/improvement in hearing loss in symptomatic infants with congenital CMV infection.[37–39] The critical trial to evaluate ganciclovir efficacy against symptomatic congenital CMV enrolled 100 infants and took >8 years to complete.[40] Infants who were >32 weeks' gestational age with confirmed congenital CMV infection with CNS involvement were randomized to receive either 6 weeks of intravenous

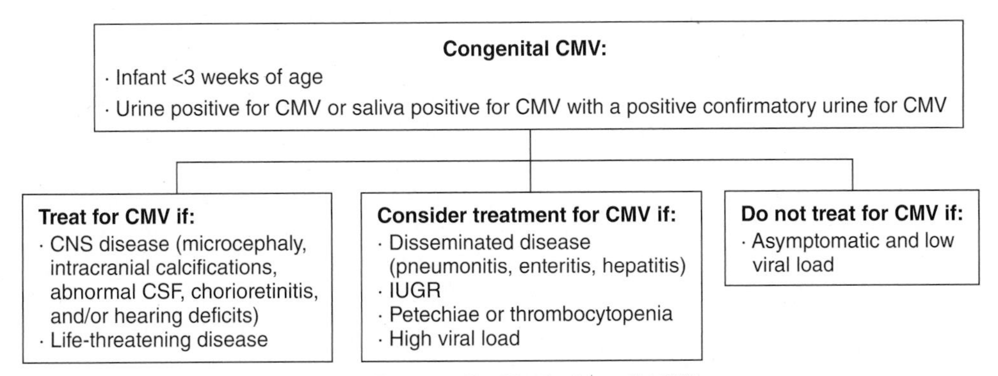

Fig. 3.1 Treatment Algorithm for Congenital CMV.

(IV) ganciclovir (6 mg/kg every 12 hours) or no treatment. CNS involvement was defined as microcephaly, intracranial calcifications, abnormal cerebrospinal fluid, chorioretinitis, and/or hearing deficits. No placebo was administered to the control group because of the ethical concerns of maintaining long-term IV access in this group. The primary endpoint was improved (or continued normal) brain stem–evoked response (BSER) in both ears between baseline and 6-month follow-up.

Although the study was limited by poor follow-up (42% of participants completed both the baseline and follow-up BSER), treatment with ganciclovir was significantly better than no treatment.[40] None (0/25) of the ganciclovir-treated infants had worsening of their hearing compared with 41% (7/17) of the no-treatment group ($P < 0.01$), and 84% (21/25) had improvement or maintained normal hearing versus 59% (10/17) in the no-treatment group ($P < 0.06$). This significant improvement continued at follow-up at >1 year but was less robust. To compare neurodevelopmental outcomes, Denver II developmental tests were performed at 6 weeks, 6 months, and 12 months. Infants treated with ganciclovir had significantly fewer developmental delays at 6 and 12 months than did untreated infants. Importantly, however, infants in the treatment group still had developmental delays compared with uninfected infants.[41]

Although these results were promising, significant side effects were associated with IV ganciclovir treatment. Neutropenia was the most significant side effect, with 63% developing grade 3 or 4 toxicity versus 21% in the no-treatment group ($P < 0.01$) and approximately 50% requiring a dose adjustment of ganciclovir.[40] There were also complications and risks associated with maintaining long-term IV access in this population (e.g., thrombus, infection, line replacement). An additional consideration is that ganciclovir can be carcinogenic and has gonadotoxicity in some animal models.[42–44]

Although ganciclovir was an effective treatment for congenital CMV, its widespread use was limited by side effects and need for long-term IV access. Thus, the CASG evaluated the pharmacokinetics of the oral prodrug of ganciclovir and valganciclovir, and found that it reached blood concentrations equivalent to those of ganciclovir at a dose of 16 mg/kg/dose twice a day.[45] There was also a reduced risk of neutropenia, with only 38% (9/24) developing grade 3 or 4 neutropenia and only two requiring a dose adjustment. In addition, the gonadotoxicity and carcinogenic effects of ganciclovir have not been seen with valganciclovir. Therefore, oral valganciclovir became the treatment of choice for congenital CMV infection.

Treatment of congenital CMV with ganciclovir or valganciclovir for 6 weeks eliminates or significantly reduces viral shedding; however, viral shedding usually returns to baseline shortly after cessation of therapy, and children can shed the virus for years.[38,43,46,47] Because many children can remain asymptomatic and may not develop SNHL or neurodevelopmental impairment until they are up to 6 years old, it was hypothesized that persistent viremia might contribute to pathogenesis and that a longer duration of therapy would improve outcomes. A randomized, placebo-controlled trial was done to address this question.

Treatment with 6 weeks of valganciclovir was compared with 6 months of valganciclovir in infants with congenital CMV with CNS involvement (as defined in previous clinical trials). Hearing was similar between the two groups at 6 months but was more likely to be improved or remain normal at 12 months in the 6-month treatment group compared with the 6-week treatment group (73% vs. 57%; $P = 0.01$), and this observation persisted at 24 months (77% vs. 64%; $P = 0.04$). Infants in the 6-month group also had significantly better neurodevelopmental outcomes, as determined using the Bayley Scales of Infant and Toddler Development, at 24 months. Interestingly, the incidence of neutropenia did not differ significantly between the two treatment groups. In the 4.5 months after valganciclovir was stopped in the 6-week treatment group, the incidence of neutropenia was 27% in the 6-week treatment group and 21% in the 6-month treatment group.[48] The investigators hypothesized that much of the neutropenia seen during CMV treatment can be attributed to congenital CMV infection rather than treatment.

These studies effectively demonstrated that infants with congenital CMV with CNS involvement have improved hearing and neurodevelopmental outcomes with antiviral treatment with valganciclovir for 6 months compared with shorter or no treatment. A subsequent study from Israel[49] treated infants who had symptomatic congenital CMV infection for 12 months and they noticed that, in most ears with mild or moderate hearing loss at birth, hearing improved in 64.9%, remained unchanged in 28.6%, and deteriorated in 6.5%. They also noticed that the benefit of treatment significantly decreased in those infants with severe hearing impairment. However, this study was limited by lack of a control group and the retrospective design.

Limitations and Future Research

As with most drug therapies, safety and efficacy studies are limited in infants, particularly premature infants. The clinical trials establishing the pharmacokinetics, safety, and efficacy of ganciclovir and valganciclovir were all limited to infants >32 weeks' gestation and >1200g in weight. There are several case studies of ganciclovir use in premature infants, with one showing the efficacy of ganciclovir followed by valganciclovir.[50–53] More studies are needed in premature infants, particularly extremely low-birth-weight infants (ELBW; <1000 g) to establish pharmacokinetics, safety, and efficacy. In addition, infants with congenital CMV with CNS disease who receive treatment should be followed long term to determine if their improvement persists as they age or if they would benefit from longer therapy, as has been observed for acyclovir treatment for congenital HSV infection.[54–56]

Still an open question is the timing of starting antiviral treatment. All of the above studies have evaluated outcomes when treatment was initiated within 1 month after birth; however, not all symptomatic newborns are diagnosed with congenital CMV within this time frame, as CNS disease may be subtle at birth. Will the benefits observed in these studies be maintained if ganciclovir or valganciclovir is started, for example, at 4 months of life? This unknown impact of late treatment for congenital CMV highlights the need for early diagnosis of congenital CMV through universal CMV screening at birth.

Summary

Infants with a diagnosis of congenital CMV that have CNS involvement should be treated with either ganciclovir (6 mg/kg IV every 12 hours) or valganciclovir (16 mg/kg by mouth every 12 hours) for a total of 6 months (Figure 3.2). Treatment should begin within the first month after birth, ideally <2 weeks. Valganciclovir should be preferentially used when the infant is safely tolerating oral intake. In infants <32 weeks' gestation or <1200g, dose adjustment may be required based on side effects or viral load.

The major risk of treatment is neutropenia, which was most pronounced with ganciclovir and in the first 6 weeks of treatment with valganciclovir. Infants should be monitored with complete blood counts, serum transaminase levels, kidney function tests, and viral load measurements during therapy. An additional consideration is that ganciclovir can be carcinogenic and have gonadotoxicity in some animal models.[42–44] These toxicities have never been shown in human studies or for valganciclovir, but the potential risk should be discussed with families. Overall, although a risk of neutropenia and theoretic risks from animal studies are associated with treatment, in this population the benefits outweigh the risks.

Congenital CMV Treatment:

Medication	Duration	Monitoring
• Ganciclovir 6 mg/kg/dose every 12 hours or • Valganciclovir 16 mg/kg/dose every 12 hours	• 6 months	Biweekly to monthly: • Complete blood count • Serum transaminase levels • Kidney function tests • CMV load (to assess for development of resistant virus and adherence)

Postnatal CMV Treatment:

Medication	Duration	Monitoring
• Ganciclovir 6 mg/kg/dose every 12 hours or • Valganciclovir 16 mg/kg/dose every 12 hours • Preterm dosing awaiting pharmacokinetic (PK) trials	• Typically at least 3 weeks, depending on clinical improvement	Frequent (weekly): • Complete blood count • Serum transaminase levels • Kidney function tests Less frequent (biweekly to monthly) • CMV load

Fig. 3.2 CMV Treatment Regimens and Monitoring.

SYMPTOMATIC CONGENITAL CMV WITHOUT CNS INVOLVEMENT AND ASYMPTOMATIC CONGENITAL CMV

Symptomatic Congenital CMV Without CNS Involvement

The randomized clinical trials addressing treatment of symptomatic congenital CMV were limited to those infants with CNS involvement at the time of diagnosis. In those infants with severe disease outside the CNS, such as pneumonitis, there are case studies documenting successful treatment with ganciclovir.[57,58] However, many children only have mild, non–life-threatening symptoms at birth (i.e., jaundice, petechiae, transient thrombocytopenia). In 2017, a European Consensus did not recommended treatment for "mild" disease, with or without detectable CMV viremia; however, the quality and strength for these recommendations were weak.[59] These guidelines, though, do advise considering treatment, after consultation with a specialist, in "moderate" disease (e.g., multiple minor findings consistent with congenital CMV but without CNS involvement). Although CNS involvement is a predictor of cognitive and motor development impairment, it is not predictive of the development of SNHL.[34,60–62] In a prospective study of 180 children diagnosed with congenital CMV, the presence of IUGR or petechiae was predictive of SNHL.[61] In addition, another study of 127 children showed that petechiae and viremia were associated with SNHL.[63] These studies suggest that some infants with symptomatic congenital CMV infection, regardless of CNS involvement, are at high risk for developing SNHL and could be considered candidates for antiviral treatment.

Asymptomatic Congenital CMV Infection

Unlike symptomatic congenital CMV infection, there are no randomized controlled trials or large clinical studies to determine if treatment of asymptomatic congenital infections reduces the risk of late hearing loss and/or improves neurodevelopmental outcomes. Most published references recommend against treating those with asymptomatic infection and instead recommend close monitoring for neurodevelopmental delay and hearing, as well as implementing early referral for ancillary services.[9,64–66] They cite the lack of evidence of the benefit of treatment and the significant risks associated with treatment; however, the majority of these recommendations were published before the availability of valganciclovir as a treatment option.

As mentioned previously, 85% to 90% of infants with congenital CMV are asymptomatic at birth, but up to 20% of those will develop neurologic impairment, most commonly SNHL.[12,13,67] The two options for treatment include (1) treating all infants with congenital infection, regardless of symptoms; and (2) determining which infants with asymptomatic congenital CMV are at high risk for neurodevelopmental impairment and treating only those high-risk infants. The difficulty lies in determining which infants who are asymptomatic at birth will go on to develop SNHL. Ideally, an accurate predictor or biomarker could be established that will determine which infants will benefit most from therapy, thereby preventing unnecessary treatment of thousands of infants. However, such a predictor or biomarker does not currently exist, and initial peripheral blood cell transcriptome profiling was not successful in defining the risk of the development of hearing loss in congenitally infected infants.[68]

The exact mechanism by which CMV causes SNHL is not clear; however, several studies suggest that direct viral cytopathology and viral-induced local inflammatory response play a role.[69,70] Pathology studies also show damage to vestibular endolymphatic systems in infected infants.[71] The progressive nature of the SNHL suggests that ongoing viral replication and damage may be responsible for part or all of the hearing loss seen. If this is true, treatment to reduce or eliminate CMV viral load should improve hearing outcomes, even in children who are asymptomatic and in particular those with high viral loads. This is similar to the theory that led to increasing the treatment duration of valganciclovir from 6 weeks to 6 months.

In fact, some studies have suggested that high plasma viral load is linked to the development of SNHL, regardless of whether the infant is symptomatic at birth.[61,63,72–74] The viral load linked to progression of SNHL in each study varied, but, in general, infants with viral loads of $<10^3$ copies/mL had no long-term complications, whereas those with viral loads $>10^5$ copies/mL were at increased risk for SNHL. These studies support the theory that high plasma viral load increases the risk for SNHL and that reducing viral load could prevent this complication. However, a post hoc analysis of two antiviral studies showed that, in infants with symptomatic congenital CMV disease treated for 6 weeks (73 infants) or 6 months (47 infants), a higher whole blood viral load before initiation of antiviral therapy had no clinically meaningful predictive value for long-term outcomes, as there was significant overlap in the amount of virus detected between groups. Further studies are needed to determine whether an infant CMV viremia measure cutoff for therapy could be validated, as well as the positive and negative predictive values of viral load, before viral load risk assessment is recommended for routine clinical use.

In the only study comparing treatment versus no treatment in asymptomatic infants with congenital CMV infection, 12 infants were treated with ganciclovir 10 mg/kg for 21 days, and 11 were observed off therapy.[75] The infants were followed for the next 4 to 10 years. Of the 18 children who completed follow-up, only two developed SNHL, and they were both in the observation group ($P = 0.18$). Although these results suggest a possible benefit of treating asymptomatic congenital CMV, the study was significantly limited by the small sample size and low follow-up rate. This study also used a shorter treatment duration than is now recommended. At this time, a phase II, open-label, single-group clinical trial is planning to evaluate 229 infants with asymptomatic congenital CMV, without SNHL and <1 month of age, who will be treated with oral valganciclovir (16 mg/kg twice daily) for 4 months. The primary objective of this study is to determine the development of SNHL at 6 months of life (ClinicalTrials.gov). Ideally, there will be more evidence-based data for future recommendations in the treatment of this group of infants affected by congenital CMV infection.

Asymptomatic Congenital CMV Infection with Isolated Hearing Loss

Another unresolved topic is the need for treatment of infants with asymptomatic congenital CMV and isolated SNHL diagnosed at birth. The recent CONCERT Study from the Netherlands treated 35 infants with oral valganciclovir or placebo (not randomized) for 6 weeks and followed them for 20 months; treatment was initiated at an average age of 8 weeks of age.[76] Preliminary results demonstrate a more common improvement in the valganciclovir group versus some deterioration or no change in the placebo group ($P = 0.044$). When infants with profound SNHL (>70 dB hearing loss) were excluded from the analysis, none of the infants receiving placebo experienced improvement and almost half deteriorated; meanwhile, most of infants treated with valganciclovir had unchanged SNHL, a small number improved, and almost none deteriorated ($P = 0.006$). Weaknesses of this study include the small sample size and the nonrandomized nature of the design, which could have led to bias in the treated versus untreated groups. A few other studies being conducted in different countries (e.g., ValEAR study in the United States, GANCIMVEAR study in France, Valgan Toddler Trial in the United Kingdom) are trying to answer this important question; all are still ongoing, and no additional preliminary data are available at this time.

Limitations and Future Research

Although studies suggest a potential benefit of treatment, a large clinical trial is needed to determine if treatment improves neurodevelopmental outcomes in infants with congenital CMV infection without overt CNS disease at birth. Importantly, it remains to be determined whether treatment of asymptomatic congenital CMV infection diagnosed at birth can prevent the development of late hearing loss or improve neurodevelopmental outcome, and there is great need for a biomarker that could predict the risk of long-term deficits in congenitally infected infants. Clearly, more studies are needed to determine which infants are at risk for neurodevelopmental impairment or if all infants with congenital CMV, regardless of presentation, would benefit from treatment.

With the implementation of routine screening for CMV by some states and institutions, this will be an increasingly more relevant and important question to answer. Universal CMV testing at birth to define this population of infants provides researchers with the perfect opportunity to study the long-term consequences of asymptomatic or symptomatic congenital CMV infection without CNS involvement and if treatment improves outcomes.

Summary

Infants with symptomatic congenital CMV without CNS involvement should be considered for treatment if they have disseminated disease, IUGR, petechiae, or a high viral load (see Figure 3.1). Physicians should consider treatment of mild or asymptomatic congenital CMV, especially those infants with a high plasma viral load. The risks and potential benefits of valganciclovir should be discussed with the parents or caregivers. The treatment dose and duration should be the same as with symptomatic congenital CMV infection.

Treatment of Postnatal CMV Infection

Routine treatment of postnatal CMV infection in immunocompetent children, including term infants, is not recommended. CMV is a self-limited infection with no known short- or long-term complications in this population. However, as described earlier, VLBW infants infected postnatally with CMV can develop a severe sepsis-like illness during an acute infection and may have an increased risk of developing BPD and neurodevelopmental impairment.[22–24,27,30]

No large trials have addressed the treatment of premature infants with postnatal CMV infection. There are several small case studies of premature infants with severe postnatal CMV infection treated with ganciclovir who showed significant clinical improvement with antiviral therapy.[21,50,51,53] In addition, in all of these studies, CMV load in plasma was eliminated or decreased by several logs. The majority of infants in these case studies had no apparent side effects from ganciclovir therapy[21,51,53]; however, in one report, therapy was discontinued after 28 days (and significant clinical improvement) in an ELBW infant secondary to neutropenia[46,50]

The more difficult question is whether premature infants with asymptomatic postnatal CMV infection would benefit from treatment. In the retrospective studies that showed an increased risk of BPD in infants with postnatal CMV infection, infants with postnatal CMV were tested at some point by their provider, presumably because they developed clinical findings that could be consistent with CMV infection.[25,27] Therefore, BPD might only be a complication in symptomatic postnatal CMV infection. However, the studies suggesting that postnatal CMV infection in VLBW infants may be associated with neurodevelopmental impairment were performed by screening all infants born to CMV-seropositive mothers at birth and following them prospectively.[21] These studies therefore represent both asymptomatic and symptomatic postnatal CMV-infected premature infants. Thus, although some sequelae appear to affect only infants with symptomatic infection, others affect both groups.

LIMITATIONS AND FUTURE RESEARCH

The full impact of postnatal CMV infection on premature infants remains unclear. A large, multicentered, prospective trial is needed to define the full incidence of disease and determine the long-term sequelae. These vulnerable infants are already at high risk for morbidity and mortality, and decreasing the contribution of CMV to their neurodevelopmental and respiratory outcome could have a significant impact. Studies are also needed to assess the role of antiviral treatment in improving the outcome of symptomatic and asymptomatic postnatal CMV infection in premature infants.

SUMMARY

Clinicians should strongly consider treating VLBW infants with severe acute disease after postnatal CMV acquisition. In these cases, treatment should consist of IV ganciclovir at a dose of 5 to 6 mg/kg IV every 12 hours for a minimum of 3 weeks, with the length of treatment depending on clinical course and viral load (see Figure 3.2). In ELBW infants, drug levels should be monitored periodically, if possible, until adequate pharmacokinetic studies are available.[77]

There is insufficient evidence at this time to recommend treatment for asymptomatic VLBW infants with postnatal CMV infection. However, studies suggest that these infants could develop long-term sequelae, and the risks associated with treatment may be less than assumed prior to the availability of valganciclovir. Further studies are needed to quantitate the risk of long-term deficits due to postnatal CMV acquisition in premature infants and determine if these could be reduced with treatment for CMV in this vulnerable population. In addition, safe strategies should be devised for prevention of breast milk–associated CMV transmission in the NICU population, such as the addition of CMV-neutralizing antibodies to maternal breast milk prior to infant feeding, allowing the full benefits of breast milk feeding while also eliminating CMV as a contributor to negative health and developmental outcomes in premature infants.

REFERENCES

1. Kenneson A, Cannon MJ. Review and meta-analysis of the epidemiology of congenital cytomegalovirus (CMV) infection. *Rev Med Virol*. 2007;17(4):253-256.
2. Manicklal S, Emery VC, Lazzarotto T, Boppana SB, Gupta RK. The "silent" global burden of congenital cytomegalovirus. *Clin Microbiol Rev*. 2013;26(1):86-102.
3. Cannon MJ, Schmid DS, Hyde TB. Review of cytomegalovirus seroprevalence and demographic characteristics associated with infection. *Rev Med Virol*. 2010;20(4):202-213.
4. Boppana SB, Rivera LB, Fowler KB, Mach M, Britt WJ. Intrauterine transmission of cytomegalovirus to infants of women with preconceptional immunity. *N Engl J Med*. 2001;344(18):1366-1371.
5. Yow MD, Williamson DW, Leeds LJ, et al. Epidemiologic characteristics of cytomegalovirus infection in mothers and their infants. *Am J Obstet Gynecol*. 1988:158(5):1189-1195.
6. Wang C, Zhang X, Bialek S, Cannon MJ. Attribution of congenital cytomegalovirus infection to primary versus non-primary maternal infection. *Clin Infect Dis*. 2011;52(2):e11-e13.
7. Malm G, Engman ML. Congenital cytomegalovirus infections. *Semin Fetal Neonatal Med*. 2007;12(3):154-159.
8. Pass RF, Fowler KB, Boppana SB, Britt WJ, Stagno S. Congenital cytomegalovirus infection following first trimester maternal infection: symptoms at birth and outcome. *J Clin Virol*. 2006;35(2):216-220.
9. Buonsenso D, Serranti D, Gargiullo L, Ceccarelli GM, Ranno O, Valentini P. Congenital cytomegalovirus infection: current strategies and future perspectives. *Eur Rev Med Pharmacol Sci*. 2012;16(7):919-935.
10. Korndewal MJ, Oudesluys-Murphy AM, Kroes ACM, van der Sande MAB, de Melker HE, Vossen ACTM. Long-term impairment attributable to congenital cytomegalovirus infection: a retrospective cohort study. *Dev Med Child Neurol*. 2017;59(12):1261-1268.
11. Dollard SC, Grosse SD, Ross DS. New estimates of the prevalence of neurological and sensory sequelae and mortality associated with congenital cytomegalovirus infection. *Rev Med Virol*. 2007;17(5):355-363.
12. Ross SA, Boppana SB. Congenital cytomegalovirus infection: outcome and diagnosis. *Semin Pediatr Infect Dis*. 2005;16(1):44-49.
13. Stagno S, Whitley RJ. Herpesvirus infections of pregnancy. Part I: Cytomegalovirus and Epstein–Barr virus infections. *N Engl J Med*. 1985;313(20):1270-1274.
14. Dahle AJ, Fowler KB, Wright JD, Boppana SB, Britt WJ, Pass RF. Longitudinal investigation of hearing disorders in children with congenital cytomegalovirus. *J Am Acad Audiol*. 2000;11(5):283-290.

15. Fowler KB, Dahl AJ, Boppana SB, Pass RF. Newborn hearing screening: will children with hearing loss caused by congenital cytomegalovirus infection be missed? *J Pediatr*. 1999;135(1):60-64.
16. Fowler KB, Stagno S, Pass RF, Britt WJ, Boll TJ, Alford CA. The outcome of congenital cytomegalovirus infection in relation to maternal antibody status. *N Engl J Med*. 1992;326(10):663-667.
17. Cannon MJ, Davis KF. Washing our hands of the congenital cytomegalovirus disease epidemic. *BMC Public Health*. 2005;5:70.
18. Smith RJ, Bale Jr JF, White KR. Sensorineural hearing loss in children. *Lancet*. 2005;365(9462):879-890.
19. Capretti MG, Lanari M, Lazzarotto T, et al. Very low birth weight infants born to cytomegalovirus-seropositive mothers fed with their mother's milk: a prospective study. *J Pediatr*. 2009;154(6):842-848.
20. de Cates CR, Gray J, Roberton NR, Walker J. Acquisition of cytomegalovirus infection by premature neonates. *J Infect*. 1994;28(1):25-30.
21. Josephson CD, Caliendo AM, Easley KA, et al. Blood transfusion and breast milk transmission of cytomegalovirus in very low-birth-weight infants: a prospective cohort study. *JAMA Pediatr*. 2014;168(11):1054-1062.
22. Brecht KF, Goelz R, Bevot A, Krägeloh-Mann I, Wilke M, Lidzba K. Postnatal human cytomegalovirus infection in preterm infants has long-term neuropsychological sequelae. *J Pediatr*. 2015;166(4):834-839.e1.
23. Lanzieri TM, Dollard SC, Josephson CD, Schmid DS, Bialek SR. Breast milk-acquired cytomegalovirus infection and disease in VLBW and premature infants. *Pediatrics*. 2013;131(6):e1937-e1945.
24. Lombardi G, Garofoli F, Manzoni P, Stronati M. Breast milk-acquired cytomegalovirus infection in very low birth weight infants. *J Matern Fetal Neonatal Med*. 2012;25(suppl 3):57-62.
25. Gunkel J, de Vries LS, Jongmans M, et al. Outcome of preterm infants with postnatal cytomegalovirus infection. *Pediatrics*. 2018;141(2):e20170635.
26. Vollmer B, Seibold-Weiger K, Schmitz-Salue C, et al. Postnatally acquired cytomegalovirus infection via breast milk: effects on hearing and development in preterm infants. *Pediatr Infect Dis J*. 2004;23(4):322-327.
27. Kelly MS, Benjamin DK, Puopolo KM, et al. Postnatal cytomegalovirus infection and the risk for bronchopulmonary dysplasia. *JAMA Pediatr*. 2015;169(12):e153785.
28. Stark A, Cantrell S, Greenberg RG, Permar SR, Weimer KED. Long-term outcomes after postnatal cytomegalovirus infection in low birthweight preterm infants: a systematic review. *Pediatr Infect Dis J*. 2021;40(6):571-581.
29. Ehrenkranz RA, Walsh MC, Vohr BR, et al. Validation of the National Institutes of Health consensus definition of bronchopulmonary dysplasia. *Pediatrics*. 2005;116(6):1353-1360.
30. Mukhopadhyay S, Meyer SA, Permar SR, Puopolo KM. Symptomatic postnatal cytomegalovirus testing among very low-birth-weight infants: indications and outcomes. *Am J Perinatol*. 2016;33(9):894-902.
31. Neuberger P, Hamprecht K, Vochem M. Case-control study of symptoms and neonatal outcome of human milk-transmitted cytomegalovirus infection in premature infants. *J Pediatr*. 2006;148(3):326-331.
32. Nijman J, de Vries LS, Koopman-Esseboom C, Uiterwaal CSPM, van Loon AM, Verboon-Maciolek MA. Postnatally acquired cytomegalovirus infection in preterm infants: a prospective study on risk factors and cranial ultrasound findings. *Arch Dis Child Fetal Neonatal Ed*. 2012;97(4):F259-F263.
33. Sawyer MH, Edwards DK, Spector SA. Cytomegalovirus infection and bronchopulmonary dysplasia in premature infants. *Am J Dis Child*. 1987;141(3):303-305.
34. Pass RF, Stagno S, Myers GJ, Alford CA. Outcome of symptomatic congenital cytomegalovirus infection: results of long-term longitudinal follow-up. *Pediatrics*. 1980;66(5):758-762.
35. Williams EJ, Gray J, Luck S, et al. First estimates of the potential cost and cost saving of protecting childhood hearing from damage caused by congenital CMV infection. *Arch Dis Child Fetal Neonatal Ed*. 2015;100(6):F501-F506.
36. Matthews T, Boehme R. Antiviral activity and mechanism of action of ganciclovir. *Rev Infect Dis*. 1988;10(suppl 3):S490-S494.
37. Trang JM, Kidd L, Gruber W, et al. Linear single-dose pharmacokinetics of ganciclovir in newborns with congenital cytomegalovirus infections. NIAID Collaborative Antiviral Study Group. *Clin Pharmacol Ther*. 1993;53(1):15-21.
38. Whitley RJ, Cloud G, Gruber W, et al. Ganciclovir treatment of symptomatic congenital cytomegalovirus infection: results of a phase II study. National Institute of Allergy and Infectious Diseases Collaborative Antiviral Study Group. *J Infect Dis*. 1997;175(5):1080-1086.
39. Zhou XJ, Gruber W, Demmler G, et al. Population pharmacokinetics of ganciclovir in newborns with congenital cytomegalovirus infections. NIAID Collaborative Antiviral Study Group. *Antimicrob Agents Chemother*. 1996;40(9):2202-2205.
40. Kimberlin DW, Lin C-Y, Sánchez PJ, et al. Effect of ganciclovir therapy on hearing in symptomatic congenital cytomegalovirus disease involving the central nervous system: a randomized, controlled trial. *J Pediatr*. 2003;143(1):16-25.
41. Oliver SE, Cloud GA, Sánchez PJ, et al. Neurodevelopmental outcomes following ganciclovir therapy in symptomatic congenital cytomegalovirus infections involving the central nervous system. *J Clin Virol*. 2009;46(suppl 4):S22-S226.
42. Faqi AS, Klug A, Merker HJ, Chahoud I. Ganciclovir induces reproductive hazards in male rats after short-term exposure. *Hum Exp Toxicol*. 1997;16(9):505-511.
43. Mareri A, Lasorella S, Iapadre G, Maresca M, Tambucci R, Nigro G. Anti-viral therapy for congenital cytomegalovirus infection: pharmacokinetics, efficacy and side effects. *J Matern Fetal Neonatal Med*. 2016;29(10):1657-1664.
44. Wutzler P, Thrust R. Genetic risks of antiviral nucleoside analogues—a survey. *Antiviral Res*. 2001;49(2):55-74.
45. Kimberlin DW, Acosta EP, Sánchez PJ, et al. Pharmacokinetic and pharmacodynamic assessment of oral valganciclovir in the treatment of symptomatic congenital cytomegalovirus disease. *J Infect Dis*. 2008;197(6):836-845.
46. Nigro G, Scholz H, Bartmann U. Ganciclovir therapy for symptomatic congenital cytomegalovirus infection in infants: a two-regimen experience. *J Pediatr*. 1994;124(2):318-322.
47. Syggelou A, Iacovidou N, Kloudas S, Christoni Z, Papaevangelou V. Congenital cytomegalovirus infection. *Ann N Y Acad Sci*. 2010;1205:144-147.
48. Kimberlin DW, Jester PM, Sánchez PJ, et al. Valganciclovir for symptomatic congenital cytomegalovirus disease. *N Engl J Med*. 2015;372(10):933-943.
49. Bilavsky E, Shahar-Nissan K, Pardo J, Attias J, Amir J. Hearing outcome of infants with congenital cytomegalovirus and hearing impairment. *Arch Dis Child*. 2016;101(5):433-438.

50. Fischer C, Meylan P, Bickle Graz M, et al. Severe postnatally acquired cytomegalovirus infection presenting with colitis, pneumonitis and sepsis-like syndrome in an extremely low birthweight infant. *Neonatology*. 2010;97(4):339-345.
51. Mehler K, Oberthuer A, Lang-Roth R, Kribs A. High rate of symptomatic cytomegalovirus infection in extremely low gestational age preterm infants of 22–24 weeks' gestation after transmission via breast milk. *Neonatology*. 2014;105(1):27-32.
52. Muller A, Eis-Hübinger AM, Brandhorst G, Heep A, Bartmann P, Franz AR. Oral valganciclovir for symptomatic congenital cytomegalovirus infection in an extremely low birth weight infant. *J Perinatol*. 2008;28(1):74-76.
53. Okulu E, Akin IM, Atasay B, Ciftçi E, Arsan S, Türmen T. Severe postnatal cytomegalovirus infection with multisystem involvement in an extremely low birth weight infant. *J Perinatol*. 2012;32(1):72-74.
54. Kimberlin DW, Lin CY, Jacobs RF, et al. Natural history of neonatal herpes simplex virus infections in the acyclovir era. *Pediatrics*. 2001;108(2):223-229.
55. Kimberlin DW, Whitley RJ, Wan W, et al. Oral acyclovir suppression and neurodevelopment after neonatal herpes. *N Engl J Med*. 2011;365(14):1284-1292.
56. Tiffany KF, Benjamin Jr DK, Palasanthiran P, O'Donnell K, Gutman LT. Improved neurodevelopmental outcomes following long-term high-dose oral acyclovir therapy in infants with central nervous system and disseminated herpes simplex disease. *J Perinatol*. 2005;25(3):156-161.
57. Hocker JR, Cook LN, Adams G, Rabalais GP. Ganciclovir therapy of congenital cytomegalovirus pneumonia. *Pediatr Infect Dis J*. 1990;9(10):743-745.
58. Vallejo JG, Englund JA, Garcia-Prats JA, Demmler GJ. Ganciclovir treatment of steroid-associated cytomegalovirus disease in a congenitally infected neonate. *Pediatr Infect Dis J*. 1994;13(3): 239-241.
59. Luck SE, Wieringa JW, Blázquez-Gamero D. Congenital cytomegalovirus: a European Expert Consensus Statement on Diagnosis and Management. *Pediatr Infect Dis J*. 2017;36(12): 1205-1213.
60. Noyola DE, Demmler GJ, Nelson CT, et al. Early predictors of neurodevelopmental outcome in symptomatic congenital cytomegalovirus infection. *J Pediatr*. 2001;138(3):325-331.
61. Rivera LB, Boppana SB, Fowler KB, Britt WJ, Stagno S, Pass RF. Predictors of hearing loss in children with symptomatic congenital cytomegalovirus infection. *Pediatrics*. 2002;110(4): 762-767.
62. Weller TH, Hanshaw JB. Virologic and clinical observations on cytomegalic inclusion disease. *N Engl J Med*. 1962;266: 1233-1244.
63. Bradford RD, Cloud G, Lakeman AD, et al. Detection of cytomegalovirus (CMV) DNA by polymerase chain reaction is associated with hearing loss in newborns with symptomatic congenital CMV infection involving the central nervous system. *J Infect Dis*. 2005;191(2):227-233.
64. Gandhi RS, Fernandez-Alvarez JR, Rabe H. Management of congenital cytomegalovirus infection: an evidence-based approach. *Acta Paediatr*. 2010;99(4):509-515.
65. James SH, Kimberlin DW. Advances in the prevention and treatment of congenital cytomegalovirus infection. *Curr Opin Pediatr*. 2016;28(1):81-85.
66. Smets K, De Coen K, Dhooge I, et al. Selecting neonates with congenital cytomegalovirus infection for ganciclovir therapy. *Eur J Pediatr*. 2006;165(12):885-890.
67. Fowler KB, Boppana SB. Congenital cytomegalovirus (CMV) infection and hearing deficit. *J Clin Virol*. 2006;35(2): 226-231.
68. Ouellette CP, Sánchez PJ, Xu Z, et al. Blood genome expression profiles in infants with congenital cytomegalovirus infection. *Nat Commun*. 2020;11(1):3548.
69. Fowler KB, McCollister FP, Dahle AJ, Boppana S, Britt WJ, Pass RF. Progressive and fluctuating sensorineural hearing loss in children with asymptomatic congenital cytomegalovirus infection. *J Pediatr*. 1997;130(4):624-630.
70. Strauss M. Human cytomegalovirus labyrinthitis. *Am J Otolaryngol*. 1990;11(5):292-298.
71. Davis LE, Johnsson LG, Kornfeld M. Cytomegalovirus labyrinthitis in an infant: morphological, virological, and immunofluorescent studies. *J Neuropathol Exp Neurol*. 1981;40(1):9-19.
72. Boppana SB, Fowler KB, Pass RF, et al. Congenital cytomegalovirus infection: association between virus burden in infancy and hearing loss. *J Pediatr*. 2005;146(6):817-823.
73. Lanari M, Lazzarotto T, Venturi V, et al. Neonatal cytomegalovirus blood load and risk of sequelae in symptomatic and asymptomatic congenitally infected newborns. *Pediatrics*. 2006;117(1): e76-e83.
74. Walter S, Atkinson C, Sharland M, et al. Congenital cytomegalovirus: association between dried blood spot viral load and hearing loss. *Arch Dis Child Fetal Neonatal Ed*. 2008;93(4): F280-F285.
75. Lackner A, Acham A, Alborno T, et al. Effect on hearing of ganciclovir therapy for asymptomatic congenital cytomegalovirus infection: four to 10 year follow up. *J Laryngol Otol*. 2009;123(4):391-396.
76. Chung PK, Schornagel F, Oudesluys-Murphy AM, et al. Targeted screening for congenital cytomegalovirus infection: clinical, audiological and neuroimaging findings. *Arch Dis Child Fetal Neonatal Ed*. 2023;108(3):302-308.
77. Sunada M, Kinoshita D, Furukawa N, et al. Therapeutic drug monitoring of ganciclovir for postnatal cytomegalovirus infection in an extremely low birth weight infant: a case report. *BMC Pediatr*. 2016;16(1):141.

Chapter 4

Neonatal Herpes Simplex Virus Infection

Nazia Kabani, MD, MSPH; David W. Kimberlin, MD

Key Points

- Herpes simplex virus (HSV) is a virus that can cause severe infection in a neonate but also has treatment options that can improve disease outcomes.
- There are three periods of acquisition of HSV: in utero, perinatal, and postnatal.
- HSV can be diagnosed via polymerase chain reaction (PCR) of blood and cerebrospinal fluid (CSF), as well as surface cultures and PCR.
- It is important to assess for disseminated HSV.
- HSV can be treated with intravenous acyclovir for management of acute disease, followed by oral acyclovir suppressive therapy.

Introduction

Of the viruses capable of infecting neonates, herpes simplex virus (HSV) is among the most severe, causing significant mortality and morbidity. Unlike many other viral pathogens, HSV is treatable using a commercially available antiviral drug: acyclovir. Neonatal HSV infection is primarily acquired in the peripartum period, which improves the likelihood that antiviral therapy can be beneficial, because viral damage is of a relatively short duration compared with injury to the developing fetal brain from viruses such as rubella, cytomegalovirus, and Zika virus, which are primarily acquired in utero. Studies conducted by the National Institute of Allergy and Infectious Diseases (NIAID) Collaborative Antiviral Study Group (CASG) over the course of four decades have advanced our knowledge of the favorable impact that antiviral therapy has on neonatal HSV disease outcomes, and many neonates now are effectively treated and experience no long-term sequelae of this potentially devastating infection.

Timing of Infection

Neonatal HSV is acquired in one of three distinct periods: in utero, perinatal, or postnatal. In most cases (~85%), neonates acquire the infection perinatally.[1] In approximately 10% of cases, neonates are infected postnatally, and in 5% the infection is acquired in utero.[1]

Risk Factors for Neonatal Infection

Risk factors that increase the likelihood of transmission from a mother with genital HSV shedding to her neonate include the following:

- Type of maternal infection (primary infection increases likelihood vs. recurrent)[2–6]
- Maternal antibody status (lower concentration of antibodies with primary infection)[6–9]
- Prolonged duration of rupture of membranes[5]
- Integrity of mucocutaneous barriers (using fetal scalp probe, incisions, etc.)[6,10,11]
- Mode of delivery (vaginal delivery increases likelihood vs. cesarean delivery)[6]

Neonates born to mothers with primary genital HSV infection near term (that is, a first episode of genital HSV infection) are at much greater risk of developing neonatal herpes than are neonates born to mothers with recurrent genital HSV infection. This increased risk is due to two factors.[2–6] First, the concentration of transplacentally acquired HSV-specific antibodies is lower in neonates born to women with primary infection.[8] In addition, these antibodies tend to be less reactive to the expressed peptides. Second, there is a larger amount of virus present in the genital tract, and virus is shed for a longer period of time in women with primary infection compared with women with recurrent HSV infection.[12] A landmark study of approximately 60,000 women in labor in the Seattle,

WA, area who did not have any symptoms of genital HSV infection at the time of delivery proved the correlation between timing of maternal infection with likelihood of neonatal HSV acquisition. Of these women, approximately 40,000 had a vaginal swab obtained within 48 hours of delivery for HSV detection (Figure 4.1).[6] Of these approximately 40,000 women, 121 women (0.3%) were identified as having asymptomatic shedding of HSV and had sera available for HSV serologic testing, thereby allowing for classification of first episodes versus recurrent maternal infections. The trial found that 57% of neonates born to mothers with primary infection (defined as infection with either HSV-1 or HSV-2 in a woman lacking antibodies to either) developed neonatal HSV, 25% of neonates born to women with first-episode nonprimary infection (defined as infection with HSV-2 in a woman lacking antibody to HSV-2 but possessing antibody to HSV-1, or vice versa) developed neonatal HSV, and only 2% of neonates born to women with recurrent HSV developed neonatal HSV (see Figure 4.1).[6] This same study also confirmed that cesarean delivery reduces the transmission of HSV to the neonate when mothers are shedding in their genital tracts, affirming the results of a previous small study published in 1971.[5] Despite this degree of protection, though, the risk of HSV transmission is not eliminated by cesarean delivery.[13,15]

Clinical Manifestations of Neonatal Infection and Disease

Neonatal HSV infection is classified based on the extent of involvement into one of three categories: disseminated disease, central nervous system (CNS) infection, or skin, eyes, and mouth (SEM) infection. Disseminated disease involves multiple organs, including but not limited to lung, liver, adrenal glands, brain, and skin. CNS disease involves the brain and can have skin lesions, as well. SEM disease is limited to just those areas. This classification is predictive of morbidity and mortality, with disseminated disease having the most significant mortality and CNS disease having the most significant morbidity.[16–22]

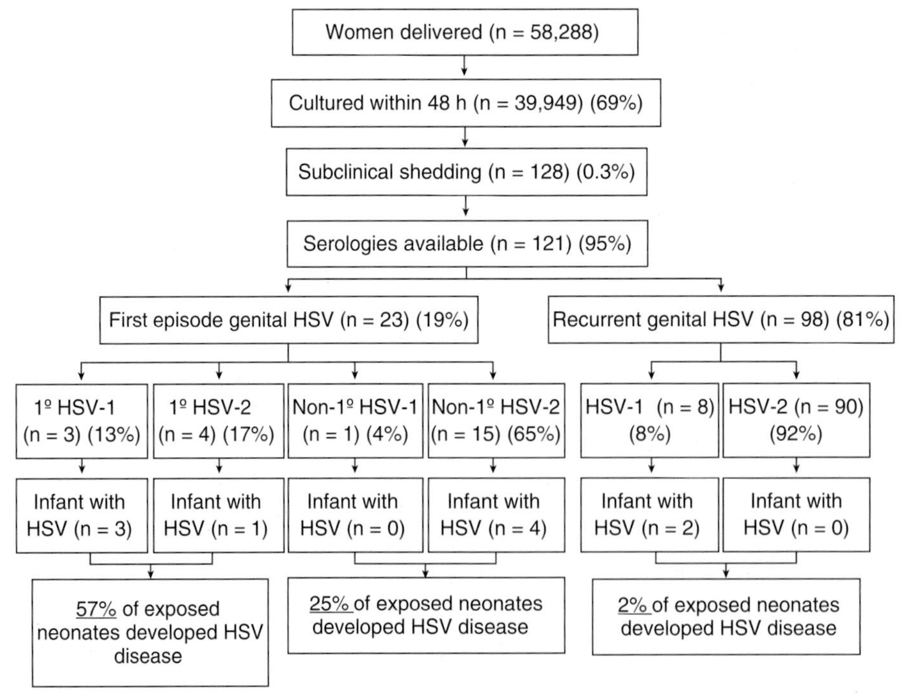

Fig. 4.1 Risk of Neonatal HSV Disease As a Function of Type of Maternal Infection. HSV, herpes simplex virus. (Adapted from Brown ZA, Wald A, Morrow RA, Selke S, Zeh J, Corey L. Effect of serologic status and cesarean delivery on transmission rates of herpes simplex virus from mother to infant. *JAMA.* 2003;289:203–209.)

Disseminated infection can manifest as severe hepatitis, disseminated intravascular coagulopathy, pneumonitis, and possibly CNS involvement (seen in 60%–75% of cases).[17,21] The mean age at presentation is around 11 days. Interestingly, over 40% of disseminated HSV disease cases do not develop skin findings during illness, which can complicate the diagnosis.[14,17,22,23]

Neonatal HSV CNS disease can present as seizures, lethargy, poor feeding, irritability, and increased fussiness, tremors, temperature instability, and bulging fontanelle. The mean age of presentation is around 16 days.[17] Around 60% to 70% of neonates with CNS disease will have skin manifestations at some point in the disease course.[17,22] Mortality is usually due to devastating brain destruction and atrophy, causing neurologic and autonomic dysfunction.

SEM disease has the best overall outcome, with virtually no mortality and with morbidity associated solely with cutaneous recurrences but no neurologic sequelae. Additionally, neonates with SEM disease are most likely to have skin lesions, facilitating diagnosis and allowing prompt initiation of antiviral treatment before the disease progresses to involve other organs, including the CNS. Presenting signs and symptoms of SEM disease include skin vesicles, fever, lethargy, and conjunctivitis.[17] Mean age of presentation is around 12 days. If SEM disease is not treated, it will likely progress to CNS or disseminated disease.[14]

Diagnosis of Neonatal HSV Disease

Because the extent of involvement varies by disease classification, the diagnosis of neonatal HSV infections requires the sampling of multiple sites:

- Swabs of mouth, nasopharynx, conjunctivae, and rectum should be obtained for HSV surface polymerase chain reaction (PCR) and, if possible, HSV culture.
- Specimens of skin vesicles should be obtained for culture and PCR.
- Cerebrospinal fluid (CSF) should be obtained for HSV PCR.
- Whole blood should be obtained for HSV PCR.
- Alanine aminotransferase should be obtained as an indicator of hepatic involvement.[24]

In past decades, the presence of red blood cells in CSF was suggestive of HSV CNS infection, likely due to relatively advanced disease due to diagnostic limitations. However, with enhanced appreciation for neonatal HSV disease and the development of more advanced imaging and diagnostic capabilities, hemorrhagic HSV encephalitis is less common, and as a result most HSV CNS CSF indices do not have significant numbers of red blood cells. Performance of whole-blood PCR adds to the other diagnostic tools but should not be used as the sole test for ruling in or ruling out neonatal HSV infection. Furthermore, viremia and DNAemia can occur in any of the three neonatal HSV disease classifications, so a positive whole-blood PCR simply rules in neonatal HSV infection but does not assist in disease classification. Of note, the performance characteristics of PCR assays on skin and mucosal surfaces, including the likelihood of false-positive results, have not been studied in neonates. Therefore, surface cultures remain the gold standard, albeit one that is not available in many locations. Other rapid diagnostic techniques include direct fluorescent antibody staining of vesicle scrapings or enzyme immunoassay detection of HSV antigens, but these are less sensitive than PCR and culture and generally should not be used. HSV isolates grown in culture or HSV DNA detected by PCR can be typed to determine whether they are HSV type 1 or HSV type 2. Chest radiographs and liver function tests can aid in the diagnosis of disseminated infection. Histologic testing is of low yield, as it has low sensitivity, and should not be used for diagnosis. Of note, all neonates with HSV disease, regardless of classification, need to have an ophthalmologic exam to look for ocular involvement. Infected neonates also should have neuroimaging studies (magnetic resonance imaging preferably, but computed tomography of the head or ultrasound are acceptable) performed to establish baseline brain anatomy.[24]

Treatment of Neonatal HSV Disease

Before antiviral therapies were available, disseminated HSV disease caused death by 1 year of age in 85% of those neonates affected. In neonates with CNS disease, the mortality was 50% (Table 4.1).[20,29] In a series of research studies conducted by the NIAID CASG between 1974 and 1997, parenteral vidarabine, low-dose acyclovir (30 mg/kg/day), and high-dose acyclovir (60 mg/kg/day) were evaluated sequentially.[18,20,25]

TABLE 4.1 Mortality and Morbidity Outcomes Among 295 Neonates With Neonatal HSV Infection, Evaluated By the National Institutes of Allergy and Infectious Diseases Collaborative Antiviral Study Group Between 1974 and 1997

	Treatment			
Extent of Disease	Placebo[20]	Vidarabine[18]	Acyclovir[18] (30 mg/kg/day)	Acyclovir[16] (60 mg/kg/day)
Disseminated disease	*n* = 13	*n* = 28	*n* = 18	*n* = 34
Dead	11 (85%)	14 (50%)	11 (61%)	10 (29%)
Alive	2 (15%)	14 (50%)	7 (39%)	24 (71%)
Normal	1 (50%)	7 (50%)	3 (43%)	15 (63%)
Abnormal	1 (50%)	5 (36%)	2 (29%)	3 (13%)
Unknown	0 (0%)	2 (14%)	2 (29%)	6 (25%)
Central nervous system infection	*n* = 6	*n* = 36	*n* = 35	*n* = 23
Dead	3 (50%)	5 (14%)	5 (14%)	1 (4%)
Alive	3 (50%)	31 (86%)	30 (86%)	22 (96%)
Normal	1 (33%)	13 (42%)	8 (27%)	4 (18%)
Abnormal	2 (67%)	17 (55%)	20 (67%)	9 (41%)
Unknown	0 (0%)	1 (3%)	2 (7%)	9 (41%)
Skin, eye, or mouth infection	*n* = 8	*n* = 31	*n* = 54	*n* = 9
Dead	0 (0%)	0 (0%)	0 (0%)	0 (0%)
Alive	8 (100%)	31 (100%)	54 (100%)	9 (100%)
Normal	5 (62%)	22 (71%)	45 (83%)	2 (22%)
Abnormal	3 (38%)	3 (10%)	1 (2%)	0 (0%)
Unknown	0 (0%)	6 (19%)	8 (15%)	7 (78%)

Adapted from Kimberlin DW. Advances in the treatment of neonatal herpes simplex infections. *Rev Med Virol.* 2001;11:157–163.

In the first of these studies, 10 days of vidarabine decreased mortality compared with placebo at 1 year both for neonates with disseminated disease (down to 50% in the vidarabine group) and for those with CNS disease (down to 14% in the vidarabine group). After comparison of low-dose acyclovir with vidarabine for 10 days, acyclovir became the primary treatment choice for neonatal HSV disease due to its favorable safety profile and its relative ease of administration (vidarabine required prolonged infusion times in large volumes of fluid). A subsequent study of high-dose acyclovir for 21 days produced further reductions in 1-year mortality, to 29% for disseminated disease (Figure 4.2) and 4% for CNS disease (Figure 4.3).[16]

This series of studies determined that neonates with neonatal HSV disease should be treated with parenteral acyclovir at a dose of 60 mg/kg/day divided into three daily doses; the dosing interval may need to be increased in premature neonates, based on their creatinine clearance.[26] The recommended treatment duration now is 21 days for neonates with disseminated or CNS disease, whereas neonates with SEM disease should be treated for 14 days.[24] All neonates with CNS HSV disease should have a repeat lumbar puncture near the end of the 21-day course of acyclovir to document that the CSF PCR is negative; if the PCR remains positive, another week of parenteral acyclovir should be administered and CSF analysis repeated in that manner until a negative CSF PCR is achieved.[17,27] In contrast, the value of serial whole-blood PCR determinations to gauge the duration of therapy has not been established, and blood PCR should not be performed after the initial testing to establish whether neonatal HSV infection exists.

The primary toxicity of higher-dose parenteral acyclovir is neutropenia.[16] Absolute neutrophil counts (ANCs) should be monitored twice weekly throughout the course of parenteral therapy. If neutropenia of <500/μL develops, either the acyclovir can be held or granulocyte colony-stimulating factor can be administered.[16]

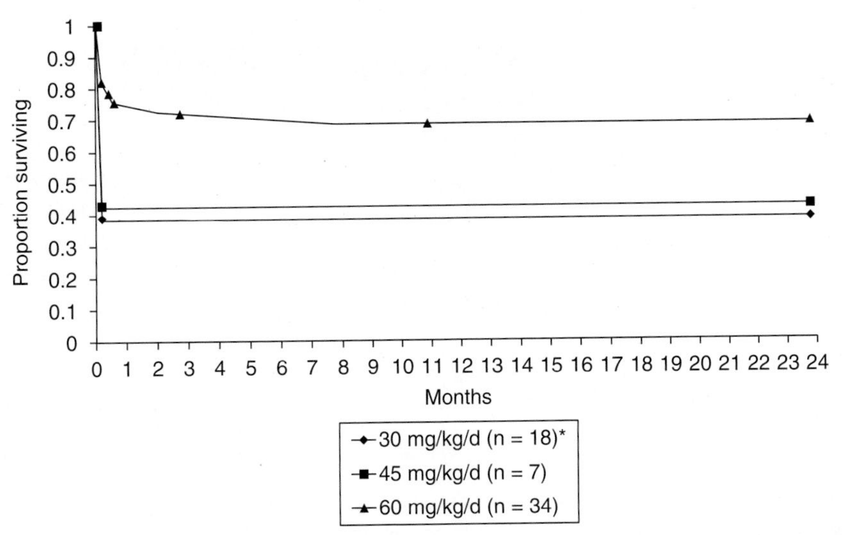

Fig. 4.2 Mortality in Patients With Disseminated Neonatal HSV Disease. (Adapted from Kimberlin DW, Lin CY, Jacobs RF, et al. Safety and efficacy of high-dose intravenous acyclovir in the management of neonatal herpes simplex virus infections. *Pediatrics.* 2001;108:230–238.)

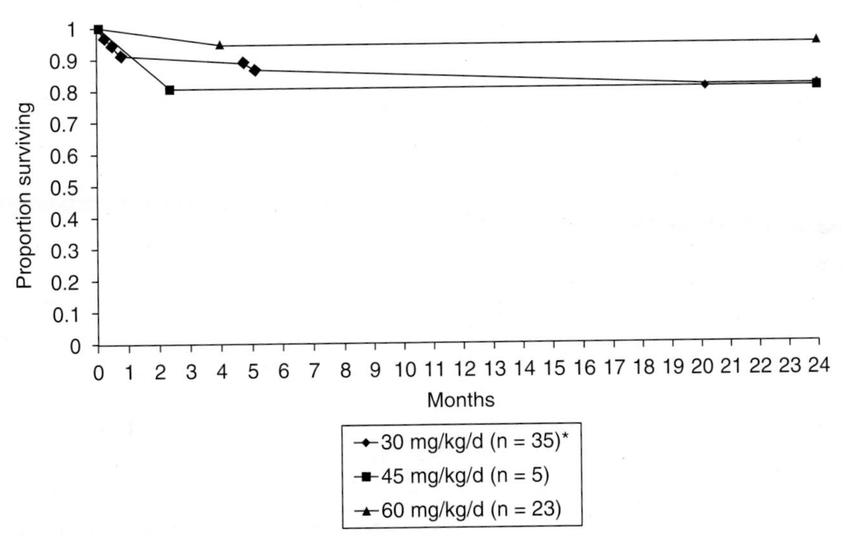

Fig. 4.3 Mortality in Patients With CNS Neonatal HSV Disease. (Adapted from Kimberlin DW, Lin CY, Jacobs RF, et al. Safety and efficacy of high-dose intravenous acyclovir in the management of neonatal herpes simplex virus infections. *Pediatrics.* 2001;108:230–238.)

Parenteral acyclovir dosing can be resumed when the ANC is >750/μL.

Oral acyclovir suppressive therapy for 6 months after acute parenteral treatment improves neurodevelopmental outcomes in neonates with CNS disease.[24] It is well known that HSV establishes latency in the sensory ganglia and occasionally reactivates and causes recurrence of disease. Reactivation may cause poor neurodevelopmental outcomes in neonates with CNS involvement. A recent study of neonates with neonatal HSV with CNS involvement compared Bayley mental developmental scores at 1 year for neonates

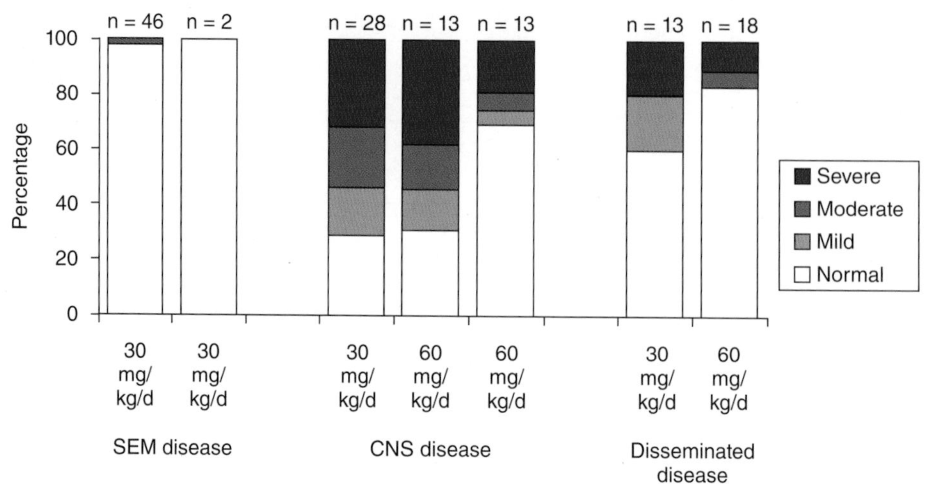

Fig. 4.4 Morbidity Among Patients With Known Outcomes After 12 Months of Life. (Adapted from Kimberlin DW, Lin CY, Jacobs RF, et al. Safety and efficacy of high-dose intravenous acyclovir in the management of neonatal herpes simplex virus infections. *Pediatrics.* 2001;108:230–238; Kimberlin DW, Whitley RJ, Wan W, et al. Oral acyclovir suppression and neurodevelopment after neonatal herpes. *N Engl J Med.* 2011;365(14):1284–1292.)

receiving suppressive therapy with acyclovir for 6 months versus neonates receiving placebo. The study found that the acyclovir group had a significantly higher mean Bayley score than the placebo group (88 vs. 68; $P = 0.046$).[28] It also demonstrated that overall neurodevelopmental outcomes were better in the acyclovir group (Figure 4.4). Suppressive acyclovir therapy also prevents skin recurrences in any classification of HSV disease.[28] Thus, neonates should receive oral acyclovir at 300 mg/m^2/dose three times daily as suppressive therapy for 6 months after the initial parenteral treatment course. This dose should be adjusted for growth monthly, and ANCs should be monitored at 2 and 4 weeks after starting therapy and then monthly thereafter while oral acyclovir is administered.[24]

Outcomes of Neonatal HSV With Treatment

Improvements in morbidity after antiviral treatment is less dramatic than improvements in mortality for neonates with disseminated disease or CNS disease. Without treatment, 50% of neonates who survived disseminated HSV disease were developing normally at 1 year of age.[20] However, with the use of higher-dose acyclovir for 21 days, the proportion of neonates developing normally at 1 year of age after disseminated HSV disease increased to 83%.[16] Similarly, for CNS HSV disease, 33% of neonates were found to develop normally at 1 year of age after 10 days of lower-dose acyclovir therapy, compared with 31% of neonates treated with higher-dose acyclovir for 21 days. With the use of 6 months of oral acyclovir therapy, though, this percentage of neonates with normal development at 1 year increased to 69%.[28] The morbidity of SEM disease also has dramatically improved since the introduction of antiviral treatment. In the pre-antiviral era, only 38% of patients with SEM disease were developing normally at 1 year of age, but with parenteral antiviral therapy this risk is eliminated (due to SEM disease not progressing to CNS or disseminated disease).[17,29]

Approach to Neonates Exposed to Active HSV Lesions at Delivery

The American Academy of Pediatrics has provided guidelines on the management of neonates born to women with active genital herpetic lesions, incorporating the most recent literature and understanding of the pathology, biology, and epidemiology of HSV infection and disease.[30] However, these recommendations are only applicable to institutions with access to PCR and quick turnaround time. They also are only for neonates of mothers with active lesions at delivery and are not applicable to neonates of mothers with asymptomatic HSV shedding.[31] Pregnant women with genital lesions at time of delivery should have viral cultures and PCR obtained from a swab of the lesion. The viral isolate or PCR amplicon should also be classified as HSV-1 or HSV-2, and the virologic result should then be compared with the type-specific serologic results from the woman obtained around the same time as the viral sample. This will allow the determination of whether she is experiencing a primary versus recurrent infection.

If a woman has a history of genital herpes prior to pregnancy and has an active lesion at delivery, this is likely to be a recurrent infection and the transmission risk to the neonate is very low (~3%).[31] At 24 hours after delivery, neonatal virology studies (e.g., HSV surface cultures and PCR, HSV blood PCR) should be collected and, if the neonate is asymptomatic, do not start acyclovir. If after 48 hours the neonate appears well and studies are negative, the neonate may be discharged home with clear education on signs and symptoms of neonatal HSV disease, as well as close follow-up with the pediatrician. However, if the surface and blood studies are positive, a full evaluation will have to be done (CSF studies including HSV PCR and serum alanine aminotransferase), and acyclovir should be started at 60 mg/kg/day in three divided doses. If these studies are negative, then treatment should be 10 days of preemptive therapy for HSV infection but not HSV disease. These neonates also should not be sent home with oral acyclovir suppression. If the full evaluation reveals evidence of HSV disease, then the neonate will need to be treated for 14 versus 21 days depending on SEM or CNS/disseminated disease. These neonates will also need repeat lumbar puncture at 21 days if they have CNS disease and will need to go home on oral suppression acyclovir therapy for 6 months.

If a woman has no known history of genital herpes prior to pregnancy and has her first genital herpes active infection at delivery, the likelihood that this is a primary infection is higher. These women are at higher risk of neonatal transmission (50%).[31] As such, at 24 hours after birth the neonate should have a full evaluation for HSV disease (see Diagnosis of Neonatal HSV Disease section, above), and intravenous acyclovir should be started while awaiting results. If the maternal serologies and virologic studies demonstrate a recurrent HSV infection, if the neonate remains asymptomatic, and if studies do not show evidence of HSV infection, then the neonate's acyclovir can be discontinued, and the neonate can be discharged home. The family should be instructed to closely monitor for signs of infection and adhere to close follow-up. However, if maternal studies are suggestive of primary infection but the neonate is asymptomatic and studies do not show infection or disease, then the neonate should be preemptively treated for 10 days with intravenous acyclovir. This is because the neonate has a high risk of progressing to infection or disease (25% to >50%).[31] Of course, if the neonate has evidence of disease, then the neonate should be fully treated and will require oral suppression therapy for 6 months, as previously noted.

Prevention of Neonatal HSV Disease

The American College of Obstetricians and Gynecologists (ACOG) recommends that a cesarean section be performed if genital lesions or prodromal symptoms are present at the time of delivery, preferably prior to rupture of membranes, to reduce the risk of neonatal HSV disease.[32] However, as mentioned earlier, neonatal HSV disease has occurred despite these precautions.[14,15] Additionally, in women with a previous diagnosis of genital herpes who do not have active lesions at delivery, a cesarean section is not indicated. An intervention currently endorsed by the ACOG to decrease cesarean section in women with recurrent genital herpes is to start oral acyclovir or valacyclovir therapy at 36 weeks of gestation. This approach has reduced the likelihood of genital lesions at the time of delivery and decreased viral detection by culture and PCR.[32] However, a case study showed that subclinical shedding is not entirely suppressed and reported eight cases of neonatal HSV disease in babies acquired from mothers on suppression therapy.[33] As such, this practice in preventing neonatal HSV disease is not fully defined.

Conclusion

Neonatal HSV disease is known to have devastating neurologic effects. Fortunately, over the past 4 decades, much has been learned regarding natural history, pathogenesis, diagnosis, and treatment of this severe infection. In the 21st century, neonatal HSV disease is treatable, and management recommendations have been standardized and implemented. As with any other area of medicine, though, information is fluid, and, as more knowledge is obtained, more questions are formed. These questions in turn drive the next series of studies, with further promise of continued advances for years to come.

REFERENCES

1. Whitley RJ, Roizman B. Herpes simplex virus infections. *Lancet*. 2001;357:1513-1518.
2. Brown ZA, Benedetti J, Ashley R, et al. Neonatal herpes simplex virus infection in relation to asymptomatic maternal infection at the time of labor. *N Engl J Med*. 1991;324:1247-1252.
3. Brown ZA, Vontver LA, Benedetti J, et al. Effects on infants of a first episode of genital herpes during pregnancy. *N Engl J Med*. 1987;317:1246-1251.
4. Corey L, Wald A. Genital herpes. In: Holmes KK, Sparling PF, Mardh PA, et al., eds. *Sexually Transmitted Diseases*. 3rd ed. New York: McGraw-Hill; 1999:285-312.
5. Nahmias AJ, Josey WE, Naib ZM, Freeman MG, Fernandez RJ, Wheeler, JH. Perinatal risk associated with maternal genital herpes simplex virus infection. *Am J Obstet Gynecol*. 1971;110:825-837.
6. Brown ZA, Wald A, Morrow RA, Selke S, Zeh J, Corey L. Effect of serologic status and cesarean delivery on transmission rates of herpes simplex virus from mother to infant. *JAMA*. 2003; 289:203-209.
7. Yeager AS, Arvin AM. Reasons for the absence of a history of recurrent genital infections in mothers of neonates infected with herpes simplex virus. *Pediatrics*. 1984;73:188-193.
8. Prober CG, Sullender WM, Yasukawa LL, Au DS, Yeager AS, Arvin AM. Low risk of herpes simplex virus infections in neonates exposed to the virus at the time of vaginal delivery to mothers with recurrent genital herpes simplex virus infections. *N Engl J Med*. 1987;316:240-244.
9. Yeager AS, Arvin AM, Urbani LJ, Kemp JA III. Relationship of antibody to outcome in neonatal herpes simplex virus infections. *Infect Immun*. 1980;29:532-538.
10. Parvey LS, Ch'ien LT. Neonatal herpes simplex virus infection introduced by fetal-monitor scalp electrodes. *Pediatrics*. 1980;65: 1150-1153.
11. Kaye EM, Dooling EC. Neonatal herpes simplex meningoencephalitis associated with fetal monitor scalp electrodes. *Neurology*. 1981;31:1045-1047.
12. Whitley RJ. Herpes simplex viruses. In: Fields BN, Knipe DM, Howley PM, et al., eds. *Fields Virology*. 3rd ed. Philadelphia, PA: Lippincott-Raven; 1996:2297-2342.
13. American College of Obstetricians and Gynecologists. ACOG practice bulletin. Management of herpes in pregnancy. Number 8 October 1999. Clinical management guidelines for obstetrician–gynecologists. *Int J Gynaecol Obstet*. 2000;68:165-173.
14. Whitley RJ, Corey L, Arvin A, et al. Changing presentation of herpes simplex virus infection in neonates. *J Infect Dis*. 1988; 158:109-116.
15. Peng J, Krause PJ, Kresch M. Neonatal herpes simplex virus infection after cesarean section with intact amniotic membranes. *J Perinatol*. 1996;16:397-399.
16. Kimberlin DW, Lin CY, Jacobs RF, et al. Safety and efficacy of high-dose intravenous acyclovir in the management of neonatal herpes simplex virus infections. *Pediatrics*. 2001;108: 230-238.
17. Kimberlin DW, Lin CY, Jacobs RF, et al. Natural history of neonatal herpes simplex virus infections in the acyclovir era. *Pediatrics*. 2001;108:223-229.
18. Whitley R, Arvin A, Prober C, et al. A controlled trial comparing vidarabine with acyclovir in neonatal herpes simplex virus infection. *N Engl J Med*. 1991;324:444-449.
19. Whitley R, Arvin A, Prober C, et al. Predictors of morbidity and mortality in neonates with herpes simplex virus infections. *N Engl J Med*. 1991;324:450-454.
20. Whitley RJ, Nahmias AJ, Soong SJ, et al. Vidarabine therapy of neonatal herpes simplex virus infection. *Pediatrics*. 1980; 66:495-501.
21. Whitley RJ. Herpes simplex virus infections. In: Remington JS, Klein JO, eds. *Infectious Diseases of the Fetus and Newborn Infants*. 3rd ed. Philadelphia, PA: WB Saunders; 1990:282-305.
22. Sullivan-Bolyai JZ, Hull HF, Wilson C, Smith AL, Corey L. Presentation of neonatal herpes simplex virus infections: implications for a change in therapeutic strategy. *Pediatr Infect Dis*. 1986;5:309-314.
23. Arvin AM, Yeager AS, Bruhn FW, Grossman M. Neonatal herpes simplex infection in the absence of mucocutaneous lesions. *J Pediatr*. 1982;100:715-721.
24. American Academy of Pediatrics. Herpes simplex. In: Kimberlin DW, Barnett ED, Lynfield R, Sawyer MH, eds. *Red Book: 2021 Report of the Committee on Infectious Diseases*. 32nd ed. Itasca, IL: American Academy of Pediatrics; 2021:407-417.
25. Whitley RJ, Yeager A, Kartus P, et al. Neonatal herpes simplex virus infection: follow-up evaluation of vidarabine therapy. *Pediatrics*. 1983;72:778-785.
26. Englund JA, Fletcher CV, Balfour Jr HH. Acyclovir therapy in neonates. *J Pediatr*. 1991;119:129-135.
27. Kimberlin DW, Lakeman FD, Arvin AM, et al. Application of the polymerase chain reaction to the diagnosis and management of neonatal herpes simplex virus disease. *J Infect Dis*. 1996;174:1162-1167.
28. Kimberlin DW, Whitley RJ, Wan W, et al. Oral acyclovir suppression and neurodevelopment after neonatal herpes. *N Engl J Med*. 2011;365(14):1284-1292.
29. Kimberlin DW. Advances in the treatment of neonatal herpes simplex infections. *Rev Med Virol*. 2001;11:157-163.
30. Kimberlin DW, Baley J, American Academy of Pediatrics Committee on Infectious Diseases, Committee on Fetus and Newborn. Guidance on management of asymptomatic neonates born to women with active genital herpes lesions. *Pediatrics*. 2013;131(2):e635-e646.
31. Pinninti SG, Kimberlin DW. Neonatal herpes simplex virus infections. *Semin Perinatol*. 2018;42(3):168-175.
32. American College of Obstetricians and Gynecologists. ACOG practice bulletin. Clinical management guidelines for obstetrician–gynecologists. Number 220 May 2020. Management of genital herpes in pregnancy. *Obstet Gynecol*. 2020;135(5):e193-e202.
33. Pinninti SG, Angara R, Feja KN, et al. Neonatal herpes disease following maternal antenatal antiviral suppressive therapy: a multicenter case series. *J Pediatr*. 2012;161(1):134-138.

Chapter 5

Antibiotic Stewardship

C. Michael Cotten, MD, MHS

Key Points

- Antibiotics are lifesaving and improve outcomes in neonatal clinical care.
- Increasing evidence in animal and human models links antibiotic exposure with alterations in the microbiome, the developing immune system, and subsequent effects on health.
- Empiric antibiotic use is linked to the emergence of infections caused by multidrug-resistant organisms and to increased risk of necrotizing enterocolitis and mortality.
- The primary goal of antibiotic stewardship programs in neonatal intensive care units is to reduce morbidity and save lives by appropriate use of antibiotics in the treatment of proven and suspected neonatal infections. A secondary goal is to reduce healthcare costs.
- Implementation of multidisciplinary antibiotic stewardship strategy may slow emergence of antibiotic resistant organisms and lead to other improved outcomes including shorter hospitalizations, and fewer adverse drug events.

Neonatologists prescribe antibiotics more than any other medication.[1,2] Because of the risk for development of antibiotic-resistant organisms, adverse drug events that may result from antibiotic exposure, the emerging evidence that antibiotics influence the developing microbiome in both term and preterm infants, and association studies linking antibiotic exposures to subsequent systemic disease, neonatologists and other stakeholders have heeded guidance from experts and more recently from more authoritative sources, such as the Centers for Disease Control and Prevention (CDC), to become better stewards of antibiotic use in the neonatal intensive care unit (NICU). Notable improvements have been associated with participation in large-scale, multicenter antibiotic stewardship efforts.[3–9] This chapter reviews early and more recent efforts to optimize antibiotic use in the NICU and highlights areas for ongoing stewardship efforts.

Antibiotic Stewardship Programs: We Were Warned

In an address to the American Association of Penicillin Producers more than 70 years ago, Alexander Fleming, the discoverer of penicillin, cautioned clinicians regarding overuse of penicillin and the emergence of organisms resistant to penicillin.[10] Approximately 40 years and dozens of approved antimicrobial compounds later, Harold Neu, a leader in infectious disease research who developed the inhibitory quotient, which reflects antimicrobial effectiveness in different tissue compartments,[11] warned of complacency regarding antibiotic use and predicted that the emergence of resistant organisms was likely to occur in community hospitals. He recommended that "antibiotic control programs, better hygiene, and improved antimicrobial activity must be adopted to limit emergence of resistance."[12]

Early Days: Reporting Emergent Resistance and Antibiotic Practice and Outcome Variation in NICUs

In the 1970s, neonatologists and infectious disease specialists recognized the high risk of infection and infection-associated mortality in the neonatal population and acknowledged the risk of emergent antibiotic resistance. Noting the emergence of resistant *Escherichia coli*, dosing recommendations for then commonly used kanamycin were changed as pharmacokinetic data from infected infants became available.[13,14] Investigators also reported variations in empirical antibiotic use, comparing practices at two Boston-area hospitals over a 4-month period. The infection rates at the two hospitals were the same, but the ratio of treated to infected infants was 15:1 at Hospital A and 28:1 at Hospital B. Hospital A's median duration of antibiotics was 7 days, and Hospital B's was 4 days. The authors provided us with a warning that resonates almost 50 years later: "The early and frequent use of antibiotics for newborn infants with suspected sepsis is warranted because of the persistent high mortality. The widespread use of antimicrobial agents is a cause for concern, however, because of the alteration of microbial flora in the treated infants and in other infants and nursery personnel."[15] This report was followed by a review article that provided guidance on empirical antibiotic choices for infants with suspected sepsis. Their guidance is applicable today, including initial therapy inclusive of coverage for the still-most common causes of early-onset sepsis, Gram-positive cocci, particularly group B *Streptococcus*, and Gram-negative enteric bacilli.[16,17] After postnatal day 4, the recommendation in 1983 was for treatment choices to include consideration for the same early-onset infection organisms, as well as acquired pathogens from the NICU environment, with a penicillin as first choice for Gram-positive organisms. The recommendation for Gram-negative coverage was that clinicians should be informed by the local infection history, as well as the antimicrobial susceptibility of organisms in the nursery, with choices being re-evaluated based on culture results.[18]

Through the 1980s and 1990s, reports of antibiotic-resistant Gram-negative organisms were emerging from NICUs.[19,20] These reports contributed to the development and testing of antibiotic policies aiming to prevent the emergence of antibiotic-resistant organisms in single centers and small numbers of nurseries. For example, in a prospective cross-over intervention trial in two identical, adjacent NICUs, colonization with bacilli resistant to the usual empirical therapy greatly increased (18-fold) when intravenous amoxicillin with cefotaxime was used as empiric therapy for early- and late-onset sepsis, compared with periods when penicillin G and tobramycin were used empirically for early-onset septicemia and flucloxacillin and tobramycin were used for late-onset septicemia; no broad-spectrum β-lactam antibiotics, such as amoxicillin and cefotaxime, were used empirically.[21] The authors concluded that their study provides solid evidence regarding the benefit of using antibiotics that have minimal impact on the mucosal environment in terms of reduced bacterial resistance.[21]

Emergence of Multicenter Reports on Antimicrobial Practice Variations

By the early 2000s, multicenter consortia were collaborating to collect data, allowing for assessments of collective practices and outcomes and better quantification of center variation in antibiotic practice. From the data collected and reported in the late 1990s and early 2000s, the challenge of infections and related mortality among the most premature infants continued, as did the evidence for higher incidence of early-onset infection for the most premature infants, the steadily high incidence of later-onset infections for premature infants in NICUs, and high incidence of mortality among infants with bloodstream infections.[22–24] As suspected, NICUs were using antibiotics often. In the first "national multicenter report" of antimicrobial use in NICUs, 31 Pediatric Prevention Network hospitals participated in two single-day point prevalence surveys of antibiotic use in 1999 and 2000. Forty-three percent of the 1582 NICU infants were on antibiotics on that single day.[25]

In 2002, the CDC launched a campaign known as 12 Steps to Prevent Antimicrobial Resistance in healthcare settings, starting with hospitalized adults. The CDC acknowledged high rates of drug-resistant infections and clinicians' suboptimal adherence to existing guidelines to prevent resistant infection. The 12 Steps effort was a multifaceted attempt to help clinicians translate guidelines into practices intended to reduce antimicrobial resistance. The campaign, which interestingly did not include the term "antibiotic stewardship," included four major strategies: (1) preventing infections, (2) diagnosing and treating infections effectively, (3) using antimicrobials wisely, and (4) preventing transmission.[26] In the first study to assess the use of the CDC's original 12 Step guidelines adapted for the NICU, investigators assessed the appropriateness of antimicrobial use in four tertiary NICUs in late 2005.[27] Antibiotic utilization information was collected for 200 infants, 50 from each of the four sites, inclusive of chart review assessing progress notes to ascertain the indications for antibiotics at two time points: initiation of each antibiotic course and continuation of the course beyond 72 hours. Indications to begin or continue could be classified as one of three possibilities: (1) empiric (treating for signs or treating a positive culture with pending susceptibility), (2) definitive (treating a pathogen with known susceptibility), or (3) prophylaxis. A course was considered inappropriate if it deviated from a CDC recommendation at initiation or continuation, or both. Clinical choices were assessed using five of the 2002 CDC recommendations listed in Table 5.1. The 200 infants in the study cohort received 323 antibiotic courses and 3344 antibiotic-days. Sixty-six percent of antibiotic course initiations were empiric, 5% were definitive, and 29% were for prophylaxis. Thirty-seven percent of continuations were for definitive treatment, 33% were empiric, and 30% were for prophylaxis. Seventy infants (35%) received at least one antibiotic course judged non-adherent to the CDC recommendations. Inappropriate use was much more commonly assessed for continuation of antibiotics (39%) compared with initiation (4%); with similar rates and reasons across the four participating sites. Vancomycin and cefazolin were the most commonly used antibiotics, and approximately a third of the uses were judged inappropriate. "Target the pathogen" was the most commonly violated CDC recommendation. Common examples of non-adherence included continuing vancomycin for methicillin-susceptible *Staphylococcus aureus* or using a carbapenem to treat a Gram-negative rod susceptible to piperacillin/tazobactam. Of note, definitions for inappropriate antibiotic use were related to changes from locally determined treatment plans. The CDC recommendations included "ask an expert," so pediatric infectious disease specialists were consulted for guidance for all infants with positive cultures. One additional caveat that may have led to an underestimate of "non-adherent use" is that courses

TABLE 5.1 CDC Recommendations for Antibiotic Stewardship and Examples of Inappropriate Use in the NICU[27]

CDC Stewardship Guidance	Examples of Inappropriate Use
Target the pathogen.	Continued use of broad-spectrum agent when a narrower spectrum agent is available Use of vancomycin for methicillin-susceptible *Staphylococcus aureus* infection Inadequate therapy Use of gentamicin for a gentamicin-resistant pathogen Continued use of two agents when a single one is adequate Use of both vancomycin and gentamicin for *Staphylococcus epidermis* bloodstream infection
Practice antimicrobial control.	Prolonged postoperative prophylaxis (e.g., cefazolin >24–48 hours) Chest tube prophylaxis (e.g., cefazolin >24–48 hours)
Treat infection not contamination or colonization.	Continued treatment of coagulase-negative *Staphylococcus* bloodstream infection with positive central venous catheter and negative peripheral blood culture in a stable infant Treatment of positive arterial line culture with negative blood cultures from other sites in a stable infant Treatment of urine culture positive for two or more organisms in a stable infant
Know when to say "NO" to antibiotics.	Initial therapy with broad-spectrum agent Use of carbapenem for empiric treatment of late-onset sepsis, without evidence of multidrug resistance or necrotizing enterocolitis (NEC) Redundant coverage Use of carbapenem *and* metronidazole for the treatment of anaerobic pathogens in NEC
Stop treatment when infection is cured or unlikely.	Prolonged duration of therapy Treatment of coagulase-negative *Staphylococcus* bloodstream infection for >10 days since last positive culture, or longer duration than indicated Treatment of *S. aureus* or Gram-negative bacilli bloodstream infections >14 days since last positive culture and/or for longer duration than indicated in the treatment plan

initiated for empiric treatment of suspected infection or continued for what was locally determined to be "culture-negative sepsis" were considered appropriate.[27] As we know, use of antibiotics for culture-negative sepsis is a topic currently receiving scrutiny.[28]

As Patel and colleagues[27] were taking their first look at the appropriateness of antibiotic use in four centers, others were collecting and reporting antibiotic practice variations and associations with morbidities from even larger NICU consortia, providing further evidence for a wide range of practice and associations between some of the variations in practice with outcomes. Clark and colleagues[29] structured the storage of medication data for retrieval and analysis warehouse derived from the daily records of tens of thousands of infants cared for in over 150 NICUs managed by the Pediatrix Medical Group (Sunrise, FL). The granular data could be used to evaluate medication use and practice variation and report associations between antibiotic use and various outcomes.[29] Investigators used the data to report associations between broad-spectrum antibiotic use (cephalosporins and carbapenems) and subsequent candidiasis in extremely premature infants.[30] Associations between exposure to cefotaxime, mostly empirical, in the first postnatal days and subsequent mortality were reported soon afterward.[29] In this large cohort, 2% of infants exposed to antibiotics had a positive culture in the first 7 postnatal days. Like the two-hospital report from Hammerschlag et al.[15] more than 20 years earlier, extreme practice variation in the use of antibiotics was noted, but in this dataset variation was reported for over 120,000 infants in over 150 NICUs submitting data between 1996 and 2004. In 15% of the NICUs, more than 50% of the infants received cefotaxime in the first postnatal days. On multivariable logistic regression, infants treated with ampicillin and cefotaxime were more likely to die than those treated with ampicillin and gentamicin (adjusted odds ratio = 1.5; 95% confidence interval, 1.4–1.7). The associations were consistent in gestational age-stratified groups (23–26 weeks', 27–30 weeks', 31–34 weeks', 35–38 weeks', and 39–42 weeks' gestation).[29]

The National Institute of Child Health and Human Development (NICHD) Neonatal Research Network (NRN) and subsequently other groups reported highly prevalent empirical antibiotic use among extremely low-birth-weight infants who had negative cultures. The duration of those empiric courses was highly variable, and there were positive associations between subsequent necrotizing enterocolitis and death with longer empirical courses.[31-35] The NRN also reported that individual and center-wide risk of candidiasis increased with higher exposure to broad-spectrum antibiotics, inclusive at the time largely of third-generation cephalosporins rather than carbapenems, similar to the findings noted from the Pediatrix Medical Group cohort.[36,37]

Large-Scale Stewardship in the NICU

Due to reports of variation in antibiotic practice, prevalent inappropriate use of antibiotics, and associations between longer-duration empirical courses and the use of empiric broad-spectrum agents (particularly third-generation cephalosporins) with outcomes, as well as the long-standing evidence regarding the emergence of antibiotic resistant organisms, larger consortiums have collaborated on implementation of more structured and supported multicenter efforts to optimize antibiotic use in the NICU.

One of the first multicenter efforts targeting antibiotic use was the Pediatrix 100,000 Babies Campaign. The Pediatrix Medical Group provides care to approximately 20% of infants in NICUs in the United States, from small community hospitals to large tertiary sites. The campaign incorporated timely data sharing as a key aspect of an eight-step model based on Kotter's eight-step process for leading organizational change.[38] The goal of the project was to change practice in Pediatrix NICUs in a number of areas, including specific mention of antibiotic stewardship, reductions in the use of cefotaxime, and reductions in the percentage of infants treated more than 3 days with ampicillin despite negative cultures. The overall goal of all the practice changes combined was to save 100,000 infants' lives.[3,38] The eight steps provide helpful structure for developing an antibiotic stewardship program in single or multicenter projects (Table 5.2). The project development began in 2007, and it was formally launched in 2009. At the time of the 100,000 Babies Campaign, 330 NICUs in over 30 states and Puerto Rico provided data to the

TABLE 5.2 **Adaptation of Kotter's Organizational Change Model Utilized in the 100,000 Babies Campaign**[38]

Concept	Kotter's Eight-Step Process	100,000 Babies Campaign Steps
Prepare	Create urgency.	Provide outcome and benchmarking data. Link participation to maintenance of certification/quality improvement.
	Create a guiding coalition.	Identify an implementation leadership team and individual champions. Enlist local and, if applicable, regional improvement champions.
	Create a vision to share.	Build on previous successes. Emphasize improvement that is practical and meaningful.
Implement	Communicate that vision.	Conduct quality summits and provide data updates to the entire NICU team.
	Remove obstacles.	Be flexible in participation. Automate, as much as possible, data collection and reports.
	Enable short-term wins.	Include simple projects and quick results.
Manage	Build on change.	Present results to peers and institution leadership. Disseminate success.
	Embed change in culture.	Maintain an ongoing emphasis on and recognition of improvement activity. Maintain an ongoing infrastructure to support improvement work.

Pediatrix data warehouse. The project amplified prior work done by Pediatrix quality-improvement leadership, and participation at all Pediatrix sites was encouraged but not mandated.[3,39] The project included surveys at sites to assess attitudes, knowledge bases, and biases among clinical staff, and the results informed educational needs, including maintenance of certification credits and project strategies. The results for infants with birth weights between 501 and 1500 g were remarkable, with decreases in cefotaxime exposures by approximately 50% and a 20% reduction in early ampicillin treatment going beyond the third postnatal day, without increases in necrotizing enterocolitis, late-onset sepsis, or mortality (Table 5.3). Multiple practices were modified, including increases in infants receiving any mother's milk and having mother's milk at discharge, as well as reductions in the use of reflux medications, dexamethasone use, ventilator days, and hypothermia at NICU admission. During the reported 7 years of the project, mortality, necrotizing enterocolitis, severe and surgical retinopathy of prematurity, and bacteremia after 3 days of life all decreased significantly.[3] As noted by Ellsbury et al.,[40–43] although other consortia were reporting successful quality-improvement efforts leading to reductions in infections, none was reporting on concurrent attempts to modify or optimize antibiotic practice.

NICUs Join the Antibiotic Stewardship Wave

In 2013, the CDC published its report on the emergence of antibiotic resistance threats.[44] The same year, an analysis appearing in the *Cochrane Database of Systematic Reviews*, entitled "Interventions to improve antibiotic prescribing practices for hospital inpatients," was updated. The aim of the article was "to evaluate the impact of interventions from the perspective of antibiotic stewardship." The meta-analyses showed that interventions targeting reductions in excessive antibiotic prescribing to inpatients reduced antimicrobial resistance or hospital-acquired infections and that interventions to increase effective prescribing can improve clinical outcome.[45] Shortly thereafter, the CDC published its first version of the recently updated report on core elements of antibiotic stewardship in 2014. The CDC report includes guidance on seven key core elements for developing successful antibiotic stewardship programs (ASPs): leadership commitment, accountability, drug expertise, action, tracking, reporting, and education.[46]

Following the article in the *Cochrane Database of Systematic Reviews*, the CDC guidance on seven key elements to antibiotic stewardship programs, and the emerging reports on variations in practice in the NRN

TABLE 5.3 Results of the 100,000 Babies Campaign: Antibiotic Process Measures and Outcomes for Infants With Birthweights 501–1500 g (2007–2013)[39]

	2007	2008	2009	2010	2011	2012	2013	*P* (Over Time)
Subjects, *N*								
	6076	6398	6272	6392	6111	6065	5893	—
Process Measures, *n* (%)								
Cefotaxime	1152 (14.3)	940 (11.1)	769 (9.2)	692 (8.2)	679 (8.1)	677 (8)	599 (7.2)	<0.0001
Early ampicillin duration of >3 days with negative cultures	2138 (35.2)	2226 (34.8)	2110 (33.6)	2096 (32.8)	1968 (32.3)	1832 (30.2)	1671 (28.4)	<0.0001
Outcome Measures, *n* (%)								
Necrotizing enterocolitis (medical and surgical)	529 (6.6)	542 (6.4)	454 (5.4)	463 (5.5)	410 (4.9)	338 (4)	323 (3.9)	<0.0001
Late-onset sepsis*	1579 (19.6)	1499 (17.7)	1360 (16.2)	1150 (13.6)	983 (11.7)	888 (10.5)	754 (9)	<0.0001
Mortality	836 (10.4)	838 (9.9)	728 (8.7)	750 (8.9)	714 (8.5)	702 (8.3)	681 (8.1)	<0.0001

*Positive blood culture was obtained >3 days after birth.

and the Pediatrix Medical Group, the California Quality Collaborative added to the information about variations in practice, reporting a 40-fold variation in antibiotic use among 52,061 infants in 127 NICUs with similar incidence of infections.[47] Following this report from a third large consortium, and in response to the CDC antibiotic stewardship initiative, the American Academy of Pediatrics Section on Perinatal and Neonatal Medicine published their "Choosing Wisely in Newborn Medicine: Five Opportunities to Improve Value." In it, they identified antibiotic therapy as an area of medication overuse and potential target for modifying practice, including "routine continuation of antibiotic therapy beyond 48 hours for initially asymptomatic infants without evidence of bacterial infection."[48] These reports and CDC recommendations were followed by the Vermont Oxford Network (VON) of Neonatal Intensive Care Units partnering with the CDC to launch the VON iNICQ Choosing Antibiotics Wisely campaign. The aim of the campaign was to decrease antibiotic overuse among the more than 140 participating VON NICUs. To provide baseline information and initiate planning for site-level ASPs, each participating site responded to a survey on the seven key domains of the CDC Core Elements of Hospital ASPs (Table 5.4). At the beginning of the project in 2016, none of the 143 participating centers was addressing all seven CDC core elements. Only 15% had commitment from leadership in place and were tracking antibiotic use rates. Six percent of the centers reported to or received reports from the National Healthcare Safety Network Antibiotic Use and Resistance Module. Sixty-two percent of centers were fortunate enough to have a pharmacist with NICU antibiotic expertise. Clearly, the results indicated that focused ASPs in NICUs that incorporated all of the CDC-recommended strategies and resources would be a challenge.[49] In the first 2 years of the project, the percentage of the participating sites implementing core elements increased in all seven domains, but only 9.9% of sites met all seven CDC core elements (Table 5.4). Although having all seven core elements in place was not achieved by many participating centers, the participating VON centers did make progress in developing processes and reducing antibiotic use. Multidisciplinary teams were formed at participating sites and expert coaching was provided up to nine times per year, including the use of web-based conferences and coaching sessions. Prevalence audits were undertaken to monitor progress on process measures and the antibiotic use rate, which was defined as the percentage of infants in the

TABLE 5.4 **CDC'S Core Elements of Hospital Antibiotic Stewardship Programs: NICU-Specific Questions for Planning Local ASPs**[48,49]

CDC Core Element	VON NICU ASP Questions	Initial	End of Year 2
Leadership commitment	Does your NICU have a formal written project plan that is used to engage senior leadership in efforts to improve antibiotic use (antibiotic stewardship)?	15.4%	68.8%
Accountability	Is there a physician leader responsible for the outcomes of stewardship activities in your NICU?	54.5%	95%
Drug expertise	Is there a pharmacist leader responsible for working to improve antibiotic use in your NICU?	61.5%	85.1%
Actions/timeout	Is there a formal procedure or process used to prompt the NICU care team to review the appropriateness of all antibiotics prescribed for infants in the NICU 48–72 hours after that initial order (e.g., "antibiotic time-out")?	21.7%	72.3%
Tracking	Does your NICU monitor antibiotic use rate (AUR), either as days of antibiotic therapy or days of antibiotic therapy per 1000 patient-days?	14.7%	78%
Reporting	Does your NICU participate in the National Healthcare Safety Network Antibiotic Use and Resistance Module?	6.3%	17.7%
Ongoing education	Does your NICU provide education to clinicians and other relevant staff on improving antibiotic prescribing?	32.9%	87.2%
Antibiotic use rate	AUR is defined as the percentage of infants in a unit receiving one or more antibiotics on the day of the audit.	16.7%	12.1%

NICU, neonatal intensive care unit.

NICU receiving one or more antibiotics on the day of the audit. In addition to the seven CDC domains, the project leadership provided four potentially better practices as more focused guidance for sites to target:

1. Demonstrate an organizational commitment and promote an organizational culture that supports appropriate antibiotic use in the NICU as a critical priority.
2. Develop, test, implement, and continually refine policies and protocols for appropriate antibiotic use in specific neonatal conditions, including suspected early- and late-onset sepsis, necrotizing enterocolitis, and surgical conditions.
3. Apply pharmacy-driven interventions designed to ensure appropriate antibiotic treatment of newborn infants.
4. Report regularly on antibiotic use and resistance in the NICU to doctors, nurses, and staff.

Each site selected the potentially better practices to guide local site-specific interventions. Importantly, all sites used quality-improvement approaches and methodologies. One important item of data collected was antibiotic use guidelines for 12 clinical categories. The prevalence of guidelines increased for all 12 categories, and the list provides a goal for sites seeking to implement and periodically update antibiotic use guidelines (Table 5.5).[6] Although not all of the categories have strong evidence supporting an approach, a recent publication provides suggested approaches based on current evidence for some of the various clinical categories.[50]

Individual VON and CDC ASPs have been subsequently reported and can provide important details of practices implemented, sustained successes, and ongoing or new challenges.[51,52] One report documented a reduction in antibiotic use rate of over 40%, and it had been sustained more than 18 months. Much of the reduction was due to practices focused on early-onset sepsis (EOS), including implementation of an evidence-based, data-derived sepsis risk calculator; implementing a 36-hour hard stop for antibiotics to assess for culture positivity; and development of guidelines for EOS evaluations among the infants born before 35 weeks' gestation.[52]

In the United States, group B *Streptococcus* has remained a significant contributor to EOS and continues to be sensitive to ampicillin, reinforcing the rationale for ampicillin for Gram-positive coverage.

TABLE 5.5 Percent of Sites Participating in CDC and VON Antibiotic Stewardship With Local Policies, Protocols, or Guidelines to Standardize the Diagnosis and Antibiotic Treatment of Common Neonatal Conditions[49]

Condition	Guideline at Start (*N* = 143 Sites)	Guideline at Finish (*N* = 141 Sites)
Maternal risk factors	53%	71.6%
Suspected or proven		
Early-onset sepsis or meningitis	44.8%	73.8%
Late-onset sepsis or meningitis	44.8%	73.8%
Ventilator-associated pneumonia	13.3%	27.7%
Central venous line infection	30.8%	48.9%
Urinary tract infection	14.0%	34.0%
Necrotizing enterocolitis	31.5%	44.7%
Surgical site infection	9.8%	19.1%
Urinary tract infection prophylaxis	19.6%	30.5%
Prophylaxis for surgery	25.2%	27.7%
Prophylaxis for fungal sepsis	35.0%	40.4%
Methicillin-resistant *Staphylococcus aureus* colonization	43.4%	51.1%

For Gram-negative coverage, gentamicin continues as the recommended first choice; however, with the emergence of resistant Gram-negative organisms, the American Academy of Pediatrics Committee on Fetus and Newborn recommendations state: "Among term newborn infants who are critically ill, the empirical addition of broader-spectrum therapy should be considered until culture results are available."[53] This recommendation is supported by a recent study that found no statistically significant advantage of one regimen over any other for the treatment of early-onset infection in newborns.[54] Although the choice of empirical treatment is important, use of the relatively recently (<10 years as of this writing) developed risk-based EOS calculator, which utilizes risk factors and assessments of clinical conditions in the first postnatal hours to derive mathematical probabilities to inform recommendations for observation, testing, and antibiotic treatment, has reduced empiric antibiotic exposures without increasing the numbers of infants who are missed by early-onset screening strategies.[55,56] Alternative strategies, based on frequent clinical assessments in the first postnatal hours and days rather than the sepsis risk calculator are also likely to effectively reduce unnecessary antibiotic exposures.[57] Both approaches are incorporated into the current recommended, acceptable practices for management of infants born at or after 35 weeks' gestation, and they have reduced the percentage of newborns empirically treated for early-onset sepsis.[53]

Although the EOS risk calculator for infants born at 35 weeks or later has had a significant impact on the care of these infants, the approach to assessment of risk and empirical antibiotic therapy for early sepsis in more preterm infants is less validated. For infants born before 35 weeks, EOS is much more common with decreasing gestational age, and the epidemiology is different, with *Escherichia coli* being the most prevalent pathogen.[16,58,59] Despite concerns with mortality, which is orders of magnitude more likely in preterm infants with EOS, and the higher prevalence of *E. coli* infections among infants of lower gestational age, an identifiable low-risk group of preterm infants appears to be a potential group to target for antibiotic stewardship efforts.[16,60,61] In one cohort study that spanned 25 years and assessed preterm infants admitted to a single NICU, 97% of the 109 infants with EOS had some combination of prolonged rupture of membranes, preterm labor, or concern for intraamniotic inflammation.[60] In another cohort of 15,000 extremely preterm infants, inclusive of 238 with EOS, those born by cesarean delivery with membrane rupture at delivery and without clinical chorioamnionitis were significantly less likely to have EOS than those with any of those conditions.[61] This low-risk group may be able to benefit from restricted antibiotic use. A double-blind, multicenter randomized clinical trial, the NICU Antibiotics and Outcomes trial (NCT03997266), is testing the risk–benefit of giving antibiotics versus placebo in the first postnatal days for low-risk infants.[62] For empiric treatment of the preterm group, the American Academy of Pediatrics Committee on Fetus and Newborn continues to recommend ampicillin and gentamicin to cover group B *Streptococcus* plus most other streptococcal and enterococcal species, as well as *Listeria*. Although most Gram-negative organisms causing external ocular infections among premature infants in the United States are ampicillin resistant, the vast majority remain sensitive to gentamicin. The authors of the Committee's recommendations acknowledge the emergence of resistant Gram-negative organisms in U.S. NICUs, saying "empirical addition of broader-spectrum antibiotic therapy may be considered until culture results are available."[63] The committee also appropriately repeated words similar to those used by Klein in his 1983 recommendations: "The choice of additional therapy should be guided by local antibiotic resistance data,"[18,63] which is still good advice that can serve as a starting point at the site level for the next generation of antibiotic stewards in the NICU.

Ongoing Challenges

The CDC-sponsored Prevention Epicenters Program has identified prevention of multidrug-resistant Gram-negative infections as a top pediatric research priority in 2020.[64] Extended-spectrum β-lactamase–producing Enterobacteriaceae and carbapenem-resistant Enterobacteriaceae are two of the most pressing Gram-negative resistance threats.[65] Epidemiologic reports from U.S. NICUs indicate a high prevalence of resistance to one or more of ampicillin, aminoglycosides, and cephalosporins among the Gram-negative bacteria causing early- and later-onset infections in NICU patients.[16,17,58,66,67] The ongoing threat from resistant organisms informs empirical antibiotic choices. In a recent comprehensive review, Flannery et al.[67] provided several guiding principles:

- Empiric antibiotic therapy [in the NICU] is typically separated by timing of suspected infection (early-onset infection and late-onset infection) and should account for local infection epidemiology and antibiotic susceptibility patterns.
- When appropriately drawn cultures are obtained and remain sterile, antibiotics should be stopped unless an alternative infection source is identified.
- As antibiotic resistance among neonatal pathogens becomes more prevalent, continuous surveillance and assessment of both neonatal antibiotic use and antibiotic susceptibility profiles are critical.

In an editorial accompanying Flannery's 2021 report on resistance, Weissman and Stoll[68] advised that vigilance and ongoing surveillance of antibiotic susceptibility of NICU pathogens are crucial. They advised, at least at present, that "the empirical regimen of ampicillin and gentamicin remains appropriate for term infants with suspected sepsis and for most preterm infants, but in the most severely ill VLBW infants, we are obliged to consider broader-spectrum antibiotics—agents that can save lives but also reshape microbial ecology at local and global levels."[68]

Actionable Items

Although antibiotic stewardship often focuses on strategies to avoid or limit antibiotic exposures, a key component of avoidance of development of resistance to antibiotics and for successful use of antibiotics to clear infections is for clinicians to use effective doses of antibiotics. NICU patients have been enrolled in multiple pharmacokinetic trials to identify the optimal dose to achieve effective drug concentrations. Much of this work has been completed by the NICHD-supported Pediatric Trials Network. These studies have informed clinicians of the need for varying dosing strategies by chronologic as well as postmenstrual age, and vigilant monitoring of the literature and U.S. Food and Drug Administration labels for antibiotics will keep clinicians up to date with regard to evidence-based dosing for the NICU population.[69–76]

Although progress has been made on limiting the administration of empirical, broad-spectrum antibiotic therapies in the NICU, particularly third-generation cephalosporins, vancomycin remains among the most commonly used antimicrobials used in NICUs.[1,2,25,27] Vancomycin is among the antibiotics most often identified as "inappropriately used."[8,27] For infants with methicillin-resistant *Staphylococcus aureus* infections, vancomycin would be considered adequate treatment. In a retrospective cohort study, inadequate empirical antibiotic therapy was associated with increased risk of mortality within 30 days of the infection.[77] In a separate retrospective cohort study of 4364 infants bacteremic with coagulase-negative *Staphylococcus*, a common bacteria identified in blood cultures obtained from preterm babies, almost two-thirds of the infants were treated empirically (before culture results were known) with vancomycin, but there was no 30-day survival advantage to having vancomycin as the initial, empirical choice before the culture results were available.[78] This combination of information, along with knowledge that coagulase-negative *Staphylococcus* is the most common cause of late-onset sepsis in premature infants, raises the question of the need for or benefit from use of empirical vancomycin as a first-line therapy in premature infants suspected of late-onset sepsis.[4,79–83]

Stewardship projects to discontinue empirical therapy with negative cultures at 48 hours or less, to use dosing strategies based on pharmacokinetic study results, and to select antibiotics based on prevalent organisms and local microbiology have successfully led to reduced use of antibiotics. Although those efforts are needed and have proven effective, NICU providers have also worked collaboratively on perhaps the most effective antibiotic stewardship intervention—decreasing neonatal infections.[84–92]

REFERENCES

1. Hsieh EM, Hornik CP, Clark RH, et al. Medication use in the neonatal intensive care unit. *Am J Perinatol*. 2014;31(9):811-821.
2. Stark A, Smith PB, Hornik CP, et al. Medication use in the neonatal intensive care unit and changes from 2010 to 2018. *J Pediatr*. 2022;240:66-71.e4.
3. Ellsbury DL, Clark RH, Ursprung R, Handler DL, Dodd ED, Spitzer AR. A multifaceted approach to improving outcomes in the NICU: the Pediatrix 100 000 Babies Campaign. *Pediatrics*. 2016;137(4):e20150389.
4. Cantey JB, Wozniak PS, Pruszynski JE, Sánchez PJ. Reducing unnecessary antibiotic use in the neonatal intensive care unit (SCOUT): a prospective interrupted time-series study. *Lancet Infect Dis*. 2016;16(10):1178-1184.
5. Schulman J, Profit J, Lee HC, et al. Variations in neonatal antibiotic use. *Pediatrics*. 2018;142(3):e20180115.
6. Dukhovny D, Buus-Frank ME, Edwards EM, et al. A collaborative multicenter QI initiative to improve antibiotic stewardship in newborns. *Pediatrics*. 2019;144(6):e20190589.
7. Greenberg RG, Chowdhury D, Hansen NI, et al. Prolonged duration of early antibiotic therapy in extremely premature infants. *Pediatr Res*. 2019;85(7):994-1000.
8. Ting JY, Paquette V, Ng K, et al. Reduction of inappropriate antimicrobial prescriptions in a tertiary neonatal intensive care unit after antimicrobial stewardship care bundle implementation. *Pediatr Infect Dis J*. 2019;38(1):54-59.
9. Prusakov P, Goff DA, Wozniak PS, et al. A global point prevalence survey of antimicrobial use in neonatal intensive care units: the no-more-antibiotics and resistance (NO-MAS-R) study. *EClinicalMedicine*. 2021;32:100727.
10. Fleming A. Speech by Alexander Fleming at a banquet in his honour by the American Association of Penicillin Producers at the Waldorf Astoria, New York, June 25, 1945. London: British Library; Add. MS 56122, ff. 232-242.
11. Ellner PD, Neu HC. The inhibitory quotient. A method for interpreting minimum inhibitory concentration data. *JAMA*. 1981;246(14):1575-1578.
12. Neu HC. The crisis in antibiotic resistance. *Science*. 1992;257(5073):1064-1073.
13. Franco JA, Eitzman DV, Baer H. Antibiotic usage and microbial resistance in an intensive care nursery. *Am J Dis Child*. 1973;126(3):318-321.
14. Howard JB, McCracken Jr GH. Reappraisal of kanamycin usage in neonates. *J Pediatr*. 1975;86(6):949-956.
15. Hammerschlag MR, Klein JO, Herschel M, Chen FC, Fermin R. Patterns of use of antibiotics in two newborn nurseries. *N Engl J Med*. 1977;296(22):1268-1269.
16. Stoll BJ, Puopolo KM, Hansen NI, et al. Early-onset neonatal sepsis 2015 to 2017, the rise of *Escherichia coli*, and the need for novel prevention strategies [published correction appears in *JAMA Pediatr*. 2021;175(2):212]. *JAMA Pediatr*. 2020;174(7):e200593.
17. Flannery DD, Puopolo KM, Hansen NI, et al. Antimicrobial susceptibility profiles among neonatal early-onset sepsis pathogens. *Pediatr Infect Dis J*. 2022;41(3):263-271.
18. Klein JO, Dashefsky B, Norton CR, Mayer J. Selection of antimicrobial agents for treatment of neonatal sepsis. *Rev Infect Dis*. 1983;5(suppl 1):S55-S64.
19. Bryan CS, John Jr JF, Pai MS, Austin TL. Gentamicin vs cefotaxime for therapy of neonatal sepsis. Relationship to drug resistance. *Am J Dis Child*. 1985;139(11):1086-1089.
20. Modi N, Damjanovic V, Cooke RW. Outbreak of cephalosporin resistant *Enterobacter cloacae* infection in a neonatal intensive care unit. *Arch Dis Child*. 1987;62(2):148-151.
21. de Man P, Verhoeven BA, Verbrugh HA, Vos MC, van den Anker JN. An antibiotic policy to prevent emergence of resistant bacilli. *Lancet*. 2000;355(9208):973-978.
22. Fanaroff AA, Wright LL, Stevenson DK, et al. Very-low-birth-weight outcomes of the National Institute of Child Health and Human Development Neonatal Research Network, May 1991

through December 1992. *Am J Obstet Gynecol*. 1995;173(5): 1423-1431.

23. Lemons JA, Bauer CR, Oh W, et al. Very low birth weight outcomes of the National Institute of Child Health and Human Development Neonatal Research Network, January 1995 through December 1996. NICHD Neonatal Research Network. *Pediatrics*. 2001;107(1):E1.
24. Stoll BJ, Hansen N, Fanaroff AA, et al. Late-onset sepsis in very low birth weight neonates: the experience of the NICHD Neonatal Research Network. *Pediatrics*. 2002;110(2 Pt 1):285-291.
25. Grohskopf LA, Huskins WC, Sinkowitz-Cochran RL, et al. Use of antimicrobial agents in United States neonatal and pediatric intensive care patients. *Pediatr Infect Dis J*. 2005;24(9):766-773.
26. Centers for Disease Control and Prevention (CDC). CDC's campaign to prevent antimicrobial resistance in health-care settings. *MMWR Morb Mortal Wkly Rep*. 2002;51(15):343.
27. Patel SJ, Oshodi A, Prasad P, et al. Antibiotic use in neonatal intensive care units and adherence with Centers for Disease Control and Prevention 12 Step Campaign to Prevent Antimicrobial Resistance. *Pediatr Infect Dis J*. 2009;28(12):1047-1051.
28. Cantey JB, Prusakov P. A proposed framework for the clinical management of neonatal "culture-negative" sepsis. *J Pediatr*. 2022;244:203-211.
29. Clark RH, Bloom BT, Spitzer AR, Gerstmann DR. Empiric use of ampicillin and cefotaxime, compared with ampicillin and gentamicin, for neonates at risk for sepsis is associated with an increased risk of neonatal death. *Pediatrics*. 2006;117(1):67-74.
30. Benjamin Jr DK, DeLong ER, Steinbach WJ, Cotton CM, Walsh TJ, Clark RH. Empirical therapy for neonatal candidemia in very low birth weight infants. *Pediatrics*. 2003;112(3 Pt 1): 543-547.
31. Cotten CM, Taylor S, Stoll B, et al. Prolonged duration of initial empirical antibiotic treatment is associated with increased rates of necrotizing enterocolitis and death for extremely low birth weight infants. *Pediatrics*. 2009;123(1):58-66.
32. Kuppala VS, Meinzen-Derr J, Morrow AL, Schibler KR. Prolonged initial empirical antibiotic treatment is associated with adverse outcomes in premature infants. *J Pediatr*. 2011; 159(5):720-725.
33. Alexander VN, Northrup V, Bizzarro MJ. Antibiotic exposure in the newborn intensive care unit and the risk of necrotizing enterocolitis. *J Pediatr*. 2011;159(3):392-397.
34. Esmaeilizand R, Shah PS, Seshia M, et al. Antibiotic exposure and development of necrotizing enterocolitis in very preterm neonates. *Paediatr Child Health*. 2018;23(4):e56-e61.
35. Cantey JB, Pyle AK, Wozniak PS, Hynan LS, Sánchez PJ. Early antibiotic exposure and adverse outcomes in preterm, very low birth weight infants. *J Pediatr*. 2018;203:62-67.
36. Benjamin Jr DK, Stoll BJ, Gantz MG, et al. Neonatal candidiasis: epidemiology, risk factors, and clinical judgment. *Pediatrics*. 2010;126(4):e865-e873.
37. Cotten CM, McDonald S, Stoll B, et al. The association of third-generation cephalosporin use and invasive candidiasis in extremely low birth-weight infants. *Pediatrics*. 2006;118(2): 717-722.
38. Kotter JP. Accelerate! *Harv Bus Rev*. 2012;90(11):44-52, 54-58, 149.
39. Bloom BT, Mulligan J, Arnold C, et al. Improving growth of very low birth weight infants in the first 28 days. *Pediatrics*. 2003;112(1 Pt 1):8-14.
40. Kaplan HC, Lannon C, Walsh MC, Donovan EF, Ohio Perinatal Quality Collaborative. Ohio statewide quality-improvement collaborative to reduce late-onset sepsis in preterm infants. *Pediatrics*. 2011;127(3):427-435.
41. Wirtschafter DD, Powers RJ, Pettit JS, et al. Nosocomial infection reduction in VLBW infants with a statewide quality-improvement model. *Pediatrics*. 2011;127(3):419-426.
42. Fisher D, Cochran KM, Provost LP, et al. Reducing central line-associated bloodstream infections in North Carolina NICUs. *Pediatrics*. 2013;132(6):e1664-e1671.
43. Lee SK, Shah PS, Singhal N, et al. Association of a quality improvement program with neonatal outcomes in extremely preterm infants: a prospective cohort study. *CMAJ*. 2014;186 (13):E485-E494.
44. Centers for Disease Control and Prevention. *Antibiotic Resistance Threats in the United States, 2013*. Available at: https://www.cdc.gov/drugresistance/pdf/ar-threats-2013-508.pdf. Accessed October 18, 2022.
45. Davey P, Brown E, Charani E, et al. Interventions to improve antibiotic prescribing practices for hospital inpatients. *Cochrane Database Syst Rev*. 2013;(4):CD003543.
46. Centers for Disease Control and Prevention (CDC). *Core Elements of Hospital Antibiotic Stewardship Programs*. Available at: https://www.cdc.gov/antibiotic-use/core-elements/hospital.html. Accessed January 20, 2023.
47. Schulman J, Dimand RJ, Lee HC, Duenas GV, Bennett MV, Gould JB. Neonatal intensive care unit antibiotic use. *Pediatrics*. 2015;135(5):826-833.
48. Ho T, Dukhovny D, Zupancic JA, Goldmann DA, Horbar JD, Pursley DM. Choosing wisely in newborn medicine: five opportunities to increase value. *Pediatrics*. 2015;136(2): e482-e489.
49. Ho T, Buus-Frank ME, Edwards EM, et al. Adherence of newborn-specific antibiotic stewardship programs to CDC recommendations. *Pediatrics*. 2018;142(6):e20174322.
50. Ting JY, Autmizguine J, Dunn MS, et al. Practice summary of antimicrobial therapy for commonly encountered conditions in the neonatal intensive care unit: a Canadian perspective. *Front Pediatr*. 2022;10:894005.
51. Makri V, Davies G, Cannell S, et al. Managing antibiotics wisely: a quality improvement programme in a tertiary neonatal unit in the UK. *BMJ Open Qual*. 2018;7(2):e000285.
52. Meyers JM, Tulloch J, Brown K, Caserta MT, D'Angio CT, Golisano Children's Hospital NICU Antibiotic Stewardship Team. A quality improvement initiative to optimize antibiotic use in a level 4 NICU. *Pediatrics*. 2020;146(5):e20193956.
53. Puopolo KM, Benitz WE, Zaoutis TE, American Academy of Pediatrics Committee on Fetus and Newborn, Committee on Infectious Diseases. Management of neonates born at ≥35 0/7 weeks' gestation with suspected or proven early-onset bacterial sepsis. *Pediatrics*. 2018;142(6):e20182894.
54. Korang SK, Safi S, Nava C, et al. Antibiotic regimens for early-onset neonatal sepsis. *Cochrane Database Syst Rev*. 2021;5(5): CD013837.
55. Escobar GJ, Puopolo KM, Wi S, et al. Stratification of risk of early-onset sepsis in newborns ≥ 34 weeks' gestation. *Pediatrics*. 2014;133(1):30-36.
56. Kuzniewicz MW, Puopolo KM, Fischer A, et al. A quantitative, risk-based approach to the management of neonatal early-onset sepsis. *JAMA Pediatr*. 2017;171(4):365-371.
57. Joshi NS, Gupta A, Allan JM, et al. Clinical monitoring of well-appearing infants born to mothers with chorioamnionitis. *Pediatrics*. 2018;141(4):e20172056.

58. Flannery DD, Akinboyo IC, Mukhopadhyay S, et al. Antibiotic susceptibility of *Escherichia coli* among infants admitted to neonatal intensive care units across the US from 2009 to 2017. *JAMA Pediatr*. 2021;175(2):168-175.
59. Schrag SJ, Farley MM, Petit S, et al. Epidemiology of invasive early-onset neonatal sepsis, 2005 to 2014. *Pediatrics*. 2016;138(6):e20162013.
60. Mukhopadhyay S, Puopolo KM. Clinical and microbiologic characteristics of early-onset sepsis among very low birth weight infants: opportunities for antibiotic stewardship. *Pediatr Infect Dis J*. 2017;36(5):477-481.
61. Puopolo KM, Mukhopadhyay S, Hansen NI, et al. Identification of extremely premature infants at low risk for early-onset sepsis. *Pediatrics*. 2017;140(5):e20170925.
62. Morowitz MJ, Katheria AC, Polin RA, et al. The NICU Antibiotics and Outcomes (NANO) trial: a randomized multicenter clinical trial assessing empiric antibiotics and clinical outcomes in newborn preterm infants. *Trials*. 2022;23(1):428.
63. Puopolo KM, Benitz WE, Zaoutis TE, American Academy of Pediatrics Committee on Fetus and Newborn, Committee on Infectious Diseases. Management of neonates born at ≤34 6/7 weeks' gestation with suspected or proven early-onset bacterial sepsis. Pediatrics. 2018;142(6):e20182896.
64. Coffin SE, Abanyie F, Bryant K, et al. Pediatric research priorities in healthcare-associated infections and antimicrobial stewardship. *Infect Control Hosp Epidemiol*. 2021;42(5):519-522.
65. Centers for Disease Control and Prevention. *Antibiotic Resistance Threats in the United States, 2019*. Available at: https://www.cdc.gov/drugresistance/pdf/threats-report/2019-ar-threats-report-508.pdf. Accessed January 20, 2023.
66. Patel SJ, Green N, Clock SA, et al. Gram-negative bacilli in infants hospitalized in the neonatal intensive care unit. *J Pediatric Infect Dis Soc*. 2017;6(3):227-230.
67. Flannery DD, Puopolo KM, Hansen NI, Sánchez PJ, Stoll BJ, Eunice Kennedy Shriver National Institute of Child Health and Human Development Neonatal Research Network. Neonatal infections: insights from a multicenter longitudinal research collaborative. *Semin Perinatol*. 2022;46(7):151637.
68. Weissman SJ, Stoll B. Ampicillin and gentamicin in infants with suspected sepsis: long live amp and gent–but for how long? *JAMA Pediatr*. 2021;175(2):131-132.
69. Smith PB, Cohen-Wolkowiez M, Castro LM, et al. Population pharmacokinetics of meropenem in plasma and cerebrospinal fluid of infants with suspected or complicated intra-abdominal infections. *Pediatr Infect Dis J*. 2011;30(10):844-849.
70. Smith PB, Cotten CM, Hudak ML, et al. Rifampin pharmacokinetics and safety in preterm and term infants. *Antimicrob Agents Chemother*. 2019;63(6):e00284-19.
71. Cohen-Wolkowiez M, Sampson M, Bloom BT, et al. Determining population and developmental pharmacokinetics of metronidazole using plasma and dried blood spot samples from premature infants. *Pediatr Infect Dis J*. 2013;32(9):956-961.
72. Salerno S, Hornik CP, Cohen-Wolkowiez M, et al. Use of population pharmacokinetics and electronic health records to assess piperacillin–tazobactam safety in infants. *Pediatr Infect Dis J*. 2017;36(9):855-859.
73. Gonzalez D, Melloni C, Yogev R, et al. Use of opportunistic clinical data and a population pharmacokinetic model to support dosing of clindamycin for premature infants to adolescents. *Clin Pharmacol Ther*. 2014;96(4):429-437.
74. Gonzalez D, Delmore P, Bloom BT, et al. Clindamycin pharmacokinetics and safety in preterm and term infants. *Antimicrob Agents Chemother*. 2016;60(5):2888-2894.
75. Le J, Poindexter B, Sullivan JE, et al. Comparative analysis of ampicillin plasma and dried blood spot pharmacokinetics in neonates. *Ther Drug Monit*. 2018;40(1):103-108.
76. Tremoulet A, Le J, Poindexter B, et al. Characterization of the population pharmacokinetics of ampicillin in neonates using an opportunistic study design. *Antimicrob Agents Chemother*. 2014;58(6):3013-3020.
77. Thaden JT, Ericson JE, Cross H, et al. Survival benefit of empirical therapy for *Staphylococcus aureus* bloodstream infections in infants. *Pediatr Infect Dis J*. 2015;34(11):1175-1179.
78. Ericson JE, Thaden J, Cross HR, et al. No survival benefit with empirical vancomycin therapy for coagulase-negative staphylococcal bloodstream infections in infants. *Pediatr Infect Dis J*. 2015;34(4):371-375.
79. Lawrence SL, Roth V, Slinger R, Toye B, Gaboury I, Lemyre B. Cloxacillin versus vancomycin for presumed late-onset sepsis in the Neonatal Intensive Care Unit and the impact upon outcome of coagulase negative staphylococcal bacteremia: a retrospective cohort study. *BMC Pediatr*. 2005;5:49.
80. Hemels MA, van den Hoogen A, Verboon-Maciolek MA, Fleer A, Krediet TG. A seven-year survey of management of coagulase-negative staphylococcal sepsis in the neonatal intensive care unit: vancomycin may not be necessary as empiric therapy. *Neonatology*. 2011;100(2):180-185.
81. Romanelli RM, Anchieta LM, Bueno E Silva AC, de Jesus LA, Rosado V, Clemente WT. Empirical antimicrobial therapy for late-onset sepsis in a neonatal unit with high prevalence of coagulase-negative *Staphylococcus*. *J Pediatr (Rio J)*. 2016;92(5):472-478.
82. Sánchez PJ, Moallem M, Cantey JB, Milton A, Michelow IC. Empiric therapy with vancomycin in the neonatal intensive care unit: let's "get smart" globally! *J Pediatr (Rio J)*. 2016;92(5):432-435.
83. Cantey JB, Anderson KR, Kalagiri RR, Mallett LH. Morbidity and mortality of coagulase-negative staphylococcal sepsis in very-low-birth-weight infants. *World J Pediatr*. 2018;14(3):269-273.
84. Horbar JD, Rogowski J, Plsek PE, et al. Collaborative quality improvement for neonatal intensive care. NIC/Q Project Investigators of the Vermont Oxford Network. *Pediatrics*. 2001;107(1):14-22.
85. Horbar JD, Edwards EM, Greenberg LT, et al. Variation in performance of neonatal intensive care units in the United States [published correction appears in *JAMA Pediatr*. 2017;171(3):306]. *JAMA Pediatr*. 2017;171(3):e164396.
86. Bizzarro MJ, Sabo B, Noonan M, et al. A quality improvement initiative to reduce central line-associated bloodstream infections in a neonatal intensive care unit. *Infect Control Hosp Epidemiol*. 2010;31(3):241-248.
87. Zachariah P, Furuya EY, Edwards J, et al. Compliance with prevention practices and their association with central line-associated bloodstream infections in neonatal intensive care units. *Am J Infect Control*. 2014;42(8):847-851.
88. Shepherd EG, Kelly TJ, Vinsel JA, et al. Significant reduction of central-line associated bloodstream infections in a network of diverse neonatal nurseries. *J Pediatr*. 2015;167(1):41-46.e63.

89. Bowen JR, Callander I, Richards R, Lindrea KB, Sepsis Prevention in NICUs Group. Decreasing infection in neonatal intensive care units through quality improvement. *Arch Dis Child Fetal Neonatal Ed.* 2017;102(1):F51-F57.
90. Salm F, Schwab F, Geffers C, Gastmeier P, Piening B. The implementation of an evidence-based bundle for bloodstream infections in neonatal intensive care units in Germany: a controlled intervention study to improve patient safety. *Infect Control Hosp Epidemiol.* 2016;37(7):798-804.
91. Greenberg RG, Kandefer S, Do BT, et al. Late-onset sepsis in extremely premature infants: 2000–2011. *Pediatr Infect Dis J.* 2017;36(8):774-779.
92. Bell EF, Hintz SR, Hansen NI, et al. Mortality, in-hospital morbidity, care practices, and 2-year outcomes for extremely preterm infants in the US, 2013-2018 [published correction appears in *JAMA.* 2022;327(21):2151]. *JAMA.* 2022;327(3): 248-263.

Chapter 6

Neonatal Fungal Infections

David A. Kaufman, MD; Hillary Liken, MD; Namrita J. Odackal, DO

Key Points

- Major risk factors for invasive *Candida* infections include extreme prematurity, a compromised gastrointestinal function or barrier, presence of a central venous catheter, and exposure to broad-spectrum antibiotics, acid suppression medications, and high-dose postnatal steroids.
- Infants at the highest risk weigh <1000 g at birth or 28 weeks' gestation, due to high mortality and the risk of neurodevelopmental impairments from infections. Preventative measures including targeted antifungal prophylaxis have lowered the incidence in this group from 5%–10% to 0%–2%.
- *Candida* pathogenesis involves exposure, adherence, and colonization, followed by infection and organ involvement. All infected infants need screening for end-organ dissemination.
- Cultures are critical to diagnosis and should include blood, urine, and cerebrospinal fluid at the time of presentation. Additionally, peritoneal cultures should be obtained in any infant with surgical necrotizing enterocolitis or bowel perforation requiring laparotomy or drainage.
- Congenital cutaneous candidiasis is an invasive infection that requires prompt recognition and evaluation, as well as systemic treatment for 14 days. Dermatologic findings of congenital cutaneous candidiasis commonly involve skin desquamation and maculopapular and/or erythematous rashes.
- Survival with candidemia is improved with central venous catheter removal. Infection-related outcomes are also improved with prompt and appropriate antifungal dosing for all infected infants and empiric therapy in high-risk infants.

How Are Invasive *Candida* Infections Defined?

Invasive *Candida* infections (ICIs) are generally defined as the presence of *Candida* species in a normally sterile body fluid or tissue.[1] Examples include bloodstream infections (BSIs), urinary tract infections (UTIs), peritonitis, meningitis, cutaneous candidiasis, and any infection of an otherwise sterile tissue, such as bones and joints. These invasive infections are frequently identified and defined based on a positive culture of blood, urine, cerebrospinal fluid (CSF), peritoneal fluid, or tissue. For congenital cutaneous candidiasis, diagnosis requires a diffuse rash with identification of *Candida* or yeast from the skin, placenta, or umbilical cord.[2]

ICIs can be classified as early onset (<72 hours after birth) or late onset (≥72 hours after birth), similar to other neonatal infections. The exception is cutaneous candidiasis, which is often specified as congenital cutaneous candidiasis (CCC) when it occurs in the first week after birth.[2] These ICIs can disseminate directly or hematogenously throughout the body, even in spite of antifungal therapy. This can lead to end-organ abscesses and damage to the heart, eyes, liver, kidneys, lungs, brain, or spleen.

How Does *Candida* Cause Invasive Infections?

Candida species represent a group of opportunistic pathogens naturally present, primarily as saprophytes, on the skin and oral and gastrointestinal (GI) mucosa, but whose presence can become pathologic due to factors related to the organism, the host, or both (Figure 6.1). This is the case in

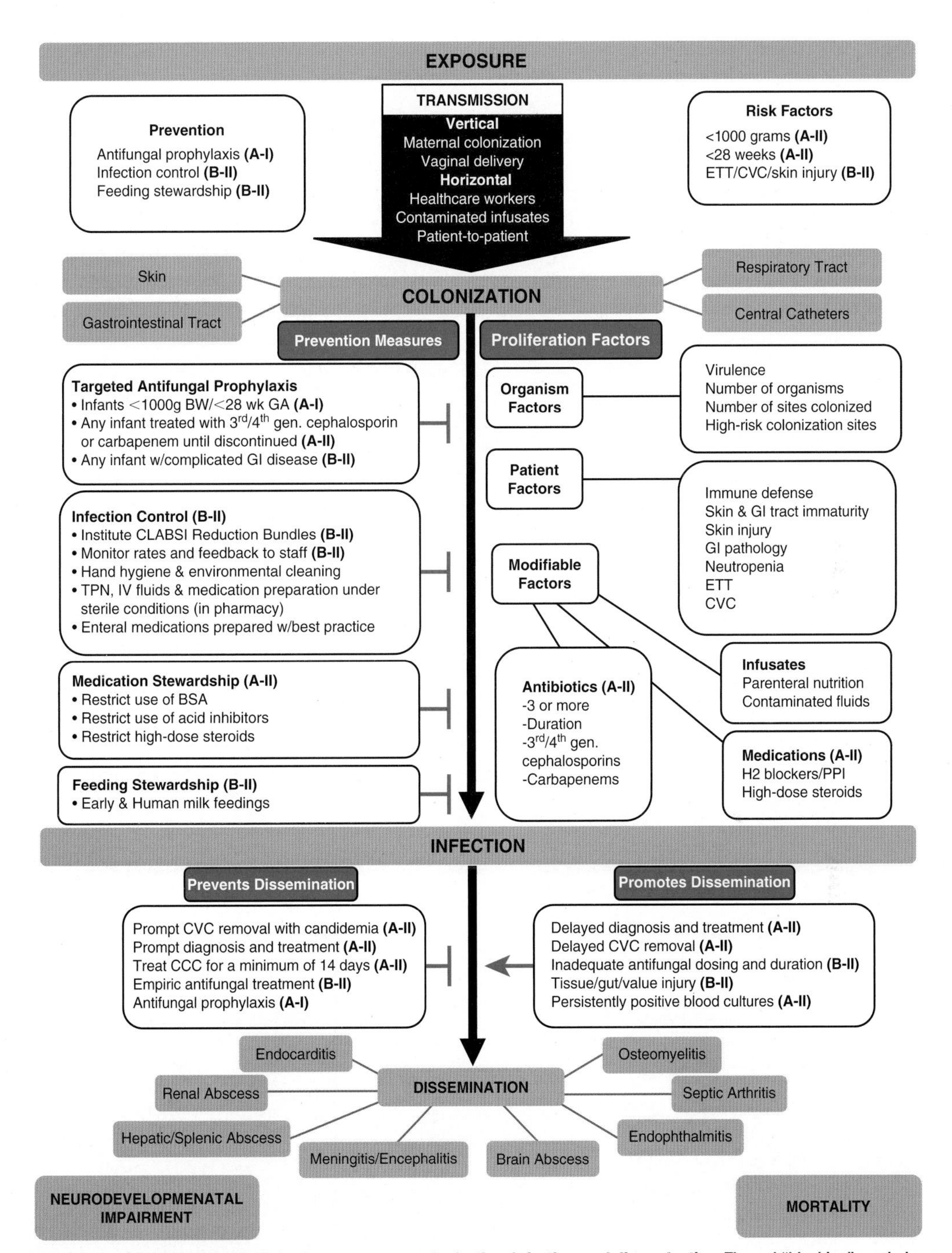

Fig. 6.1 Pathogenesis of invasive *Candida* infections: exposure, colonization, infection, and dissemination. The red "blocking" symbol represents factors that decrease or prevent the risk of ICI; the green arrows indicate factors increasing risk, some of which are modifiable. *BCx,* blood culture; *CVC,* central venous catheter; *EON,* early-onset neutropenia; *ET,* endotracheal tube; *IV,* intravenous; *VLBW,* very low birth weight. *High-risk colonization sites, including CVC, ET, and urine. Level of evidence is based on the U.S. Public Health Service Grading System for ranking recommendations in clinical guidelines, where the strength of recommendation and levels of evidence include *A,* good evidence; *B,* moderate evidence; *C,* poor evidence; *I,* at least one randomized clinical trial; *II,* at least one well-designed but nonrandomized trial; and *III,* expert opinions based on experience or limited clinical reports.

infants, who have distinct immune system function with little or no adaptive and minimal innate immunity. Additionally, critical barriers to organisms (e.g., skin, respiratory tract) are breached with intravenous catheters and/or endotracheal tubes. As an opportunistic organism, *Candida* species can also lead to infections if the host is exposed to a large number of organisms and/or when *Candida* can proliferate easily. Proliferation is favorable under certain conditions, such as diminished immunity, when antibiotics eradicate competitive flora or H_2 blockers decrease stomach acidity.

What Are Predisposing Factors for ICIs in the Neonatal Intensive Care Unit?

ICIs are of special concern in premature infants, with early gestational age being the greatest risk factor. Understanding why this population is susceptible, as well as other potential risk factors, is helpful in identifying infants most at risk for infection and potential candidates for preventative measures (Figures 6.1 and 6.2).

PREMATURITY

The more premature the infant, the more underdeveloped the immune system and the barrier defenses and the greater the likelihood of procedures, antibiotic exposures, and use of other medications contributing to colonization and ICIs.

COLONIZATION

Local colonization of the skin or mucosal surfaces can lead to ICIs, with *Candida* penetrating epidermal barriers to infect underlying tissue or directly invading the bloodstream and spreading hematogenously. Very-low-birth-weight (VLBW; <1500 g at birth) infants are more susceptible to colonization with *Candida* and are at a higher risk of progression to an invasive infection. Colonization is inversely correlated with gestational age and birth weight. In the first weeks after birth, >50% of extremely low-birth-weight (ELBW; <1000 g at birth) and 25% to 50% of VLBW infants are colonized, compared with 5% to 10% of full-term infants.[1] Colonization during the first 2 weeks of life occurs primarily on the skin and in the gastrointestinal tract, including the rectum and oropharynx, followed a week or two later by respiratory tract colonization in high-risk infants.[3] Progression to infection occurs in approximately one of four colonized infants, influenced by both the number and location of colonized sites in premature infants. Colonization of three or more sites or at a high-risk site (urine, catheter tips, drains, and surgical devices) is more likely to be associated with progression to an ICI.[4–9]

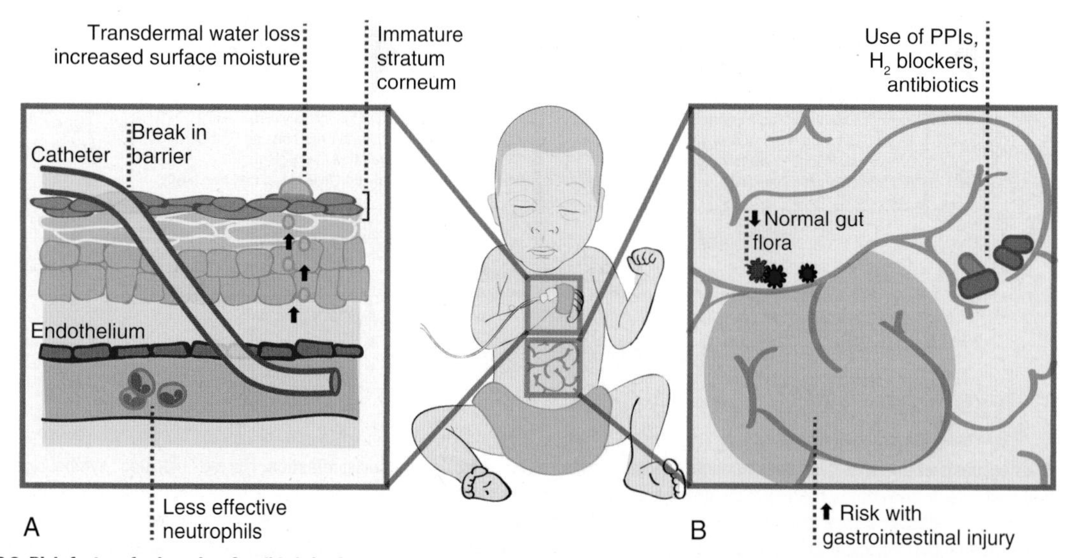

Fig. 6.2 Risk factors for invasive *Candida* infections. (A) Effects of immature skin, neutrophil function and central venous catheter. (B) Gastrointestinal tract predisposing factors. *PPIs,* proton-pump inhibitors.

Colonization can occur by way of vertical transmission from the mother or horizontal transmission from nosocomial sources. Early colonization (≤1 week of age) is more often attributed to maternal sources, with an increased risk for early *Candida albicans* colonization in premature infants born vaginally. Horizontal transmission occurs from healthcare workers, family, and medical interventions. In a prospective trial studying fungal colonization in six neonatal intensive care units (NICUs), 29% of healthcare workers had hand cultures positive for *Candida* species, with nearly the same percentage of infants (23%) having mucosal colonization.[10] Although *C. albicans* was the more common fungal isolate in all NICU patients, *C. parapsilosis* was the most common species isolated from the hands of NICU staff.[10] *C. parapsilosis* colonization is also associated with receiving parenteral nutrition.

IMMUNE SYSTEM

Immaturity of the immune system includes the physical barriers with regard to controlling colonization and preventing infection is evident in the underdeveloped skin, gut, and respiratory tract (Figure 6.2). For example, at 26 weeks' gestation, the stratum corneum is composed of only three cell layers and produces a thin keratin layer, compared with 15 layers with a thick keratin overlying layer in term infants (Figure 6.2A). Premature infants have a multitude of deficient immune cellular functions and reduced protein production. Neutrophils are one of the most important components in the initial response of the innate immune system to *Candida* infections, both through direct phagocytosis and through neutrophil extracellular trap formation. Premature infants have neutrophils with lower chemotaxis, fewer phagocytosing pathogens and producing NETs as compared to adults.

GUT MICROBIOME

Like the immune system, the gut microbiota play an important role in suppressing *Candida* colonization and preventing invasive infection. The intestinal microbiota of premature infants are different and less diverse in composition than those of term infants. In one study, probiotics (*Lactobacillus reuteri* and *L. rhamnosus*) showed significantly lower *Candida* stool colonization compared with the control premature infants, whereas lactoferrin with and without *L. rhamnosus* decreased ICIs without changing *Candida* colonization, potentially preventing translocation.[11,12] Analysis of randomized controlled trials has been complex, with benefits found for infants 1000 to 1500 g but not for the highest risk infants (<1000 g). Specifically for preventing ICI, probiotics may alter colonization but not the incidence of ICI.[13]

MEDICATIONS

Certain medications, including antibiotics, histamine-2 antagonists, and postnatal corticosteroids, increase the risk of ICIs (Figure 6.2B). Longer antibiotic duration, administering two or more antibiotics, third- and fourth-generation cephalosporin, and carbapenem antibiotics are associated with increased risk of ICIs.[14] Dexamethasone and high-dose hydrocortisone (>1 mg/kg/day) are associated with increased risk. Although ELBW infants are at high risk, exposure to hydrocortisone alone at 1 mg/kg/day with a weaning schedule did not further increase the high incidence of ICIs (9% in the hydrocortisone group vs. 10% in the control group).[15]

LINES, TUBES, AND FEEDINGS

Use of central venous catheters (Figure 6.2A) and endotracheal tubes increases the risk of ICIs in infants.[16] Infants who receive larger amounts of expressed milk from their mothers generally have fewer infections, but a decrease in ICIs has not been demonstrated.[1] These studies have not controlled whether the milk was fresh or frozen. Freezing then thawing human milk is associated with a reduction of protective components such as maternal white blood cells, lactoferrin, immunoglobulin A, and lysozyme. Studies of pasteurized donor human milk have not demonstrated a decrease in infections of any type.[17] Prospective epidemiologic studies have found that infants who are not able to or do not receive enteral feedings by 3 days after birth are more likely to develop an ICI.[14]

GASTROINTESTINAL PATHOLOGY AND ABDOMINAL SURGERY

GI pathology (Figure 6.2B) is associated with an increased risk for ICI in infants with tracheoesophageal fistula, gastroschisis, omphalocele, Hirschsprung disease, intestinal atresias, or necrotizing enterocolitis (NEC).[18,19]

What Factors Contribute to the Virulence of *Candida*?

BIOFILM FORMATION

C. albicans, *C. parapsilosis*, and other *Candida* species are able to form biofilms, which can promote invasion and resist killing by antifungal therapy (see Figure 6.3A). These biofilms adhere to medical devices and prevent the penetration of antifungals. This trait explains in part the need to remove central venous catheters to clear candidemia and improve outcomes.[20]

EVADING THE HOST IMMUNE SYSTEM

C. albicans has defense mechanisms to evade the normal human immune response, making it especially dangerous to immunocompromised premature infants (see Figure 6.3B). *C. albicans* can conceal its surface structures from the host immune system, and phagocytes have difficulty recognizing *C. albicans* because its hyphae contain surface proteins that mimic complement receptors. The fungus also degrades cell surface complement C3b, which reduces immune recognition and, after phagocytosis, can lead to macrophage rupture.[21]

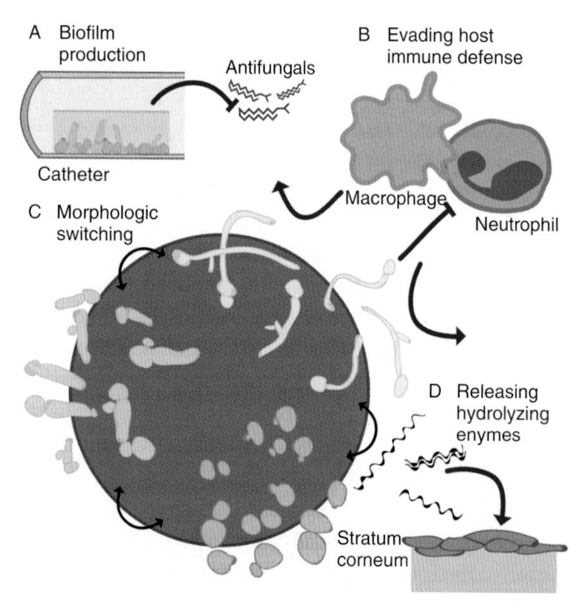

Fig. 6.3 ***Candida*** **virulence factors.** (A) Biofilm formation. (B) Evading host immune system. (C) Morphologic switching. (D) Hydrolyzing enzymes.

MORPHOLOGIC SWITCHING

Morphologic switching reflects the ability of *C. albicans* to take on both yeast and filamentous forms (hyphae and pseudohyphae) (see Figure 6.3C). Changes between these forms are triggered by environmental factors, such as pH, temperature, and the presence of amino acids. Animal studies have found that infection with wild-type strains, capable of both yeast and filamentous forms, had the greatest mortality when compared with infection with either the filamentous-only or the yeast-only forms.[22] The yeast form facilitates cell and tissue invasion. Inside human cells, the filamentous formation increases destruction and evades the host's immune response.[22,23]

HYDROLYZING ENZYMES

C. albicans produces hydrolyzing enzymes, including proteases, phospholipases, and lipases, that enable *C. albicans* to digest epithelial cells and invade host tissue (see Figure 6.3D). The phospholipase enzymes, such as phospholipase B (*caPLB1*), are important in penetrating host cells. Secreted aspartic proteases (SAPs) are another group of enzymes that enable *Candida* to progress from colonization to invasive infection. SAPs break down different proteins, including keratin and collagen, making them advantageous in invading host tissues. SAPs are produced by most *Candida* species, except for *C. glabrata*, with *C. albicans* producing the highest amounts.

TOXINS

C. albicans can also produce toxins that add to its virulence. Candidalysin is a cytolytic peptide toxin that directly damages epithelial membranes and stimulates a proinflammatory cytokine response.[24]

Which Organisms Cause ICIs in the NICU?

The *Candida* species that predominates in the NICU depends on timing of infection, etiology, and whether or not the infant is receiving antifungal prophylaxis. CCC and early-onset ICI infections are due to *C. albicans* in 90% of cases. In late-onset ICIs in infants not receiving antifungal prophylaxis, the majority in the NICU are due to the species *C. albicans* (~50%) and *C. parapsilosis*, followed by *C. glabrata*.[20,25,26] For infants on antifungal prophylaxis, ICIs are rare and more commonly due to *C. parapsilosis* and *C. glabrata*.[9,25,27–29] Infections due to *C. tropicalis*, *C. lusitaniae*, *C. krusei*, *C. guillermondii*, and other species occur less frequently independent of prophylaxis. *C. albicans* is the most pathogenic of the *Candida* species, with mortality two to three times higher than other *Candida* species.[30] This pathogenicity is attributed to the virulence factors of *C. albicans* described earlier.

What Is the Incidence of ICIs in the NICU?

There is variation in the incidence of ICIs in different NICUs. The considerable variation in the incidence of ICIs is based on infant demographics, including gestational age or birth-weight cutoffs for resuscitation of extremely premature infants and practices related to feeding, medication, and antibiotic use by the individual NICUs. NICUs that do not resuscitate infants <24 weeks have a lower incidence of ICIs in infants <1000 g compared with centers caring for infants at 22 and 23 weeks' gestation. For more mature infants, the number of infants cared for with NEC, gastroschisis, and other complex GI diseases influences the incidence of ICIs. Finally, infection control practices and use of antifungal prophylaxis are other major factors affecting the incidence of ICIs.[31] Antifungal prophylaxis is associated with an incidence of 0% to 1% even at the lowest gestational ages and among the highest-risk infants.[9,29,32]

Few studies include all types of ICIs as defined earlier and are largely limited to the incidence of *Candida* BSIs and/or meningitis. In the absence of antifungal prophylaxis, the incidence of ICI in ELBW infants is around 10% and exceeds 20% in those at <25 weeks' gestation. *Candida* UTIs occur in 3% to 4% of ELBW infants.[9,16] Meningitis and peritonitis (often complicating focal bowel perforation and surgical NEC) may be seen in an additional 1% to 2% of ELBWs.[16,33]

Examining candidemia alone, the largest report to date is from 128 U.S. NICUs using National Nosocomial Infections Surveillance system data from 1995 to 2004 (N = 130,523 infants).[34] Despite limitations resulting from data accrual during an era when antifungal prophylaxis and other preventative measures were being introduced, among ELBW infants the median NICU-specific infection incidence was 7.5%, but 25% of NICUs had an incidence of 13.5% or higher. The pooled mean candidemia incidence for infants of birth weights of <1000 g, 1001 to 1500 g, 1501 to 2500 g, and >2501 g were 5.1%, 1.3%, 0.36%, and 0.3%, respectively.

What Is the Neurodevelopmental Impairment Impact and Survival Among Infants Who Develop ICIs and What Factors Can Improve These Outcomes?

Neurodevelopmental impairment (NDI) or delay is a common long-term complication of ICIs, even in the absence of documented fungal meningitis. In ELBW infants, NDI was reported in 57% of infants with candidemia and 53% of infants with *Candida* meningitis.[19,20,35,36] Empiric therapy on the day cultures are sent or initiating prompt antifungal therapy within 2 days of the blood culture may help decrease NDI. Studies have demonstrated improved outcomes when antifungals were started promptly when cultures become positive (within 2 days of when the blood culture was obtained) and a decrease in the combined outcome of NDI or death with empiric antifungal therapy started the day cultures were sent.[20,36] Most importantly, prevention via antifungal prophylaxis and infection control measures eliminates ICI as a cause of NDI.

IS SURVIVAL DIFFERENT BETWEEN CANDIDEMIA AND CANDIDURIA IN PREMATURE INFANTS?

Mortality is high in premature infants with candiduria as well as candidemia. In a study of ELBW infants, all-cause mortality was 28% for *Candida* BSI, 26% for *Candida* UTI, 50% for other sterile sites (meningitis and peritonitis), and 57% if two or more culture sites were involved (BSI + UTI or UTI + meningitis).[16] Attributable mortality (the difference between infants with ICIs and noninfected infants) was 20%.

WHAT FACTORS AFFECT SURVIVAL?

Survival is higher in larger infants. Infants weighing >1000 g with ICIs had a much lower mortality of 2%.[37] The *Candida* species causing the infection also affects survival. *C. albicans* is more virulent than other *Candida* species. In VLBW infants, *Candida*-associated mortality was 44% in infants with *C. albicans* compared with 19% for infants with *C. parapsilosis*.[30]

HOW CAN SURVIVAL BE IMPROVED?

Survival is improved in candidemia cases with prompt removal of a central venous catheter.[16] Additionally, empiric antifungal therapy and prompt treatment when *Candida* has been identified from culture aid in improving survival alone and the combined outcome of survival and NDI.[36]

What Is the Most Common Skin Finding With CCC and How Is It Diagnosed and Managed?

CCC presents most commonly at birth but can occur within the first week. Dermatologic findings include desquamating, maculopapular, papulopustular, and/or erythematous rashes. Findings in a recent study found that desquamation (scaling, peeling, flaking, or exfoliation) was the most common presentation (Figure 6.4).[2] CCC can occur with or without dissemination, such as pneumonia or BSI. Without prompt identification and treatment, dissemination to the blood, urine, or CSF can occur, with incidence ranging from 11% in term infants to 33% in infants 1000 to 2500 g and 66% in ELBW infants.[38] Skin biopsies demonstrate a high burden of yeast, with invasion into the epidermis and dermis with inflammation and injury, including granulomas, focal necrosis, and hemorrhage. For these reasons, preterm and term infants should be treated promptly at the time of rash

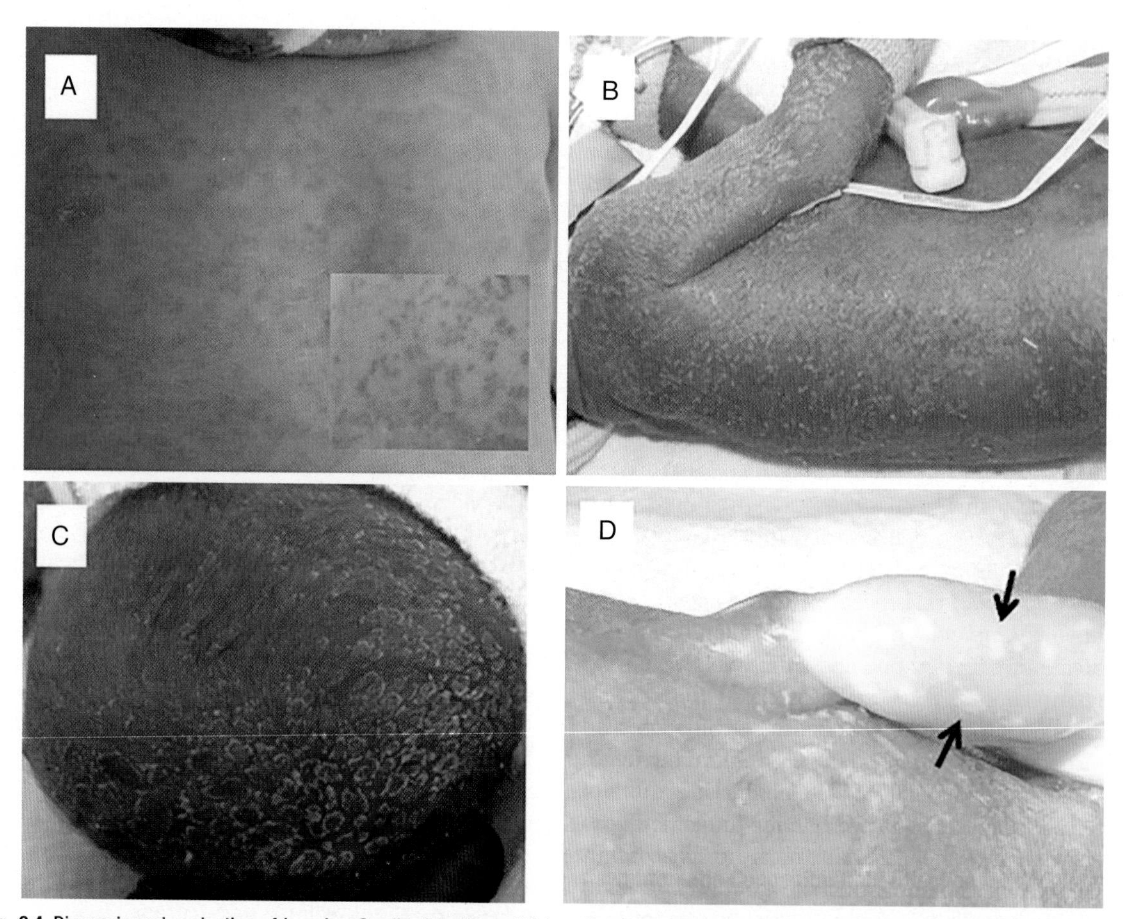

Fig. 6.4 Diagnosis and evaluation of invasive *Candida* infections. *ICI,* invasive *Candida* infection; *CVC,* central venous catheter; *US,* ultrasound; *MRI,* magnetic resonance imaging; *EOD,* end-organ dissemination; *NEC,* necrotizing enterocolitis. If bowel disease is present or part of the infant's history, such as NEC or focal bowel perforation, then a complete abdominal US for abscess should be performed.

presentation with systemic antifungal therapy and for a minimum of 14 days (Figure 6.4). Delaying systemic treatment, solitary use of topical therapy (nystatin), or treating for <10 days are associated with *Candida* dissemination to the bloodstream.[2]

Diagnosis of CCC is made by the presence of a diffuse CCC rash involving major skin areas of the body, extremities, and face or scalp, as well as funisitis, presenting in the first week (≤7 days), with identification of *Candida* species or yeast from (1) skin or mucous membrane cultures, (2) placenta staining or cultures, or (3) umbilical cord staining or cultures.

When evaluating a diffuse CCC rash in the first week of life, aerobic skin cultures for both fungal and bacterial organisms should be obtained to identify the source of infection. Examination of the umbilical cord for yellow plaques and placenta can aid in the diagnosis, as well. Both should be sent for specific fungal staining and aerobic culture. Additionally, blood culture, urine culture if older than 48 hours, and CSF if no rash on the back is present, should be performed. Most experts would defer the lumbar puncture if there is cutaneous involvement on the back due to invasion into the dermis and risk of introducing *Candida* into the CSF. Empiric antifungal therapy should be started pending culture results. Differential diagnoses include staphylococcal and other bacterial and fungal skin infections. In certain cases when the rash could be due to bacterial and fungal pathogens, empiric staphylococcal and fungal empiric coverage should be initiated pending culture results.

CUTANEOUS CANDIDIASIS

Cutaneous (or mucocutaneous) candidiasis (CC) presents as a diffuse rash with similar skin manifestations as CCC but occurs later, at 8 or more days after birth. In the era before antifungal prophylaxis, the incidence was ~8% in VLBW infants.[1] Risk factors include extreme prematurity, vaginal birth, postnatal steroids, and hyperglycemia. Similar to CCC, CC in premature infants is an invasive infection of the skin and will disseminate if not systemically treated. Aerobic skin cultures for both fungal and bacterial organisms must be obtained to identify the nature of the infection. Additionally, blood and urine cultures, plus a lumbar puncture if no rash on the back is present, should be performed. Empiric systemic therapy should be started at the time of skin presentation, and treatment should be continued for a minimum of 14 days in premature infants.

How Long Are Blood Cultures Positive With Candidemia?

Compared with bacteremia, candidemia is associated with prolonged positivity of blood cultures with a median of 3 days even in the absence of end-organ dissemination.[20]

SIGNS OF CANDIDEMIA

Signs of *Candida* bloodstream infections are similar to those with bacteremia, with candidemia having some unique patterns related to thrombocytopenia (Table 6.1).[39] VLBW infants with candidemia (as well as those with Gram-negative bacteremia) have lower initial platelet counts, lower platelet nadirs, and a greater duration of thrombocytopenia compared with those with Gram-positive sepsis.[34] The percentage decrease from baseline at presentation is also greater with candidemia (50%) compared with Gram-positive infection. Among the *Candida* species, *C. albicans* and

TABLE 6.1 Presenting Signs of Candidemia in VLBW Infants

Frequently Present (>50%)	Less Common
Thrombocytopenia <100,000/µL	Hypotension
Immature-to-total neutrophil ratio ≥ 0.2	Hyperglycemia
(1-3)-Beta-D-glucan >125 pg/dL	Neutrophilia
↑ Apnea and/or bradycardia	Metabolic acidosis
↑ Oxygen requirement	Lethargy and/or hypotonia
↑ Assisted ventilation	Gastrointestinal signs
	Neutropenia

C. parapsilosis present with lower platelet counts and more apnea compared with *C. glabrata*.[1] Most importantly, candidemia can be associated with disseminated disease (see Figure 6.1). Evaluation of the cardiac, renal, ophthalmologic, and central nervous systems is warranted even if there is only one blood culture positive for *Candida*. These can be performed at presentation or 5 to 7 days into treatment. Reevaluation for end-organ dissemination should occur with persistent candidemia (>5 to 7 days).

WHAT IS THE MOST COMMON SITE FOR END-ORGAN DISSEMINATION WITH CANDIDEMIA?

Candida endocarditis and infected vascular thrombi, the most common complications of candidemia (>5%), are associated with higher mortality than candidemia alone.[40] Central vascular catheters are a risk factor, as local trauma to valvular, endocardial, or endothelial tissue leads to thrombus formation and infection at the time of insertion and/or at any time while in situ. When antifungal therapy alone is unsuccessful in resolving the endocarditis or thrombus, thrombolytic or anticoagulation therapy has been used in some cases, but the suitability of these measures depends on the infant's gestational age and accompanying conditions.

By the time an ICI becomes clinically apparent, *Candida* often has disseminated to form abscesses in tissues, organs, or body fluids. The adherence properties of *Candida* predispose to endocarditis, endophthalmitis, dermatitis, peritonitis, osteomyelitis, and septic arthritis. Fungal abscesses may form in the heart, CNS, kidneys, liver, spleen, skin, bowel, and peritoneum (see Figures 6.1 and 6.5). One meta-analysis (1979–2002) found the incidence of endocarditis to be 5%; renal involvement, 5%; CNS abscesses, 4%; and endophthalmitis, 3%.[40] End-organ dissemination is higher in ELBW infants and in infants with persistent candidemia for >5 to 7 days.[34]

End-organ dissemination is reduced by prompt removal of central vascular catheters and initiation of antifungal therapy as soon as blood cultures become positive. In addition, antifungal prophylaxis, empiric therapy, optimal antifungal dosing, and improved culturing techniques and diagnostics have contributed to a decline in the incidence of end-organ dissemination.[9,20,27]

What Screening Is Needed to Diagnose End-Organ Dissemination for Each Site of ICI?

Screening for dissemination depends on the site of infection (see Figure 6.5). With documented candidemia, initial screening for end-organ dissemination should include an echocardiogram, renal ultrasound, cranial ultrasound, and ophthalmologic examination. If there is significant bowel pathology such as NEC or focal bowel perforation, a complete abdominal ultrasound should be performed to rule out peritoneal, liver, or splenic involvement. If signs of septic arthritis (joint swelling) or osteomyelitis (swelling or immobility) are present, a clinical diagnosis can be made and antifungal treatment provided for 4 to 6 weeks. Joint aspiration may help with diagnosis in the absence of candidemia. Evaluation with bone scan or magnetic resonance imaging (MRI) may help define the extent of involvement, but imaging should not be used to rule out joint or bone involvement in infants if clinically apparent. If candidemia persists, end-organ dissemination is even more likely, and the initial screening tests should be repeated along with additional surveillance after 5 to 7 days, including (1) ultrasound at the location of the tip of any prior central catheters for infected thrombus, (2) complete abdominal ultrasound for abscesses (laparotomy is sometimes considered for high clinical suspicion), and (3) cranial ultrasound or MRI to detect brain dissemination. Abscesses that are amenable to drainage or surgery should be removed.

What Are Risk Factors for Renal Candidiasis?

Candida infection of the kidneys may result from an ascending UTI via the urethra or via direct seeding from the bloodstream. Colonization and proliferation are augmented by proteinuria, nitrogenous compounds, acidic pH (premature infant urine is alkalotic), hydrophobic *Candida* cells, and the presence of Enterobacteriaceae such as *Escherichia coli*. SAPs and phospholipases play a role in the renal system as well, attacking structural and immunologic defenses leading to tissue injury and invasion.[41] Risk factors for candiduria include vaginal birth, lower mean birth weight and gestational age, male gender, and prolonged initial courses of empiric antibiotic therapy.[42]

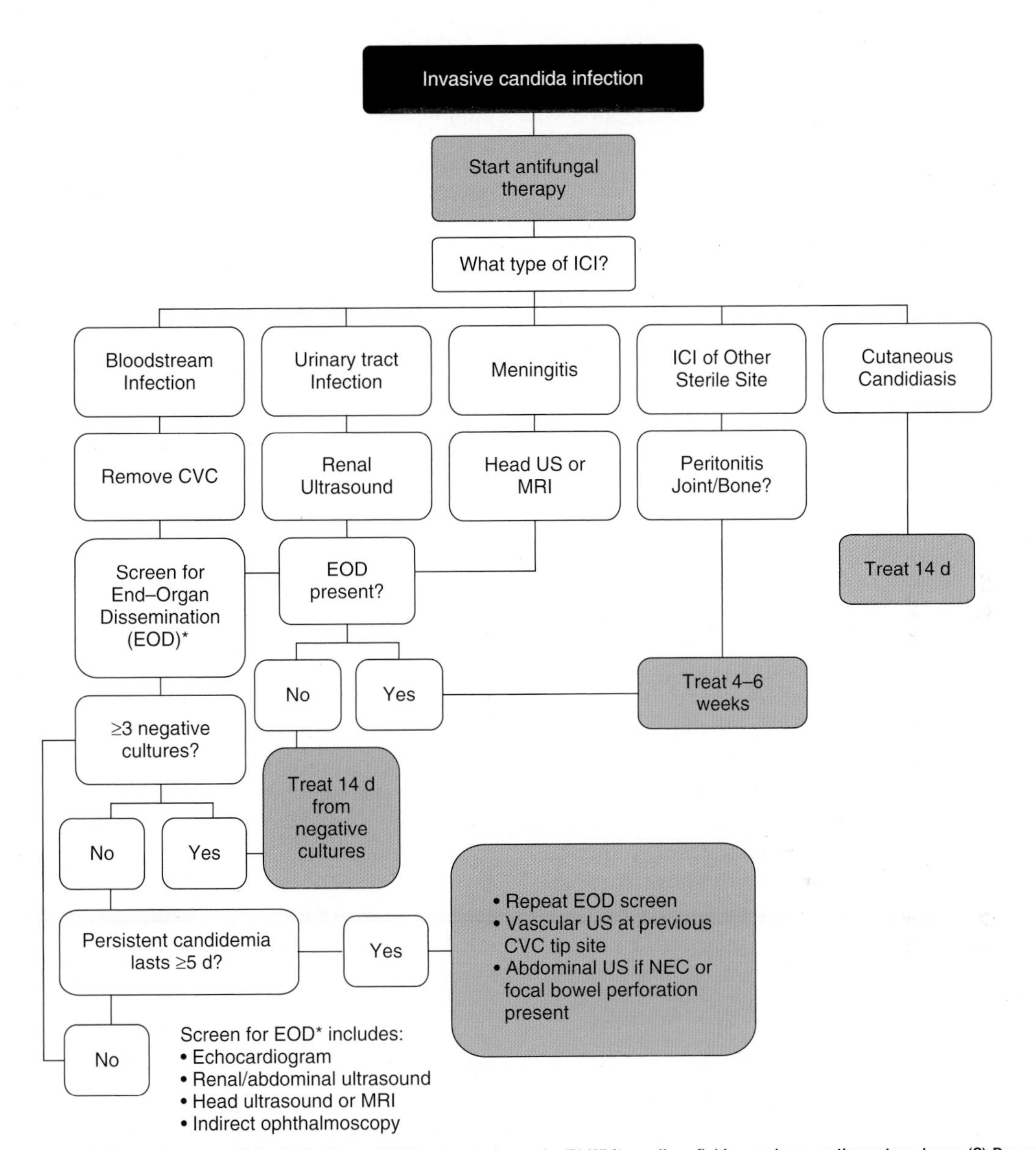

Fig. 6.5 Congenital cutaneous candidiasis findings. (A) Maculopapular rash. (B) White–yellow flaking rash on erythematous base. (C) Dry, cracking scaly rash. (D) Funisitis shown as white–yellow plaques (arrows identifying two examples) of the umbilical cord. *ICI*, invasine candida infection; *US*, ultrasound; *MRI*, magnetic resonance imaging; *CVC*, central venous catheter; *NEC*, necrotizing enterocolitis

HOW COMMON ARE *CANDIDA* UTIs FOR ELBW INFANTS AND HOW ARE THEY MANAGED?

Late-onset sepsis evaluations should include a urine culture obtained via sterile catheterization.[43] Infection is most commonly defined as growth of ≥10,000 CFU/mL from a sterile catheterization or ≥1000 CFU/mL in urine obtained by suprapubic bladder aspiration. Some experts and studies have not found colony counts to be useful in diagnosis; instead, they have found that the presence of any *Candida* in the urine is associated with significant infection and outcomes.[16,42] *Candida* UTIs may occur alone or in conjunction with *Candida* sepsis. Other researchers have considered lower CFUs not to be an infection but rather colonization at a high-risk site, and preemptive treatment could be considered. Empiric antifungal therapy should be started with subsequent sepsis evaluations if urine colonization is known pending culture results. UTIs and sepsis have similar presentations. Elevated creatinine levels without other causes may be another sign of a UTI. Renal ultrasonography is warranted for all *Candida* UTIs to evaluate for abscess formation. In the absence of antifungal prophylaxis, candiduria can occur in up to 2.4% of VLBW and 6% of ELBW infants.[1,9,16]

WITH *CANDIDA* URINARY TRACT INFECTION, WHAT PERCENTAGE OF INFANTS HAVE RENAL DISSEMINATION?

Renal fungal abscess formation may occur in infants with candiduria via an ascending infection or dissemination to the kidneys with candidemia.[41] In previous eras, renal abscesses developed in as high as 58% of infants with candiduria ± candidemia, whereas a more recent study from 2004 to 2007 found the incidence to be 0% (0/23 evaluated) with candiduria alone and 22% (2/9) with multiple sites of *Candida* infection.[42] Between these two study periods, antifungal prophylaxis, pharmacokinetic and safety studies of appropriate initial antifungal dosing (e.g., amphotericin B deoxycholate at 1 mg/kg compared with 0.25 mg/kg in the previous era), and increased empiric antifungal therapy may have attenuated formation of renal abscesses. These studies have small numbers but suggest that in infants with candiduria prompt initial antifungal therapy has improved outcomes, so renal imaging should be performed at presentation and repeated in cases with persistent candiduria.

Can Meningitis and Central Nervous System Involvement Occur Without Candidemia?

Meningitis, encephalitis, or abscess formation may complicate candidemia or occur separately. Because 50% of meningitis cases occur without documented candidemia, lumbar puncture at the time of sepsis evaluation before the initiation of antifungal therapy is important, as CSF cell counts and chemistries often are not abnormal with CNS infections in studies with a mixture of lumbar punctures performed before and after antifungal treatments. This may be due to the timing of the lumbar puncture, the neonatal host response, or the location of the CNS infection (spinal fluid vs. brain tissue).

WHAT IS THE RISK FOR CNS ABSCESS FORMATION WITH MENINGITIS?

In cases of candidemia or CNS fungal disease, neuroimaging (ultrasonography or MRI) is needed to evaluate for abscess formation. Abscess formation occurs in approximately 4% of candidemia and 33% of meningitis cases.[1] Animal studies have demonstrated CNS involvement in cases of fungal sepsis.[44] Ultrasonography can be performed initially and continues to improve in quality, but it is not as sensitive as MRI. Studies have also found an association between ICI and periventricular leukomalacia in premature infants, possibly related to the release of cytokines that may damage the periventricular white matter.

Is It More Common for *Candida* Peritonitis to Occur with Focal Bowel Perforation or NEC?

Candida peritonitis can complicate both focal bowel perforation and NEC. If exploratory laparotomy or drains are placed, cultures should be obtained to determine what organisms are present. Peritonitis may initially present with or without erythema as part of abdominal symptomatology. Identification of pathogens in the peritoneal cavity is critical to appropriate management of bowel perforation or peritonitis and to prevent abscess formation. *Candida* species are the predominant organism causing peritonitis in 44% of focal bowel perforation cases and in 15% of the perforated NEC cases in infants not receiving antifungal prophylaxis.[33] Although radiographs are the most common study identifying bowel perforation, some cases may be missed, and ultrasound or exploratory laparotomy may be necessary if clinically indicated.

Studies in the era before antifungal prophylaxis demonstrated candidemia complicating 16% of cases of NEC.[1] Culture of the rectum, stool, or oral flora in infants with diagnosis of NEC should be performed to evaluate for the presence of *Candida* species or yeast. If *Candida* is isolated, systemic antifungal therapy should be initiated in addition to the antibacterial treatment of the NEC.[45] This may not be needed in infants who have been on antifungal prophylaxis since birth.

Is Preemptive Treatment Indicated If Candida Is Isolated From an Endotracheal Culture?

Pneumonia remains a difficult diagnosis in ventilated infants with chronic lung disease, as radiologic findings of infection, atelectasis, fluid, and scarring are often similar. Respiratory tract colonization usually occurs 1 to 2 weeks after skin and GI colonization and is associated with a high risk for ICI.[9] Preemptive treatment has been shown to prevent candidemia dissemination in intubated ELBW infants when *Candida* is detected in the lungs by culture, polymerase chain reaction (PCR), or *Candida* mannan antigen.[46,47]

Endophthalmitis and Retinopathy of Prematurity

Endophthalmitis presents most commonly as an intraocular dissemination from the bloodstream but also could be a rare complication of retinopathy of prematurity surgery or local trauma. Endophthalmitis progresses from a chorioretinal lesion that subsequently elevates and breaks free in the vitreous, appearing as a white fluffy ball. It can present as solitary or multiple yellow–white elevated lesions in the posterior retina and vitreous. The clear cell-free vitreous becomes hazy due to an influx of inflammatory cells. Endophthalmitis incidence has decreased significantly, likely due to more rapid diagnosis, treatment, and prevention of ICIs. Even in the absence of visible retinal abscesses or chorioretinitis, *Candida* sepsis increases the risk for severe retinopathy of prematurity, and screening for retinal pathology, if not already indicated by gestational age or birth weight criteria, is recommended in premature infants with candidemia.

Who Are High-Risk Infants for Whom Antifungal Prophylaxis Could Be Considered?

High-risk infants who benefit from targeted antifungal prophylaxis have a combination of risk factors, including the degree of immaturity of the immune system, which can be defined by gestational age at birth; the presence of invasive vascular devices or endotracheal tubes, which can easily become and stay colonized; a disease process that favors *Candida* colonization; and the time period during which they are receiving infusions or medications that facilitate the proliferation of *Candida* (parenteral nutrition, antibiotics, and to a lesser extent postnatal steroids and acid inhibitors).

The optimal approach involves infant-focused prevention based on specific risk factors for ICIs. Although centers may vary in overall incidence, at the lowest gestational ages individual risk factors drive ICI risk. In addition to incidence, it is important to factor in the mortality and long-term neurodevelopmental impairment of ICIs, which occur in 75% of ELBW infants.[16,48] Based on ICI incidence alone in the absence of antifungal prophylaxis, the approximate number that must be treated for infants <25 weeks' gestation is 1 in 5; for 25 weeks' gestation, 1 in 10; and, for 26 and 27 weeks' gestation, 1 in 20.[16] From randomized placebo controlled trials, meta-analyses, and *Cochrane Reviews*, antifungal prophylaxis with fluconazole has demonstrated efficacy and safety without the emergence of resistance when used to target infants based on risk factors during their highest risk time period in premature infants.[9,25,27,29,32,49–51] Two other risk factors and groups are worth noting. Complex GI diseases such as gastroschisis, stage 2 or greater NEC, and Hirschsprung disease while infants are requiring parenteral nutrition, central venous access, and/or antibiotics put the infants at a high risk for ICIs.[18,52] Additionally, when treatment for infections in any NICU patient necessitates using third- or fourth-generation cephalosporins or carbapenems, the risk for ICI is significantly increased.[16] Guidance for fluconazole prophylaxis for high-, moderate-, and low-risk infants considering specific factors for when they become high risk for ICI, as well as *Candida*-related mortality and morbidity, are summarized in Table 6.2. Standardizing care with the development of center guidelines for antifungal prophylaxis yields optimal outcomes in prevention.

What Is the Average Time Required to Identify Candida From Culture?

The best method for diagnosing ICIs remains culture of blood, urine, CSF, and peritoneal fluid or other sterile body fluids. Obtaining sufficient blood culture

TABLE 6.2 Targeted Antifungal Prophylaxis for Preventing Invasive *Candida* Infections

	High Risk (Infants With High Mortality and Neurodevelopmental Impairment From ICIs)	Moderate Risk (Infants with Significant Mortality and Neurodevelopmental Impairment From ICIs)	Low Risk (Infants With Low Mortality From ICIs)
Level of evidence	Grade A-I	Grade A-I	Grade B-II
Birth weight	<750 g	750–999 g	≥1000 g
Gestational age	≤25 weeks' gestation	26 and 27 weeks' gestation	≥28 weeks' gestation
With the addition of risk factors	*One or more of the following:* Central venous catheter Parenteral nutrition Third-/fourth-generation cephalosporins/carbapenems >2 days of antibiotics Complex GI disease	*One or more of the following:* Third-/fourth-generation cephalosporins/carbapenems Complex GI disease or *Two or more of the following:* Central venous catheter Parenteral nutrition >5 days of antibiotics	*One or more of the following:* >2 days of Third-/fourth-generation cephalosporins/carbapenems Complex GI disease
High-risk time period	While CVC is in place or receiving parenteral nutrition or antibiotics	While CVC is in place or receiving parenteral nutrition or antibiotics	While CVC is in place or receiving parenteral nutrition or antibiotics
Dosing	3 or 6 mg/kg IV fluconazole twice a week		
Azole-resistance prevention	Limit length of prophylaxis to high-risk time period. For systemic treatment (empiric, suspected, and proven) of ICIs, use amphotericin B or non-azole antifungals. Use twice-weekly dosing of fluconazole prophylaxis.		

Level of evidence is based on the U.S. Public Health Service Grading System for ranking recommendations in clinical guidelines, where the strength of recommendation and levels of evidence include *A*, good evidence; *B*, moderate evidence; *C*, poor evidence; *I*, at least one randomized clinical trial; *II*, at least one well-designed but nonrandomized trial; and *III*, expert opinions based on experience or limited clinical reports. Complex GI disease includes patients with stage ≥2 necrotizing enterocolitis, gastroschisis, or Hirschsprung disease with significant disease requiring (or is expected to require) no enteral feedings and/or on antibiotics for ≥7 days. *IV*, intravenous; *CVC*, central venous catheter; *ICI*, invasive candida infection.

volumes (≥1 mL) and performing urine and CSF fluid cultures at the time of evaluation for sepsis remain critical to making prompt diagnosis. Aerobic cultures detect *Candida* but are not good for the detection of other fungi. Although neonatal infections may have low colony counts, they are above the detection limit of newer blood culture methods. On average, neonatal blood cultures demonstrate the growth of *Candida* by 37 hours, and 97% of blood cultures are positive by 72 hours.[53] Prior antifungal therapy does affect time to positivity. Clinical diagnosis has greatly improved, as laboratories have become more skilled at culturing *Candida*, identifying *Candida* species, and performing susceptibility testing. Although some in vitro studies found a lack of growth of *Candida* in blood cultures, clinical neonatal studies have demonstrated high reliability when appropriate culture volumes and methods are used. The frequent occurrence of multiple positive blood cultures also aids in the diagnosis of candidemia. In NICU patients, from 1989 to 1999, 97% of 110 ICIs were diagnosed by cultures; only three infants were not diagnosed until autopsy.[54]

How Good Are the Newer Laboratory Diagnostic Adjunctive Tests?

Adjunctive laboratory tests have not replaced cultures, but they can be useful in identifying high-risk infants who would benefit from early empiric antifungal therapy (pending culture results) and in monitoring response to antifungal therapy. PCR and fungal cell wall polysaccharides such as (1-3)-beta-D-glucan (BDG) and mannan can be extremely helpful in detecting non-bloodstream infections and determining the need for extension of treatment.[1] They are currently not better than cultures in identifying true ICIs, and costs per yield are high if included in each infection evaluation. As the multiplex PCR test is being utilized in some centers, future research will help guide its potential usefulness.

BDG levels are helpful if there is uncertainty in deciding the need for empiric antifungal therapy and in following response to therapy as levels decrease over time with antifungal therapy. Various cutoff points have been recommended for interpreting BDG levels in infants. Serum BDG levels are higher in infants with ICI: 364 pg/mL (interquartile range [IQR], 131–976) versus 89 pg/mL (IQR, 30–127) in noninfected infants. These levels decrease significantly with antifungal therapy, to 58 pg/mL (IQR, 28–81).[55,56] The cutoff for BDG should be higher (>125 pg/mL) for infants than adults (>80 pg/mL) due to the effect that colonization and other infections (Gram-negative and coagulase-negative *Staphylococcus*) may have on BDG levels. BDG levels in infants infected with coagulase-negative staphylococci were found to be 116 pg/mL (IQR, 46–128) and 118 pg/mL (IQR, 52–304) in infants without bacteremia.[55,56] One challenge is that BDG can be elevated to the same degree with fungal colonization as with ICI, and studies have not critically examined this effect. Infants colonized at certain high-risk sites (e.g., the respiratory tract) may benefit from empiric treatment.[46,47] One study used mannan levels ≥0.5 ng/mL in endotracheal lavage aspirates as a criterion for preemptive treatment and significantly decreased ICI.[47] Further study of preemptive treatment at certain BDG levels may be beneficial. BDG may also give false-positive results after transfusion of blood products in adults and infants.[55] A study of 133 VLBW infants found BDG to be higher in transfused (red blood cells or fresh frozen plasma) infants (170 pg/mL; IQR, 65–317) compared with non-transfused infants (57 pg/mL; IQR, 34–108; $P < 0.001$).[55]

Another method that may help with the decision to start early empiric therapy is direct fluorescent assay in buffy coat.[57] This test is a fluorescent stain that binds to structures containing cellulose and chitin. This diagnostic test has been successfully used for identifying hyphae and spores and may help with rapid diagnosis and antifungal treatment, as results may be obtained within 1 to 2 hours.

Molecular techniques, including PCR and DNA microarray technology, may identify fungi and their antifungal susceptibilities more quickly and with higher sensitivity than is possible with blood cultures. Fungal PCR to detect the gene for 18S ribosomal RNA in premature infants has yielded promising results. PCR is useful when fungal infection suspicion is high despite negative cultures. PCR can detect candidemia and non-bloodstream infections, including *Candida* peritonitis or candiduria, as well as previous *Candida* infections and endotracheal colonization.[58] Similar to adjunctive tests, the ability of PCR to distinguish infection from colonization has not been critically studied.

Other markers of fungal disease include anti-*Candida* antibodies, D-arabinitol (a *Candida* metabolite), and fungal chitin synthase. These markers are similarly challenging to study, as they may be present with bloodstream infections, non-bloodstream infections, or colonization alone.

Are Cases of Mold Infections on the Rise?

Aspergillosis and mucormycosis are filamentous fungi or mold infections that can cause severe infections in extremely premature infants. As more infections at the lower gestational ages are surviving, there are more case reports in the literature, but more study is needed. *Aspergillus* most often presents as a cutaneous infection and not as pulmonary or disseminated disease. Voriconazole or an echinocandin should be the first-line agent indicated in neonatal aspergillosis A cases. The cutaneous manifestations of molds (Figure 6.6) compared to *Candida* are summarized in Table 6.3.

Molds are ubiquitous, but environmental contamination such as dust and soil from hospital construction or air systems can carry spores that may settle in wounds or be inhaled. Prevention includes scheduled cleaning of the ventilation systems and proper control of dust during NICU repairs or construction.

Mucormycosis initially presents as a black rimmed lesion or eschar at the site of local trauma, a covered area, or the back.[59] Increased risk is seen with extreme prematurity, neutropenia, or postnatal steroid exposure. Local trauma can include sites of intravenous catheter infiltrates and NEC. Prompt diagnosis and

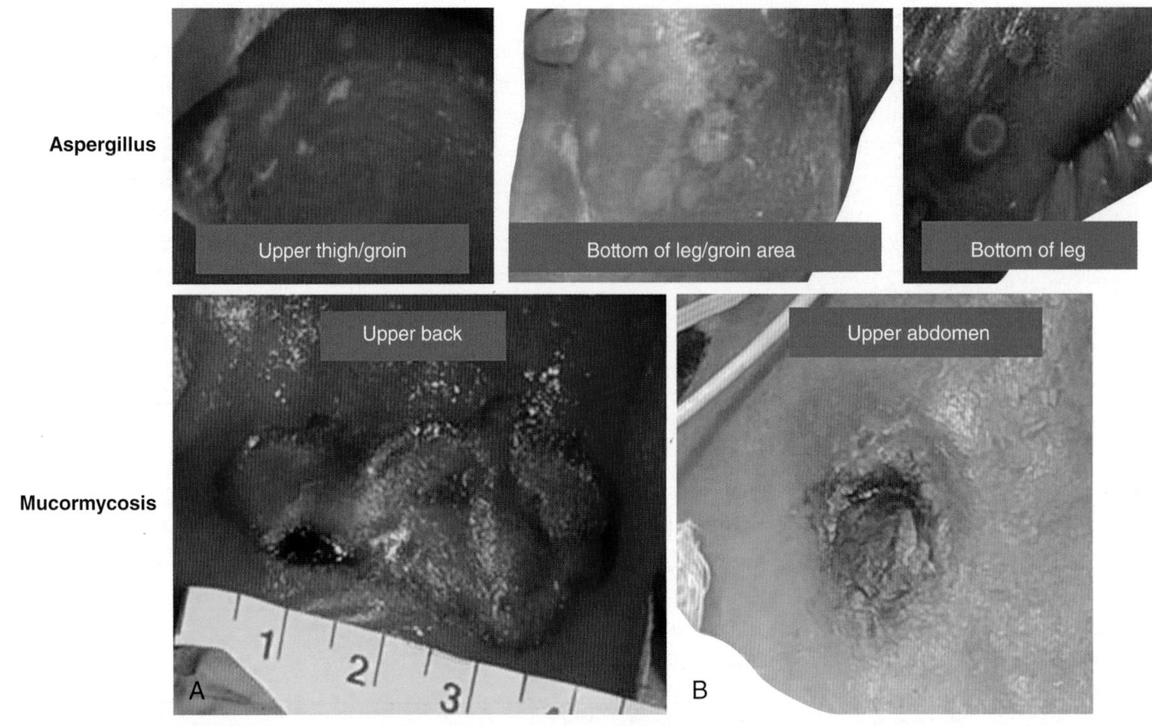

Fig. 6.6 Cutaneous mold infection examples. *Aspergillus* infection progresses from small, white powder-like lesions to circular yellow indurated lesions with an erythematous ring and inflamed target lesion. Two examples of mucormycosis: (A) Amorphous inflamed yellow–tan lesion with dark eschar border, and (B) black eschar with an erythematous ring at a previously covered area.

TABLE 6.3 Cutaneous Mold and *Candida* Infections in Neonates

	Aspergillosis (*Aspergillus fumigatus*)	Mucormycosis (*Rhizopus* and *Mucor* Species)	Candidiasis (*Candida* Species)
Dermatologic findings	Small, white, powder-like rashes Yellow crusted lesions Yellow ulceration areas Dark scab-like lesions Target lesions	Initially begins as erythema and induration progressing to necrosis leading to a black eschar Black rimmed lesion or eschar at the site of a covered area, back, or local trauma	Desquamation (scaling, peeling, flaking, or exfoliation) Maculopapular, papulopustular, and/or erythematous rashes
Evaluation	Culture (aerobic or fungal) or biopsy	Fungal culture or biopsy	Culture (aerobic or fungal)
Diagnosis	Dichotomously branched and septate hyphae, identified by 10% KOH wet prep or Gomori methenamine-silver nitrate stain	Broad non-septate or pauciseptate hyphae that become twisted and ribbon-like and branch at right angles from the parent hyphae; pauciseptate (few septa) differentiates from aspergillosis	Yeast cells and pseudohyphae can be found with Gram, calcofluor white, or fluorescent antibody stains; microscopic examination of 10% to 20% KOH prep or Gomori methenamine-silver nitrate stain
Treatment (start empirically at presentation of rash/lesions)	Voriconazole, echinocandins	Amphotericin B (surgical debridement if medical management is not effective)	Amphotericin B and other susceptible antifungals

amphotericin B (and at times surgical debridement) attenuate ulceration and necrosis and improve survival. A high degree of suspicion is needed, and a tissue biopsy is often needed to diagnose these right-angle branched non-septated hyphae. Mortality from the infection without prompt diagnosis and treatment can be as high as 61%.

REFERENCES

1. Kaufman D, Fairchild KD. Clinical microbiology of bacterial and fungal sepsis in very-low-birth-weight infants. *Clin Microbiol Rev*. 2004;17(3):638-680.
2. Kaufman DA, Coggins SA, Zanelli SA, Weitkamp J-H. Congenital cutaneous candidiasis: prompt systemic treatment is associated with improved outcomes in neonates. *Clin Infect Dis*. 2017;64(10):1387-1395.
3. Kaufman DA, Gurka MJ, Hazen KC, Boyle R, Robinson M, Grossman LB. Patterns of fungal colonization in preterm infants weighing less than 1000 grams at birth. *Pediatr Infect Dis J*. 2006;25(8):733-737.
4. Manzoni P, Farina D, Antonielli d'Oulx E, Leonessa ML, Gomirato G, Arisio R. An association between anatomic site of *Candida* colonization and risk of invasive candidiasis exists also in preterm neonates in neonatal intensive care unit. *Diagn Microbiol Infect Dis*. 2006;56(4):459-460.
5. Manzoni P, Farina D, Leonessa M, et al. Risk factors for progression to invasive fungal infection in preterm neonates with fungal colonization. *Pediatrics*. 2006;118(6):2359-2364.
6. Manzoni P, Farina D, Galletto P, et al. Type and number of sites colonized by fungi and risk of progression to invasive fungal infection in preterm neonates in neonatal intensive care unit. *J Perinat Med*. 2007;35(3):220-226.
7. Manzoni P, Farina D, Monetti C, et al. Early-onset neutropenia is a risk factor for *Candida* colonization in very low-birth-weight neonates. *Diagn Microbiol Infect Dis*. 2007;57(1):77-83.
8. Manzoni P, Stolfi I, Pugni L, et al. A multicenter, randomized trial of prophylactic fluconazole in preterm neonates. *N Engl J Med*. 2007;356(24):2483-2495.
9. Kaufman D, Boyle R, Hazen KC, Patrie JT, Robinson M, Donowitz LG. Fluconazole prophylaxis against fungal colonization and infection in preterm infants. *N Engl J Med*. 2001; 345(23):1660-1666.
10. Saiman L, Ludington E, Dawson JD, et al. Risk factors for *Candida* species colonization of neonatal intensive care unit patients. *Pediatr Infect Dis J*. 2001;20(12):1119-1124.
11. Manzoni P, Meyer M, Stolfi I, et al. Bovine lactoferrin supplementation for prevention of necrotizing enterocolitis in very-low-birth-weight neonates: a randomized clinical trial. *Early Hum Dev*. 2014;90(suppl 1):S60-S65.
12. Romeo MG, Romeo DM, Trovato L, et al. Role of probiotics in the prevention of the enteric colonization by *Candida* in preterm newborns: incidence of late-onset sepsis and neurological outcome. *J Perinatol*. 2011;31(1):63-69.
13. Hu HJ, Zhang GQ, Zhang Q, Shakya S, Li ZY. Probiotics prevent candida colonization and invasive fungal sepsis in preterm neonates: a systematic review and meta-analysis of randomized controlled trials. *Pediatr Neonatol*. 2017;58(2):103-110.
14. Benjamin DK, Smith PB, Arrieta A, et al. Safety and pharmacokinetics of repeat-dose micafungin in young infants. *Clin Pharmacol Ther*. 2010;87(1):93-99.
15. Watterberg KL, Gerdes JS, Cole CH, et al. Prophylaxis of early adrenal insufficiency to prevent bronchopulmonary dysplasia: a multicenter trial. *Pediatrics*. 2004;114(6):1649-1657.
16. Benjamin DK, Stoll BJ, Gantz MG, et al. Neonatal candidiasis: epidemiology, risk factors, and clinical judgment. *Pediatrics*. 2010;126(4):e865-e873.
17. Meier P, Patel A, Esquerra-Zwiers A. Donor human milk update: evidence, mechanisms, and priorities for research and practice. *J Pediatr*. 2017;180:15-21.
18. Feja KN, Wu F, Roberts K, et al. Risk factors for candidemia in critically ill infants: a matched case-control study. *J Pediatr*. 2005;147(2):156-161.
19. Barton M, O'Brien K, Robinson JL, et al. Invasive candidiasis in low birth weight preterm infants: risk factors, clinical course and outcome in a prospective multicenter study of cases and their matched controls. *BMC Infect Dis*. 2014;14:327.
20. Benjamin DK, Stoll BJ, Fanaroff AA, et al. Neonatal candidiasis among extremely low birth weight infants: risk factors, mortality rates, and neurodevelopmental outcomes at 18 to 22 months. *Pediatrics*. 2006;117(1):84-92.
21. Krysan DJ, Sutterwala FS, Wellington M. Catching fire: *Candida albicans*, macrophages, and pyroptosis. *PLoS Pathog*. 2014; 10(6):e1004139.
22. Bendel CM, Hess DJ, Garni RM, Henry-Stanley M, Wells CL. Comparative virulence of *Candida albicans* yeast and filamentous forms in orally and intravenously inoculated mice. *Crit Care Med*. 2003;31(2):501-507.
23. Cleary IA, Reinhard SM, Lazzell AL, et al. Examination of the pathogenic potential of *Candida albicans* filamentous cells in an animal model of haematogenously disseminated candidiasis. *FEMS Yeast Res*. 2016;16(2):fow011.
24. Moyes DL, Wilson D, Richardson JP, et al. Candidalysin is a fungal peptide toxin critical for mucosal infection. *Nature*. 2016;532(7597):64-68.
25. Aliaga S, Clark RH, Laughon M, et al. Changes in the incidence of candidiasis in neonatal intensive care units. *Pediatrics*. 2014;133(2):236-242.
26. Chitnis AS, Magill SS, Edwards JR, Chiller TM, Fridkin SK, Lessa FC. Trends in *Candida* central line-associated bloodstream infections among NICUs, 1999–2009. *Pediatrics*. 2012; 130(1):e46-e52.
27. Kaufman D, Boyle R, Hazen KC, Patrie JT, Robinson M, Grossman LB. Twice weekly fluconazole prophylaxis for prevention of invasive *Candida* infection in high-risk infants of <1000 grams birth weight. *J Pediatr*. 2005;147(2):172-179.
28. Autmizguine J, Smith PB, Prather K, et al. Effect of fluconazole prophylaxis on *Candida* fluconazole susceptibility in premature infants. *J Antimicrob Chemother*. 2018;73(12):3482-3487.
29. Ericson JE, Kaufman DA, Kicklighter SD, et al. Fluconazole prophylaxis for the prevention of candidiasis in premature infants: a meta-analysis using patient-level data. *Clin Infect Dis*. 2016;63(5):604-610.
30. Stoll BJ, Hansen N, Fanaroff AA, et al. Late-onset sepsis in very low birth weight neonates: the experience of the NICHD Neonatal Research Network. *Pediatrics*. 2002;110(2 Pt 1):285-291.
31. Chang YJ, Choi IR, Shin WS, Lee JH, Kim YK, Park MS. The control of invasive *Candida* infection in very low birth weight infants by reduction in the use of 3rd generation cephalosporin. *Korean J Pediatr*. 2013;56(2):68-74.

32. Kaufman DA, Morris A, Gurka MJ, Kapik B, Hetherington S. Fluconazole prophylaxis in preterm infants: a multicenter case-controlled analysis of efficacy and safety. *Early Hum Dev*. 2014;90(suppl 1):S87-S90.
33. Coates EW, Karlowicz MG, Croitoru DP, Buescher ES. Distinctive distribution of pathogens associated with peritonitis in neonates with focal intestinal perforation compared with necrotizing enterocolitis. *Pediatrics*. 2005;116(2):e241-e246.
34. Guida JD, Kunig AM, Leef KH, McKenzie SE, Paul DA. Platelet count and sepsis in very low birth weight neonates: is there an organism-specific response? *Pediatrics*. 2003;111(6 Pt 1):1411-1415.
35. Barton M, Shen A, O'Brien K, et al. Early-onset invasive candidiasis in extremely low birth weight infants: perinatal acquisition predicts poor outcome. *Clin Infect Dis*. 2017;64(7):921-927.
36. Greenberg RG, Benjamin DK, Gantz MG, et al. Empiric antifungal therapy and outcomes in extremely low birth weight infants with invasive candidiasis. *J Pediatr*. 2012;161(2):264-269.e2.
37. Zaoutis TE, Heydon K, Localio R, Walsh TJ, Feudtner C. Outcomes attributable to neonatal candidiasis. *Clin Infect Dis*. 2007; 44(9):1187-1193.
38. Darmstadt GL, Dinulos JG, Miller Z. Congenital cutaneous candidiasis: clinical presentation, pathogenesis, and management guidelines. *Pediatrics*. 2000;105(2):438-444.
39. Fanaroff AA, Korones SB, Wright LL, et al. Incidence, presenting features, risk factors and significance of late onset septicemia in very low birth weight infants. The National Institute of Child Health and Human Development Neonatal Research Network. *Pediatr Infect Dis J*. 1998;17(7):593-598.
40. Benjamin DK, Poole C, Steinbach WJ, Rowen JL, Walsh TJ. Neonatal candidemia and end-organ damage: a critical appraisal of the literature using meta-analytic techniques. *Pediatrics*. 2003;112(3 Pt 1):634-640.
41. Fisher JF, Kavanagh K, Sobel JD, Kauffman CA, Newman CA. *Candida* urinary tract infection: pathogenesis. *Clin Infect Dis*. 2011;52(suppl 6):S437-S451.
42. Wynn JL, Tan S, Gantz MG, et al. Outcomes following candiduria in extremely low birth weight infants. *Clin Infect Dis*. 2012;54(3):331-339.
43. Aviles-Otero N, Ransom M, Weitkamp J, et al. Urinary tract infections in very low birthweight infants: a two-center analysis of microbiology, imaging and heart rate characteristics. *J Neonatal Perinatal Med*. 2021;14(2):269-276.
44. Hope WW, Mickiene D, Petraitis V, et al. The pharmacokinetics and pharmacodynamics of micafungin in experimental hematogenous *Candida* meningoencephalitis: implications for echinocandin therapy in neonates. *J Infect Dis*. 2008;197(1):163-171.
45. Hegde A, Kaufman DA. *Antifungal Prophylaxis in High-Risk Neonates with Complex Gastrointestinal Disease (NEC and Gastroschisis)*. Available at: https://www.pas-meeting.org/past-programs/. Accessed April 28, 2018.
46. Vendettuoli V, Tana M, Tirone C, et al. The role of *Candida* surveillance cultures for identification of a preterm subpopulation at highest risk for invasive fungal infection. *Pediatr Infect Dis J*. 2008;27(12):1114-1116.
47. Posteraro B, Sanguinetti M, Boccia S, et al. Early mannan detection in bronchoalveolar lavage fluid with preemptive treatment reduces the incidence of invasive *Candida* infections in preterm infants. *Pediatr Infect Dis J*. 2010;29(9):844-848.
48. Kimberlain DW, Barnett ED, Lynfield R, Sawyer MH, eds. Candidiasis. In: *Red Book: 2021–2024 Report of the Committee on Infectious Diseases*. 32nd ed. Itasca, IL: American Academy of Pediatrics; 2021.
49. Benjamin DK, Hudak ML, Duara S, et al. Effect of fluconazole prophylaxis on candidiasis and mortality in premature infants: a randomized clinical trial. *JAMA*. 2014;311(17): 1742-1749.
50. Cleminson J, Austin N, McGuire W. Prophylactic systemic antifungal agents to prevent mortality and morbidity in very low birth weight infants. *Cochrane Database Syst Rev*. 2015;(10): CD003850.
51. Weitkamp JH, Ozdas A, LaFleur B, Potts AL. Fluconazole prophylaxis for prevention of invasive fungal infections in targeted highest risk preterm infants limits drug exposure. *J Perinatol*. 2008;28(6):405-411.
52. De Rose DU, Santisi A, Ronchetti MP, et al. Invasive *Candida* infections in neonates after major surgery: current evidence and new directions. *Pathogens*. 2021;10(3):319.
53. Pappas PG, Kauffman CA, Andes DR, et al. Clinical practice guideline for the management of candidiasis: 2016 update by the Infectious Diseases Society of America. *Clin Infect Dis*. 2016;62(4):e1-e50.
54. Noyola DE, Fernandez M, Moylett EH, Baker CJ. Ophthalmologic, visceral, and cardiac involvement in neonates with candidemia. *Clin Infect Dis*. 2001;32(7):1018-1023.
55. Goudjil S, Chazal C, Moreau F, Leke A, Kongolo G, Chouaki T. Blood product transfusions are associated with an increase in serum (1-3)-beta-d-glucan in infants during the initial hospitalization in neonatal intensive care unit (NICU). *J Matern Fetal Neonatal Med*. 2017;30(8):933-937.
56. Cornu M, Goudjil S, Kongolo G, et al. Evaluation of the (1,3)-β-d-glucan assay for the diagnosis of neonatal invasive yeast infections. *Med Mycol*. 2018;56(1):78-87.
57. Higareda-Almaraz MA, Loza-Barajas H, Maldonado-González JG, Higareda-Almaraz E, Benítez-Godínez V, Murillo-Zamora E. Usefulness of direct fluorescent in buffy coat in the diagnosis of *Candida* sepsis in neonates. *J Perinatol*. 2016;36(10): 874-877.
58. Tirodker UH, Nataro JP, Smith S, LasCasas L, Fairchild KD. Detection of fungemia by polymerase chain reaction in critically ill neonates and children. *J Perinatol*. 2003;23(2): 117-122.
59. Murphy J, Yost CC, Short S, Alashari M, Chan B. B. Black eschar on a 4-day-old preterm infant. *NeoReviews*. 2018;19(9): e564-e568.

Chapter 7

When to Perform Lumbar Puncture in Infants at Risk for Meningitis in the Neonatal Intensive Care Unit

Ashley Stark, MD, MS; Rachel G. Greenberg, MD, MB, MHS

Key Points

- Meningitis occurs most commonly in the neonatal period and is associated with significant morbidity and mortality.
- Of infants with meningitis, 15% to 38% have negative blood cultures. Selective evaluation of infants with culture-proven bacteremia can result in missed diagnoses of meningitis.
- Routine lumbar puncture in well-appearing infants evaluated because of maternal risk factors is not recommended.
- Lumbar puncture can be deferred or omitted from early-onset sepsis evaluation in premature infants with respiratory distress syndrome.
- Lumbar puncture should be performed as part of the evaluation of infants with suspected late-onset infection.
- Lumbar puncture should be deferred in severely ill infants with cardiorespiratory compromise, although empiric therapy should be considered if meningitis is strongly suspected.
- Repeat lumbar punctures in infants receiving adequate antibiotic therapy and showing clinical improvement are not recommended.
- Lumbar punctures performed with ultrasound guidance may improve procedural success, particularly in smaller premature infants.

Introduction

The neonatal period is the most common time in life for the presentation of bacterial meningitis, with an estimated incidence of approximately 0.3 per 1000 live births in developed countries[1,2] and 0.8 per 1000 life births in underdeveloped countries.[3] However, this figure is likely an underestimate, as 30% to 70% of infants who undergo sepsis evaluation do not have a lumbar puncture (LP) performed.[4,5] In developed countries, mortality from meningitis ranges between 10% and 15% for term infants[6] and reaches 25% in premature infants.[7] In underdeveloped countries, mortality ranges from 40% to 58%.[8] Although associated mortality has decreased over time, long-term morbidity remains high.[9,10] Identification of meningitis in infants by clinical examination can be difficult, as early signs are often subtle and nonspecific. Examination of the cerebrospinal fluid (CSF) is essential for diagnosis, identification of pathogens, and appropriate choice of therapy.[11]

The role of the LP as part of the diagnostic evaluation of neonatal sepsis, especially in premature infants in the first 72 hours after birth, remains controversial.[12] The incidence of meningitis among asymptomatic infants with antepartum risk factors for infection alone[13–17] and premature infants with respiratory distress but no other signs of sepsis[18–20] is extremely low. However, 20% to 30% of infants with culture-proven early-onset sepsis (EOS) have concomitant bacterial meningitis.[21,22] Furthermore, about 15% to 38% of infants with confirmed meningitis have negative blood cultures,[4,21,23–25] suggesting that negative blood cultures cannot exclude meningitis in a sick infant. Therefore, selective evaluation of infants with culture-proven bacteremia results in missed cases of meningitis. Clinicians must additionally account for the variability of the presenting signs of meningitis based on birth weight and gestational age.[3] Initial signs of meningitis in the neonate may include temperature instability, lethargy, apnea, and bradycardia, which are nonspecific and often subtle; more classic meningitic signs such as fever, irritability, seizures, and bulging fontanelle are often seen later in the course of meningitis and in infants weighing >2500 g.[3]

In infants under evaluation for early- and late-onset sepsis, an LP is not performed in approximately 30% to 70% of infants, respectively.[4,5] The most common reasons for deferring an LP include the low incidence of neonatal meningitis, especially in the first 72 hours after birth in infants at risk for sepsis[13–15,18–20]; the low yield of the procedure[16,17,26,27]; the risk of complications[28–33]; and the fact that very-low-birth-weight (VLBW) infants (<1500 g birth weight) often have respiratory and cardiovascular compromise with the procedure.[4] However, there are advantages to obtaining an LP promptly. Diagnosing meningitis has implications in management and prognosis, as the duration of therapy has to be increased, and antimicrobial agents with higher degrees of central nervous system (CNS) penetration should be used.[34,35] Initiation of empiric antimicrobial therapy before LP may result in CSF sterilization, leading to underdiagnosis or in unnecessarily prolonged treatment when the possibility of meningitis cannot be excluded.[36] A delay or failure to diagnose meningitis is associated with inappropriate choice in spectrum and duration of antibiotic therapy, partially treated meningitis, increased mortality, and neurologic sequelae.[37]

Increased Susceptibility to Meningitis in Premature Infants

Bacteria can enter the CNS by (1) "receptor-mediated" transcellular movement through meningeal endothelial cells, (2) disruption of intracellular junctions of the cerebral microvasculature, or (3) transport across the blood–brain barrier within leukocytes.[10,38] Infants, especially premature infants, have a number of host defense impairments that increase their vulnerability to serious bacterial, fungal, and viral infections of the CNS, and they lack protective maternal antibodies, which do not cross the placenta until after 32 weeks gestational age.[3,39] Studies in fetal and neonatal animals have demonstrated immaturity and increased permeability of the blood–brain barrier,[40] which is reflected in the elevated CSF protein content of the premature infant.[41] Premature infants are also more likely to have foreign devices such as endotracheal tubes, arterial and venous catheters, and intraventricular devices, placing them at increased risk of invasive infections.[42]

Accumulating evidence links intrauterine and postnatal neonatal infections with adverse neurodevelopmental outcomes in premature infants.[43–47] Exposure of the immature brain, and particularly the white matter, to inflammatory mediators causing cytotoxic injury is associated with increased risk for abnormal cognitive and motor functioning.[48] VLBW infants with meningitis are more likely to have major neurologic disability (45% vs. 11%) and subnormal (<70) Mental Developmental Index results (38% vs. 14%) compared with uninfected infants.[49]

Role of LP in the Evaluation of Early-Onset Sepsis

The Centers for Disease Control and Prevention defines EOS as blood or CSF culture-proven infection within the first week after birth.[50] In hospitalized premature infants, EOS has also been defined as culture-proven infections occurring within the first 3 days after birth.[51,52] The incidence of EOS in the United States is estimated to be 0.8 to 1 per 1000 live births, with the highest incidence among the most premature infants.[5,53–56] Due to widespread implementation of intrapartum antibiotic prophylaxis, the incidence of EOS has declined among term infants; however, whether or not there is a similar decrease in the incidence for premature infants remains unclear.[53] Group B *Streptococcus* (GBS) remains the most frequent isolated pathogen associated with EOS in the United States and other developed countries among term infants, and *Escherichia coli* has emerged as the most common cause in VLBW infants.[5,51,55–57] Among infants with early-onset GBS disease, the most commonly identified syndromes are bacteremia without focus (83%), pneumonia (9%), and meningitis (7%).[58] Collection of CSF via LP is needed to rule out meningitis; however, its role in infants with suspected EOS remains controversial, and clinical practice varies greatly by center.[59]

The yield of CSF cultures in asymptomatic infants who undergo evaluation due to perinatal risk factors for infection is extremely low in the first few days after birth.[13,16,17,27] In a retrospective review of 3423 asymptomatic full-term infants evaluated because of maternal risk factors for infection in the first 7 days after birth, no cases of meningitis were observed.[13] A prospective study of 712 asymptomatic infants who underwent LP during the first week after birth for suspected sepsis found nine positive CSF cultures (13%); however, only one infant had concomitant bacteremia and a clinical course consistent with meningitis, and the remaining cases were considered contaminants.[17] Consistent with these findings, a review of 506 infants at risk for infection or with suspected sepsis found no cases of meningitis among 263 infants who underwent LP within the first 72 hours after birth.[27] However, the incidence of positive CSF cultures increases with advancing postnatal age; after 7 days of age, the incidence of meningitis in infants evaluated for sepsis may be as high as 10%.[27] Conversely, a retrospective review of 169,849 infants born in U.S. Army hospitals during a 5-year period identified 43 cases of meningitis in the first 72 hours after birth. Of these 43 cases, five occurred in premature infants with respiratory distress syndrome (RDS), eight were born at term with no specific CNS symptoms and negative blood cultures, and three had positive blood cultures but were asymptomatic.[37] Those findings were worrisome because it suggested that meningitis can occur in infants with negative blood cultures who appeared completely well; however, the retrospective nature of that case series makes that observation uncertain. Taking the available evidence into account, it is likely safe to omit routine LPs in well-appearing infants evaluated because of maternal risk factors (Table 7.1).

TABLE 7.1 Role of LP in Infant Sepsis Evaluation

Study	Population	Results	Conclusions
Johnson et al., 1997[13]	Full-term infants with suspected sepsis in the first 7 days after birth (*N* = 5135)	11/1712 (0.6%) symptomatic infants had meningitis. 0/3423 asymptomatic infants had meningitis.	LP is unnecessary in asymptomatic full-term infants.
Fielkow et al., 1991[16]	Infants with LP in the first 7 days after birth (*N* = 1073)	13/789 (1.6%) symptomatic infants had meningitis. 0/284 asymptomatic infants had meningitis.	LP is not indicated in asymptomatic infants evaluated for sepsis because of maternal risk factors, including chorioamnionitis.
Schwersenski et al., 1991[17]	Infants with LP in the first 7 days after birth (*N* = 712) Infants with LP after 7 days after birth (*N* = 114)	1/712 (0.1%) infants with suspected sepsis had meningitis with concomitant culture-proven bacteremia. 4/114 (3.5%) infants with suspected sepsis had meningitis. 3/114 (2.6%) had concomitant culture-proven bacteremia.	Incidence of coexistent meningitis and sepsis in the first 7 days after birth is extremely low. Routine LPs in asymptomatic infants with risk factors for infection in the first 7 days after birth are not justified. Incidence of coexistent meningitis and sepsis after the first week after birth is 2.6%. Yield of LPs is higher when performed for specific indications after 7 days after birth.
Ajayi and Mokuolu, 1997[27]	Infants with suspected sepsis in the first 72 hours, between 72 hours and 7 days, and after 7 days after birth (*N* = 506)	0/263 had meningitis in the first 72 hours. 9/115 (8%) had meningitis between 72 hours and 7 days after birth. 13/128 (10%) had meningitis after 7 days after birth.	Changing to a selective approach did not result in missed cases of meningitis in the first 72 hours after birth. LPs should be reserved for infants with bacteremia or CNS signs in the evaluation of EOS. CSF yield increases with age.

Continued

TABLE 7.1 Role of LP in Infant Sepsis Evaluation—cont'd

Study	Population	Results	Conclusions
Wiswell et al., 1995[37]	Infants at 29–42 weeks' gestation with culture-proven meningitis in the first 72 hours after birth (*N* = 43)	5/43 (12%) premature infants with RDS. 3/43 (7%) asymptomatic term infants with bacteremia. 8/43 (19%) term infants with no CNS symptoms and negative BC.	Using selective criteria to perform LPs in the first 72 hours resulted in delayed or missed diagnoses of meningitis in 37% of the cases.
Eldadah et al., 1987[19]	Infants at 23 and 40 weeks' gestation with RDS and suspected sepsis in the first 24 hours after birth (*N* = 238)	17/238 (7%) infants had culture-proven bacteremia. 0/203 infants had meningitis.	Risks of LP may exceed benefits in infants with RDS and no specific signs of CNS infection.
Hendricks-Muñoz and Shapiro, 1990[18]	Infants at ≤34 weeks' gestation with suspected sepsis in the first 6 hours after birth (*N* = 1390)	32/1390 (2.3%) infants had culture-proven sepsis. 0/1390 had meningitis or partially treated meningitis in the first 24 hours. 112/123 infants with initial negative BC developed LOS (38% cases of meningitis).	Omission of LP in early sepsis evaluation in premature infants does not result in missed diagnosis of meningitis in the first 24 hours after birth. LP is essential in the evaluation of LOS.
Weiss et al., 1991[20]	Infants at ≤36 weeks' gestation with RDS who underwent LP in the first day after birth (*N* = 1495)	4/1495 (0.3%) infants had meningitis. 3/1495 (0.2%) had concomitant culture-proven bacteremia.	LP should be performed in selected cases in premature infants with RDS.
Kumar et al., 1995[60]	Infants with LP for suspected sepsis (*N* = 169)	5/148 (3.3%) symptomatic infants had meningitis with no culture-proven bacteremia. 0/21 asymptomatic infants had meningitis evaluated for maternal risk factors.	LP may be omitted in asymptomatic infants with risk factors but should be performed in infants with clinical sepsis.
Stoll et al., 2004[4]	VLBW infants with suspected sepsis after 72 hours after birth (*N* = 9641)	134/9641 (1.4%) infants had meningitis. 89/134 (66%) infants with meningitis had culture-proven bacteremia.	Meningitis may be underdiagnosed. LP should be part of LOS evaluation among VLBW infants.

BC, blood culture; *LOS*, late-onset sepsis.

Similarly, the incidence of meningitis in premature infants with RDS is low.[19,20] In a retrospective review of 238 infants born between 23 and 40 weeks' gestation admitted with RDS and evaluated for suspected sepsis within the first 24 hours after birth, no cases of meningitis were found among 203 CSF cultures collected.[19] The authors suggested reserving LPs for infants with RDS with positive blood cultures or infants with other concomitant signs after 24 hours of age, such as hypothermia or hyperthermia, poor feeding, or specific CNS signs. Supporting a selective approach in premature infants with RDS, only four cases of proven early-onset meningitis were found among 1495 infants at 27 to 36 weeks' gestation who were admitted with respiratory distress and evaluated for sepsis with an LP within the first 24 hours after birth.[20] Another retrospective case review of 1390 premature infants who were ≤34 weeks' gestation and evaluated for sepsis identified 32 infants with bacteremia in the first 6 hours after birth but no missed cases of meningitis (confirmed by autopsy in infants who died).[18] Therefore, deferring or omitting LP from EOS evaluation in premature infants with RDS when the clinician believes that the infant's signs correspond to a noninfectious condition is a reasonable approach (see Table 7.1).

Current recommendations by the American Academy of Pediatrics (AAP) Committee on Fetus and Newborn suggest performing an LP as part of the evaluation of EOS in (1) infants with bacteremia, (2) infants with signs of infection when clinically stable, (3) infants with suspected bacteremia based on laboratory findings, and (4) infants with clinical deterioration despite initial antibiotic treatment.[12]

Role of LP in the Evaluation of Late-Onset Sepsis

Late-onset sepsis (LOS), sepsis occurring after postnatal day 3,[61,62] occurs most commonly among VLBW infants with a median age of infection on postnatal day 18.[57] The incidence of LOS in developed countries is three per 1000 live births[57] and varies inversely with gestational age and birth weight and across clinical centers.[63–66] The incidence of LOS in VLBW infants ranges from 21% to 41%.[62,65] Risk factors for LOS include long-term mechanical ventilation, presence of central lines, absence of early breast milk feeding, prolonged administration of parenteral nutrition, surgical intervention, and increased length of stay.[63] Gram-positive organisms are the most commonly isolated pathogens in LOS (63%–78%), with coagulase-negative staphylococci accounting for the majority of episodes, followed by Gram-negative organisms (19%–25%), including *Escherichia coli* (5%–8%) and *Klebsiella* spp. (5%–6%).[4,61,65] With advances in neonatal care improving the survival of extremely premature infants, invasive candidiasis has become an increasingly important cause of morbidity and mortality, affecting approximately 9% of VLBW and extremely low-birth-weight infants during hospitalization. Among infants in this population who develop invasive candidiasis, 20% die and 50% of survivors have severe neurodevelopmental impairment.[67–69] About 5% to 9% of candidemic premature infants develop *Candida* meningitis.[67,68]

Meningitis is more common in infants evaluated for LOS compared with infants evaluated for EOS.[17,27] A fivefold increase in the yield of LP has been observed after the first week after birth.[17] Among infants with late-onset GBS disease, up to 27% may present with meningitis.[58,70] However, the role of LP as part of the evaluation of LOS, and particularly among VLBW infants, is controversial, and clinical practice varies (see Table 7.1). A survey of 69 Australian neonatologists found that only 51% of practitioners performed routine LPs in premature infants with suspected LOS.[71] Some authors have suggested a selective approach to inclusion of LP in the evaluation of LOS, limiting the procedure to infants with neurologic signs, absence of signs of specific organ infection, bacteremia, and the presence of risk factors such as central lines, mechanical ventilation, and VLBW.[72] However, there is considerable evidence that meningitis after 72 hours of age may occur in the absence of a positive blood culture, as approximately one-third of infants with bacterial meningitis[4,23–25,57] and one-half of infants with *Candida* meningitis[68,73] have negative blood cultures.

An LP might be considered part of the routine evaluation of suspected LOS for the following reasons: (1) the clinical presentation of meningitis is indistinguishable from that of sepsis; (2) meningitis may occur in the absence of a positive blood culture; (3) the incidence of Gram-negative or fungal organisms is higher in LOS with increased risk of poor outcomes; (4) late-onset infection due to GBS is more likely to be associated with meningitis; and (5) meningitis is more common in infants evaluated for LOS compared with EOS. Failure to perform an LP in VLBW infants with suspected LOS may result in missed or partially treated cases of meningitis. In this highly vulnerable population, with increased severity of illness and mortality, the risk of potentially devastating outcomes from not performing an LP may be greater than the potential benefit of avoiding an LP.[4,34,74–77] However, some clinicians recommend a more selective approach to LP in infants with suspected LOS to include any infant with a positive blood culture, infants with clinical signs or laboratory data suggestive of sepsis, and infants who do not respond to conventional antibiotic therapy in the usual fashion.

Role of LP in Viral Meningitis

Although most cases are benign, some viral CNS infections may result in increased morbidity and mortality if not properly diagnosed and treatment is not initiated promptly.[78] Enterovirus infection is the most common cause of viral meningitis in young infants and children, particularly during summer and early fall outbreaks.[79,80] Although most cases are benign and self-limited, recent case series have linked neonatal enteroviral infections with periventricular leukomalacia,[81,82] and infants with enterovirus myocarditis have shown an increased risk of mortality.[83–85] The clinical presentation of enteroviral sepsis and meningitis is nonspecific and may resemble bacterial sepsis or meningitis.[86] CSF analysis by reverse transcription–polymerase chain reaction is an efficient method for diagnosing enteroviral meningitis, regardless of CSF profile, particularly in infants ≤3 months of age.[87–90]

Neonatal herpes simplex virus (HSV) infection occurs in one out of every 3200 live births in the United States[91] and is associated with significant mortality and long-term sequelae among survivors, including seizures, psychomotor retardation, spasticity, and learning disabilities.[92,93] The disease can present in three different patterns: (1) 25% of cases involve multiple visceral organs, with or without CNS compromise (disseminated disease); (2) 30% have CNS disease, with or without skin, eye, or mouth involvement; and (3) 45% are localized to the skin, eye, or mouth.[94] HSV infection should always be considered in infants with suspected sepsis, particularly if they fail to improve after 48 hours of antibiotic therapy with persistently negative bacterial cultures.[94,95] The AAP Committee on Infectious Diseases recommends considering HSV infection in infants with fever, irritability, and abnormal CSF findings, particularly in the presence of seizures. CSF polymerase chain reaction (PCR) is the method of choice for documenting CNS disease in infants with suspected HSV infection.[96–98] Approximately half of all infants with HSV infection have CNS involvement (CNS-isolated disease or disseminated disease with CNS involvement).[99] Given that only 20% of infants with disseminated HSV infection and 50% of infants with CNS disease develop cutaneous vesicles, an LP should be performed for detection of HSV DNA in the CSF in any infant with a suspected HSV infection.[100]

Asymptomatic infants born to mothers with visible genital lesions characteristic of HSV and no previous history of genital HSV should undergo evaluation with HSV CSF PCR at 24 hours of age.[101] However, HSV CSF PCR in infants born to mothers with a previous history of genital HSV is only indicated when surface cultures or the blood or surface PCR result is positive.[101]

Clinicians should consider HSV infection in the differential diagnosis of any acutely ill infant and have a low threshold to perform an LP, as the outcome depends on early diagnosis and prompt antiviral therapy.[99] Because persistent HSV DNA detection in the CSF by PCR after completion of antiviral therapy is associated with increased risk of death or moderate to severe neurologic impairment,[96,101,102] all infants with confirmed HSV CNS disease should undergo a repeat LP at the end of treatment to document CSF clearance, and intravenous antiviral therapy should be continued if the CSF PCR remains positive.[99,103] Although a positive PCR is highly predictive of HSV infection, a negative result does not eliminate the possibility of CNS disease, and in cases in which HSV cannot be ruled out antiviral therapy should be initiated or continued.[102,104]

Risks Associated With LP in Newborn Infants

Concerns about the dangers of LP, particularly in a population with cardiovascular or respiratory instability, are the most common reasons for deferring or omitting the procedure.[4] Studies in animal models have shown an association between performance of an LP during bacteremia and later development of meningitis, possibly due to bacterial invasion of the subarachnoid space after microtrauma.[105,106] However, observational studies in infants and children found that the incidence of meningitis was not significantly different between patients with bacteremia who underwent an LP and those without a diagnostic LP.[107,108] Therefore, an LP in an infant with suspected bacteremia should not be omitted for theoretical concerns of inducing meningitis, as the risk of missing the diagnosis of meningitis is higher than the possibility of meningeal infection derived from the procedure.[109] Although infectious complications are rare, repeated LPs have been associated with lumbar epidural abscess and vertebral osteomyelitis in premature infants with posthemorrhagic hydrocephalus.[30]

Transtentorial or transforaminal herniation resulting from raised intracranial pressure after LP is a potential risk[31,32,110]; however, this event is rare in the neonatal period due to the increased compliance of the neonatal skull in the setting of open fontanelles.[111,112] Rare cases of infants presenting with uncal or cerebellar herniation are related to other concomitant disease processes that increase intracranial pressure, such as galactosemia[113] and large cerebral infarcts.[114]

LPs may be associated with later development of epidermoid spinal tumors through the iatrogenic implantation of epidermal fragments into the spinal canal during the procedure,[33,115] especially when performed with a needle with no stylet.[116,117] To avoid this risk, some authors recommend using the smallest needle available with the stylet in place until the skin is punctured.[117,118]

Intramedullary or epidural hemorrhage is a rare but serious complication of LP in infants and children that can cause severe neurologic sequelae such as paraplegia,[119] but it usually occurs in the presence of coagulopathy[120,121] and can result from injury to the conus medullaris in premature infants.[122] Recent imaging techniques have demonstrated that CSF leakage into the epidural space after LP is common in infants and reveals a characteristic sonographic appearance.[123] Among 33 infants who underwent LP during the first 21 days after birth, 21 cases of CSF leakage were identified by spinal sonography. Although obliteration of the subarachnoid space may occur when the fluid collection is extensive, complete resorption was observed in all cases with no evident sequelae.

LPs performed in the first three postnatal days may be associated with severe intraventricular hemorrhage (IVH) in premature infants.[124] There are many plausible explanations for the link between LPs and IVH, including fluctuations in cerebral blood flow secondary to head position during LP procedure, loss of CSF volume, and transient alterations in pO_2 and pCO_2.[124] One study of 106,461 VLBW infants showed that grade III and IV IVH was higher for infants who underwent LP in the first three days of life with adjusted odds ratios of 2.64 on postnatal day 0, 2.21 on postnatal day 1, 1.55 on postnatal day 2, and 2.25 on postnatal day 3.[124] Another study assessing the complication rate of LPs in term and preterm infants reported two out of 204 infants with IVH within 72 hours after LP.[125] Both instances of IVH were considered low grade, and one was diagnosed in the setting of severe septic shock, calling into question whether the LP was directly associated with the resultant IVH.[125] Further research is needed to further elucidate whether an LP is simply a marker of severe illness or is independently associated with an increased risk of IVH.

Hypoxemia and clinical deterioration can occur in infants undergoing an LP, especially in those who are premature and VLBW with respiratory insufficiency.[28,126–128] Although drops in mean transcutaneous pO_2 may occur with each of the three most commonly used positions for an LP (lateral flexed, lateral extended, and upright positions), the decrease in oxygenation is more prominent in the flexed position, leading some authors to recommend the upright or modified flexed position with neck extension in infants.[28,128] Best practices for positioning during neonatal LPs and early versus late stylet removal are currently being investigated by the NeoCLEAR study group; study results and recommendations will be forthcoming.[129] Desaturation events are most likely to occur in infants of lower gestational age and those requiring either non-invasive respiratory support or mechanical ventilation at the time of the LP.[125] Preoxygenation before the LP has been recommended by some authors[127]; however, excessive oxygen administration may lead to increased morbidities (e.g., retinopathy of prematurity) and should not be routinely used.[130–132]

In addition to the increased risk of complications in premature infants, performing an LP in this population can be technically challenging due to the small anatomic structures. However, successful access of the subarachnoid space has been reported in small infants in the setting of administration of spinal anesthesia.[133–136] In technically challenging cases, the upright position facilitates the procedure, as it provides the largest interspinous space for the vast majority of infants and can be performed safely.[134,137]

Role of Ultrasound in Performing LPs

The use of ultrasound (US) has been recently incorporated into many procedures performed in the NICU, including LPs.[138] The anatomical landmarks for LP can be difficult to assess clinically, particularly in infants, and US can increase the clinician's confidence in appropriate landmarks.[139,140] US may be additionally helpful in VLBW and extremely low-birth-weight infants, as they tend to have less vertebral ossification, thus allowing for better visualization of the spinal canal.[141] However, whether US increases first time and overall success in addition to reducing the incidence of traumatic LPs remains to be fully elucidated.[125,141,142] US may also have utility in detecting neonatal meningitis in the absence of LP, as one study suggests spinal US findings of debris, septations, and decreased spinal cord pulsations have a sensitivity of 67% and specificity of 92% in infants with meningitis.[143]

Are There Any Contraindications to Performing an LP in the Newborn Infant?

Although thrombocytopenia is a significant risk factor for spinal hemorrhages,[144] reports in infants are scarce, and evidence supporting the appropriate platelet count threshold before inserting a needle or catheter is lacking.[145] To alleviate the risk of bleeding related to the procedure, thrombocytopenia may be corrected with platelet transfusion before the LP or epidural anesthesia. Studies in thrombocytopenic children with oncologic diseases requiring routine LPs reported no procedure-related hemorrhage with platelet counts $<50 \times 10^9$/L.[146–148] Currently, the National Institute for Health and Care Excellence (NICE) guidelines on the management of blood transfusions recommend considering prophylactic platelet transfusions to raise the platelet count above 50×10^9/L in patients who are having invasive procedures.[149] Unless thrombocytopenia is profound ($<50 \times 10^9$/L), performing an LP in thrombocytopenic infants is likely safe, and delaying the procedure is not justified.

Skin infection near the site of puncture can increase the risk of spreading the infection with the needle from adjacent soft tissue into the bone, resulting in osteomyelitis.[150–152] Therefore, performing an LP over an area of infection is not recommended. LP should be deferred in severely ill infants with cardiorespiratory compromise, as it may produce hypoxemia and further clinical deterioration.[11] The 2010 NICE clinical guidelines on recognition, diagnosis, and management of bacterial meningitis in children recommend delaying LP when contraindications are present until they no longer exist. In all cases, the decision to perform an LP should not delay the initiation of antibiotic therapy.[153]

LPs in the Setting of Antibiotic Exposure: Are They Useful?

CSF cultures are the gold standard for the diagnosis of meningitis, but interpretation of LP results can be challenging. A significant number of infants are exposed to intrapartum or empiric antibiotics before LP, which can reduce the yield of CSF cultures and obscure the diagnosis of meningitis.[23,36,154] In a retrospective review including 128 children and infants from 1 day to 16 years of age with suspected or confirmed bacterial meningitis, parenteral exposure to third-generation cephalosporins before the performance of an LP resulted in CSF sterilization of meningococcus within 2 hours and pneumococcus within 4 to 10 hours of initiation of therapy.[36] Similarly, CSF cultures may be "falsely negative" in infants born to mothers who received intrapartum antibiotics for chorioamnionitis or GBS colonization. Many antimicrobial agents (including penicillin and ampicillin) cross the placenta, reaching the fetal circulation. Intrapartum antibiotics may interfere with the growth of bacteria and increase the likelihood of false-negative cultures.[23,37,50] The low yield of CSF cultures in the setting of antibiotic exposure may result in an inability to adjust therapy based on antimicrobial susceptibility or unnecessarily prolonged treatment if the possibility of bacterial meningitis cannot be excluded. However, delaying antimicrobial therapy has been associated with short-term morbidity, including seizures, subdural effusions, hemiparesis, and long-term neurologic impairments.[155] To avoid this situation, clinicians often rely on CSF parameters rather than cultures to determine the likelihood of meningitis. However, reference ranges of CSF parameters and those indicative of neonatal meningitis are the subject of debate and may be affected by several factors such as gestational age, postnatal age, antibiotic exposure, and traumatic taps.[156] The mean white blood cell (WBC) count in healthy, uninfected preterm or term infants in most studies is <10 cells/mm^3,[24,157–160] CSF protein concentrations in uninfected term infants are usually <100 mg/dL, and premature infants show higher values that vary inversely with gestational and postnatal age.[159–163] CSF glucose concentrations in normoglycemic and noninfected infants are usually between 70% and 80% of the serum level and increase with each month after birth,[12,161] with no significant differences between preterm and term infants[159,164]; values are lower in infants with meningitis.[24] CSF parameters collected from the largest cohort to date of premature infants demonstrated a poor positive predictive value (PPV) of WBC count, protein, and glucose levels for the diagnosis of meningitis (4%–10%).[24] Consistent with these findings, CSF glucose and protein values were highly variable in a study including 9111 near-term and term infants with and without meningitis. In addition, meningitis occurred in the presence of normal CSF parameters. Therefore, no single value was found useful to exclude the diagnosis of meningitis.[25] Based on these data, CSF parameters, either alone or in combination, have poor sensitivity and poor PPV for diagnosis of meningitis in both preterm and term infants in the absence of CSF cultures.

CSF parameters were studied among a cohort of 13,495 infants who underwent at least one LP for the evaluation of EOS and LOS due to GBS.[23] Infants with culture-proven GBS meningitis showed an increase in WBC count (271 cells/mm^3 vs. 6 cells/mm^3) and protein levels (322 mg/dL vs. 114 mg/dL) and a decrease in glucose concentrations (13 mg/dL vs. 49 mg/dL) compared with infants without meningitis. Because GBS meningitis also occurred among infants exposed to intrapartum prophylaxis and in the setting of negative blood cultures (20%), clinicians should not disregard the risk of GBS disease in the setting of intrapartum antibiotic prophylaxis or when blood cultures are negative for GBS.[23]

The interpretation of the CSF WBC count in infants exposed to antibiotics is also complicated by the possibility of traumatic LPs, which occurs in up to 50% of cases.[165,166] When the CSF is contaminated with more than 10×10^9/L red cells, CSF WBC counts tend to be lower than predicted by calculations based on the red blood cell (RBC) to WBC ratio, disguising a true leukocytosis and masking the diagnosis of meningitis.[167] Although adjusting WBC counts based on CSF and peripheral RBC counts overestimates the number of WBCs originating from the peripheral blood and underestimates CSF WBCs, potentially leading to missed cases of meningitis,[165] the observed-to-predicted ratio, obtained by dividing the observed CSF WBC by the predicted CSF WBC, may help identify cases of meningitis despite CSF abnormalities in the setting of a traumatic LP.[168,169]

In summary, prenatal or empiric antibiotic exposure may decrease the sensitivity of CSF cultures, increasing the likelihood of false-negative results that can result in missed cases of meningitis. CSF parameters in the neonatal population are highly variable and may be further compromised by antibiotic exposure, as well as traumatic taps. Although some CSF values are suggestive of meningitis, the PPV is poor, and meningitis can occur in the presence of normal WBC, protein, and glucose counts. Therefore, CSF cultures remain the gold standard for diagnosis even in the setting of antibiotic exposure and traumatic taps.

Emerging Role of the BioFire FilmArray

Recent advances in PCR technology may allow for earlier diagnosis of meningitis via the BioFire FilmArray (BFA), which can detect 14 different pathogens including cytomegalovirus, enterovirus, herpes simplex viruses 1 and 2, human herpes virus 6, human parechovirus, varicella zoster virus, *Cryptococcus neoformans/Cryptococcus gattii*, *Escherichia coli* K1, *Haemophilus influenza*, *Listeria monocytogenes*, *Neisseria meningitidis*, and *Streptococcus agalactiae*.[170] Several studies have evaluated the efficacy of the BFA in the clinical setting.[170–172] The BFA demonstrated 100% sensitivity for nine of its 14 analytes (*Cryptococcus gattii*, *Escherichia coli* K1, *Haemophilus influenza*, *Streptococcus pneumoniae*, CMV, HSV-1, HSV-2, human parechovirus, and varicella zoster virus), 95.7% for enteroviruses, and 85.7% for human herpesvirus 6, and the specificity for all analytes was >99.2%.[170] The BFA requires significantly less CSF volume than traditional methods of testing, has the potential to decrease antibiotic and antiviral exposure as its turnaround time is much shorter (1–3 hours) in comparison to standard cultures (24–48 hours), and decreases length of stay.[170,173–177] Currently, there are no known studies of its use in premature infants. However, given its emerging advantages over conventional detection of meningitis, as it can be used effectively in the setting of pretreatment with antibiotics, it is likely that the BFA will play a larger role in the detection of neonatal meningitis.

Repeating LPs in Infants With Meningitis: Is It Necessary?

Repeating an LP during therapy in an infant with culture-proven meningitis has been the subject of debate. Some experts have recommended repeating LP in all patients 24 to 48 hours after initiation of antibiotic therapy to document CSF sterilization, as persistence of positive cultures despite treatment may result in a greater risk of complications and poor outcomes.[178,179] The rationale for repeating CSF examinations has been well documented. A cohort study including 118 infants with culture-proven meningitis and repeat CSF cultures reported that clearance of infection occurred between 2 and 7 days after antibiotics were begun for different organisms. The presence of a second positive culture and persistent elevated WBC is associated with increased mortality.[180,181] With the emergence of antibiotic-resistant bacterial strains, a repeat LP might also be useful to guide antibiotic therapy in infants with no clinical improvement after 48 hours of appropriate antibiotic therapy.[182] Because rapid progression of meningitis has been observed, some authors have suggested that repeating an LP may be justified when the first CSF culture is negative but the clinical picture and other laboratory tests are discordant.[183–186] However, published recommendations do not support repeating the LP routinely.[153,187] The AAP Diagnosis and Management of Meningitis guidelines recommend repeating CSF examination in infants with no clinical evidence of improvement by 24 to 72 hours after the beginning of therapy.[187] In agreement with this, the NICE in 2010 issued guidelines on the management of meningitis and discouraged repeat LPs in infants who are receiving adequate antibiotic therapy and show clinical improvement. Furthermore, they do not recommend an LP before discontinuing therapy if the infant is clinically well.[153] Clinical practice appears to adhere to these guidelines; a survey among 109 pediatricians and neonatologists indicated that the majority of practitioners (82%) did not repeat LPs and preferred a more selective approach based on the clinical findings in the infant.[188]

LPs are sometimes performed after treatment of meningitis to confirm cure by CSF normalization. Different criteria have been proposed for the assessment of CSF findings in the setting of repeated LPs at the end of antibiotic therapy ranging from normal to "acceptable" cell counts, protein, and glucose levels.[189] However, several authors have demonstrated that, despite efficient antibiotic therapy, CSF pleocytosis and abnormally elevated protein concentration are commonly observed when treatment is discontinued.[189–191] Among infants with meningitis who cleared the infection and had at least one abnormal value at the time of the last positive culture, only 4% were found to eventually normalize CSF WBC counts, protein, and glucose levels.[181] Because the ranges of glucose and protein levels and cell counts at the end of treatment vary widely, CSF findings may lead to unnecessary intervention in uninfected infants while failing to recognize those still infected.[189,192] In one study, 44% of infants with bacterial meningitis underwent repeat LPs at the discretion of the treating physician, with those infected with a Gram-negative bacteria being more likely to undergo repeat LPs.[180] A retrospective study that included 165 infants >1 month of age with end-of-treatment LPs found that 13 infants with no late complications or relapse were considered treatment failures based on "abnormal" findings in CSF, leading to additional courses of antibiotics, repeated LPs, and more hospital days. In addition, two patients who had signs consistent with complications of their meningitis had reassuring end-of-treatment CSF findings.[189] Consistent with these findings, a review of 47 children between 2 months and 15 years of age with culture-proven meningitis showed that persistence of CSF abnormalities was not associated with complications of the disease but with prolonged antibiotic treatment beyond 13 days.[192] Based on this evidence, the performance of LP at the end of treatment as a "test of cure" or to define length of therapy is not recommended. The single exception, as mentioned in previous sections, is in the diagnosis of HSV meningitis.

LPs in Infants With Intraventricular Drainage Device–Associated Infection

Posthemorrhagic hydrocephalus is a major complication of intracranial hemorrhage in premature infants associated with significant morbidity and mortality, as well as poor neurodevelopmental outcomes among survivors.[193–195] Two temporary devices are commonly used before the permanent insertion of a ventriculoperitoneal shunt. The ventricular reservoir or ventricular access device is a CSF reservoir connected to a catheter inserted into the ventricles that allows decompression of the ventricular system by serial tapping, and the ventriculosubgaleal shunt consists of a large subgaleal pocket connected to a ventricular catheter that allows continuous CSF diversion.[196]

Infection is a common complication of intraventricular drainage devices (IVDDs), with a reported incidence between 8% and 11%.[197–199] Risk factors include prematurity,[200,201] gestational age at procedure,[197] and previous meningitis.[197,201] Shunt infections are a major source of morbidity and economic burden, with greater need for additional surgical procedures and longer hospital stays.[202,203] They are associated with neurodevelopmental disability[195] and a mortality rate that approaches 10%.[204]

In a cohort of 9704 infants who underwent LP, which included 181 infants with either a ventriculoperitoneal shunt or CSF reservoir placement, no significant differences were observed in WBC counts or protein and glucose levels between those with or without drainage devices.[205] As noted earlier, CSF values in infants with devices were not useful in identifying infants with meningitis. Although CSF eosinophilia was previously considered a marker of infection in infants with IVDDs,[206] recent reports have found no clinical significance in the rise of this parameter for the diagnosis of infection.[205,207] In a case-control study of infants at <34 weeks' gestation with CSF reservoirs who underwent serial taps (5- to 8-day intervals), there was a wide variation in all CSF parameters in infants with negative or positive cultures with abnormal values even in the absence of infection.[199] In addition, the percentages of CSF neutrophils and protein were higher at insertion and declined significantly with subsequent taps, whereas RBC count, glucose, and proportion of lymphocytes and eosinophils showed no significant changes. The authors found that cutoff values of CSF WBC counts of >42 cells/mm^3 and protein >250 mg/dL in later taps after the insertion of IVDDs may result in a sensitivity of almost 90%. However, CSF testing from IVDD in the absence of suspected infection is not recommended due to the limited diagnostic value.[199,205] Moreover, routine culture of shunt components removed at revision in the absence of clinical infection is not recommended, as evidence shows that bacteriologically positive cultures in asymptomatic infants in the majority of cases represents a contaminant and has no therapeutic implications.[208]

Summary

Meningitis is associated with significant morbidity and mortality in the neonatal population. CSF culture obtained via LP is the gold-standard method for the diagnosis of meningitis, and early initiation of antibiotic treatment is paramount to reduce mortality and poor neurodevelopmental outcomes. The most common reason for not performing an LP is that the perceived low incidence of meningitis does not justify the risk of the procedure in an infant with respiratory or cardiovascular compromise. However, despite potential adverse events, LP is not associated with increased mortality. Although clinical practice varies, the current recommendation is to perform an LP routinely in all infants with bacteremia or neurologic signs/symptoms in the neonatal intensive care unit, regardless of gestational age, with suspected EOS or LOS. Before performing an LP, the infant must be clinically stable (Figure 7.1). Repeating the LP during treatment is only justified if there is no clinical evidence of improvement 24 to 72 hours after initiation of therapy, and it is not recommended at the end of treatment to confirm cure in bacterial meningitis.

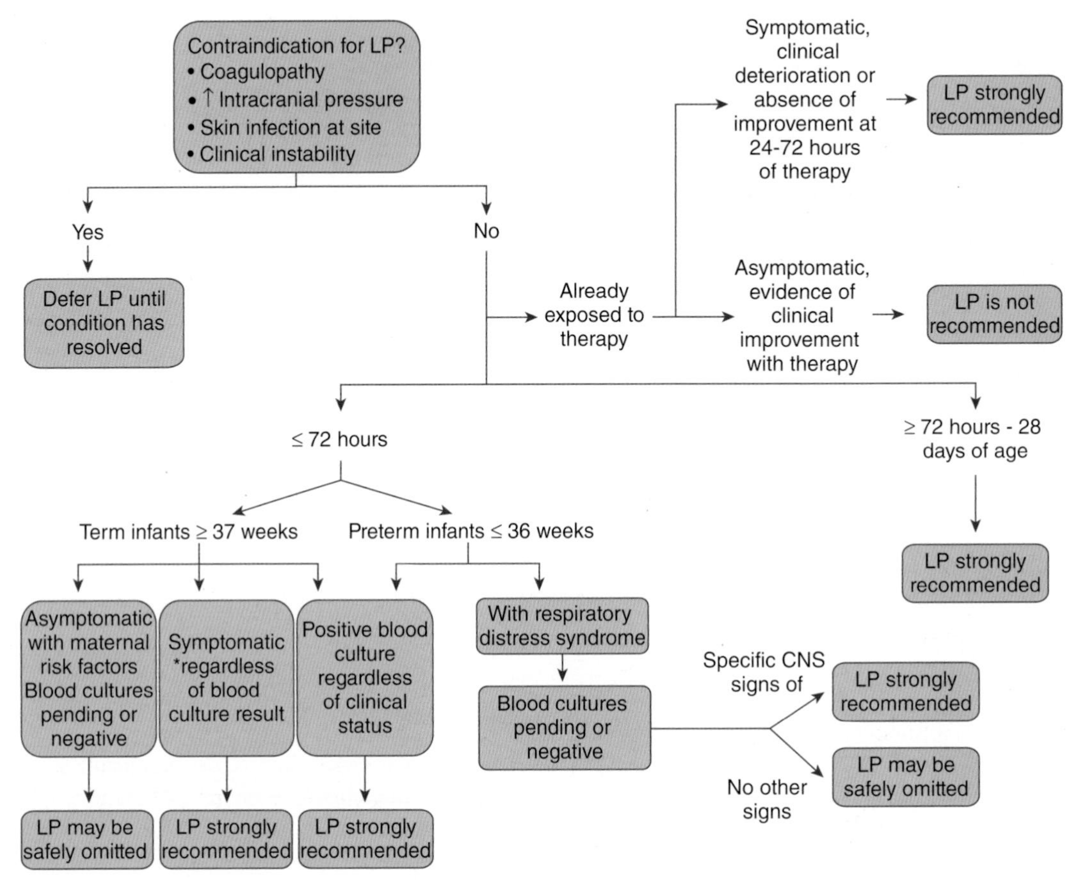

Fig. 7.1 Summary of recommendations of performance of lumbar puncture (LP) in the evaluation of infants at risk for meningitis. (*Symptoms include fever or hypothermia, irritability, hypotonia, poor feeding, apnea, hypotension, seizures, and bulging anterior fontanel.)

REFERENCES

1. Heath PT, Okike IO. Neonatal bacterial meningitis: an update. *Paediatr Child Health*. 2010;20:526-530.
2. Okike IO, Johnson AP, Henderson KL, et al. Incidence, etiology, and outcome of bacterial meningitis in infants aged <90 days in the United Kingdom and Republic of Ireland: prospective, enhanced, national population-based surveillance. *Clin Infect Dis*. 2014;59(10):e150-e157.
3. Aleem S, Greenberg RG. When to include a lumbar puncture in the evaluation for neonatal sepsis. *NeoReviews*. 2019;20(3): e124-e134.
4. Stoll BJ, Hansen N, Fanaroff AA, et al. To tap or not to tap: high likelihood of meningitis without sepsis among very low birth weight infants. *Pediatrics*. 2004;113(5):1181-1186.
5. Stoll BJ, Hansen NI, Sánchez PJ, et al. 2. *Pediatrics*. 2011; 127(5):817-826.
6. Heath PT, Okike IO, Oeser C. Neonatal meningitis: can we do better? *Adv Exp Med Biol*. 2011;719:11-24.
7. Gaschignard J, Levy C, Romain O, et al. Neonatal bacterial meningitis: 444 cases in 7 years. *Pediatr Infect Dis J*. 2011;30(3): 212-217.
8. Thaver D, Zaidi AK. Burden of neonatal infections in developing countries: a review of evidence from community-based studies. *Pediatr Infect Dis J*. 2009;28(suppl 1):S3-S9.
9. de Louvois J, Halket S, Harvey D. Neonatal meningitis in England and Wales: sequelae at 5 years of age. *Eur J Pediatr*. 2005; 164(12):730-734.
10. Polin RA, Harris MC. Neonatal bacterial meningitis. *Semin Neonatol*. 2001;6(2):157-172.
11. Riordan FA, Cant AJ. When to do a lumbar puncture. *Arch Dis Child*. 2002;87(3):235-237.
12. Polin RA. Management of neonates with suspected or proven early-onset bacterial sepsis. *Pediatrics*. 2012;129(5):1006-1015.
13. Johnson CE, Whitwell JK, Pethe K, Saxena K, Super DM. Term newborns who are at risk for sepsis: are lumbar punctures necessary? *Pediatrics*. 1997;99(4):E10.
14. Mecredy RL, Wiswell TE, Hume RF. Outcome of term gestation neonates whose mothers received intrapartum antibiotics for suspected chorioamnionitis. *Am J Perinatol*. 1993;10(5): 365-368.
15. Ray B, Mangalore J, Harikumar C, Tuladhar A. Is lumbar puncture necessary for evaluation of early neonatal sepsis? *Arch Dis Child*. 2006;91(12):1033-1035.

16. Fielkow S, Reuter S, Gotoff SP. Cerebrospinal fluid examination in symptom-free infants with risk factors for infection. *J Pediatr*. 1991;119(6):971-973.
17. Schwersenski J, McIntyre L, Bauer CR. Lumbar puncture frequency and cerebrospinal fluid analysis in the neonate. *Am J Dis Child*. 1991;145(1):54-58.
18. Hendricks-Muñoz KD, Shapiro DL. The role of the lumbar puncture in the admission sepsis evaluation of the premature infant. *J Perinatol*. 1990;10(1):60-64.
19. Eldadah M, Frenkel LD, Hiatt IM, Hegyi T. Evaluation of routine lumbar punctures in newborn infants with respiratory distress syndrome. *Pediatr Infect Dis J*. 1987;6(3):243-246.
20. Weiss MG, Ionides SP, Anderson CL. Meningitis in premature infants with respiratory distress: role of admission lumbar puncture. *J Pediatr*. 1991;119(6):973-975.
21. Visser VE, Hall RT. Lumbar puncture in the evaluation of suspected neonatal sepsis. *J Pediatr*. 1980;96(6):1063-1067.
22. Hoque MM, Ahmed AS, Chowdhury MA, Darmstadt GL, Saha SK. Septicemic neonates without lumbar puncture: what are we missing? *J Trop Pediatr*. 2006;52(1):63-65.
23. Ansong AK, Smith PB, Benjamin DK, et al. Group B streptococcal meningitis: cerebrospinal fluid parameters in the era of intrapartum antibiotic prophylaxis. *Early Hum Dev*. 2009;85 (suppl 10):S5-S7.
24. Smith PB, Garges HP, Cotton CM, Walsh TJ, Clark RH, Benjamin Jr DK. Meningitis in preterm neonates: importance of cerebrospinal fluid parameters. *Am J Perinatol*. 2008;25(7): 421-426.
25. Garges HP, Moody MA, Cotten CM, et al. Neonatal meningitis: what is the correlation among cerebrospinal fluid cultures, blood cultures, and cerebrospinal fluid parameters? *Pediatrics*. 2006;117(4):1094-1100.
26. MacMahon P, Jewes L, de Louvois J. Routine lumbar punctures in the newborn—are they justified? *Eur J Pediatr*. 1990;149(11): 797-799.
27. Ajayi OA, Mokuolu OA. Evaluation of neonates with risk for infection/suspected sepsis: is routine lumbar puncture necessary in the first 72 hours of life? *Trop Med Int Health*. 1997; 2(3):284-288.
28. Weisman LE, Merenstein GB, Steenbarger JR. The effect of lumbar puncture position in sick neonates. *Am J Dis Child*. 1983;137(11):1077-1079.
29. Teele DW, Dashefsky B, Rakusan T, Klein JO. Meningitis after lumbar puncture in children with bacteremia. *N Engl J Med*. 1981;305(18):1079-1081.
30. Bergman I, Wald ER, Meyer JD, Painter MJ. Epidural abscess and vertebral osteomyelitis following serial lumbar punctures. *Pediatrics*. 1983;72(4):476-480.
31. Addy DP. When not to do a lumbar puncture. *Arch Dis Child*. 1987;62(9):873-875.
32. Slack J. Coning and lumbar puncture. *Lancet*. 1980;2(8192): 474-475.
33. Potgieter S, Dimin S, Lagae L, et al. Epidermoid tumours associated with lumbar punctures performed in early neonatal life. *Dev Med Child Neurol*. 1998;40(4):266-269.
34. McIntyre P, Isaacs D. Lumbar puncture in suspected neonatal sepsis. *J Paediatr Child Health*. 1995;31(1):1-2.
35. Adams-Chapman I, Bann CM, Das A, et al. Neurodevelopmental outcome of extremely low birth weight infants with *Candida* infection. *J Pediatr*. 2013;163(4):961-967.e3.
36. Kanegaye JT, Soliemanzadeh P, Bradley JS. Lumbar puncture in pediatric bacterial meningitis: defining the time interval for recovery of cerebrospinal fluid pathogens after parenteral antibiotic pretreatment. *Pediatrics*. 2001;108(5):1169-1174.
37. Wiswell TE, Baumgart S, Gannon CM, Spitzer AR. No lumbar puncture in the evaluation for early neonatal sepsis: will meningitis be missed? *Pediatrics*. 1995;95(6):803-806.
38. Pong A, Bradley JS. Bacterial meningitis and the newborn infant. *Infect Dis Clin North Am*. 1999;13(3):711-733, viii.
39. Camacho-Gonzalez A, Spearman PW, Stoll BJ. Neonatal infectious diseases: evaluation of neonatal sepsis. *Pediatr Clin North Am*. 2013;60(2):367-389.
40. Saunders NR, Dreifuss JJ, Dziegielewska KM, et al. The rights and wrongs of blood–brain barrier permeability studies: a walk through 100 years of history. *Front Neurosci*. 2014;8:404.
41. Bauer CH, New MI, Miller JM. Cerebrospinal fluid protein values of premature infants. *J Pediatr*. 1965;66:1017-1022.
42. Edwards M. Postnatal bacterial infections. In: Martin R, Fanaroff AA, Walsh MC, eds. *Fanaroff and Martin's Neonatal-Perinatal Medicine: Diseases of the Fetus and Infant*. 9th ed. Philadelphia, PA: Elsevier; 2011:793-830.
43. Dammann O, Leviton A. Brain damage in preterm newborns: might enhancement of developmentally regulated endogenous protection open a door for prevention? *Pediatrics*. 1999;104 (3 Pt 1):541-550.
44. Perlman JM. White matter injury in the preterm infant: an important determination of abnormal neurodevelopment outcome. *Early Hum Dev*. 1998;53(2):99-120.
45. Jacobsson B. Infectious and inflammatory mechanisms in preterm birth and cerebral palsy. *Eur J Obstet Gynecol Reprod Biol*. 2004;115(2):159-160.
46. Schlapbach LJ, Aebischer M, Adams M, et al. Impact of sepsis on neurodevelopmental outcome in a Swiss National Cohort of extremely premature infants. *Pediatrics*. 2011;128(2): e348-e357.
47. Mitha A, Foix-L'Hélias L, Arnaud C, et al. Neonatal infection and 5-year neurodevelopmental outcome of very preterm infants. *Pediatrics*. 2013;132(2):e372-e380.
48. Adams-Chapman I, Stoll BJ. Neonatal infection and long-term neurodevelopmental outcome in the preterm infant. *Curr Opin Infect Dis*. 2006;19(3):290-297.
49. Doctor BA, Newman N, Minich NM, Taylor HG, Fanaroff AA, Hack M. Clinical outcomes of neonatal meningitis in very-low birth-weight infants. *Clin Pediatr (Phila)*. 2001;40(9):473-480.
50. Verani JR, McGee L, Schrag SJ. Prevention of perinatal group B streptococcal disease—revised guidelines from CDC, 2010. *MMWR Recomm Rep*. 2010;59(RR-10):1-36.
51. Stoll BJ, Hansen N, Fanaroff AA, et al. Changes in pathogens causing early-onset sepsis in very-low-birth-weight infants. *N Engl J Med*. 2002;347(4):240-247.
52. Hornik CP, Fort P, Clark RH, et al. Early and late onset sepsis in very-low-birth-weight infants from a large group of neonatal intensive care units. *Early Hum Dev*. 2012;88(suppl 2):S69-S74.
53. Puopolo KM, Benitz WE, Zaoutis TE. Management of neonates born at ≤34 6/7 weeks' gestation with suspected or proven early-onset bacterial sepsis. *Pediatrics*. 2018;142(6):e20182896.
54. Weston EJ, Pondo T, Lewis MM, et al. The burden of invasive early-onset neonatal sepsis in the United States, 2005–2008. *Pediatr Infect Dis J*. 2011;30(11):937-941.
55. Polcwiartek LB, Smith PB, Benjamin DK, et al. Early-onset sepsis in term infants admitted to neonatal intensive care units (2011–2016). *J Perinatol*. 2021;41(1):157-163.
56. Stoll BJ, Puopolo KM, Hansen NI, et al. Early-onset neonatal sepsis 2015 to 2017, the rise of *Escherichia coli*, and the need

for novel prevention strategies. *JAMA Pediatr*. 2020;174(7):e200593.
57. Vergnano S, Menson E, Kennea N, et al. Neonatal infections in England: the NeonIN surveillance network. *Arch Dis Child Fetal Neonatal Ed*. 2011;96(1):F9-F14.
58. Phares CR, Lynfield R, Farley MM, et al. Epidemiology of invasive group B streptococcal disease in the United States, 1999–2005. *JAMA*. 2008;299(17):2056-2065.
59. Patrick SW, Schumacher RE, Davis MM. Variation in lumbar punctures for early onset neonatal sepsis: a nationally representative serial cross-sectional analysis, 2003–2009. *BMC Pediatr*. 2012;12:134.
60. Kumar P, Sarkar S, Narang A. Role of routine lumbar puncture in neonatal sepsis. *J Paediatr Child Health*. 1995;31(1):8-10.
61. Shane AL, Stoll BJ. Neonatal sepsis: progress towards improved outcomes. *J Infect*. 2014;68(suppl 1):S24-S32.
62. Stoll BJ, Hansen N, Fanaroff AA, et al. Late-onset sepsis in very low birth weight neonates: the experience of the NICHD Neonatal Research Network. *Pediatrics*. 2002;110(2 Pt 1):285-291.
63. Boghossian NS, Page GP, Bell EF, et al. Late-onset sepsis in very low birth weight infants from singleton and multiple-gestation births. *J Pediatr*. 2013;162(6):1120-1124.e1.
64. Tsai MH, Hsu JF, Chu SM, et al. Incidence, clinical characteristics and risk factors for adverse outcome in neonates with late-onset sepsis. *Pediatr Infect Dis J*. 2014;33(1):e7-e13.
65. Greenberg RG, Kandefer S, Do BT, et al. Late-onset sepsis in extremely premature infants: 2000–2011. *Pediatr Infect Dis J*. 2017;36(8):774-779.
66. Chu A, Hageman JR, Schreiber M, Alexander K. Antimicrobial therapy and late onset sepsis. *NeoReviews*. 2012;13(2):e94-e102.
67. Kilpatrick R, Scarrow E, Hornik C, Greenberg RG. Neonatal invasive candidiasis: updates on clinical management and prevention. *Lancet Child Adolesc Health*. 2022;6(1):60-70.
68. Benjamin Jr DK, Stoll BJ, Fanaroff AA, et al. Neonatal candidiasis among extremely low birth weight infants: risk factors, mortality rates, and neurodevelopmental outcomes at 18 to 22 months. *Pediatrics*. 2006;117(1):84-92.
69. Benjamin Jr DK, Stoll BJ, Gantz MG, et al. Neonatal candidiasis: epidemiology, risk factors, and clinical judgment. *Pediatrics*. 2010;126(4):e865-e873.
70. Jordan HT, Farley MM, Craig A, et al. Revisiting the need for vaccine prevention of late-onset neonatal group B streptococcal disease: a multistate, population-based analysis. *Pediatr Infect Dis J*. 2008;27(12):1057-1064.
71. Joshi P, Barr P. The use of lumbar puncture and laboratory tests for sepsis by Australian neonatologists. *J Paediatr Child Health*. 1998;34(1):74-78.
72. Flidel-Rimon O, Leibovitz E, Eventov Friedman S, Juster-Reicher A, Shinwell ES. Is lumbar puncture (LP) required in every workup for suspected late-onset sepsis in neonates? *Acta Paediatr*. 2011;100(2):303-304.
73. Cohen-Wolkowiez M, Smith PB, Mangum B, et al. Neonatal *Candida* meningitis: significance of cerebrospinal fluid parameters and blood cultures. *J Perinatol*. 2007;27(2):97-100.
74. Zea-Vera A, Turín CG, Rueda MS, et al. [Use of lumbar puncture in the evaluation of late-onset sepsis in low birth weight neonates]. *Rev Peru Med Exp Salud Publica*. 2016;33(2):278-282.
75. Malbon K, Mohan R, Nicholl R. Should a neonate with possible late onset infection always have a lumbar puncture? *Arch Dis Child*. 2006;91(1):75-76.
76. Millichap J. Lumbar puncture in late onset neonatal infection. *Pediatr Neurol Briefs*. 2006;20(1):6-7.
77. Kaul V, Harish R, Ganjoo S, Mahajan B, Raina SK, Koul D. Importance of obtaining lumbar puncture in neonates with late onset septicemia a hospital based observational study from north-west India. *J Clin Neonatol*. 2013;2(2):83-87.
78. Norris CM, Danis PG, Gardner TD. Aseptic meningitis in the newborn and young infant. *Am Fam Physician*. 1999;59(10):2761-2770.
79. Romero JR, Newland JG. Viral meningitis and encephalitis: traditional and emerging viral agents. *Semin Pediatr Infect Dis*. 2003;14(2):72-82.
80. March B, Eastwood K, Wright IM, Tilbrook L, Durrheim DN. Epidemiology of enteroviral meningoencephalitis in neonates and young infants. *J Paediatr Child Health*. 2014;50(3):216-220.
81. Verboon-Maciolek MA, Utrecht FG, Cowan F, Govaert P, van Loon AM, de Vries LS. White matter damage in neonatal enterovirus meningoencephalitis. *Neurology*. 2008;71(7):536.
82. Callen J, Paes BA. A case report of a premature infant with coxsackie B1 meningitis. *Adv Neonatal Care*. 2007;7(5):238-247.
83. Schlapbach LJ, Ersch J, Balmer C, et al. Enteroviral myocarditis in neonates. *J Paediatr Child Health*. 2013;49(9):E451-E454.
84. Freund MW, Kleinveld G, Krediet TG, van Loon AM, Verboon-Maciolek MA. Prognosis for neonates with enterovirus myocarditis. *Arch Dis Child Fetal Neonatal Ed*. 2010;95(3):F206-F212.
85. Morriss Jr FH, Lindower JB, Bartlett HL, et al. Neonatal enterovirus infection: case series of clinical sepsis and positive cerebrospinal fluid polymerase chain reaction test with myocarditis and cerebral white matter injury complications. *AJP Rep*. 2016;6(3):e344-e351.
86. Hawkes MT, Vaudry W. Nonpolio enterovirus infection in the neonate and young infant. *Paediatr Child Health*. 2005;10(7):383-388.
87. Hysinger EB, Mainthia R, Fleming A. Enterovirus meningitis with marked pleocytosis. *Hosp Pediatr*. 2012;2(3):173-176.
88. Mulford WS, Buller RS, Arens MQ, Storch GA. Correlation of cerebrospinal fluid (CSF) cell counts and elevated CSF protein levels with enterovirus reverse transcription-PCR results in pediatric and adult patients. *J Clin Microbiol*. 2004;42(9):4199-4203.
89. Graham AK, Murdoch DR. Association between cerebrospinal fluid pleocytosis and enteroviral meningitis. *J Clin Microbiol*. 2005;43(3):1491.
90. Klein-Kremer A, Nir V, Eias K, Nir R-R, Yakubov R, Gershon K. Clinical investigation: the presence of viral meningitis without pleocytosis among pediatric patients. *Open J Pediatr*. 2014;4(4):276-282.
91. Brown ZA, Wald A, Morrow RA, Selke S, Zeh J, Corey L. Effect of serologic status and cesarean delivery on transmission rates of herpes simplex virus from mother to infant. *JAMA*. 2003;289(2):203-209.
92. Overall Jr JC. Herpes simplex virus infection of the fetus and newborn. *Pediatr Ann*. 1994;23(3):131-136.
93. Rudnick CM, Hoekzema GS. Neonatal herpes simplex virus infections. *Am Fam Physician*. 2002;65(6):1138-1142.
94. Martin R, Fanaroff, AA, Walsh, MC, eds. *Fanaroff and Martin's Neonatal-Perinatal Medicine: Diseases of the Fetus and Infant*. 9th ed. Philadelphia, PA: Elsevier; 2011.

95. Amel Jamehdar S, Mammouri G, Sharifi Hoseini MR, et al. Herpes simplex virus infection in neonates and young infants with sepsis. *Iran Red Crescent Med J*. 2014;16(2):e14310.
96. Malm G, Forsgren M. Neonatal herpes simplex virus infections: HSV DNA in cerebrospinal fluid and serum. *Arch Dis Child Fetal Neonatal Ed*. 1999;81(1):F24-F29.
97. Anderson NE, Powell KF, Croxson MC. A polymerase chain reaction assay of cerebrospinal fluid in patients with suspected herpes simplex encephalitis. *J Neurol Neurosurg Psychiatry*. 1993;56(5):520-525.
98. Rowley AH, Whitley RJ, Lakeman FD, Wolinsky SM. Rapid detection of herpes-simplex-virus DNA in cerebrospinal fluid of patients with herpes simplex encephalitis. *Lancet*. 1990;335(8687):440-441.
99. Kimberlin DW, Lin CY, Jacobs RF, et al. Natural history of neonatal herpes simplex virus infections in the acyclovir era. *Pediatrics*. 2001;108(2):223-229.
100. Malm G. Neonatal herpes simplex virus infection. *Semin Fetal Neonatal Med*. 2009;14(4):204-208.
101. Kimberlin DW, Baley J. Guidance on management of asymptomatic neonates born to women with active genital herpes lesions. *Pediatrics*. 2013;131(2):e635-e646.
102. Kimberlin DW, Lakeman FD, Arvin AM, et al. Application of the polymerase chain reaction to the diagnosis and management of neonatal herpes simplex virus disease. National Institute of Allergy and Infectious Diseases Collaborative Antiviral Study Group. *J Infect Dis*. 1996;174(6):1162-1167.
103. Kimberlin D. Herpes simplex virus, meningitis and encephalitis in neonates. *Herpes*. 2004;11(suppl 2):65a-76a.
104. Troendle-Atkins J, Demmler GJ, Buffone GJ. Rapid diagnosis of herpes simplex virus encephalitis by using the polymerase chain reaction. *J Pediatr*. 1993;123(3):376-380.
105. Petersdorf RG, Swarner DR, Garcia M. Studies on the pathogenesis of meningitis. II. Development of meningitis during pneumococcal bacteremia. *J Clin Invest*. 1962;41(2):320-327.
106. Weed LH, Wegeforth P, Ayer JB, et al. The production of meningitis by release of cerebrospinal fluid: during an experimental septicemia: preliminary note. *JAMA*. 1919;72(3):190-193.
107. Pray L. Lumbar puncture as a factor in the pathogenesis of meningitis. *Am J Dis Child*. 1941;62:295-308.
108. Eng RH, Seligman SJ. Lumbar puncture-induced meningitis. *JAMA*. 1981;245(14):1456-1459.
109. Williams J, Lye DC, Umapathi T. Diagnostic lumbar puncture: minimizing complications. *Intern Med J*. 2008;38(7):587-591.
110. Harper JR, Lorber J, Hillas Smith G, Bower BD, Eykyn SJ. Timing of lumbar puncture in severe childhood meningitis. *Br Med J (Clin Res Ed)*. 1985;291(6496):651-652.
111. Davies PA, Rudd PT. Neonatal meningitis. *Clin Devel Med*. 1994;132:83.
112. Polin RA, Yoder MC, eds. *Workbook in Practical Neonatology*. 5th ed. Philadelphia, PA: Elsevier; 2015.
113. Kalay S, Oztekin O, Tezel G, Demirtaş H, Akçakuş M, Oygûr N. Cerebellar herniation after lumbar puncture in galactosemic newborn. *AJP Rep*. 2011;1(1):43-46.
114. Thibert RL, Burns JD, Bhadelia R, Takeoka M. Reversible uncal herniation in a neonate with a large MCA infarct. *Brain Dev*. 2009;31(10):763-765.
115. Ziv ET, Gordon McComb J, Krieger MD, Skaggs DL. Iatrogenic intraspinal epidermoid tumor: two cases and a review of the literature. *Spine (Phila Pa 1976)*. 2004;29(1):E15-E18.
116. Batnitzky S, Keucher TR, Mealey Jr J, Campbell RL. Iatrogenic intraspinal epidermoid tumors. *JAMA*. 1977;237(2):148-150.
117. Shaywitz BA. Epidermoid spinal cord tumors and previous lumbar punctures. *J Pediatr*. 1972;80(4):638-640.
118. Halcrow SJ, Crawford PJ, Craft AW. Epidermoid spinal cord tumour after lumbar puncture. *Arch Dis Child*. 1985;60(10):978-979.
119. Adler MD, Comi AE, Walker AR. Acute hemorrhagic complication of diagnostic lumbar puncture. *Pediatr Emerg Care*. 2001;17(3):184-188.
120. Faillace WJ, Warrier I, Canady AI. Paraplegia after lumbar puncture. In an infant with previously undiagnosed hemophilia A. Treatment and peri-operative considerations. *Clin Pediatr (Phila)*. 1989;28(3):136-138.
121. Cromwell LD, Kerber C, Ferry PC. Spinal cord compression and hematoma: an unusual complication in a hemophiliac infant. *AJR Am J Roentgenol*. 1977;128(5):847-849.
122. Tubbs RS, Smyth MD, Wellons JC III, Oakes WJ. Intramedullary hemorrhage in a neonate after lumbar puncture resulting in paraplegia: a case report. *Pediatrics*. 2004;113(5):1403-1405.
123. Kiechl-Kohlendorfer U, Unsinn KM, Schlenck B, Trawöger R, Gassner I. Cerebrospinal fluid leakage after lumbar puncture in neonates: incidence and sonographic appearance. *AJR Am J Roentgenol*. 2003;181(1):231-234.
124. Testoni D, Hornik CP, Guinsburg R, et al. Early lumbar puncture and risk of intraventricular hemorrhage in very low birth weight infants. *Early Hum Dev*. 2018;117:1-6.
125. Bedetti L, Lugli L, Marrozzini L, et al. Safety and success of lumbar puncture in young infants: a prospective observational study. *Front Pediatr*. 2021;9:692652.
126. Sun S, Vangvanichyakorn K, Aranda Z, Ruiz N, Levine R. 1447 harmful effect of lumbar puncture in newborn infants. *Pediatr Res*. 1981;15:684.
127. Fiser DH, Gober GA, Smith CE, Jackson DC, Walker W. Prevention of hypoxemia during lumbar puncture in infancy with preoxygenation. *Pediatr Emerg Care*. 1993;9(2):81-83.
128. Gleason CA, Martin RJ, Anderson JV, Carlo WA, Sanniti KJ, Fanaroff AA. Optimal position for a spinal tap in preterm infants. *Pediatrics*. 1983;71(1):31-35.
129. Marshall ASJ, Sadarangani M, Scrivens A, et al. Study protocol: NeoCLEAR: neonatal champagne lumbar punctures every time - an RCT: a multicentre, randomised controlled 2 × 2 factorial trial to investigate techniques to increase lumbar puncture success. *BMC Pediatr*. 2020;20(1):165.
130. Weinberger B, Laskin DL, Heck DE, Laskin JD. Oxygen toxicity in premature infants. *Toxicol Appl Pharmacol*. 2002;181(1):60-67.
131. Shahzad T, Radajewski S, Chao CM, Bellusci S, Ehrhardt H. Pathogenesis of bronchopulmonary dysplasia: when inflammation meets organ development. *Mol Cell Pediatr*. 2016;3(1):23.
132. Hartnett ME. Pathophysiology and mechanisms of severe retinopathy of prematurity. *Ophthalmology*. 2015;122(1):200-210.
133. Williams RK, Abajian JC. High spinal anaesthesia for repair of patent ductus arteriosus in neonates. *Paediatr Anaesth*. 1997;7(3):205-209.
134. Webster AC, McKishnie JD, Kenyon CF, Marshall DG. Spinal anaesthesia for inguinal hernia repair in high-risk neonates. *Can J Anaesth*. 1991;38(3):281-286.
135. Nickel US, Meyer RR, Brambrink AM. Spinal anesthesia in an extremely low birth weight infant. *Paediatr Anaesth*. 2005;15(1):58-62.

136. Libby A. Spinal anesthesia in preterm infant undergoing herniorrhaphy. *AANA J*. 2009;77(3):199-206.
137. Öncel S, Günlemez A, Anik Y, Alvur M. Positioning of infants in the neonatal intensive care unit for lumbar puncture as determined by bedside ultrasonography. *Arch Dis Child Fetal Neonatal Ed*. 2013;98(2):F133-F135.
138. Miller LE, Stoller JZ, Fraga MV. Point-of-care ultrasound in the neonatal ICU. *Curr Opin Pediatr*. 2020;32(2):216-227.
139. Baxter B, Evans J, Morris R, et al. Neonatal lumbar puncture: are clinical landmarks accurate? *Arch Dis Child Fetal Neonatal Ed*. 2016;101(5):F448-F450.
140. Kim S, Adler DK. Ultrasound-assisted lumbar puncture in pediatric emergency medicine. *J Emerg Med*. 2014;47(1): 59-64.
141. Stoller JZ, Fraga MV. Real-time ultrasound-guided lumbar puncture in the neonatal intensive care unit. *J Perinatol*. 2021;41(10):2495-2498.
142. Olowoyeye A, Fadahunsi O, Okudo J, Opaneye O, Okwundu C. Ultrasound imaging versus palpation method for diagnostic lumbar puncture in neonates and infants: a systematic review and meta-analysis. *BMJ Paediatr Open*. 2019;3(1):e000412.
143. Nepal P, Sodhi KS, Saxena AK, Bhatia A, Singhi S, Khandelwal N. Role of spinal ultrasound in diagnosis of meningitis in infants younger than 6 months. *Eur J Radiol*. 2015;84(3): 469-473.
144. Evans RW. Complications of lumbar puncture. *Neurol Clin*. 1998;16(1):83-105.
145. Estcourt LJ, Ingram C, Doree C, Trivella M, Stanworth SJ. Use of platelet transfusions prior to lumbar punctures or epidural anaesthesia for the prevention of complications in people with thrombocytopenia. *Cochrane Database Syst Rev*. 2016;(5): CD011980.
146. Foerster MV, Pedrosa FDPR, da Fonseca TCT, Couceiro TCDM, Lima LC. Lumbar punctures in thrombocytopenic children with cancer. *Paediatr Anaesth*. 2015;25(2):206-210.
147. Veen JJ, Vora AJ, Welch JC. Lumbar puncture in thrombocytopenic children. *Br J Haematol*. 2004;127(2):233-234; author reply 234-235.
148. Howard SC, Gajjar A, Ribeiro RC, et al. Safety of lumbar puncture for children with acute lymphoblastic leukemia and thrombocytopenia. *JAMA*. 2000;284(17):2222-2224.
149. Pasquali SK, Sanders SP, Li JS. Oral antihypertensive trial design and analysis under the pediatric exclusivity provision. *Am Heart J*. 2002;144(4):608-614.
150. Wald ER. Risk factors for osteomyelitis. *Am J Med*. 1985; 78(6B):206-212.
151. Findlay L, Kemp FH. Osteomyelitis of the spine following lumbar puncture. *Arch Dis Child*. 1943;18(94):102-105.
152. Feinbloom RI, Halaby FA. Acute pyogenic spondylitis in infancy. A case report to emphasize the potential risk in lumbar puncture. *Clin Pediatr (Phila)*. 1966;5(11):683-684.
153. NICE. *Meningitis (Bacterial) and Meningococcal Septicaemia in Under 16s: Recognition, Diagnosis and Management*. London: National Institute for Health and Care Excellence; 2015.
154. Feldman WE. Effect of prior antibiotic therapy on concentrations of bacteria in CSF. *Am J Dis Child*. 1978;132(7):672-674.
155. Lebel MH, McCracken Jr GH. Delayed cerebrospinal fluid sterilization and adverse outcome of bacterial meningitis in infants and children. *Pediatrics*. 1989;83(2):161-167.
156. Srinivasan L, Harris MC, Shah SS. Lumbar puncture in the neonate: challenges in decision making and interpretation. *Semin Perinatol*. 2012;36(6):445-453.
157. Byington CL, Kendrick J, Sheng X. Normative cerebrospinal fluid profiles in febrile infants. *J Pediatr*. 2011;158(1):130-134.
158. Kestenbaum LA, Ebberson J, Zorc JJ, Hodinka RL, Shah SS. Defining cerebrospinal fluid white blood cell count reference values in neonates and young infants. *Pediatrics*. 2010;125(2): 257-264.
159. Nascimento-Carvalho CM, Moreno-Carvalho OA. Normal cerebrospinal fluid values in full-term gestation and premature neonates. *Arq Neuropsiquiatr*. 1998;56(3A):375-380.
160. Ahmed A, Hickey SM, Ehrett S, et al. Cerebrospinal fluid values in the term neonate. *Pediatr Infect Dis J*. 1996;15(4): 298-303.
161. Mukherjee G, Waris R, Rechler W, et al. Determining normative values for cerebrospinal fluid profiles in infants. *Hosp Pediatr*. 2021;11(9):930-936.
162. Shah SS, Ebberson J, Kestenbaum LA, Hodinka RL, Zorc JJ. Age-specific reference values for cerebrospinal fluid protein concentration in neonates and young infants. *J Hosp Med*. 2011;6(1):22-27.
163. Bonadio WA, Stanco L, Bruce R, Barry D, Smith D. Reference values of normal cerebrospinal fluid composition in infants ages 0 to 8 weeks. *Pediatr Infect Dis J*. 1992;11(7):589-591.
164. Srinivasan L, Shah SS, Padula MA, Abbasi S, McGowan KL, Harris MC. Cerebrospinal fluid reference ranges in term and preterm infants in the neonatal intensive care unit. *J Pediatr*. 2012;161(4):729-734.
165. Greenberg RG, Smith PB, Cotten CM, Moody MA, Clark RH, Benjamin Jr DK. Traumatic lumbar punctures in neonates: test performance of the cerebrospinal fluid white blood cell count. *Pediatr Infect Dis J*. 2008;27(12):1047-1051.
166. Schreiner RL, Kleiman MB. Incidence and effect of traumatic lumbar puncture in the neonate. *Dev Med Child Neurol*. 1979;21(4):483-487.
167. Osborne JP, Pizer B. Effect on the white cell count of contaminating cerebrospinal fluid with blood. *Arch Dis Child*. 1981;56(5):400-401.
168. Bonadio WA, Smith DS, Goddard S, Burroughs J, Khaja G. Distinguishing cerebrospinal fluid abnormalities in children with bacterial meningitis and traumatic lumbar puncture. *J Infect Dis*. 1990;162(1):251-254.
169. Mazor SS, McNulty JE, Roosevelt GE. Interpretation of traumatic lumbar punctures: who can go home? *Pediatrics*. 2003;111(3):525-528.
170. Leber AL, Everhart K, Balada-Llasat JM, et al. Multicenter evaluation of BioFire FilmArray meningitis/encephalitis panel for detection of bacteria, viruses, and yeast in cerebrospinal fluid specimens. *J Clin Microbiol*. 2016;54(9):2251-2261.
171. Hanson KE, Slechta ES, Killpack JA, et al. Preclinical assessment of a fully automated multiplex PCR panel for detection of central nervous system pathogens. *J Clin Microbiol*. 2016;54(3): 785-787.
172. Tansarli GS, Chapin KC. Diagnostic test accuracy of the BioFire® FilmArray® Meningitis/Encephalitis panel: a systematic review and meta-analysis. *Clin Microbiol Infect*. 2020;26(3):281-290.
173. Blaschke AJ, Holmberg KM, Daly JA, et al. Retrospective evaluation of infants aged 1 to 60 days with residual cerebrospinal fluid (CSF) tested using the FilmArray Meningitis/Encephalitis (ME) panel. *J Clin Microbiol*. 2018;56(7):e00277-18.
174. Stark A, Peterson J, Weimer K, Hornik C. Postnatally acquired CMV meningitis diagnosed via BioFire FilmArray: a case report. *J Neonatal Perinatal Med*. 2021;14(3):445-450.

175. Chang D, Okulicz JF, Nielsen LE, White BK. A tertiary care center's experience with novel molecular meningitis/encephalitis diagnostics and implementation with antimicrobial stewardship. *Mil Med*. 2018;183(1-2):e24-e27.
176. Eichinger A, Hagen A, Meyer-Bühn M, Huebner J. Clinical benefits of introducing real-time multiplex PCR for cerebrospinal fluid as routine diagnostic at a tertiary care pediatric center. *Infection*. 2019;47(1):51-58.
177. Nabower AM, Miller S, Biewen B, et al. Association of the FilmArray Meningitis/Encephalitis panel with clinical management. *Hosp Pediatr*. 2019;9(10):763-769.
178. MacDonald MG, Seshia M, Mullett M, eds. *Avery's Neonatology: Pathophysiology and Management of the Newborn*. 5th ed. Philadelphia, PA: Lippincott, Williams & Wilkins; 1999.
179. Heath PT, Nik Yusoff NK, Baker CJ. Neonatal meningitis. *Arch Dis Child Fetal Neonatal Ed*. 2003;88(3):F173-F178.
180. Ting JY, Roberts A, Khan S, et al. Predictive value of repeated cerebrospinal fluid parameters in the outcomes of bacterial meningitis in infants <90 days of age. *PLoS ONE*. 2020;15(8): e0238056.
181. Greenberg RG, Benjamin Jr DK, Cohen-Wolkowiez M, et al. Repeat lumbar punctures in infants with meningitis in the neonatal intensive care unit. *J Perinatol*. 2011;31(6):425-429.
182. Tunkel AR, Scheld WM. Issues in the management of bacterial meningitis. *Am Fam Physician*. 1997;56(5):1355-1362.
183. Kindley AD, Harris F. Repeat lumbar puncture in the diagnosis of meningitis. *Arch Dis Child*. 1978;53(7):590-592.
184. Rapkin RH. Repeat lumbar punctures in the diagnosis of meningitis. *Pediatrics*. 1974;54(1):34-37.
185. Fischer GW, Brenz RW, Alden ER, Beckwith JB. Lumbar punctures and meningitis. *Am J Dis Child*. 1975;129(5):590-592.
186. Heckmatt JZ. Coliform meningitis in the newborn. *Arch Dis Child*. 1976;51(8):569-575.
187. Klein JO, Feigin RD, McCracken Jr GH. Report of the task force on diagnosis and management of meningitis. *Pediatrics*. 1986;78(5 Pt 2):959-982.
188. Agarwal R, Emmerson AJ. Should repeat lumbar punctures be routinely done in neonates with bacterial meningitis? Results of a survey into clinical practice. *Arch Dis Child*. 2001;84(5): 451-452.
189. Durack DT, Spanos A. End-of-treatment spinal tap in bacterial meningitis. Is it worthwhile? *JAMA*. 1982;248(1):75-78.
190. Chartrand SA, Cho CT. Persistent pleocytosis in bacterial meningitis. *J Pediatr*. 1976;88(3):424-426.
191. Bonadio WA, Smith D. Cerebrospinal fluid changes after 48 hours of effective therapy for *Hemophilus influenzae* type B meningitis. *Am J Clin Pathol*. 1990;94(4):426-428.
192. Jacob J, Kaplan RA. Bacterial meningitis. Limitations of repeated lumbar puncture. *Am J Dis Child*. 1977;131(1):46-48.
193. Murphy BP, Inder TE, Rooks V, et al. Posthaemorrhagic ventricular dilatation in the premature infant: natural history and predictors of outcome. *Arch Dis Child Fetal Neonatal Ed*. 2002;87(1):F37-F41.
194. Adams-Chapman I, Hansen NI, Stoll BJ, Higgins R. Neurodevelopmental outcome of extremely low birth weight infants with posthemorrhagic hydrocephalus requiring shunt insertion. *Pediatrics*. 2008;121(5):e1167-e1177.
195. Resch B, Gedermann A, Maurer U, Ritschl E, Müller W. Neurodevelopmental outcome of hydrocephalus following intra-/periventricular hemorrhage in preterm infants: short- and long-term results. *Childs Nerv Syst*. 1996;12(1):27-33.
196. Robinson S. Neonatal posthemorrhagic hydrocephalus from prematurity: pathophysiology and current treatment concepts. *J Neurosurg Pediatr*. 2012;9(3):242-258.
197. Spader HS, Hertzler DA, Kestle JR, Riva-Cambrin J. Risk factors for infection and the effect of an institutional shunt protocol on the incidence of ventricular access device infections in preterm infants. *J Neurosurg Pediatr*. 2015;15(2): 156-160.
198. Drake JM, Kestle JR, Milner R, et al. Randomized trial of cerebrospinal fluid shunt valve design in pediatric hydrocephalus. *Neurosurgery*. 1998;43(2):294-303; discussion 303-305.
199. Bajaj M, Lulic-Botica M, Natarajan G. Evaluation of cerebrospinal fluid parameters in preterm infants with intraventricular reservoirs. *J Perinatol*. 2012;32(10):786-790.
200. Bruinsma N, Stobberingh EE, Herpers MJ, Vles JS, Weber BJ, Gavilanes DA. Subcutaneous ventricular catheter reservoir and ventriculoperitoneal drain-related infections in preterm infants and young children. *Clin Microbiol Infect*. 2000;6(4): 202-206.
201. McGirt MJ, Zaas A, Fuchs HE, George TM, Kaye K, Sexton DJ. Risk factors for pediatric ventriculoperitoneal shunt infection and predictors of infectious pathogens. *Clin Infect Dis*. 2003;36(7):858-862.
202. Kanik A, Sirin S, Kose E, Eliacik K, Anil M, Helvaci M. Clinical and economic results of ventriculoperitoneal shunt infections in children. *Turk Neurosurg*. 2015;25(1):58-62.
203. Morina Q, Kelmendi F, Morina A, Morina D, Bunjaku D. Ventriculoperitoneal shunt complications in a developing country: a single institution experience. *Med Arch*. 2013;67(1): 36-38.
204. Vinchon M, Dhellemmes P. Cerebrospinal fluid shunt infection: risk factors and long-term follow-up. *Childs Nerv Syst*. 2006;22(7):692-697.
205. Lenfestey RW, Smith PB, Moody MA, et al. Predictive value of cerebrospinal fluid parameters in neonates with intraventricular drainage devices. *J Neurosurg*. 2007;107(suppl 3): 209-212.
206. Wiersbitzky SK, Ahrens N, Becker T, Panzig B, Abel J, Stenger RD. The diagnostic importance of eosinophil granulocytes in the CSF of children with ventricular-peritoneal shunt systems. *Acta Neurol Scand*. 1998;97(3):201-203.
207. Lan CC, Wong TT, Chen SJ, Liang ML, Tang RB. Early diagnosis of ventriculoperitoneal shunt infections and malfunctions in children with hydrocephalus. *J Microbiol Immunol Infect*. 2003;36(1):47-50.
208. Steinbok P, Cochrane DD, Kestle JR. The significance of bacteriologically positive ventriculoperitoneal shunt components in the absence of other signs of shunt infection. *J Neurosurg*. 1996;84(4):617-623.

Chapter 8

Perinatal and Neonatal Considerations in COVID-19

Alejandra Barrero-Castillero, MD, MPH

Key Points

- The incidence of COVID-19 in newborns is low; however, COVID-19 can still cause severe illness and complications.
- Evidence related to the COVID-19 pandemic and perinatal and neonatal care continues to evolve, but many unanswered questions remain.
- Pregnant and non-pregnant individuals have similar manifestations of COVID-19 symptoms, but pregnant individuals are at increased risk for severe COVID-19–associated illness; risk is reduced with vaccination.
- Perinatal transmission of SARS-CoV-2 from mothers to their infants is most likely via environmental exposure to aerosolized droplets of viral particles after birth.
- Clinical practices to reduce the transmission have changed throughout the pandemic.
- The COVID-19 pandemic has exposed and magnified disparities deeply rooted in structural racism and socioeconomic inequality that must be addressed when caring for mothers and their newborns.

Introduction

Severe acute respiratory syndrome coronavirus 2 (SARS-CoV-2) is a ribonucleic acid (RNA) respiratory virus responsible for the coronavirus disease 2019 (COVID-19) pandemic. The pandemic's global health crisis continues to challenge countries and public health organizations worldwide.[1,2] COVID-19 was first reported and described in Wuhan, Hubei Province, China, in December 2019.[3,4] Since then, World Health Organization (WHO) data indicate that there have been over 600 million cases globally and over 6 million deaths worldwide. Most deaths have come from the United States (>93 million cases).[5] In adults, including pregnant individuals, symptoms range from asymptomatic through mild influenza-like symptoms to severe respiratory illness, multiple organ failure, and death.[3,4,6] Perinatal and postnatal transmission is low, particularly when appropriate precautions are met.[7–9] Signs of neonatal disease have most commonly ranged from asymptomatic to mildly symptomatic; although relatively rare, the risk of infants acquiring the infection and developing complications is still considerable.[9–12] Severe COVID-19 in pregnancy has been associated with an increased risk of stillbirth, preterm delivery, fetal growth restriction, and cesarean delivery.[13,14] The COVID-19 pandemic has additionally exposed and magnified racial and ethnic health disparities deeply rooted in structural racism and socioeconomic inequality that must be addressed when caring for mothers and their newborns.[15–17] As the rate of infection worldwide continues to change, and scientific evidence continues to evolve, this chapter includes recommendations and important perinatal and neonatal considerations in COVID-19.

SARS-COV-2 ORIGIN

SARS-CoV-2 is an RNA respiratory virus, part of the Coronaviridae family, and is responsible for the COVID-19 pandemic.[2,18] Coronaviruses have been described since the 1960s and have been responsible for causing other pandemics, including SARS-CoV in 2003 and Middle East respiratory syndrome coronavirus (MERS-CoV) in 2012. However, coronavirus is most commonly known for being the agent responsible for the common cold.[3,17–20]

SARS-CoV-2 most likely originated through a zoonotic event, meaning that the infection was likely transmitted from animals to humans. In this case, the virus naturally evolved and most likely spread from a bat to humans or through an intermediate reservoir (possibly a pangolin).[4,19,21] Given that SARS-CoV-2 has a high rate of genetic mutations, there have been many variants identified in different parts of the world, including Delta and Omicron, which are the predominant variants in the United States.[22]

VIRAL CELL ENTRY

The SARS-CoV-2 virus core has a viral capsid with a receptor-binding domain of the SARS-CoV-2 spike (S) glycoprotein that enables binding to the human cell-surface protein angiotensin-converting enzyme 2 (ACE2) on the host cell and initiates viral entry. The S glycoprotein is cleaved by the host protease transmembrane serine protease 2 (TMPRSS-2), allowing the virus to enter the cell cytoplasm by either endocytosis or fusion.[17,23,24] Once inside the cell, the single-stranded viral RNA is replicated into a large polyprotein cleaved by a viral protease into smaller pieces of viral RNA. The viral RNA and proteins are then packed into a nucleocapsid and assembled into a new virion released with new viral copies to infect the host further.[25,26] Given that ACE2 is mainly expressed in the epithelial surfaces in upper and lower airways (also found in other tissues such as the small intestine, brain, blood vessels, and muscle), SARS-CoV-2 causes mainly respiratory illness.[27] The expression of ACE2 and TMPRSS2 in children's airway epithelia is lower compared with adults.[28] These findings, in addition to an immature immune system, likely contribute to the decreased rate of infection and transmission in children, as well as to a milder clinical course.[28,29]

MODE OF TRANSMISSION

Perinatal transmission of SARS-CoV-2 is most commonly via environmental exposure to aerosolized droplets of viral particles after birth and not via the transplacental route.[17,30,31] Other possible evaluated routes include vertical transmission via the placenta, contact with infected secretions during delivery, and breast milk. Although there have been a few positive cases of neonates born to individuals with SARS-CoV-2 right after delivery, there is not enough evidence to support vertical transmission.[7,30,32] SARS-CoV-2 has not yet been isolated from breast milk, but there are a few case reports of viral RNA detection; the latter does not demonstrate potential for transmission by this route, however.[33] In systematic reviews, the percentage of positive tests among neonates born to positive SARS-CoV-2 individuals (as a proxy for perinatal transmission) range from 1% to 9.1%, with no difference between vaginal and cesarean births.[7–9,34,35] The rates vary depending on the study size, timing of publication before and after implementation of maternal surveillance testing, different waves of the pandemic, and different variant peaks.[7] For this reason, the true incidence of neonatal test positivity is unknown.[7] In a multicenter cohort in Massachusetts, the leading risk factor for neonatal test positivity was "maternal social vulnerability."

Prenatal and Obstetrical Considerations

Pregnant and non-pregnant individuals have similar manifestations of COVID-19 symptoms, but pregnant individuals are at increased risk for severe COVID-19–associated illness.[7] Immunologic and physiologic adaptive alterations during pregnancy, including diaphragm elevation and increased heart rate and oxygen consumption, may increase the risk for more severe illness and complications, particularly in respiratory infections.[13,14,36,37] In addition to more severe illness, symptomatic pregnant and recently pregnant people with COVID-19 are at increased risk for hospitalization, admission to the intensive care unit, need for mechanical ventilation, need for extracorporeal membrane oxygenation, and death compared with non-pregnant individuals of reproductive age.[13,37,38] Some complications have been associated with the increased predisposition to hypercoagulability and thrombotic changes in the placenta that may predispose to abnormal oxygenation and adverse perinatal outcomes, including stillbirth.[39] For example, there is an increased prevalence of decidual arteriopathy and other features of maternal vascular malperfusion that may compromise perfusion of the maternal and fetal vasculature.[39,40] Cases of stillbirth have been associated with extensive histological changes with placentitis (marked intervillositis with a mixed inflammatory infiltrate and massive perivillous fibrinoid deposition with trophoblast damage).[41] More studies are needed to clarify the impact of SARS-CoV-2 infection on the physiology of pregnancy, the placenta, and resultant fetal complications.

COVID-19 VACCINATION DURING PREGNANCY AND LACTATION

On December 11, 2020, the U.S. Food and Drug Administration (FDA) released an "Emergency Use Authorization" for the first COVID-19 vaccine for adult use.[42] Despite pregnant individuals being initially excluded from the phase 3 COVID-19 vaccine trials, organizations around the world, including the American College of Obstetricians and Gynecologists (ACOG), the Society for Maternal-Fetal Medicine, and the Centers for Disease Control and Prevention (CDC) strongly recommend that pregnant and lactating individuals be vaccinated against COVID-19, given increased morbidity and mortality from COVID-19 infection.[38,43,44] Vaccination in pregnancy is a safe and effective measure to reduce the risk of complications of COVID-19, and it is recommended that all pregnant and lactating individuals be vaccinated and boosted against COVID-19 regardless of the type of vaccine (including the new bivalent booster protecting for the SARS-CoV-2 Omicron variant) and timing during pregnancy.[32,45] In countries where there are other approved vaccines (e.g., ChAdOx1-S/nCoV-19 [recombinant] vaccine, which is a replication-deficient adenoviral vector vaccine), the recommendation is to receive mRNA vaccines (i.e., Pfizer or Moderna) given the greater availability of safety data on mRNA vaccines than for the adenoviral vaccine.[46] The WHO recommends using the adenoviral vector vaccine in pregnant individuals only when the benefits of vaccination outweigh the potential risks.[47] Recent studies have shown that receipt of a COVID-19 mRNA vaccine results in a robust maternal humoral response that benefits the fetus.[45] Vaccine-elicited antibodies are found in infant cord blood, likely due to maternal immunoglobulin G antibodies crossing the placenta to achieve relatively high titers in the fetus, as well as in breast milk. Vaccinated pregnant and nonpregnant individuals developed cross-reactive antibody responses and T-cell responses against SARS-CoV-2 variants of concern.[45] Given that newborns have an immature immune system, immunity transferred from the placenta via vaccination in pregnancy is essential, mainly to protect the first 6 months of life until the infant becomes eligible to receive COVID-19 vaccination. More longitudinal follow-up data on passive immunity in newborns of vaccinated mothers are necessary.

PRENATAL CARE

The ACOG recommends that all pregnant individuals receive the standard components of prenatal care.[48] During an acute SARS-CoV-2 infection fetal management should be similar to the care provided for any critically ill pregnant person (continuous fetal monitoring in viable fetuses). Table 8.1 describes the antenatal and postnatal recommendations with some adaptations in the setting of COVID-19.

USE OF ANTENATAL CORTICOSTEROIDS IN COVID-19

Evidence suggests that dexamethasone in hospitalized patients with COVID-19 decreases the 28-day mortality in those receiving invasive mechanical ventilation.[55] Thus, ACOG recommends that SARS-CoV-2 status should not alter decision-making regarding antenatal corticosteroid administration. ACOG recommends a course of anten-al steroids for all pregnant individuals at risk for preterm delivery within 7 days with fetuses less than 33 6/7 weeks' gestational age, as well as for late preterm pregnancies 34 0/7 to 36 6/7 weeks' gestational age with no' prior course of steroids administered.[56] Pregnant individuals with SARS-CoV-2 that meet criteria for the use of antenatal corticosteroids for fetal lung maturity should receive standard doses of dexamethasone as follows:

- Initiate with dexamethasone (6 mg intravenous, every 12 hours for four doses) for fetal maturation.
- Continue with the course of treatment for maternal COVID-19 with dexamethasone (6 mg daily, oral or intravenous) for 10 days or until discharge (whichever comes first).[56]

DELIVERY ROOM AND IMMEDIATE POSTNATAL CONSIDERATIONS

COVID-19 has altered the delivery and immediate postnatal experience, with numerous measures in place that have changed throughout the pandemic to

TABLE 8.1 Antenatal and Postnatal Recommendations With Some Adaptations in the Setting of COVID-19

Routine prenatal care	COVID-19 and routine immunizations during pregnancy continue to be essential during the COVID-19 pandemic with no specific timing around the COVID-19 vaccine.[44] ACOG supports the use of telehealth in obstetrics and gynecology and encourages physicians to become familiar with this new technology.[49] General considerations are recommended to avoid exposure to COVID-19 and help prevent the spread (routine hygiene practices and safety measures, including social distancing, limiting contact, and wearing masks), particularly in unvaccinated individuals.
Management of pregnancy complications in patients with SARS-CoV-2	If a pregnancy is complicated by critical illness, the woman should ideally be cared for at a Level III or IV hospital with obstetric services and an adult ICU.[80] COVID-19 status alone is not necessarily a reason to transfer non-critically ill pregnant women with suspected or confirmed COVID-19, but care location planning should be based on the levels of maternal and neonatal care. In December 2021, the FDA issued emergency authorization for pregnant individuals with mild to moderate COVID-19 to receive treatment with Paxlovid (nirmatrelvir tablets and ritonavir tablets).[51]
Postnatal care	Birthing parents with COVID-19 and newborns may room-in according to standard care practices (unless the mother is acutely ill with COVID-19 and is unable to care for the infant safely).[52] Delayed cord clamping and skin-to-skin care in the delivery room should continue per usual center practice in addition to the use of masks.[52] Breastfeeding is strongly recommended as the best feeding choice. Good hand hygiene and the use of masks while breastfeeding is encouraged. Data show that postnatal infections are equally seen in breastfed and formula-fed infants.[32] SARS-CoV-2 RNA has occasionally been found in breast milk after recent infection; however, it has no pathological significance and does not represent any risk for disease transmission to infants.[53] The AAP strongly recommends continuing routine screening and infant care, including newborn screening, hearing screening, and critical congenital heart defect screening, unless community circumstances related to the pandemic require necessary adjustments.[54]
Psychosocial support	Given that pregnant and recently pregnant individuals are at risk of COVID-19–related psychosocial stress, it is recommended that institutions offer mental health or social work services or referrals to additional resources, particularly for patients who are experiencing difficulties related to the COVID-19 pandemic (e.g., housing and food insecurity, mental health disorders). ACOG recommends that all pregnant women get screened for postpartum depression, using the Edinburg Postnatal Depression Scale.

protect the safety of pregnant individuals, caregivers, and newborns. Initial care practices varied, based on experience with other perinatally transmitted viruses, along with an incomplete understanding of the disease pathogenesis and SARS-CoV-2 viral spread. These practices included recommending separation of the mother–infant dyad (i.e., no skin-to-skin care in the delivery room, no rooming-in, and restriction of direct breastfeeding by mothers with known SARS-CoV-2 infection).[31,57,58] In some cases, elective cesarean deliveries were recommended. Separation policies aimed to protect infants from potential harm but did not account for the psychosocial and clinical impact of separation.[17,31] Table 8.1 describes the postnatal recommendations with some adaptations in the setting of COVID-19 based on accumulated evidence from the WHO, American Academy of Pediatrics (AAP), and CDC.[52]

Neonatal COVID-19 Diagnosis and Management

The rate of perinatal acquisition among neonates born to individuals positive for SARS-CoV-2 is low compared to rates in adults and older children.[7,17,29] Death in the newborn period directly attributable to perinatal infection with SARS-CoV-2 is extremely rare in the United States.[52] Despite the low perinatal and postnatal incidence in contrast to older children and adults, COVID-19 can cause severe illness in infants and children, particularly those less than 5 years old who were not eligible for COVID-19 vaccination until recently.[22,59] During the Omicron peak in early 2022 in the United States, there were five times more hospitalizations in children less than 4 years old than during the Delta peak.[22] This hospitalization increase was even greater in infants less than 6 months old. For that reason, vaccination is recommended to all eligible persons (6 months old and older, including pregnant individuals) to reduce the risk for severe disease.[22,59,60] To date, there is no FDA-approved vaccine for infants less than 6 months of age.[59] In addition to the risk of neonatal infection, maternal infection is associated with increased perinatal morbidity and complications, including an increased risk of preterm birth.[32,52]

DIAGNOSTIC TESTING FOR COVID-19 IN NEWBORNS

Infants with symptoms consistent with COVID-19 and infants who are asymptomatic but had close contact with confirmed or suspected COVID-19 infection (a person under investigation) should be tested. Close contact is defined as a distance of less than 6 feet for a cumulative total of 15 minutes over 24 hours. There are three types of tests available to diagnose COVID-19 in infants:[61,62]

1. Nucleic acid amplification tests (NAATs), reverse transcription–polymerase chain reaction (RT-PCR) tests on respiratory specimens (nasopharyngeal swabs, nasal swabs, saliva, and lower respiratory tract in intubated patients),[63] are the gold standard for diagnosing SARS-CoV-2 infection, with superior sensitivity and a good turnaround time of 24 to 48 hours. Positive RT-PCR confirms the diagnosis of SARS-CoV-2 infection but can remain positive for weeks after the onset of infection. False-negative RT-PCR can occur. If there is a high suspicion of COVID-19, repeating the test is recommended if initial testing is negative.[9]
2. Antigen tests involve viral protein detection via nasopharyngeal or nasal swabs. Overall, they are less sensitive than NAATs. Sensitivity is highest in symptomatic individuals within 5 to 7 days of symptom onset. They are accessible and convenient, as they can be done at home or point of care.
3. Serology tests utilize serum antibody detection to identify prior infection (or infection at least 3 to 4 weeks prior). Serology tests have variable sensitivity and specificity, and cross-reactivity with other coronaviruses has been reported. Immunoglobulin (Ig)G or IgM presence does not define when infection occurred, but IgG might help identify active infection.

CHARACTERISTICS OF NEONATES WITH COVID-19

Thanks to several national, regional, and local surveillance programs collecting epidemiological data on mother–infant dyads since the beginning of the pandemic, including the National Registry for Surveillance and Epidemiology of Perinatal COVID-19 Infection, CDC Surveillance for Emerging Threats to Mothers and Babies Network, Vermont Oxford Network, and MedNAX, we now know and continue to identify trends in disease, epidemiology, and the impact of SARS-CoV-2 infection on maternal and infant health.[9] It remains unclear why neonates mainly experience mild symptoms and have lower mortality rates.[64,65] Early in the pandemic, several studies reported a lower risk of infection and milder symptoms in infected infants. Clinical presentations of neonates infected with SARS-CoV-2 vary greatly, ranging from asymptomatic carriers to critical illness. Most cases (84%) were found in infants tested due to maternal COVID-19 infection. Of the positive cases, about 20% were asymptomatic.[66] The symptomatic neonates most commonly present with respiratory distress (40%), fever (32%), and feeding intolerance (24%).[66] Laboratory tests show nonspecific findings, including increased white blood cell count and increased serum levels of creatinine phosphokinase, liver enzymes, C-reactive protein, and procalcitonin. Small case series from China in 2020 described two term neonates with significant complications, including disseminated intravascular coagulation and multi-organ dysfunction, resulting in neonatal death.[66] Most recently, there have been reports of more severe disease in infants with the Delta variant rising within the population (Delta: SARS-CoV-2 B.1.617.2).[11,12] In a registry from the Turkish Neonatal Society, among 176 neonates (<28 days of age) from 44 neonatal intensive care units who acquired SARS-CoV-2 infection after discharge from the birth hospital, symptoms included fever (64%), feeding intolerance (26%), cough (22%), tachypnea (19%), diarrhea (8%), irritability (7%), and rash (2%).[67] The median length of stay was 9 days; 25% required ventilatory support, and the most common complication was myocarditis (5.7%), showing that disease in the neonates who required hospitalization can be severe.[67]

CHARACTERISTICS OF NEONATES WITH LATE-ONSET COVID-19

Data on neonates with SARS-CoV-2 outside the perinatal period are minimal. Late-onset COVID-19 usually manifests 2 to 3 weeks after birth, with family members or close contacts as the source. Clinical symptoms are the same as those of early-onset COVID-19.[68]

MULTISYSTEM INFLAMMATORY SYNDROME IN NEONATES

A rare but serious COVID-19 complication similar to Kawasaki disease has been described in children. Multisystem inflammatory syndrome in children (MIS-C) is manifested as a post-infectious immune-mediated condition usually seen 3 to 5 weeks after COVID-19. It is associated with coronary artery aneurysms, cardiac dysfunction, and multiorgan inflammatory manifestations.[69,70] It has not been widely described in neonates and there are no standardized diagnostic criteria. Neonates born to COVID-19-positive mothers may present with a multisystem inflammatory syndrome in neonates (MIS-N). Infants described in case series with unexplained signs of multisystem inflammation, cardiac dysfunction, prolonged QTc, coronary dilation, and thrombosis who were born to mothers with a history of suspected or confirmed COVID-19 are suspected of having MIS-N.[11] MIS-N compared to MIS-C not only results from SARS-CoV-2 infection in the infant but may also follow maternal SARS-CoV-2 infection.[64] MIS-N is hypothesized to be caused by the transplacental transfer of SARS-CoV-2 antibodies or antibodies developed in the neonate after infection with SARS-CoV-2.[11] More data are needed to describe the diagnostic criteria and evaluate potential therapies, such as intravenous immunoglobulin and steroids.

COVID-19 IN PRETERM INFANTS

Few studies have described SARS-CoV-2 in preterm infants. The most common clinical signs include hyperglycemia and bone marrow dysfunction (i.e., leukopenia or leukocytosis).[12] A case report of a 26-week preterm neonate described the new development of streaky infiltrates on chest radiography following the acquisition of SARS-CoV-2 infection but no changes in baseline respiratory support.[71]

MANAGEMENT OF INFANTS WITH COVID-19

Management of SARS-CoV-2 infection in neonates is mainly supportive, including respiratory support, oxygen, close monitoring of fluid status and electrolyte balance, and empiric antibiotics if there is suspected bacterial co-infection. In addition to supportive therapy, remdesivir, an RNA-dependent inhibitor of RNA polymerase in coronaviruses, is approved for use via an emergency drug authorization by the FDA with no minimum age.[72] Intravenous remdesivir has been used safely and effectively in infants under 5 days of age in Ebola trials and, most recently, for neonatal COVID-19. No severe adverse drug reactions have been reported, except for elevated liver enzymes and, occasionally, diarrhea, rash, renal impairment, and hypotension.[73,74] Additionally, oral absorption is poor, so there is likely limited absorption in neonates from breast milk of mothers who may be on the agent.[74]

In hospitalized infants, placement in a single-patient isolation room is recommended. Staff and providers should follow the infection prevention interventions to reduce transmission of SARS-CoV-2, including hand hygiene, environmental disinfection, and appropriate personal protective equipment, particularly during aerosol-generating procedures.[75]

MANAGEMENT OF INFANTS BORN TO INDIVIDUALS WITH SUSPECTED OR CONFIRMED COVID-19

Initial AAP guidelines in 2020 at the onset of the COVID-19 pandemic recommended temporary separation of the mother and newborn due to the risk of perinatal and postnatal exposure.[52] Evidence suggests that the risk of infection during birth hospitalization can be diminished if appropriate precautions to protect infants from maternal secretions are taken. To date, the AAP recommends that mothers and well newborn infants should room-in. If the mother is acutely ill and unable to take care of the infant, then temporary separation should be considered and discussed with the family.[52] If the infant requires intensive care (e.g., due to prematurity), the infant should be admitted to a single-patient isolation room with negative pressure, if available, and tested within the first 72 hours after birth. Infants who have been in contact with an infected parent after birth need infection control precautions for 10 days after the last maternal–infant contact.[52]

Ethical and Psychosocial Considerations

Families with COVID-19 are at greater risk for stress, anxiety, and depression and may require specialized and individualized teaching, counseling, and support during the newborns' admission and after discharge. Another indirect burden and long-term impact of the COVID-19 pandemic on children is orphanhood and caregiver loss, which is considered an adverse childhood experience that may result in a profound long-term impact on health and well-being for children.[76] As of 2022, excess mortality data from the WHO found that more than 10.5 million children worldwide have lost one or both parents during the pandemic.[77] In the United States, over 140,000 children have lost a primary or secondary caregiver to COVID-19, with significant disparities in associated deaths across racial and ethnic groups (1.1 to 4.5 risk of loss higher among Black and Hispanic children compared to non-Hispanic White children).[78] Hispanic and non-Hispanic Black pregnant individuals have been disproportionately affected by SARS-CoV-2 infection during pregnancy.[13] The COVID-19 pandemic has additionally exposed and magnified racial and ethnic health disparities deeply rooted in structural racism and socioeconomic inequality that must be addressed when caring for mothers and their newborns.[15–17]

REFERENCES

1. World Health Organization. *Coronavirus Disease 2019 (COVID-19): Situation Report 50*. 2020. Available at: https://www.who.int/docs/default-source/coronaviruse/situation-reports/20200310-sitrep-50-covid-19.pdf. Accessed January 24, 2023.
2. Li Q, Guan X, Wu P, et al. Early transmission dynamics in Wuhan, China, of novel coronavirus-infected pneumonia. *N Engl J Med*. 2020;382(13):1199-1207.
3. Wu F, Zhao S, Yu B, et al. A new coronavirus associated with human respiratory disease in China. *Nature*. 2020;579(7798):265-269.
4. Zhou P, Yang XL, Wang XG, et al. A pneumonia outbreak associated with a new coronavirus of probable bat origin. *Nature*. 2020;579(7798):270-273.
5. World Health Organization. *WHO Coronavirus (COVID-19) Dashboard*. Available at: https://covid19.who.int. Accessed September 1, 2022.
6. Huang C, Wang Y, Li X, et al. Clinical features of patients infected with 2019 novel coronavirus in Wuhan, China. *Lancet*. 2020;395(10223):497-506.
7. Angelidou A, Sullivan K, Melvin PR, et al. Association of maternal perinatal SARS-CoV-2 infection with neonatal outcomes during the COVID-19 pandemic in Massachusetts. *JAMA Netw Open*. 2021;4(4):e217523.
8. Martínez-Perez O, Vouga M, Cruz Melguizo S, et al. Association between mode of delivery among pregnant women with COVID-19 and maternal and neonatal outcomes in Spain. *JAMA*. 2020;324(3):296-299.
9. AAP Section on Neonatal–Perinatal Medicine. *NPC-19 Registry*. Available at: https://my.visme.co/view/ojq9qq8e-npc-19-registry. Accessed January 24, 2023.
10. Yu Y, Chen P. Coronavirus disease 2019 (COVID-19) in neonates and children from China: a review. *Front Pediatr*. 2020;8:287.
11. Molloy EJ, Nakra N, Gale C, Dimitriades VR, Lakshminrusimha S. Multisystem inflammatory syndrome in children (MIS-C) and neonates (MIS-N) associated with COVID-19: optimizing definition and management [published online ahead of print September 1, 2022]. *Pediatr Res*. Available at: https://doi.org/10.1038/s41390-022-02263-w.
12. Boly TJ, Reyes-Hernandez ME, Daniels EC, Kibbi N, Bermick JR, Elgin TG. Hyperglycemia and cytopenias as signs of SARS-CoV-2 delta variant infection in preterm infants. *Pediatrics*. 2022;149(6):e2021055331.
13. Ellington S, Strid P, Tong VT, et al. Characteristics of women of reproductive age with laboratory-confirmed SARS-CoV-2 infection by pregnancy status - United States, January 22–June 7, 2020. *MMWR Morb Mortal Wkly Rep*. 2020;69(25):769-775.
14. Vlachodimitropoulou Koumoutsea E, Vivanti AJ, Shehata N, et al. COVID-19 and acute coagulopathy in pregnancy. *J Thromb Haemost*. 2020;18(7):1648-1652.
15. Webb Hooper M, Nápoles AM, Pérez-Stable EJ. COVID-19 and racial/ethnic disparities. *JAMA*. 2020;323(24):2466-2467.

16. Evans MK. Covid's color line —infectious disease, inequity, and racial justice. *N Engl J Med*. 2020;383(5):408-410.
17. Barrero-Castillero A, Beam KS, Bernardini LB, et al. COVID-19: neonatal–perinatal perspectives. *J Perinatol*. 2021;41(5):940-951.
18. Tyrrell DA, Bynoe ML. Cultivation of viruses from a high proportion of patients with colds. *Lancet*. 1966;1(7428):76-77.
19. Flores-Vega VR, Monroy-Molina JV, Jiménez-Hernández LE, Torres AG, Santos-Preciado JI, Rosales-Reyes R. SARS-CoV-2: evolution and emergence of new viral variants. *Viruses*. 2022;14(4):653.
20. Cui J, Li F, Shi ZL. Origin and evolution of pathogenic coronaviruses. *Nat Rev Microbiol*. 2019;17(3):181-192.
21. Holmes EC, Goldstein SA, Rasmussen AL, et al. The origins of SARS-CoV-2: a critical review. *Cell*. 2021;184(19):4848-4856.
22. Marks KJ, Whitaker M, Agathis NT, et al. Hospitalization of infants and children aged 0–4 years with laboratory-confirmed COVID-19—COVID-NET, 14 states, March 2020–February 2022. *MMMR Morb Mortal Wkly Rep*. 2022;71(11):429-436.
23. Letko M, Marzi A, Munster V. Functional assessment of cell entry and receptor usage for SARS-CoV-2 and other lineage B betacoronaviruses. *Nat Microbiol*. 2020;5(4):562-569.
24. Ou X, Liu Y, Lei X, et al. Characterization of spike glycoprotein of SARS-CoV-2 on virus entry and its immune cross-reactivity with SARS-CoV. *Nat Commun*. 2020;11(1):1620.
25. Ziegler CGK, Allon SJ, Nyquist SK, et al. SARS-CoV-2 receptor ACE2 is an interferon-stimulated gene in human airway epithelial cells and is detected in specific cell subsets across tissues. *Cell*. 2020;181(5):1016-1035.e19.
26. Sungnak W, Huang N, Bécavin C, et al. SARS-CoV-2 entry factors are highly expressed in nasal epithelial cells together with innate immune genes. *Nat Med*. 2020;26(5):681-687.
27. Li MY, Li L, Zhang Y, Wang XS. Expression of the SARS-CoV-2 cell receptor gene ACE2 in a wide variety of human tissues. *Infect Dis Poverty*. 2020;9(1):45.
28. Heinonen S, Helve O, Andersson S, Janér C, Süvari L, Kaskinen A. Nasal expression of SARS-CoV-2 entry receptors in newborns. *Arch Dis Child Fetal Neonatal Ed*. 2022;107(1):95-97.
29. Carsetti R, Quintarelli C, Quinti I, et al. The immune system of children: the key to understanding SARS-CoV-2 susceptibility? *Lancet Child Adolesc Health*. 2020;4(6):414-416.
30. Fenizia C, Biasin M, Cetin I, et al. Analysis of SARS-CoV-2 vertical transmission during pregnancy. *Nat Commun*. 2020;11(1):5128.
31. Tomori C, Gribble K, Palmquist AEL, Ververs MT, Gross MS. When separation is not the answer: breastfeeding mothers and infants affected by COVID-19. *Matern Child Nutr*. 2020;16(4):e13033.
32. Jamieson DJ, Rasmussen SA. An update on COVID-19 and pregnancy. *Am J Obstet Gynecol*. 2022;226(2):177-186.
33. Chambers C, Krogstad P, Bertrand K, et al. Evaluation for SARS-CoV-2 in breast milk from 18 infected women. *JAMA*. 2020;324(13):1347-1348.
34. Dumitriu D, Emeruwa UN, Hanft E, et al. Outcomes of neonates born to mothers with severe acute respiratory syndrome coronavirus 2 infection at a large medical center in New York City. *JAMA Pediatr*. 2021;175(2):157-167.
35. Verma S, Bradshaw C, Auyeung NSF, et al. Outcomes of maternal–newborn dyads after maternal SARS-CoV-2. *Pediatrics*. 2020;146(4):e2020005637.
36. Mor G, Cardenas I. The immune system in pregnancy: a unique complexity. *Am J Reprod Immunol*. 2010;63(6):425-433.
37. Dashraath P, Wong JLJ, Lim MXK, et al. Coronavirus disease 2019 (COVID-19) pandemic and pregnancy. *Am J Obstet Gynecol*. 2020;222(6):521-531.
38. Zambrano LD, Ellington S, Strid P, et al. Update: characteristics of symptomatic women of reproductive age with laboratory-confirmed SARS-CoV-2 infection by pregnancy status - United States, January 22–October 3, 2020. *MMWR Morb Mortal Wkly Rep*. 2020;69(44):1641-1647.
39. Shanes ED, Mithal LB, Otero S, Azad HA, Miller ES, Goldstein JA. Placental pathology in COVID-19. *Am J Clin Pathol*. 2020;154(1):23-32.
40. Baergen RN, Heller DS, Goldstein JA. Placental pathology in COVID-19. *Am J Clin Pathol*. 2020;154(2):279.
41. Konstantinidou AE, Angelidou S, Havaki S, et al. Stillbirth due to SARS-CoV-2 placentitis without evidence of intrauterine transmission to fetus: association with maternal risk factors. *Ultrasound Obstet Gynecol*. 2022;59(6):813-822.
42. U. S. Food and Drug Administration. *FDA Takes Key Action in Fight Against COVID-19 by Issuing Emergency Use Authorization for First COVID-19 Vaccine*. Available at: https://www.fda.gov/news-events/press-announcements/fda-takes-key-action-fight-against-covid-19-issuing-emergency-use-authorization-first-covid-19. Accessed August 21, 2022.
43. Panagiotakopoulos L, Myers TR, Gee J, et al. SARS-CoV-2 infection among hospitalized pregnant women: reasons for admission and pregnancy characteristics - eight U.S. health care centers, March 1–May 30, 2020. *MMWR Morb Mortal Wkly Rep*. 2020;69(38):1355-1359.
44. Oliver SE, Gargano JW, Marin M, et al. The Advisory Committee on Immunization Practices' interim recommendation for use of Pfizer-BioNTech COVID-19 vaccine - United States, December 2020. *MMWR Morb Mortal Wkly Rep*. 2020;69(50):1922-1924.
45. Collier ARY, McMahan K, Yu J, et al. Immunogenicity of COVID-19 mRNA vaccines in pregnant and lactating women. *JAMA*. 2021;325(23):2370-2380.
46. Royal College of Obstetricians and Gynaecologists. *COVID-19 Vaccines, Pregnancy and Breastfeeding*. Available at: https://www.rcog.org.uk/guidance/coronavirus-covid-19-pregnancy-and-women-s-health/vaccination/covid-19-vaccines-pregnancy-and-breastfeeding-faqs/. Accessed January 25, 2023.
47. World Health Organization. *AstraZeneca ChAdOx1-S/nCoV-19 [recombinant], COVID-19 Vaccine*. Available at: https://www.who.int/publications/m/item/chadox1-s-recombinant-covid-19-vaccine. Accessed January 25, 2023.
48. American College of Obstetricians and Gynecologists. *COVID-19 FAQs for Obstetricians–Gynecologists, Obstetrics*. Available at: https://www.acog.org/clinical-information/physician-faqs/covid-19-faqs-for-ob-gyns-obstetrics. Accessed January 25, 2023.
49. DeNicola N, Grossman D, Marko K, et al. Telehealth interventions to improve obstetric and gynecologic health outcomes: a systematic review. *Obstet Gynecol*. 2020;135(2):371-382.
50. American College of Obstetricians and Gynecologists. Levels of maternal care: obstetric care consensus no. 9. *Obstet Gynecol*. 2019;134(2):e41-e55.
51. National Institutes of Health. *Coronavirus Disease 2019 (COVID-19) Treatment Guidelines*. Available at: https://www.covid19treatmentguidelines.nih.gov/. Accessed January 25, 2023.
52. American Academy of Pediatrics. *FAQs: Management of Infants Born to Mothers with Suspected or Confirmed COVID-19*.

Available at: https://www.aap.org/en/pages/2019-novel-coronavirus-covid-19-infections/clinical-guidance/faqs-management-of-infants-born-to-covid-19-mothers/. Accessed January 25, 2023.
53. Krogstad P, Contreras D, Ng H, et al. No infectious SARS-CoV-2 in breast milk from a cohort of 110 lactating women. *Pediatr Res*. 2022;92(4):1140-1145.
54. American Academy of Pediatrics. *Guidance on Newborn Screening during COVID-19*. Available at: https://www.aap.org/en/pages/2019-novel-coronavirus-covid-19-infections/clinical-guidance/guidance-on-newborn-screening-during-covid-19/. Accessed January 25, 2023.
55. Horby P, Lim WS, Emberson JR, et al. Dexamethasone in hospitalized patients with Covid-19. *N Engl J Med*. 2021;384(8):693-704.
56. Committee on Obstetric Practice. Committee opinion no. 713: antenatal corticosteroid therapy for fetal maturation. *Obstet Gynecol*. 2017;130(2):e102-e109.
57. Chen D, Yang H, Cao Y, et al. Expert consensus for managing pregnant women and neonates born to mothers with suspected or confirmed novel coronavirus (COVID-19) infection. *Int J Gynaecol Obstet*. 2020;149(2):130-136.
58. Wyckoff AS. *AAP Issues Guidance on Infants Born to Mothers with Suspected or Confirmed COVID-19*. Available at: https://publications.aap.org/aapnews/news/6713?autologincheck=redirected. Accessed January 25, 2023.
59. Centers for Disease Control and Prevention. *Stay Up to Date with COVID-19 Vaccines Including Boosters*. Available at: https://www.cdc.gov/coronavirus/2019-ncov/vaccines/stay-up-to-date.html?s_cid=11747:cdc up to date vaccine:sem.ga:p:RG:GM:gen:PTN:FY22. Accessed January 25, 2023.
60. Centers for Disease Control and Prevention. *COVID-19 Vaccines While Pregnant or Breastfeeding*. Available at: https://www.cdc.gov/coronavirus/2019-ncov/vaccines/recommendations/pregnancy.html. Accessed January 25, 2023.
61. Weissleder R, Lee H, Ko J, Pittet MJ. COVID-19 diagnostics in context. *Sci Transl Med*. 2020;12(546):eabc1931.
62. Cheng MP, Papenburg J, Desjardins M, et al. Diagnostic testing for severe acute respiratory syndrome-related coronavirus 2: a narrative review. *Ann Intern Med*. 2020;172(11):726-734.
63. Corman VM, Landt O, Kaiser M, et al. Detection of 2019 novel coronavirus (2019-nCoV) by real-time RT-PCR. *Euro Surveill*. 2020;25(3):2000045.
64. Pawar R, Gavade V, Patil N, et al. Neonatal multisystem inflammatory syndrome (MIS-N) associated with prenatal maternal SARS-CoV-2: a case series. *Child (Basel)*. 2021;8(7):572.
65. Ryan L, Plötz FB, van den Hoogen A, et al. Neonates and COVID-19: state of the art: Neonatal Sepsis series. *Pediatr Res*. 2022;91(2):432-439.
66. Liguoro I, Pilotto C, Bonanni M, et al. SARS-COV-2 infection in children and newborns: a systematic review. *Eur J Pediatr*. 2020;179(7):1029-1046.
67. Akin IM, Kanburoglu MK, Tayman C, et al. Epidemiologic and clinical characteristics of neonates with late-onset COVID-19: 1-year data of Turkish Neonatal Society. *Eur J Pediatr*. 2022;181(5):1933-1942.
68. Lakshminrusimha S, Hudak ML, Dimitriades VR, Higgins RD. Multisystem inflammatory syndrome in neonates following maternal SARS-CoV-2 COVID-19 infection. *Am J Perinatol*. 2022;39(11):1166-1171.
69. Godfred-Cato S, Bryant B, Leung J, et al. COVID-19-associated multisystem inflammatory syndrome in children - United States, March–July 2020. *MMWR Morb Mortal Wkly Rep*. 2020;69(32):1074-1080.
70. Feldstein LR, Tenforde MW, Friedman KG, et al. Characteristics and outcomes of US children and adolescents with multisystem inflammatory syndrome in children (MIS-C) compared with severe acute COVID-19. *JAMA*. 2021;325(11):1074-1087.
71. Piersigilli F, Carkeek K, Hocq C, et al. COVID-19 in a 26-week preterm neonate. *Lancet Child Adolesc Health*. 2020;4(6):476-478.
72. U.S. Food and Drug Administration. *Coronavirus (COVID-19) Update: FDA Issues Emergency Use Authorization for Potential COVID-19 Treatment*. Available at: https://www.fda.gov/news-events/press-announcements/coronavirus-covid-19-update-fda-issues-emergency-use-authorization-potential-covid-19-treatment. Accessed January 25, 2023.
73. Mulangu S, Dodd LE, Davey RTJ, et al. A randomized, controlled trial of Ebola virus disease therapeutics. *N Engl J Med*. 2019;381(24):2293-2303.
74. National Institute of Child Health and Human Development. *Drugs and Lactation Database (LactMed®)*. Bethesda, MD: National Library of Medicine; 2006.
75. Centers for Disease Control and Prevention. *Isolation and Precautions for People with COVID-19*. Available at: https://www.cdc.gov/coronavirus/2019-ncov/your-health/isolation.html. Accessed January 25, 2023.
76. Felitti VJ, Anda RF, Nordenberg D, et al. Relationship of childhood abuse and household dysfunction to many of the leading causes of death in adults: the adverse childhood experiences (ACE) study. *Am J Prev Med*. 1998;14(4):245-258.
77. Hillis S, N'konzi JPN, Msemburi W, et al. Orphanhood and caregiver loss among children based on new global excess COVID-19 death estimates. *JAMA Pediatr*. 2022;176(11):1145-1148.
78. Hillis SD, Blenkinsop A, Villaveces A, et al. COVID-19-associated orphanhood and caregiver death in the United States [published online ahead of print October 7, 2021]. *Pediatrics*. Available at: https://doi.org/10.1542/peds.2021-053760.

Chapter 9

Congenital Syphilis

Shelley M. Lawrence, MD, MS

Key Points

- The incidence of syphilis in the United States has been increasing since 2012.
- The two leading causes of missed congenital syphilis prevention opportunities are the lack of adequate maternal syphilis treatment despite a timely diagnosis and absence of prenatal care and subsequent maternal syphilis testing.
- Although reverse screening algorithms have been adopted in many healthcare settings, traditional screening methods utilizing a quantitative rapid plasma reagin (RPR) test remains the standard of care for pregnant women and newborns.
- *Treponema pallidum* remains highly sensitive to penicillin, and healthcare providers should follow established treatment algorithms for infected individuals.

Introduction

Before the microbiologic era, venereal diseases were poorly distinguished from one another. Because the mother's infection usually remained undiagnosed, fetal syphilis was thought to occur during conception by transmission through the father's sperm.[1] Although Gaspard Torella first described the neonatal form of syphilis in 1497, it was not until the mid-16th century that maternal transmission of *Treponema pallidum* was considered in the pathogenesis of congenital syphilis (CS).[1] Before the introduction of penicillin in the early- to mid-1940s, CS was routinely treated with mercurial compounds, which were administered orally to "wet nurses" or rubbed onto women's nipples to indirectly treat breastfed infants.[2]

Although appropriate screening and treatment protocols currently exist for *T. pallidum* infection, syphilis remains a menace to public health. In the United States, the number of syphilis cases has increased since 2000, when the fewest cases were reported to the Centers for Disease Control and Prevention (CDC) since the pre-penicillin era.[3–5] As a direct consequence, the annual number of CS cases has also risen each year since 2012 (Figure 9.1).[6] The most recent CDC report (2020) documented a total of 2,148 cases of CS were reported, including 122 syphilitic stillbirths, 27 infant deaths, and a national rate of 57.3 cases per 100,000 live births.[6] This rate represents a 15% increase relative to 2019 and a 254% rise compared to 2016,[6] so the incidence of CS has now nearly matched that of group B streptococcal neonatal sepsis (0.52 per 1000 live births in 2019).[7]

Although affected pregnancies may end prematurely, most infants born to syphilitic mothers appear normal and are without clinical or laboratory evidence of infection at birth.[8–10] If left untreated, however, these children will develop manifestations of disease months to years later, including lifelong physical and neurologic impairments.[11,12] Importantly, interventions to improve the coverage and effect of syphilis screening during pregnancy could reduce syphilis-associated stillbirth and perinatal death by 50% worldwide.[10,13] The two leading causes of missed CS prevention opportunities cited by the CDC were the lack of adequate maternal syphilis treatment despite a timely diagnosis (40.2%), followed by an absence of prenatal care and subsequent syphilis testing (36.3%). These missed opportunities require immediate correction to attenuate the rise of syphilis in the United States.[6,12]

A 2019 investigation by Umapathi and colleagues[14] also documented significant independent risk factors for CS. In a review of 5912 CS-related hospitalizations in the United States between 2009 and 2016, these investigators found that African American ethnicity, public insurance/uninsured, low socioeconomic status, geographic location (south and west hospital regions), prematurity, and low birth weight contributed

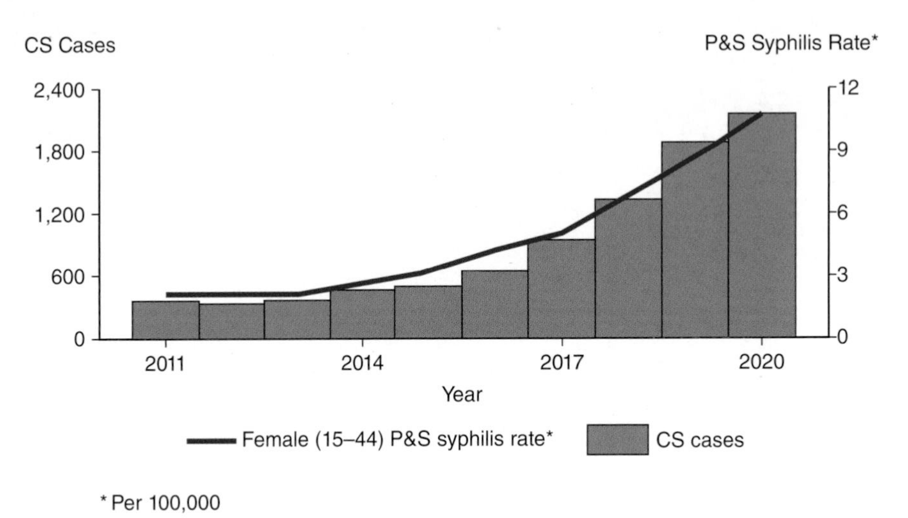

Fig. 9.1 Congenital syphilis—reported cases by year of birth and rates of primary and secondary syphilis among females 15 to 44 years old in the United States (2010–2019). ACRONYMS: *CS*, congenital syphillis; *P&S*, primary and secondary syphillis.

to an increased incidence of CS. The rate of in-hospital deaths associated with CS was 0.54% (32 deaths among 5912 hospitalizations), and the mean length of stay was higher for infants with CS than those without CS (12.38 ± 0.10 days vs. 3.42 ± 0.1 days). Moreover, the economic burden of CS more than doubled throughout the study after adjustments were made for inflation ($120,665,203 in 2016 vs. $54,290,310 in 2009), for a total estimated cost of $345 million over the 7-year study period. Although the CDC mandates reporting of CS cases to its national database,[12] the number of hospitalizations recorded in the study was significantly higher than those reported to the CDC.[8] These authors suggested that the lack of CDC active surveillance for sexually transmitted infections, including CS, may have accounted for this difference.

Racial disparities are vitally important to the rise of CS, as minority populations have substantially higher rates for all reportable sexually transmitted diseases (i.e., chlamydia, gonorrhea, and the highly infectious primary and secondary stages of syphilis).[6] In 2019, non-Hispanic Blacks comprised 30.6% of all syphilis cases (almost five times the rate among White individuals), although they make up only 12.5% of the U.S. population.[6] In high syphilis morbidity regions of the southern United States, failure to provide adequate maternal treatment (37.0%) for Black and Hispanic mothers was the leading cause for missed prevention opportunities for CS, and lack of timely prenatal care (31.6%) was a primary factor for White mothers. In the western regions of the United States, racial/ethnic differences were less pronounced, with >41% of mothers failing to receive timely prenatal care and >29% failing to receive adequate treatment despite an early syphilis diagnosis.[12] Therefore, early diagnosis and treatment of syphilis in all women are necessary to prevent serious, lasting economic and long-term complications associated with congenital *T. pallidum* infection.[11,15]

Treponema Pallidum

In 1905, the etiology of syphilis was identified by Berlin zoologist Fritz Schaudinn and dermatologist Erich Hoffmann, who initially called the organism *Spirochaeta pallida* but renamed it as *Treponema* later that year.[1,16] *T. pallidum* is a member of the Spirochaetaceae family, which is known to cause "endemic treponematoses," such as bejel (*T. pallidum* subsp. *endemicum*), yaws (*T. pallidum* subsp. *pertenue*), and pinta (*T. carateum*), in addition to vector-borne Lyme disease (*Borrelia burgdorferi*) and relapsing fever (*Borrelia hermsii*).[17] Unique restriction sites in genes that encode TpN15 and Gpd provide a genetic method for differentiating the syphilis spirochete from other causes of human nonvenereal treponematoses.[18]

T. pallidum, one of the smallest characterized prokaryotes, is composed of a 1.14-Mb genome that encodes 1041 putative proteins.[19] As such, this pathogen is a prime example of an organism that has undergone genome reduction to increase its efficiency but at the expense of becoming highly dependent on its host for the majority of its essential metabolic processes.[20,21] This transformation makes the study of *T. pallidum* challenging because it is incredibly fragile and cannot survive outside of a mammalian host nor be grown with routine culture techniques.[17,22] Even though the genomic sequence of *T. pallidum* does not reveal any obvious classical virulent factors that account for clinical signs and symptoms of syphilis infection, this organism produces several lipoproteins that may induce the expression of host inflammatory mediators through recognition by toll-like receptor 2.[23]

The survival of *T. pallidum* is dependent on two key mechanisms: (1) its capacity to evade the host immune responses, and (2) its highly invasive potential.[17] *T. pallidum* can invade many anatomic sites considered "immune privileged" due to decreased surveillance by sentry innate immune cells, including the placenta, eye, and central nervous system (CNS).[24] By avoiding host immune detection, *T. pallidum* can establish chronic infections in quiescent environments that may subsequently facilitate the seeding of nonprivileged tissues.[24] Therefore, the development of symptomatic late syphilis is suspected to occur in some individuals from poorly defined factors that induce *T. pallidum* organisms to begin dividing at higher rates. This unregulated proliferation leads to a minimum number of organisms (or "critical antigenic mass") needed to trigger a host pro-inflammatory immune response.[22,24]

The host adaptive immune response produces strongly reactive antibodies directed against many *T. pallidum* proteins.[25,26] These antibodies, however, do not readily bind to the outer membrane of intact treponemes, prompting experts to propose that the *T. pallidum* surface is nonantigenic.[24,27,28] Outer membrane proteins, encoded by 12 *tpr* genes, also exhibit a phenomenon known as phase variation of expression regulation. This differential gene expression means that *T. pallidum* can downregulate the expression of outer membrane proteins for which a host immune response has been mounted, while simultaneously upregulating the expression of new Tprs.[17,24] This genetic-based evasion technique may further contribute to the establishment of chronic infection.[24,29]

Transmission

T. pallidum is generally transmitted through direct contact with a syphilitic chancre located on the external genitals, vagina, rectum, anus, mouth, or lips. The highest person-to-person transmission rates are observed in the highly infectious early stages of syphilis, especially secondary syphilis.[8,15,30] The average time between syphilis acquisition and the start of the first symptom is 21 days (range, 10–90 days).[31] *T. pallidum* can traverse the fetal membranes to gain access to the amniotic fluid, resulting in fetal infection in nearly 75% of analyzed specimens from women with early syphilis.[8,32,33] Vertical transmission increases as the stage of pregnancy advances but can occur at any time during gestation.[8]

Women with late latent syphilis and low titers may transmit the infection to their offspring(s), although at substantially less risk.[8,30] In 2002, Sheffield and colleagues[34] reported vertical transmission results from Parkland Memorial Hospital in Dallas, TX, between 1988 and 1998, with rates of 29%, 59%, 50%, and 13% in mothers with primary, secondary, early latent, and late latent infections, respectively. Moreover, in 1950, Ingraham and colleagues[35] showed that, among 220 women with untreated syphilis of less than 4 years' duration, 41% of their infants were born alive but had CS, 25% were stillborn, 14% died in the neonatal period, 2% had low birth weight but no evidence of syphilis, and only 18% were normal full-term infants without CS.

Risk factors for syphilis transmission in pregnant mothers include young age, multiple sexual partners, low socioeconomic and educational status, unstable housing or homelessness, methamphetamine or heroin abuse, sex in conjunction with drug use or transactional sex, late entry into prenatal care (i.e., first visit during the second trimester or later) or no prenatal care, inadequate treatment of sexual partners, unprotected sex, a previous history of sexually transmitted infections, and incarceration of the woman or her partner.[12,30,36–40] The recent rise in U.S. syphilis cases is also attributed to an outbreak of infection among men having sex with men, which may relate to an increase in unsafe sexual behavior due to improved antiretroviral treatment for human immunodeficiency virus (HIV).[30]

Clinical Significance and Outcomes

In 1990, national reporting guidelines were revised and broadened by the CDC. The case definition of CS was modified to include all liveborn and stillborn infants, irrespective of clinical findings, who had reactive serologic tests for syphilis and were delivered to women with untreated or inadequately treated syphilis (Table 9.1).[15,41] This change resulted in a four- to fivefold increase in reported cases of CS when compared to the previously used Kaufman criteria, which included only infants with clinical, laboratory, or radiologic abnormalities.[8,42] In reproductive-aged females, syphilis has risen more than 172% between 2015 and 2019 and is accompanied by a >291% increase in the incidence of CS.[30] In 2019, CS rates were sixfold

TABLE 9.1 CDC Case Definition of Congenital Syphilis With Early and Late Clinical Manifestations

2015 CDC Case Definitions of CS

A. *Probable cases of CS*: If the infant is born to a woman who was untreated or inadequately treated, regardless of signs in the infant, or an infant or child who has a reactive nontreponemal test for syphilis (VDRL, RPR, or equivalent serologic methods) AND any one of the following:[15]
   1. Any evidence of CS on physical examination
   2. Any evidence of CS on radiographs of long bones
   3. A reactive CSF VDRL test
   4. In a nontraumatic lumbar puncture, an elevated CSF WBC count or protein (without other cause), with the following suggested parameters for abnormal CSF WBC count and protein values:
      a. During the first 30 days of life, a CSF WBC count of >15/mm^3 or a CSF protein >120 mg/dL.
      b. After the first 30 days of life, a CSF WBC count of >5/mm^3 or a CSF protein > 40 mg/dL regardless of CSF serology; the treating clinician should be consulted to interpret the CSF values for the specific patient.

B. *Syphilitic stillbirth*: A fetal death that occurs after a 20-week gestation or in which the fetus weighs greater than 500 g and the mother had untreated or inadequately treated syphilis at delivery. Adequate treatment is defined as completion of a penicillin-based regimen, in accordance with CDC treatment guidelines, appropriate for the stage of infection, and initiated 30 or more days before delivery.

C. *Confirmed CS*: A case that is laboratory confirmed.

Early Signs of CS	Late Signs of CS
Clinically observed ~ 2–10 weeks after birth or within the first 2 years of life	Clinically observed in the first 2 decades of life
Rhinitis ("snuffles")	Saddle nose deformity
Hepatosplenomegaly	Hutchinson's teeth
Fever	Mulberry molars
Pneumonitis	Olympian brow
Rash	Higouménakis' sign
Lymphadenopathy	Saber shins
Ascites	Clutton joints
Hematologic	Scaphoid scapula
Nephropathy	Ophthalmic complications
Periostitis and osteochondritis	Eighth-nerve deafness
Neurosyphilis	Neurosyphilis

The CDC defines congenital syphilis as an infection with *T. pallidum* in a fetus or infant acquired during pregnancy from a mother with untreated or inadequately treated syphilis.[12] *CDC*, Centers for Disease Control and Prevention; *VDRL*, Venereal Disease Research Laboratory; *RPR*, rapid plasma reagin; *CS*, congenital syphilis; *CSF*, cerebrospinal fluid; *WBC*, white blood cell.

higher among infants born to American Indian or Alaska Native mothers, fourfold greater for those born to Black mothers, and twofold greater for those born to Hispanic or Latino mothers (155, 106, and 65 cases per 100,000 live births, respectively) compared with White mothers (22 cases per 100,000 live births).[31]

A recent 2016 review of CS cases in the United States reported that, among 2508 pregnant women with syphilis, approximately 88% received prenatal care at least 30 days before delivery, 89.4% were tested for syphilis at least 30 days before delivery, and 76.9% received an adequate treatment regimen beginning at least 30 days before delivery.[43] These authors estimated that 1928 potential CS cases (75%) were successfully averted during this reporting period, ranging between 55.0% and 92.3% in states that recorded at least 10 syphilis cases among pregnant women. Although most CS cases were found to be averted, these authors found considerable geographic variation in syphilis cases and significant gaps in delivering timely prenatal care, syphilis testing, and adequate treatment to pregnant women diagnosed with syphilis. The most common factors contributing to these gaps were (1) failure of timely initiation of appropriate therapy to pregnant women with positive syphilis test results, and (2) newly acquired syphilitic infections among pregnant women who had tested negative for syphilis infection earlier in pregnancy. Inadequate treatment regimens (i.e., nonpenicillin therapy) or failure to complete prescribed antibiotic courses in syphilitic pregnant women were less common, but not insignificant, causes of CS in this patient cohort.

CS can present with *early signs*, which may be present at birth or appear within the first 2 years of life, or with *late signs*, which arise within the first 2 decades (Table 9.2).[44] The most common early signs of CS

TABLE 9.2 Treatment Recommendations for Congenital Syphilis According to Test Results[30]

Scenario	Test Results	Physical Examination	Recommended Evaluation	Recommended Treatment
Confirmed proven or highly probable	Serum quantitative nontreponemal serologic titer fourfold greater than the mother's titer at delivery *or* Positive darkfield test or PCR of the placenta, cord, lesion, or body fluids *or* Positive silver stain of the placenta	Abnormal or consistent with CS	CSF analysis for VDRL, cell count, and protein CBC with differential and platelet count Long-bone radiographs Other tests as clinically indicated*	Aqueous crystalline penicillin G 100,000–150,000 U/kg/day administered as 50,000 U/kg/dose IV every 12 hours during the first 7 days of life and every 8 hours of life thereafter for a total of 10 days *or* Procaine penicillin G 50,000 U/kg/dose IM in a single daily dose for 10 days
Possible	Serum quantitative nontreponemal serologic titer equal to or less than fourfold the mother's titer at delivery and one of the following: 1. The mother was not treated, inadequately treated, or has no documentation of having received treatment. 2. The mother was treated with a regimen other than penicillin. 3. The mother received the recommended regimen but treatment was initiated at <30 days prior to delivery.	Normal	CSF analysis for VDRL, cell count, and protein CBC with differential and platelet count Long-bone radiographs†	Aqueous crystalline penicillin G 100,000–150,000 U/kg/day administered as 50,000 U/kg/dose IV every 12 hours during the first 7 days of life and every 8 hours of life thereafter for a total of 10 days *or* Procaine penicillin G 50,000 U/kg/dose IM in a single daily dose for 10 days *or* Benzathine penicillin G 50,000 U/kg/dose IM in a single dose‡

Continued

TABLE 9.2 Treatment Recommendations for Congenital Syphilis According to Test Results[30]—cont'd

Scenario	Test Results	Physical Examination	Recommended Evaluation	Recommended Treatment
Less likely	Serum quantitative nontreponemal serologic titer equal to or less than fourfold the mother's titer at delivery and *both* of the following are true: 1. The mother was treated during pregnancy, treatment was appropriate for the infection stage, and the treatment regimen was initiated ≥ 30 days prior to delivery. 2. The mother has no evidence of reinfection or relapse.	Normal	No evaluation is necessary	Benzathine penicillin G 50,000 U/kg/dose IM in a single dose If follow-up and close serologic follow-up every 2–3 months for 6 months is certain for infants whose mother's nontreponemal titers decline at least fourfold after therapy for early syphilis or remained stable for low-titer, latent syphilis (i.e., VDRL < 1:2 or RPR < 1:4), then may consider not treating the newborn.
Not likely	Serum quantitative nontreponemal serologic titer equal to or less than fourfold the mother's titer at delivery and *both* of the following are true: 1. The mother's treatment was adequate before pregnancy. 2. The mother's nontreponemal serologic titer remained low and stable before and during pregnancy and at delivery (e.g., VDRL < 1:2 or RPR < 1:4)	Normal	No evaluation is necessary	No treatment is required; however, any neonate with reactive nontreponemal tests should be followed serologically to ensure the nontreponemal test returns to negative. Benzathine penicillin G 50,000 U/kg/dose in a single IM injection might be considered, particularly if follow-up is uncertain and the neonate has a reactive nontreponemal test.

CS, congenital syphilis; *PCR*, polymerase chain reaction; *CSF*, cerebrospinal fluid; *CBC*, complete blood count; *IV*, intravenous; *IM*, intramuscular; *VDRL*, Venereal Disease Research Laboratory; *RPR*, rapid plasma reagin.

*Other clinically indicated tests may include a chest radiograph, liver function tests, neuroimaging, ophthalmologic examination, and auditory brainstem response.

†This regimen is not necessary if a 10-day course of parental therapy is administered.

‡The recommended evaluation (i.e., CSF analysis, long-bone radiographs, and CBC with platelet count) should be normal and follow-up certain before deciding on this treatment course. If any portion of the workup is abnormal or not performed, if CSF analysis cannot be interpreted because of blood contamination, or if follow-up is uncertain, a 10-day course of penicillin G is required. Also, mothers with early syphilis should have a 10-day course of penicillin G administered due to the high risk of CS.

include hepatosplenomegaly, rash, fever, neurosyphilis, pneumonitis, rhinitis ("snuffles"), generalized lymphadenopathy, and ascites. Early manifestations of CS usually become apparent 2 to 10 weeks after birth. Syphilitic rhinitis is usually the first symptom to be recognized and is observed in up to 50% of newborns with CS.[24] Jaundice and elevated serum transaminases and alkaline phosphatase associated with syphilitic hepatitis may transiently worsen after the initiation of penicillin therapy.[8,44,45] Hepatosplenomegaly is generally caused by either extracellular hematopoiesis or hepatitis and may take months to resolve.[8] Hematologic findings may include (1) leukocytosis, (2) Coombs-negative hemolytic anemia that may persist for weeks after treatment, and (3) thrombocytopenia that may present clinically as petechiae and purpura and may be the sole manifestation of congenital infection.[8,15,45–47] Nephropathy has also been described in cases of CS and may present in two forms: (1) nephrotic syndrome and (2) acute glomerulonephritis.

Nonetheless, both forms have their basis in the deposition of immune complexes within the glomerular basement membrane[48,49] and present with proteinuria and/or hematuria.[8]

Syphilitic pemphigus, a characteristic fluid-filled, bullous skin eruption, may be present at birth or develop over the first few weeks of life with peeling, eventual crusting, and wrinkling of the skin.[8,44] Vesiculobullous lesions may be preceded by oval, maculopapular skin lesions (reminiscent of secondary syphilis) that may become copper-colored with desquamation over a period of 1 to 3 weeks and occur primarily on the palms and soles. Additional skin manifestations are condylomata lata, or white, flat, raised plaques, which may occur on mucocutaneous areas (i.e., perioral, perianal, lips, tongue, palate, and fissures around the lips, nares, or anus) and are rare manifestations of CS infection.[8,44] Contact precautions must be strictly enforced when handling infants with skin lesions or nasal discharge, as the resulting fluid contains large quantities of spirochetes that are highly infectious and readily spread by contact.[8,44]

Periostitis and osteochondritis are also common findings that may be observed in well-appearing infants with CS at birth.[8] Radiographic abnormalities are generally symmetric and involve the long bones (humerus, tibia, and femur), ribs, and skull, with the lower extremities being involved more often than the upper extremities.[8] Osteochondritis involves the metaphysis and is visualized by routine radiographic techniques around 5 weeks after fetal infection.[8] Bone lesions may be painful and result in epiphyseal dislocation with refusal to move the involved extremity (pseudoparalysis of Parrot)[8,23,26] or lead to subepiphyseal fracture.[50] Wimberger sign describes bilateral demineralization and osseous destruction of the proximal medial tibial metaphysis.[8] Even without appropriate antibiotic therapy, spontaneous resolution of bone lesions is observed during the first 6 months of life and occurs irrespective of disease severity.[8,44,45]

In contrast to their term counterparts, preterm infants were found by Chinese investigators to present more often with the characteristic skin rash (36.2% vs. 9.7%; $P < 0.001$), hepatomegaly (51.7% vs. 25%; $P = 0.02$), splenomegaly (32.8% vs. 15.4%; $P = 0.02$), PRP titer $\geq$ 1:8 (96.6% vs. 70.8%; $P < 0.001$), thrombocytopenia (43.1% vs. 23.6%; $P = 0.018$), elevated C-reactive protein (65.5% vs. 36.5%; $P = 0.002$), and abnormal long-bone X-ray results (94.6% vs. 68.1%; $P < 0.001$).[51] Mothers who delivered preterm infants were less likely to receive treatment for syphilis (15.5% vs. 40.3%; $P = 0.003$) and more often opted for withdrawal of care (31% vs.12.5%; $P = 0.036$) due to the unaffordable cost and the high prevalence of co-morbidities and long-term neurodevelopmental impairments observed in survivors of severe cases of CS.[51] After infancy, CS and acquired syphilis may be difficult to distinguish, as clinical signs may not be obvious and stigmata have not yet developed.[15] Although maternal antibodies can complicate the interpretation of serologic tests in infants <6 months of age, reactive tests past 18 months are considered to reflect the status of the infant.[15]

Late signs of CS will manifest in 40% of untreated neonates with CS and are caused by persistent inflammation from chronic *T. pallidum* infection. Characteristic findings include the following:[44,52]

- Saddle-nose deformity caused by snuffles-related nasal cartilage destruction
- Hutchinson's teeth resulting from perinatal syphilitic vasculitis, which damages the developing tooth buds and presents clinically as widely spaced, notched, and peg-shaped upper central incisors
- Mulberry molars where the first lower molars are multi-cuspid
- Perforation of the hard palate
- Olympian brow resulting from prolonged periostitis and frontal bossing
- Higouménakis' sign, which is caused by thickening of the sternoclavicular portion of the clavicle
- Saber shins due to anterior bowing of the mid-tibias
- Clutton joints, which present as symmetric, painless, and sterile synovial effusions and primarily involve the knees of children between 8 to 15 years of age
- Scaphoid scapula

Corneal scarring, glaucoma, optic nerve atrophy, and interstitial keratitis (onset at age 5 to 20 years) may also be observed, as well as eighth-nerve deafness due to osteochondritis of the otic capsule, which develops in 3% of untreated CS cases and usually begins with high-frequency hearing loss between ages 8 and 10 years.[44,53] The Hutchinson triad is characterized by Hutchinson's teeth, interstitial keratitis, and eighth-nerve deafness. The sequelae of syphilitic rhinitis includes a short maxilla with high-arched palate and rhagades, which are spoke-like scars from fissures.[8,44] Although infants with late signs of CS are not considered infectious, treatment during pregnancy or within the first 3 months of life will prevent the development of these characteristic lesions.[8,44]

Invasion of the CNS by *T. pallidum* (or neurosyphilis) occurs in about 23% to 60% of infants with clinical, laboratory, or radiographic signs of CS.[8,39,54] Moreover, neurosyphilis affects an estimated 8% of asymptomatic infants with CS born to mothers with untreated early syphilis.[44] Most cases of neonatal neurosyphilis are asymptomatic. If left untreated at birth, however, acute leptomeningitis may develop within the first few months of life and present with a bulging fontanelle and splitting of sutures, emesis, and enlarging head circumference with impaired neuropsychomotor development, resulting in irreversible neurologic sequelae.[30,39] Alternatively, chronic meningovascular neurosyphilis may lead to progressive hydrocephalus, cranial nerve palsies, cerebral infarction, paralysis, seizure disorder, and neurodevelopmental regression.[8,44]

In a recent study from Brazil, no newborn diagnosed with neurosyphilis exhibited radiographic abnormalities of long bones, but CSF analyses showed that 42.8% (9/21) had high protein (>150 mg/dL), 28.6% (6/21) had a high number of leukocytes (>25 leukocytes/mm^3 CSF), and 28.6% (6/21) showed a positive Venereal Disease Research Laboratory (VDRL) test result. Although laboratory testing may help support the diagnosis of neurosyphilis, no single test can be used to diagnose neurosyphilis in all instances.[30] Current diagnostic assays that are considered specific for neurosyphilis, such as a positive cerebrospinal fluid VDRL, have a relatively low sensitivity[55–58] due to the passive transfer of nontreponemal immunoglobulin G (IgG) antibodies from the serum into the CSF.[8,30] This concept was demonstrated by Michelow and coworkers,[54] who calculated a sensitivity and specificity of (1) a reactive CSF VDRL test result (53% and 90%), (2) pleocytosis (38% and 88%), and (3) elevated protein content (56% and 78%).

A Canadian study conducted between 2002 and 2010 further reported that nearly a quarter of CS survivors exhibited a neurologic disability, including speech–language delay, blindness, microcephaly, and/or neurodevelopmental delay.[59] Thus, if clinical, laboratory, and/or radiographic evaluation supports a diagnosis of CS, therapy effective against CNS infection is warranted, irrespective of the results of the CSF analysis.[8] Close neurodevelopmental assessments and early referral to intervention services are also strongly recommended for all infants diagnosed with or treated for CS.

Diagnosis

Because *T. pallidum* is challenging to grow in culture, the diagnosis of syphilis infection is established by observing spirochetes in body fluids or tissue and is suggested by serologic test results. *T. pallidum* is very difficult to visualize using light microscopy but may be identified by darkfield microscopy, polymerase chain reaction (PCR) testing, and fluorescent antibody or silver staining of mucocutaneous lesions, nasal discharge, vesicular fluid, amniotic fluid, placenta, umbilical cord, or tissue obtained at autopsy.[8] Routine syphilis screening typically employs two protocols (Figure 9.2).[60] The first is traditional screening that utilizes nontreponemal testing, such as the RPR and VDRL tests, with reflex to treponemal analysis, including the enzyme immunoassay/chemiluminescence immunoassay (EIA/CIA), *T. pallidum* particle agglutination test (TP-PA), and/or fluorescent treponemal antibody absorption (FTA-ABS) tests. The second protocol is reverse sequence screening that employs treponemal analysis with reflex to nontreponemal testing.

Since 2010, syphilis testing in the United States has primarily transitioned to reverse sequence screening, beginning with EIA/CIA analysis.[10,30] Although this algorithm is more time and cost effective for high-volume laboratories,[61] it is associated with an ~14% to 40% false-positive rate.[15] This error in testing necessitates that a second treponemal test be completed to assist clinical decision-making. Because the reverse sequence algorithm for syphilis testing is a broad-based approach, initial antibody tests can identify persons who were previously treated for syphilis,

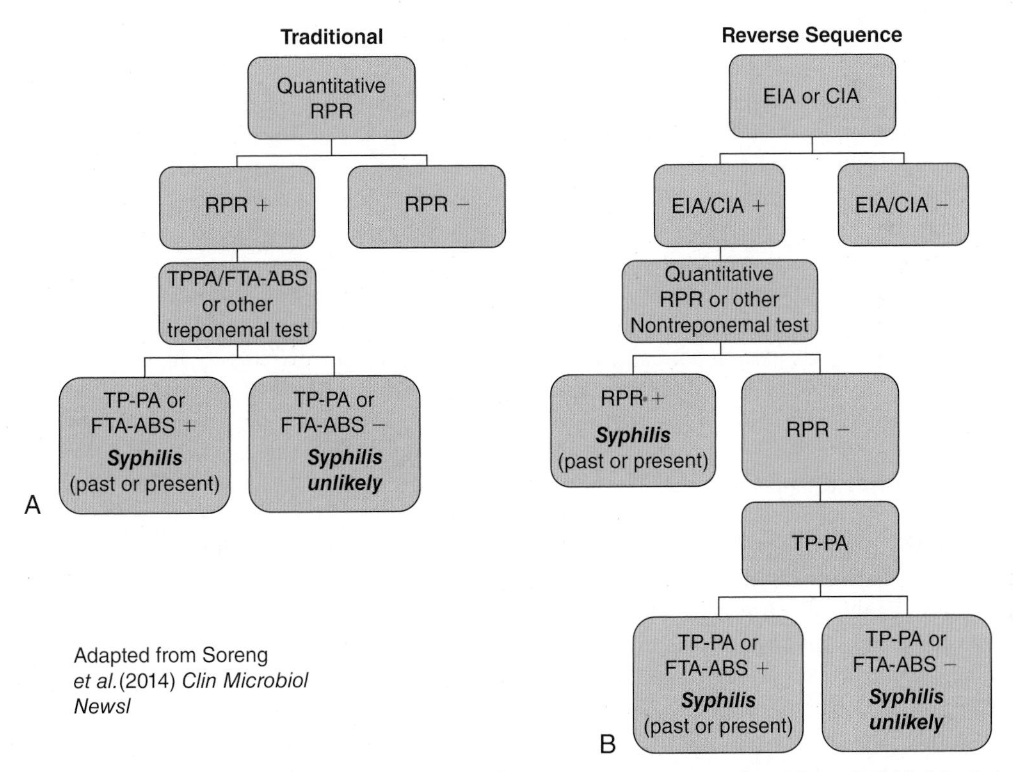

Fig. 9.2 Traditional versus reverse sequence testing algorithms for syphilis screening. (Adapted from Soreng K, Levy R, Fakile Y. Serologic testing for syphilis: benefits and challenges of a reverse algorithm. *Clin Microbiol Newsl.* 2014;36:195–202.)

those with untreated or incompletely treated syphilis, and those with false-positive test results with a low likelihood of infection.[30,61]

Adoption of reverse sequence screening may also complicate the evaluation of CS. If initial tests are negative, no further investigation is generally required. However, if an infant has a positive EIA/CIA result, then the diagnosis can only be inferred because maternal nontreponemal and treponemal IgG antibodies are transferred transplacentally to the fetus. Therefore, this immunologic occurrence can complicate the interpretation of reactive syphilis serologic tests in infants up to 18 months of age.[8,30]

Persons with a positive treponemal screening test should have a standard quantitative nontreponemal test with titer performed reflexively by the laboratory to guide patient management decisions. For example, if the EIA/CIA is positive, a quantitative RPR test should be performed. If the RPR test is positive, then the patient is determined to have syphilis, either past or present. If the nontreponemal test is negative (i.e., discrepant), then the laboratory should perform a treponemal test different from the one used for initial testing, preferably a TP-PA test or treponemal assay based on different antigens than the original test, to adjudicate the results of the initial test. Because RPR and VDRL tests measure the patient's antibody response to nontreponemal antigens, these tests lack specificity. Although treponemal-specific tests (TP-PA or FTA-ABS) are technically simple to perform, these tests are labor intensive and require subjective interpretation by laboratory personnel.[62] Conversely, the RPR and VDRL tests are subject to the prozone phenomenon (false-negative result in the presence of high antibody titer) and may also be falsely negative in early infection.[10,30] Although additional confirmatory testing may lead to delays in diagnosis and treatment, no single test is currently commercially available that enables accurate, rapid, inexpensive, and simple widespread testing for syphilis infection.[63]

Both treponemal and nontreponemal tests can produce nonreactive results in recently acquired syphilis infections, with ~20% of tests being negative during the primary stage of syphilis.[15] Treponemal antibodies usually do not appear until 1 to 4 weeks after the chancre, leading to false-negative results if employing RPR or EIA/CIA screening methods.[62] Up to 40% of adults and 80% of pregnant women may have discordant results (reactive EIA/CIA, nonreactive RPR test, and nonreactive TP-PA test), which are more common in populations with low syphilis prevalence, suggesting a false-positive EIA/CIA screen.[8,64,65] Moreover, about half of pregnant women with discordant results will have a subsequent negative EIA/CIA test result after delivery, which further supports the occurrence of false positivity.[8,65] In some patients, humoral antibodies against cardiolipin, a nonspecific human antigen that cross-reacts with *T. pallidum* antigens, may also cause false-positive test results. When serologic tests do not correspond with clinical findings of presumptive primary syphilis, secondary syphilis, latent syphilis, or CS, empiric treatment is recommended for those with risk factors for syphilis, and the use of other tests (i.e., placental or tissue biopsy for histology and immunostaining and PCR of any lesions) should be considered.[30]

Most people who have a positive treponemal test will have a reactive test for the remainder of their lives, irrespective of disease severity or the completion of appropriate treatment regimens. Only 15% to 25% of patients will become serologically nonreactive after 2 to 3 years if treated during the primary stage of syphilis infection.[66] Because treponemal antibody titers do not predict treatment response, they should not be used for this purpose.[30] The same nontreponemal test, however, should be performed on the mother and her infant so that accurate comparisons can be made.[8] False-positive nontreponemal test results can be associated with multiple medical conditions and factors unrelated to syphilis, including other infections (e.g., HIV), autoimmune conditions, vaccinations, injection drug use, pregnancy, and older age.[67,68] Because more rare *T. pallidum* subspecies (i.e., *pertenue*, *endemicum*, *bejel*, and *carateum*) are morphologically identical, share high DNA homology, and are closely related antigenically to the subspecies *pallidum*, they may also produce reactive syphilis test results but are not transmitted perinatally and do not cause neurologic disease.[15,44]

Pregnant women or newborns with a reactive nontreponemal test should always receive a treponemal test to confirm a syphilis diagnosis (i.e., traditional algorithm or RPR test). Sequential serologic tests for a patient should be performed using the same testing method (VDRL or RPR tests) and preferably be completed by the same laboratory. Even though VDRL and RPR tests are equally valid assays, quantitative results from the two tests cannot be directly compared with each other because the methods are different, and RPR titers are frequently slightly higher than VDRL titers. The unusual finding of an infant's serum quantitative nontreponemal serologic titer that is fourfold higher (or equivalent to a change of two dilutions, such as from 1:8 to 1:32) than the mother's titer is confirmatory of congenital infection.[10,30,69] However, the absence of such a finding does not exclude a CS diagnosis, as most infants with CS have nontreponemal serologic titers that are the same or one to two dilutions less than the maternal titer.[8]

Routine screening of umbilical cord blood is not recommended because it can become contaminated with maternal blood and yield a false-positive test result. Conversely, Wharton's jelly within the umbilical cord can yield a false-negative test result.[30] Because passively transferred maternal antibodies can persist for more than 15 months, treponemal testing (i.e., TP-PA and EIA/CIA) on neonatal serum is not recommended due to the difficulty of interpreting results. Commercially available IgM tests are also not recommended and provide little value in diagnosing CS.[30,70]

No mother or newborn should leave the hospital without maternal serologic status documentation at least once during pregnancy. Pregnant women living in communities with high rates of syphilis and women at high risk for syphilis acquisition during pregnancy should have serologic testing performed during the first prenatal visit within the first trimester of pregnancy and repeated twice during the third trimester at 28 weeks of gestation and delivery. Any woman who has a fetal death after 20 weeks of gestation should also be tested for syphilis.[30] Despite these recommendations from the CDC, eight states still have no prenatal screening requirements, and only 14 have third-trimester mandates. Of those with third-trimester mandates, four direct screening at birth and six have screening requirements if the mother had increased risk factors for infection.[30,71] Repeat syphilis screening in the third trimester of pregnancy, however, was shown to reduce maternal and neonatal adverse outcomes in the United States compared with single first-trimester testing.[72] More specifically, these investigators projected an annual cost savings of $52 million, with 41 fewer cases of CS, the prevention of 27 neonatal and infant deaths, and the avoidance of 73 intrauterine fetal deaths each year by adding third-trimester maternal syphilis screening.

If maternal syphilis is diagnosed and treated at or before 24 weeks of gestation, serologic titers should not be repeated before 8 weeks after treatment (i.e., at 32 weeks of gestation), but they should be repeated at delivery. Titers should be repeated sooner if reinfection or treatment failure is suspected. For syphilis diagnosed and treated after 24 weeks of gestation, serologic titers should be repeated only at delivery.[30] Histologic examination of the placenta shows that the organ is usually large, pale, friable, and thickened with hypercellular villi that demonstrate acute and chronic inflammatory inflammation and proliferative fetal vascular changes. Histopathologic features include necrotizing funisitis, villous enlargement, and acute villitis.[8,73] Erythroblastosis was more common in stillborn infants with CS than all liveborn infants (odds ratio= 16; 95% confidence interval, 1–370).[73] Spirochetes can also be found in the umbilical vessel walls.[4,44,73] Placental and umbilical cord histopathology should be performed on every case of suspected syphilis.[8,73] The addition of histologic evaluation to conventional diagnostic evaluations has improved the detection rate for CS from 67% to 89% in liveborn infants and 91% to 97% in stillborn infants.[73]

Treatment

When penicillin became available in 1943, Lentz and Ingraham began to treat pregnant women and infected neonates with the new drug in Philadelphia.[1,74] Whereas maternal treatment was highly effective, the deaths of three of nine infants were thought to be caused by complications of CS, rather than exposure to the new antimicrobial agent. However, a year later, these authors discovered that administration of penicillin to syphilitic persons, including newborns, could result in an adverse immunologic response, known as the Jarisch–Herxheimer reaction, with 34 "reactions" recorded among 69 infants who were treated with penicillin.[75] A follow-up study by Holzel and colleagues[76] in 1956 found 14 deaths among 32 infants treated during the first 3 months of life, and the Jarisch–Herxheimer reaction was listed as a contributory cause of seven deaths. This reaction is observed in approximately 40% to 45% of women treated for syphilis, especially during the second half of pregnancy.[77,78] This condition, which typically occurs within the first 24 hours of treatment, is caused by the acute and unregulated release of host proinflammatory cytokines, triggered by the death of large numbers of *T. pallidum* spirochetes following exposure to effective antimicrobials.[79,80] Clinical signs and symptoms include fever, tachypnea, tachycardia, hypotension, skin rash, and cardiovascular collapse that may result in death. Because preterm uterine contractions and fetal distress have been reported, hospital admission for initial maternal syphilis treatment is advisable.[78,81,82] Corticosteroid therapy has not been shown to alter or prevent the reaction, and treatment usually consists of supportive care only.[8] This reaction is now rare in the treatment of CS.

In 1990, the CDC and American Academy of Pediatrics (AAP) recommended that all infants whose mothers had untreated or inadequately treated syphilis at delivery be diagnosed with CS and treated with penicillin, even if the infants appeared to be asymptomatic (Table 9.1).[83] Treatment decisions for *suspected* CS in newborns, however, are usually based on syphilis identification in the mother, as well as evaluation of maternal history and ongoing risk factors; adequacy of maternal and sex partner treatment; presence of clinical, laboratory, or radiographic evidence of syphilis in the neonate; and direct comparison of maternal (at delivery) and neonatal titers using identical nontreponemal serologic testing (i.e., RPR or VDRL tests).[30]

Newborns with confirmed CS should receive either aqueous crystalline penicillin G (50,000 U/kg intravenously every 12 hours for the first week of age, followed by every 8 hours beyond 7 days of age) for 10 days or aqueous procaine penicillin G (50,000 U/kg intramuscularly once daily for 10 days) (Table 9.2). If more than 1 day of therapy is missed, the entire course should be restarted. Because insufficient data exist regarding the use of ampicillin, a full 10 days of penicillin should be administered even if the newborn received ampicillin for empiric coverage for possible sepsis.[8] Conversely, a complete evaluation consisting of cerebrospinal fluid (CSF) analysis, long-bone radiographs, and complete blood count (CBC) with differential and platelet counts should be performed to guide optimal therapy for neonates who have a normal physical examination and a serum quantitative nontreponemal serologic titer less than fourfold the maternal titer and one of the following: (1) mother was not treated, inadequately treated, or has no documentation of having received treatment; (2) mother was treated with a non-penicillin G regimen[84]; or (3) mother received recommended treatment <4 weeks before delivery.[8] If all of these studies are normal, then the neonate can receive a single intramuscular (IM) injection of benzathine penicillin G (BPG; 50,000 U/kg).[85] However, if a 10-day treatment with parenteral penicillin therapy is planned, an extensive workup is unnecessary.[8] Additional studies, including chest radiographs, liver function tests, cranial imaging, ophthalmologic examination, and hearing evaluations, should be done as clinically indicated.[30] Normal neonates born to mothers adequately treated during pregnancy and greater than 4 weeks before delivery should be considered as a "close contact" and receive a single IM injection of BPG (50,000 U/kg). An extensive evaluation is not recommended for these patients.[8,30,34,86] Neonates with suspected or proven CS can be cared for using only standard precautions. If the infant has cutaneous lesions or mucous membrane involvement, then contact precautions with gloves should be instituted until 24 hours of treatment have been completed.[8]

Because *T. pallidum* undergoes a very low rate of division during latent disease, a prolonged course of penicillin is necessary to prevent treatment failure for late latent syphilis (>1 year duration), tertiary syphilis, and latent syphilis of unknown duration.[4] Certain penicillin preparations may not penetrate sequestered sites where *T. pallidum* can reside, including the CNS and aqueous humor, so appropriate penicillin preparation selection is important for the eradication of infection. Combinations of benzathine penicillin, procaine penicillin, and oral penicillin preparations are not efficacious for treating syphilis. Parenteral penicillin G is the only therapy with documented efficacy for syphilis during pregnancy, and pregnant women who report penicillin allergy should be desensitized and treated with penicillin at the stage of infection.[30] Treatment failures are most likely to occur with later gestational age at treatment, shorter treatment-delivery intervals (<30 days), high maternal titers, and earlier stages of disease, particularly with secondary syphilis.[87–89] If follow-up is not likely, women with an isolated reactive treponemal test and without a history of treated syphilis should be treated according to the syphilis stage.[30] Most women will not achieve a fourfold reduction in titers before delivery, although this does not indicate treatment failure.[90] A fourfold increase in titer after treatment (e.g., from 1:8 to 1:32) that is sustained for >2 weeks, however, is concerning for reinfection or treatment failure.[30] Adequate maternal syphilis treatment is vital, with 2008 and 2012 WHO data showing reductions in fetal deaths or stillbirths of 82% following appropriate treatment of *T. pallidum* infection; in preterm and low-birth-weight deliveries, 65%; in neonatal deaths, 80%; and in clinical disease in newborns, 97%.[91]

Special Considerations

SYPHILIS AND MATERNAL HIV INFECTION

All pregnant women who have syphilis and their sexual partners should be tested for coinfection with HIV, although infants born to mothers coinfected with syphilis and HIV do not require different evaluation, therapy, or follow-up.[8,30,92] Similarly, any neonate at risk for CS should receive a full evaluation and HIV testing. Placental inflammation from CS infection might increase the risk for perinatal transmission of HIV, with some evidence suggesting the direct involvement of *T. pallidum* in facilitating HIV infection and progression. Incorporating antiretroviral therapy per current HIV guidelines might improve clinical outcomes among persons coinfected with HIV and syphilis and attenuate concerns about the adequate treatment of syphilis in persons with HIV virologic suppression.[30,93,94]

EVALUATION AND TREATMENT OF INFANTS AND CHILDREN ≥1 MONTH OF AGE WITH CONGENITAL SYPHILIS

Older infants and children ≥1 month old who are identified as having reactive serologic tests for syphilis should be examined thoroughly and have maternal serology and records reviewed to assess whether they have congenital or acquired syphilis.[8,30] In extremely early or incubating syphilis cases, all maternal serologic tests might be negative at the time of delivery, with infection remaining undetected until the diagnosis is made later in the infant or child. Any infant or child at risk for CS should receive a full evaluation and testing for HIV infection.[30] Additional testing should include CSF analysis for VDRL testing, cell count, and protein, as well as a complete CBC and platelet counts. Other tests should be performed as clinically indicated (i.e., long-bone radiographs, chest radiograph, liver function tests, abdominal ultrasound, ophthalmologic examination, neuroimaging, and auditory brainstem response).[8,30]

Completed physical examinations and serologic testing (i.e., RPR or VDRL) should occur every 3 months until the test becomes nonreactive or there is a fourfold titer reduction. If the titers rise at any point for more than 2 weeks or do not decrease fourfold after 12 to 18 months, the patient should have CSF analysis with VDRL titers and receive a 10-day course of parenteral penicillin G in coordination with infectious disease consultation.[30] Treponemal tests, including EIA, CIA, and TP-PA, should not be used to evaluate treatment response in neonates and infants because maternal IgG treponemal antibodies might persist for >15 months after delivery. Infants or children whose initial CSF evaluations are abnormal do not need repeat lumbar puncture unless their serologic titers do not decrease fourfold after 12 to 18 months.[30] After 18 months of follow-up, abnormal CSF indices that persist and cannot be attributed to other ongoing illnesses indicate that retreatment is needed for possible neurosyphilis and should be managed in consultation with an expert.[30]

INTERNATIONAL ADOPTEE, IMMIGRANT, AND/OR REFUGEE CHILDREN

In countries where treponemal infections (i.e., yaws or pinta) are endemic, children may have reactive nontreponemal and treponemal serologic tests because these diagnostics cannot distinguish among the different subspecies of *T. pallidum*. Due to the possibility of syphilis infection (*T. pallidum* subspecies *pallidum*) in these children, a complete evaluation for CS should be completed.[30] If the workup (including CSF examination) is normal, the child may receive three weekly doses of BPG (50,000 U/kg body weight IM).[30] Alternatively, a 10-day course of intravenous (IV) aqueous penicillin G followed by a single dose of BPG (50,000 U/kg body weight IM up to the adult dose of 2.4 million U) can be considered for those with a normal workup and CSF findings.[30]

PENICILLIN SHORTAGES

Despite exposure to penicillin for >70 years, *T. pallidum* remains completely sensitive to this antibiotic. Standard treatment with BPG is highly effective for treating all stages of uncomplicated syphilis, and IV aqueous crystalline penicillin G or IM procaine penicillin (plus probenecid) are effective for patients with CNS involvement.[17,30] The manufacturing of BPG, however, is an unattractive business model because the drug is expensive to make but commands a market price of pennies per dose because it is an older antibiotic that is now off-patent. This aspect has led to market exits, inflexible production cycles, and minimum order quantities that have all been found to affect BPG supply.[95] Today, just four companies produce the active pharmaceutical ingredient for penicillin: one in Austria and three in China.[95] At least five companies abandoned the global penicillin market within the last 10 years in search of a more profitable drug.[95]

When IV or IM penicillin preparations are unavailable or cannot be tolerated, IV ampicillin or parenteral ceftriaxone can be used with caveats (see https://www.cdc.gov/std/treatment-guidelines/penicillin-allergy.htm).[30] The use of oral antibiotics, such as azithromycin or other macrolides, is not recommended for treatment or prophylaxis of syphilis due to rising *T. pallidum* resistance to this drug class.[17,30] Pediatric patients who receive alternative antibiotics for the treatment of CS require close clinical monitoring to detect and treat complications from possible inadequate treatment and to identify and evaluate alternative maternal and CS treatment regimens in advance of future penicillin shortages.[96]

Follow-Up

All neonates treated for CS should receive complete follow-up examinations and serologic testing (i.e., RPR or VDRL) every 2 to 3 months until a nonreactive test is obtained.[30] If a neonate was not treated for CS because the diagnosis was considered less or not likely due to suspected passive transfer of maternal IgG antibodies, serologic titers should decrease by 3 months of age and be nonreactive by 6 months of age, and no further evaluations are necessary. If the nontreponemal test remains reactive at 6 months, then the infant is likely infected and requires syphilis treatment.[30] Neonates with a negative nontreponemal test at birth and whose mothers were seroreactive at delivery should be retested at 3 months of age to rule out serologically negative incubating CS at the time of birth.[30] If nontreponemal serologic titers persist at 6 to 12 months of age, the infant should be re-evaluated (including CSF examination) and managed in consultation with an infectious disease expert, as retreatment with a 10-day course of a penicillin G regimen might be indicated. Neonates treated for CS do not require a CSF examination unless RPR or VDRL titers persist at 6 to 12 months of age, even if initial CSF values were abnormal. Persistent nontreponemal titers and CSF abnormalities, however, should be managed in consultation with an expert.[30]

If nontreponemal titers remain the same or increase fourfold at any time after 12 to 18 months of age, the child should receive a full evaluation and be re-treated with parental penicillin G for 10 days. Titers that remain reactive beyond 18 months of age confirm a diagnosis of CS, as no passively transferred maternal IgG antibodies should be present.[30] As many as 30% of children with confirmed CS and who received appropriate treatment with penicillin have nonreactive treponemal tests at >18 months of age. If the child was not previously treated, treatment for late CS is indicated. If the infant is found to have abnormal CSF findings, then repeat lumbar punctures for CSF analysis should be completed at 6 months after therapy. A reactive CSF VDRL test result or an abnormal protein content or cell count that cannot be attributed to other ongoing illnesses at that time is an indication for retreatment.[8]

Summary

In 2017, the CDC released *Call to Action: Let's Work Together to Stem the Tide of Rising Syphilis*,[63,97] with important actionable items such as the development of novel point of care tests for the accurate and timely diagnosis of syphilis. This document also calls explicitly for public health departments to take action to reduce CS by (1) partnering with healthcare providers; (2) working with state and local sexually transmitted disease and maternal–child health programs; (3) conducting partner services and increasing screening, prioritizing pregnant women; (4) partnering with patient advocacy groups; and (5) improving CS surveillance. A national CS prevention strategy must prioritize interventions that target the root cause of missed opportunities while maximizing the impact of finite resources.[12]

Rates of CS closely mirror those of primary and secondary syphilis. In the US, syphilis cases in reproductive aged females has risen more than 414% in the last decade, which is accompanied by a > 500% surge in the incidence of congenital syphilis (CS).[4,12] Preventing CS requires eliminating the barriers to family planning and prenatal care, ensuring syphilis screening at the first prenatal visit with rescreening at 28 weeks' gestation and delivery (as indicated), and providing appropriate and timely treatment for pregnant women with syphilis.[12,30] No mother or newborn should leave the hospital without the maternal serologic syphilis status documented at least once during the pregnancy.[8] Syphilis is a potentially eradicable disease, but this can be achieved only with sustained international will and cooperation to fund the necessary screening and treatment programs.[98] In the United States, the re-emergence of syphilis has been met by a biomedical research landscape with limited human and financial resources. Few researchers and clinicians with interests in syphilis remain, and attracting new talent to this field has been challenging due to the difficulty in working with *T. pallidum* and the successful attainment of research funding to sustain their careers.[99] Recruitment of researchers, with proportional increases in research funding and engagement of industry/funding partnerships for syphilis diagnostics and vaccine development are all necessary if eradicating syphilis is to be realized.[17]

REFERENCES

1. Obladen M. Curse on two generations: a history of congenital syphilis. *Neonatology.* 2013;103:274-280.
2. Swediaur FX. *A Comprehensive Treatise Upon the Symptoms, Consequences, Nature, and Treatment of Venereal, or Syphilitic, Diseases.* Vol. 2. London: Longman, Hurst, Rees, Orme, and Brown; 1819: 109-115.
3. Braxton J, Davis D, Emerson B, et al. *Sexually Transmitted Disease Surveillance 2017.* Atlanta, GA: Centers for Disease Control and Prevention, National Center for HIV/AIDS, Viral Hepatitis, STD, and TB Prevention; 2018.
4. Bowen V, Braxton J, Davis D, et al. *Sexually Transmitted Disease Surveillance 2018.* Atlanta, GA: Centers for Disease Control and Prevention, National Center for HIV/AIDS, Viral Hepatitis, STD, and TB Prevention; 2019.

5. Peterman TA, Su J, Bernstein KT, et al. Syphilis in the United States: on the rise? *Expert Rev Anti Infect Ther.* 2015;13:161-168.
6. Centers for Disease Control and Prevention. *Sexually Transmitted Disease Surveillance 2019*. Atlanta, GA: Centers for Disease Control and Prevention, National Center for HIV/AIDS, Viral Hepatitis, STD, and TB Prevention; 2021.
7. Centers for Disease Control and Prevention, Emerging Infections Program Network. *Active Bacterial Core Surveillance Report, Group B Streptococcus, 2019*. Atlanta, GA: Centers for Disease Control and Prevention; 2021.
8. Cooper JM, Sanchez PJ. Congenital syphilis. *Semin Perinatol.* 2018;42:176-184.
9. Dorfman DH, Glaser JH. Congenital syphilis presenting in infants after the newborn period. *N Engl J Med.* 1990;323:1299-1302.
10. Heston S, Arnold S. Syphilis in children. *Infect Dis Clin North Am.* 2018;32:129-144.
11. Kimberlin D, Brady M, Jackson M, et al. Syphilis. In: Kimberlin DW, Long SS, Brady MT, Jackson MA, eds. *Red Book 2018: Report of the Committee on Infectious Diseases*. Itasca, IL: American Academy of Pediatrics; 2018:773-788.
12. Kimball A, Torrone E, Miele K, et al. Missed opportunities for prevention of congenital syphilis - United States, 2018. *MMWR Morb Mortal Wkly Rep.* 2020;69:661-665.
13. Hawkes S, Matin N, Broutet N, Low N. Effectiveness of interventions to improve screening for syphilis in pregnancy: a systematic review and meta-analysis. *Lancet Infect Dis.* 2011;11:684-691.
14. Umapathi KK, Thavamani A, Chotikanatis K. Incidence trends, risk factors, mortality and healthcare utilization in congenital syphilis-related hospitalizations in the United States: a nationwide population analysis. *Pediatr Infect Dis J.* 2019;38:1126-1130.
15. Centers for Disease Control and Prevention, Division of Health Informatics and Surveillance. *Congenital Syphilis (Treponema pallidum) 2015 Case Definition*. Available at: https://ndc.services.cdc.gov/case-definitions/congenital-syphilis-2015/. Accessed January 25, 2023.
16. Schaudinn FR, Hoffmann E. Vorl ufiger Bericht über das Vorkommen von Spirochaeten in syphilitischen Krankheitsprodukten und bei Papillomen. *Arbeiten aus dem Kaiserlichen Gesundheitsamte.* 1905;22:527-534.
17. Cameron CE, Lukehart SA. Current status of syphilis vaccine development: need, challenges, prospects. *Vaccine.* 2014;32:1602-1609.
18. Centurion-Lara A, Castro C, Castillo R, Shaffer JM, Van Voorhis WC, Lukehart SA. The flanking region sequences of the 15-kDa lipoprotein gene differentiate pathogenic treponemes. *J Infect Dis.* 1998;177:1036-1040.
19. Fraser CM, Norris SJ, Weinstock GM, et al. Complete genome sequence of *Treponema pallidum*, the syphilis spirochete. *Science.* 1998;281:375-388.
20. Walker EM, Arnett JK, Heath JD, Norris SJ. *Treponema pallidum* subsp. *pallidum* has a single, circular chromosome with a size of approximately 900 kilobase pairs. *Infect Immun.* 1991;59:2476-2479.
21. Walker EM, Howell JK, You Y, et al. Physical map of the genome of *Treponema pallidum* subsp. *pallidum* (Nichols). *J Bacteriol.* 1995;177:1797-1804.
22. Turner TB, Hollander DH. Biology of the treponematoses based on studies carried out at the International Treponematosis Laboratory Center of the Johns Hopkins University under the auspices of the World Health Organization. *Monogr Ser World Health Organ.*1957;(35):3-266.
23. Lien E, Sellati TJ, Yoshimura A, et al. Toll-like receptor 2 functions as a pattern recognition receptor for diverse bacterial products. *J Biol Chem.* 1999;274:33419-33425.
24. Lafond RE, Lukehart SA. Biological basis for syphilis. *Clin Microbiol Rev.* 2006;19:29-49.
25. Baker-Zander SA, Hook III EW, Bonin P, Handsfield HH, Lukehart SA. Antigens of *Treponema pallidum* recognized by IgG and IgM antibodies during syphilis in humans. *J Infect Dis.* 1985;151:264-272.
26. Norris SJ, Sell S. Antigenic complexity of *Treponema pallidum*: antigenicity and surface localization of major polypeptides. *J Immunol.* 1984;133:2686-2692.
27. Deacon WE, Falcone VH, Harris A. A fluorescent test for treponemal antibodies. *Proc Soc Exp Biol Med.* 1957;96:477-480.
28. Penn CW, Rhodes JG. Surface-associated antigens of *Treponema pallidum* concealed by an inert outer layer. *Immunology.* 1982;46:9-16.
29. Leader BT, Hevner K, Molini BJ, Barrett LK, Van Voorhis WC, Lukehart SA. Antibody responses elicited against the *Treponema pallidum* repeat proteins differ during infection with different isolates of *Treponema pallidum* subsp. *pallidum*. *Infect Immun.* 2003;71:6054-6057.
30. Workowski KA, Bachmann LH, Chan PA, et al. Sexually transmitted infections treatment guidelines, 2021. *MMWR Recomm Rep.* 2021;70:1-187.
31. Centers for Disease Control and Prevention. *Syphilis - CDC Detailed Fact Sheet*. Available at: https://www.cdc.gov/std/syphilis/stdfact-syphilis-detailed.htm. Accessed January 25, 2023.
32. Nathan L, Bohman VR, Sanchez PJ, Leos NK, Twickler DM, Wendel Jr GD. In utero infection with *Treponema pallidum* in early pregnancy. *Prenat Diagn.* 1997;17:119-123.
33. Nathan L, Twickler DM, Peters MT, Sánchez PJ, Wendel Jr GD. Fetal syphilis: correlation of sonographic findings and rabbit infectivity testing of amniotic fluid. *J Ultrasound Med.* 1993;12:97-101.
34. Sheffield JS, Sanchez PJ, Morris G, et al. Congenital syphilis after maternal treatment for syphilis during pregnancy. *Am J Obstet Gynecol.* 2002;186:569-573.
35. Ingraham Jr NR. The value of penicillin alone in the prevention and treatment of congenital syphilis. *Acta Derm Venereol Suppl (Stockh).* 1950;31:60-87.
36. Biswas HH, Chew Ng RA, Murray EL, et al. Characteristics associated with delivery of an infant with congenital syphilis and missed opportunities for prevention-California, 2012 to 2014. *Sex Transm Dis.* 2018;45:435-441.
37. Slutsker JS, Hennessy RR, Schillinger JA. Factors contributing to congenital syphilis cases - New York City, 2010–2016. *MMWR Morb Mortal Wkly Rep.* 2018;67:1088-1093.
38. DiOrio D, Kroeger K, Ross A. Social vulnerability in congenital syphilis case mothers: qualitative assessment of cases in Indiana, 2014 to 2016. *Sex Transm Dis.* 2018;45:447-451.
39. Ribeiro ADDC, Dan CS, Santos ADS, Croda J, Simionatto S. Neurosyphilis in Brazilian newborns: a health problem that could be avoided. *Rev Inst Med Trop Sao Paulo.* 2020;62:e82.
40. Korenromp EL, Mahiane SG, Nagelkerke N, et al. Syphilis prevalence trends in adult women in 132 countries - estimations using the Spectrum Sexually Transmitted Infections model. *Sci Rep.* 2018;8:11503.
41. Centers for Disease Control and Prevention. *Syphilis (Treponema pallidum) 1990 Case Definition*. Available at: https://ndc.services.cdc.gov/case-definitions/syphilis-1990/. Accessed January 25, 2023.

42. Cohen DA, Boyd D, Prabhudas I, Mascola L. The effects of case definition in maternal screening and reporting criteria on rates of congenital syphilis. *Am J Public Health.* 1990;80:316-317.
43. Kidd S, Bowen VB, Torrone EA, Bolan G. Use of national syphilis surveillance data to develop a congenital syphilis prevention cascade and estimate the number of potential congenital syphilis cases averted. *Sex Transm Dis.* 2018;45:S23-S28.
44. Woods CR. Congenital syphilis-persisting pestilence. *Pediatr Infect Dis J.* 2009;28:536-537.
45. Wilkinson RH, Heller RM. Congenital syphilis: resurgence of an old problem. *Pediatrics.* 1971;47:27-30.
46. Berry MC, Dajani AS, Resurgence of congenital syphilis. *Infect Dis Clin North Am.* 1992;6:19-29.
47. Mascola L, Pelosi R, Blount JH, Binkin NJ, Alexander CE, Cates Jr W. Congenital syphilis. Why is it still occurring? *JAMA.* 1984;252:1719-1722.
48. Hill LL, Singer DB, Falletta J, Stasney R. The nephrotic syndrome in congenital syphilis: an immunopathy. *Pediatrics.* 1972;49:260-266.
49. Yuceoglu AM, Sagel I, Tresser G, Wasserman E, Lange K. The glomerulopathy of congenital syphilis. A curable immune-deposit disease. *JAMA.* 1974;229:1085-1089.
50. Jacobs K, Vu DM, Mony V, Sofos E, Buzi N. Congenital syphilis misdiagnosed as suspected nonaccidental trauma. *Pediatrics.* 2019;144:e20191564.
51. Zhou Q, Wang L, Chen C, Cao Y, Yan W, Zhou W. A case series of 130 neonates with congenital syphilis: preterm neonates had more clinical evidences of infection than term neonates. *Neonatology.* 2012;102:152-156.
52. Borella L, Goobar JE, Clark GM. Synovitis of the knee joints in late congenital syphilis. Clutton's joints. *JAMA.* 1962;180:190-192.
53. Cooper JM, Porter M, Bazan JA, Nicholson LM, Sánchez PJ. Re-emergence of congenital syphilis in Ohio. *Pediatr Infect Dis J.* 2018;37:1286-1289.
54. Michelow IC, Wendel Jr GD, Norgard MV, et al. Central nervous system infection in congenital syphilis. *N Engl J Med.* 2002;346:1792-1798.
55. Lithgow KV, Cameron CE. Vaccine development for syphilis. *Expert Rev Vaccines.* 2017;16:37-44.
56. Smith BC, Simpson Y, Morshed MG, et al. New proteins for a new perspective on syphilis diagnosis. *J Clin Microbiol.* 2013;51:105-111.
57. Sena AC, White BL, Sparling PF. Novel *Treponema pallidum* serologic tests: a paradigm shift in syphilis screening for the 21st century. *Clin Infect Dis.* 2010;51:700-708.
58. Causer LM, Kaldor JM, Fairley CK, et al. A laboratory-based evaluation of four rapid point-of-care tests for syphilis. *PLoS ONE.* 2014;9:e91504.
59. Verghese VP, Hendson L, Singh A, Guenette T, Gratrix J, Robinson JL. Early childhood neurodevelopmental outcomes in infants exposed to infectious syphilis in utero. *Pediatr Infect Dis J.* 2018;37:576-579.
60. Lin JS, Eder M, Bean S. *Screening for Syphilis Infection in Pregnant Women: A Reaffirmation Evidence Update for the U.S. Preventive Services Task Force.* Rockville, MD: Agency for Healthcare Research and Quality; 2018.
61. Ortiz DA, Shukla MR, Loeffelholz MJ. The traditional or reverse algorithm for diagnosis of syphilis: pros and cons. *Clin Infect Dis.* 2020;71:S43-S51.
62. Morshed M. Current trend on syphilis diagnosis: issues and challenges. *Adv Exp Med Biol.* 2014;808:51-64.
63. Centers for Disease Control and Prevention. *Call to Action: Let's Work Together to Stem the Tide of Rising Syphilis in the United States.* Available at: https://www.cdc.gov/std/syphilis/Syphilis-CalltoActionApril2017.pdf. Accessed January 25, 2023.
64. Centers for Disease Control and Prevention (CDC). Discordant results from reverse sequence syphilis screening—five laboratories, United States, 2006–2010. *MMWR Morb Mortal Wkly Rep.* 2011;60:133-137.
65. Mmeje O, Chow JM, Davidson L, Shieh J, Schapiro JM, Park IU. Discordant syphilis immunoassays in pregnancy: perinatal outcomes and implications for clinical management. *Clin Infect Dis.* 2015;61:1049-1053.
66. Centers for Disease Control and Prevention (CDC). Syphilis testing algorithms using treponemal tests for initial screening—four laboratories, New York City, 2005–2006. *MMWR Morb Mortal Wkly Rep.* 2008;57:872-875.
67. Nandwani R, Evans DT. Are you sure it's syphilis? A review of false positive serology. *Int J STD AIDS.* 1995;6:241-248.
68. Tuddenham S, Katz SS, Ghanem KG. Syphilis laboratory guidelines: performance characteristics of nontreponemal antibody tests. *Clin Infect Dis.* 2020;71:S21-S42.
69. Tong ML, Lin LR, Liu LL, et al. Analysis of 3 algorithms for syphilis serodiagnosis and implications for clinical management. *Clin Infect Dis.* 2014;58:1116-1124.
70. Kelly M, Hendry S, Norton R. The utility of the syphilis enzyme immunoassay IgM in the diagnosis of congenital syphilis. *Diagn Microbiol Infect Dis.* 2020;98:115152.
71. Centers for Disease Control and Prevention (CDC), Division of STD Prevention (DSTDP). *State Statutory and Regulatory Language Regarding Prenatal Syphilis Screenings in the United States, 2018.* Washington, DC: U.S. Department of Health and Human Services (HHS); 2020.
72. Hersh AR, Megli CJ, Caughey AB. Repeat screening for syphilis in the third trimester of pregnancy: a cost-effectiveness analysis. *Obstet Gynecol.* 2018;132:699-707.
73. Sheffield JS, Sánchez PJ, Wendel Jr GD, et al. Placental histopathology of congenital syphilis. *Obstet Gynecol.* 2002;100:126-133.
74. Lentz JW. Penicillin in the prevention and treatment of congenital syphilis. *JAMA.* 1944;126:408-413.
75. Platou RV, Allan Jr JH, Ingraham NR, et al. Early congenital syphilis; treatment of two hundred and fifty-two patients with penicillin. *JAMA.* 1947;133:10-16.
76. Holzel A. Jarisch-Herxheimer reaction following penicillin treatment of early congenital syphilis. *Br J Vener Dis.* 1956;32:175-180.
77. Myles TD, Elam G, Park-Hwang E, Nguyen T. The Jarisch-Herxheimer reaction and fetal monitoring changes in pregnant women treated for syphilis. *Obstet Gynecol.* 1998;92:859-864.
78. Uku A, Albujasim Z, Dwivedi T, Ladipo Z, Konje JC. Syphilis in pregnancy: the impact of "the Great Imitator." *Eur J Obstet Gynecol Reprod Biol.* 2021;259:207-210.
79. Hori H, Sato Y, Shitara T. Congenital syphilis presenting as Jarisch-Herxheimer reaction at birth. *Pediatr Int.* 2015;57:299-301.
80. Wang C, He S, Yang H, Liu Y, Zhao Y, Pang L. Unique manifestations and risk factors of Jarisch-Herxheimer reaction during treatment of child congenital syphilis. *Sex Transm Infect.* 2018;94:562-564.
81. Klein VR, Cox SM, Mitchell MD, Wendel Jr GD. The Jarisch-Herxheimer reaction complicating syphilotherapy in pregnancy. *Obstet Gynecol.* 1990;75:375-380.

82. Rac MWF, Greer LG, Wendel Jr GD. Jarisch-Herxheimer reaction triggered by group B *Streptococcus* intrapartum antibiotic prophylaxis. *Obstet Gynecol.* 2010;116:552-556.
83. Zenker P. New case definition for congenital syphilis reporting. *Sex Transm Dis.* 1991;18:44-45.
84. Zhou P, Qian Y, Xu J, Gu Z, Liao K. Occurrence of congenital syphilis after maternal treatment with azithromycin during pregnancy. *Sex Transm Dis.* 2007;34:472-474.
85. Paryani SG, Vaughn AJ, Crosby M, Lawrence S. Treatment of asymptomatic congenital syphilis: benzathine versus procaine penicillin G therapy. *J Pediatr.* 1994;125:471-475.
86. Rac MW, Revell PA, Eppes CS. Syphilis during pregnancy: a preventable threat to maternal-fetal health. *Am J Obstet Gynecol.* 2017;216:352-363.
87. Conover CS, Rend CA, Miller Jr GB, Schmid GP. Congenital syphilis after treatment of maternal syphilis with a penicillin regimen exceeding CDC guidelines. *Infect Dis Obstet Gynecol.* 1998;6:134-137.
88. Plotzker RE, Murphy RD, Stoltey JE. Congenital syphilis prevention: strategies, evidence, and future directions. *Sex Transm Dis.* 2018;45:S29-S37.
89. Alexander JM, Sheffield JS, Sánchez PJ, Mayfield J, Wendel Jr GD. Efficacy of treatment for syphilis in pregnancy. *Obstet Gynecol.* 1999;93:5-8.
90. Rac MW, Bryant SN, McIntire DD, et al. Progression of ultrasound findings of fetal syphilis after maternal treatment. *Am J Obstet Gynecol.* 2014;211:426.e1-6.
91. Blencowe H, Cousens S, Kamb M, Berman S, Lawn JE. Lives Saved Tool supplement detection and treatment of syphilis in pregnancy to reduce syphilis related stillbirths and neonatal mortality. *BMC Public Health.* 2011;11:S9.
92. Rodriguez PJ, Roberts DA, Meisner J, et al. Cost-effectiveness of dual maternal HIV and syphilis testing strategies in high and low HIV prevalence countries: a modelling study. *Lancet Glob Health.* 2021;9:e61-e71.
93. Ghanem KG, Moore RD, Rompalo AM, Erbelding EJ, Zenilman JM, Gebo KA. Neurosyphilis in a clinical cohort of HIV-1-infected patients. *AIDS.* 2008;22:1145-1151.
94. Ghanem KG, Moore RD, Rompalo AM, Erbelding EJ, Zenilman JM, Gebo KA. Antiretroviral therapy is associated with reduced serologic failure rates for syphilis among HIV-infected patients. *Clin Infect Dis.* 2008;47:258-265.
95. Araujo RS, Souza ASS, Braga JU. Who was affected by the shortage of penicillin for syphilis in Rio de Janeiro, 2013–2017? *Rev Saude Publica.* 2020;54:109.
96. Rocha AFB, Araújo MAL, Taylor MM, Kara EO, Broutet NJN. Treatment administered to newborns with congenital syphilis during a penicillin shortage in 2015, Fortaleza, Brazil. *BMC Pediatr.* 2021;21:166.
97. Hsu KK. Congenital syphilis: time for a national prevention program. *Sex Transm Dis.* 2017;44:503-504.
98. Woods CR. Syphilis in children: congenital and acquired. *Semin Pediatr Infect Dis.* 2005;16:245-257.
99. Kersh EN, Lukehart, SA. Biomedical research priorities for modern syphilis clinical management, diagnosis, and vaccines: overview and commentary for Unit 1. *Sex Transm Dis.* 2018;45:S7-S9.

Chapter **10**

Gonococcal Eye Prophylaxis—Are Mandates Still Justified?

Margaret R. Hammerschlag, MD; Susannah Franco, PharmD

Key Points

- Neonatal ocular prophylaxis for prevention of gonococcal ophthalmia was first introduced by Credé in 1881.
- Gonococcal ophthalmia became and still is very uncommon due to the introduction in the 1950s of prenatal screening for *Neisseria gonorrhoeae* and treatment of pregnant women.
- Erythromycin ophthalmic ointment is the only preparation available for neonatal ocular prophylaxis in the United States.
- Neonatal ocular prophylaxis with erythromycin ophthalmic ointment does not prevent chlamydial ophthalmia, which was the major cause of ophthalmia neonatorum through the 1990s.
- Data on the efficacy of erythromycin ophthalmic ointment for prevention of gonococcal ophthalmia are limited and difficult to assess in settings where prenatal screening is part of routine prenatal care.

Introduction

Credé reported in 1881 that the instillation of 2% silver nitrate drops into the eyes of newborn infants reduced the incidence of gonococcal ophthalmia neonatorum.[1] However, much has changed over the 140 years since this study was published. At the beginning of the 20th century, before expectant mothers were being screened for sexually transmitted infections (STIs), the term ophthalmia neonatorum was, for all practical purposes, synonymous with gonococcal conjunctivitis. As neonatal conjunctivitis came under control with silver nitrate prophylaxis, the importance of another form of ophthalmia neonatorum, inclusion blennorrhea (later identified as being due to *Chlamydia trachomatis*), was noted. The relationship between maternal genital infection and conjunctivitis of the newborn with inclusion bodies within epithelial cells was established by Thygeson and Stone in 1942.[2] Penicillin first became available to treat patients in the 1950s,[3] which allowed for the treatment of gonococcal infection. Gonococcal ophthalmia became and still is very uncommon due to the introduction of prenatal screening for *Neisseria gonorrhoeae* and treatment of pregnant women.[4] *C. trachomatis* was the most common cause of neonatal conjunctivitis in the United States in the latter half of the 20th century before the Centers for Disease Control and Prevention (CDC) recommended routine prenatal screening of pregnant women for *C. trachomatis* in 1993,[5] which has resulted in a dramatic decrease in perinatal chlamydial infection, including conjunctivitis, in the United States.[6] Currently, erythromycin ophthalmic ointment is the only preparation available for neonatal ocular prophylaxis in the United States.[6] Tetracycline ophthalmic ointment is no longer manufactured, and silver nitrate has not been available for over 2 decades. Many hospitals in the United States had switched to erythromycin ophthalmic ointment by the 1980s. Neonatal ocular prophylaxis with erythromycin is also specifically mandated by law in many states. However, neonatal ocular prophylaxis with erythromycin or tetracycline ophthalmic ointment does not prevent chlamydial ophthalmia.[6]

The CDC and the U.S. Preventive Services Task Force (USPSTF) currently recommend neonatal ocular prophylaxis with erythromycin ophthalmic ointment primarily for prevention of gonococcal ophthalmia.[7,8] Several countries in Europe (e.g., United Kingdom, Germany, Norway, Sweden, Denmark) have discontinued universal ocular prophylaxis and others offer parental choice.[9,10] The World Health Organization (WHO) still recommends neonatal ocular prophylaxis for the prevention of both gonococcal and chlamydial ophthalmia.[11] In 2015, the Canadian Pediatric Society recommended discontinuation of routine neonatal ocular prophylaxis in Canada, with an emphasis on enhanced prenatal screening for gonorrhea and *C. trachomatis*.[12]

Given the changed epidemiology of ophthalmia neonatorum in the United States and the impact of prenatal screening and treatment of pregnant women for *N. gonorrhoeae*, the question of whether mandates for ocular prophylaxis for the prevention of neonatal gonococcal ophthalmia in the United States are still necessary should be reevaluated.

Macrolide Resistance in *N. gonorrhoeae*

Erythromycin is the oldest macrolide antibiotic, a broad-spectrum class of antibiotics that exhibits its bacteriostatic action by binding to the 50S ribosomal subunit, which prevents translocation of the peptidyl-tRNA, interacting with the 23S rRNA and blocking the peptide exit channel in the 50S ribosomal subunits; this causes the incomplete release of polypeptides from the ribosomes and ultimately inhibits protein synthesis.[13–15] Bacterial resistance mechanisms against erythromycin and other macrolide antibiotics are thought to be genetic via modification of the 23S rRNA subunit by rRNA methylases, which block the binding of macrolides to the 23S rRNA, or through specific nucleotide alterations in 23S rRNA. Another theorized resistance mechanism is an overexpression of efflux pumps, especially the MtrCDE efflux pump.[13]

Genes encoding rRNA methylase, referred to as macrolide–lincosamide–streptogramin B resistance genes, or *erm* genes, have been identified in strains of *N. gonorrhoeae* since the 1990s. These genes confer high levels of resistance to erythromycin.[13,15] High-level resistance of *N. gonorrhoeae* to azithromycin has been associated with a single point mutation in all four copies of the 23S rRNA A2059G gene and with Mtr mutations. A study published in 1990 found that 14% of 300 *N. gonorrhoeae* strains from Canada and Kenya exhibited the Mtr phenotype, which decreased susceptibility to azithromycin fourfold.[13,16,17]

N. gonorrhoeae has developed resistance to the majority of antibiotics used for treatment in adults, including penicillin, tetracycline, fluoroquinolones, and sulfonamides.[8,18] Because of the increasing resistance of *N. gonorrhoeae* to azithromycin, including high-level resistance, a single 2-g dose of azithromycin was no longer recommended for treatment of gonococcal infections in the 2015 CDC Sexually transmitted Diseases Treatment Guidelines.[19] After its introduction in the 1980s, azithromycin was the only macrolide antibiotic recommended for the treatment of gonococcal infections. Azithromycin is eight times more active against *N. gonorrhoeae* compared to erythromycin.[13,16] Because erythromycin has never been strongly recommended for gonococcal treatment, with scarce reports of its use in combination with rifampin, no recent data on the susceptibility of *N. gonorrhoeae* to erythromycin exist.[8,20–22] Whether antibiotic resistance decreases the efficacy of 0.5% erythromycin ophthalmic ointment prophylaxis against gonococcal ophthalmia neonatorum is unknown, but speculation can be made based on azithromycin susceptibility data.

Azithromycin resistance has been surveilled since 1992 in the United States. Azithromycin can be used as a surrogate for macrolide resistance in gonococcal conjunctivitis, as class resistance is typically exhibited. If *N. gonorrhoeae* is resistant to azithromycin, it is likely to be more resistant to erythromycin.[13] The Australian Gonococcal Surveillance Program (AGSP) has monitored *N. gonorrhoeae* resistance since 1981; *N. gonorrhoeae* is considered resistant to azithromycin when the minimum inhibitory concentration (MIC) is ≥1 mg/L.[23] The AGSP 2019 report indicated that 4.6% of gonococcal isolates were resistant to azithromycin and that resistance had been increasing in Australia since 2012.[23]

Slaney et al.[16] analyzed 300 strains of *N. gonorrhoeae* in Canada and Kenya and found that the MICs to azithromycin and erythromycin were 0.25 mg/L and 2 mg/L, respectively. In 1997, Young et al.[24] reported two isolates of *N. gonorrhoeae* of the same serotype and auxotype (1B6/NR), meaning their genetic make-up and growth response patterns are comparable, with similar antibiograms (other than erythromycin and azithromycin susceptibilities) in a 13-year-old boy before and 3 weeks after a single 1-g dose of azithromycin. Pretreatment MICs were 0.125 mg/L to azithromycin and 1 mg/L to erythromycin. After one dose of azithromycin, MICs were 3 mg/L to azithromycin and 32 mg/L to erythromycin, indicating that macrolide resistance developed after treatment. The long half-life of azithromycin, which is beneficial in the treatment of chlamydial infections, may lead to resistance in *N. gonorrhoeae* by selecting for resistance-associated mutations in the 23S rRNA gene.[24] The continued use of azithromycin since these reports probably further increased macrolide resistance to *N. gonorrhoeae*.

Nucleic acid amplification testing is preferred over bacterial culture and antimicrobial susceptibility testing (AST) for gonococcal infection diagnosis. Because of this, very few clinical microbiology labs perform AST for gonococci. The Gonococcal Isolate Surveillance Project (GISP), established in 1986, provides some insight on macrolide resistance in the United States. A small number of *N. gonorrhoeae* isolates are collected monthly from over 20 sexually transmitted disease (STD) clinics and sent to the CDC for antibiotic resistance testing. The Clinical and Laboratory Standards Institute defines gonococcal isolates as being resistant to azithromycin at MIC >1 mg/L.[17,25] Within the GISP, *N. gonorrhoeae* is considered resistant to azithromycin when the MIC is ≥2 mg/L. In 2013 and 2014, 0.6% and 2.5% of *N. gonorrhoeae* isolates, respectively, were resistant to azithromycin. In 2018, 4.6% of *N. gonorrhoeae* isolates were resistant to azithromycin; in 2019, 5.1% were resistant.[17,25] WHO currently recommends a combination of intramuscular (IM) ceftriaxone and 1 g of azithromycin, but these recommendations were last updated in 2016.[11] The 2021 CDC Sexually Transmitted Infections Treatment Guidelines dropped the recommendation for dual treatment with 1 g of azithromycin and increased the dose of ceftriaxone to 500 mg.[7] This dual therapy was initially introduced to mitigate a possible development of resistance to ceftriaxone, but it may have contributed to the development of azithromycin resistance, as 1 g of azithromycin was probably subtherapeutic for treatment of gonorrhea. Although ceftriaxone resistance is rare, gonococcal resistance to azithromycin continues to increase globally.[20,26] Another CDC-supported initiative, Strengthening the United States Response to Resistant Gonorrhea (SURRG), involves eight U.S. jurisdictions and collects specimens for culture and AST from patients at STD and community clinics in California, Colorado, Indiana, Hawaii, New York, North Carolina, Washington, and Wisconsin.[27] Over 10,000 gonococcal isolates were collected in 2018 and 2019, 11% of which had MICs ≥ 2 mg/L.[27] Data from Indiana from May 2017 through December 2018 collected via the GISP and SURRG initiatives tested over 1000 *N. gonorrhoeae* isolates via ETEST. Of these isolates, 4.8% exhibited resistance (MIC ≥ 2 mg/L), and 1.4% exhibited high-level azithromycin resistance, defined as MIC ≥256 mg/L.[17] Other countries with extensive surveillance have reported increasing antibiotic resistance rates of *N. gonorrhoeae* in recent years.[7] From 2011 to 2015, Canada reported increased resistance of *N. gonorrhoeae* to erythromycin (32.4%) and azithromycin (4.7%).[18] Germany also reported increased resistance of *N. gonorrhoeae* isolates to azithromycin; 20.7% of isolates from January through May of 2021 had MICs >1 mg/L.[26]

Macrolide Pharmacokinetic Considerations in Treatment of Gonococcal Conjunctivitis

Very little data exist on the pharmacokinetics of including erythromycin and azithromycin, macrolides in neonates. Macrolides exhibit concentration-dependent activity.[21,28] Importantly, the MICs of antibiotics can vary by body site. Erythromycin reaches high concentrations in the eye when administered via ophthalmic ointment, but the concentration reached in the conjunctiva, how long it remains, and if the concentration can overcome resistance are unknown.[7,12,14] A case report of two adults with gonococcal conjunctivitis described the AST of five *N. gonorrhoeae* strains between 2003 and 2013 in Japan performed using ETEST. Susceptibility to erythromycin decreased over the 10-year period; the maximum MICs to erythromycin and azithromycin were 1 mg/L and 0.25 mg/L, respectively. The authors concluded that the erythromycin concentrations reached in the conjunctiva may not surpass the MIC.[29]

Erythromycin ophthalmic ointment, administered topically to the eyes, has limited penetration into eyelid tissue despite prolonged contact with the eyelid, eye, and blood–eye barrier.[14] Other potential barriers to drug delivery that may contribute to inadequate neonatal ocular prophylaxis with 0.5% erythromycin ophthalmic ointment include tear turnover and drainage, nasolacrimal drainage, and blinking.[30] Tear secretions are decreased in preterm infants but are similar to adults by term age, so term neonates specifically may be exposed to decreased levels of erythromycin and preterm neonates are better able to retain a high ophthalmic concentration.[31]

Barriers in the anterior eye segment, including the corneal epithelium, stroma, and blood–aqueous barrier, also limit drug entry into the eye, which has not been studied in infants but would theoretically hold true for them. Pre-corneal loss after topical ophthalmic administration, reported to be up to 80%, may decrease the bioavailability of erythromycin, which is compounded by its limited absorption through the corneal epithelium.[31] It is also unknown what transporters exist in the conjunctiva and how the transporters affect permeation.[32] Topical administration may not be appropriate for erythromycin, which is only active at high concentrations based on its pharmacokinetic index of efficacy.[32]

Azithromycin and erythromycin are both lipophilic, meaning they readily penetrate across cellular membranes and into tissues (including the conjunctiva), resulting in a relatively high volume of distribution compared to hydrophilic drugs. Although the lipophilicities of these two macrolides have not been compared, we can infer based on the volume of distribution (V_d) of azithromycin (31.1 L/kg) and the V_d of erythromycin (0.64 L/kg) that erythromycin is far less able to penetrate into body tissues. This is further illustrated by reports of the detection of azithromycin in body sites up to 4 weeks after a single oral dose.[28] Whereas the V_d values for both drugs are likely higher in infants due to their higher percentage of body fat, how their pharmacokinetic and pharmacodynamic data apply to ophthalmic formulations is unclear.

Another difference between azithromycin and erythromycin is that azithromycin is only 7% protein bound at high concentrations due to saturation of the binding sites. Conversely, erythromycin is consistently about 85% protein bound. This means far less free drug is available for pharmacologic action against gonococci compared to azithromycin.[28] Unfortunately, how to apply these concepts from the plasma to the eye is challenging, as protein binding in the eye is not well understood. Drug efficacy varies by site of infection, which is important when considering the evidence for gonococcal treatment with azithromycin, and there is a lack of evidence for erythromycin based on systemic administration for sexually transmitted disease.

The degree to which erythromycin can be absorbed across membranes can be additionally measured by the degree of ionization, or the pK_a. The pK_a of erythromycin is 7.87, meaning that 50% of the drug will be nonionized and therefore more lipophilic and absorbable into tissues at a pH of 7.87. The pH of the eye is 7.11, slightly lower than that of the blood.[28,33] The extent of ionization of a drug is affected by the pH of the tissues in which it is distributed, so we can consider the degree of ionization to be slightly more in the eye versus the blood, which would mean that erythromycin is less lipid soluble and less able to permeate across cellular membranes when administered topically versus systemically. The higher topically administered dose may enable adequate concentrations in the conjunctiva regardless of these pharmacokinetic considerations. However, limited evidence suggests topical erythromycin may not achieve concentrations above the MIC, which is necessary for eradication of *N. gonorrhoeae*.[29]

Although we do not know what concentration is reached in the eye, it can be inferred that erythromycin is significantly less pharmacologically active in the plasma and the eye compared to azithromycin. Again, how to apply this to neonatal ocular prophylaxis is less clear, but it further illustrates that erythromycin has no place in the management of *N. gonorrhoeae* infections. Azithromycin, which is much more active, is no longer recommended for treatment of gonococcal infections. These physiologic limitations, in addition to resistance of *N. gonorrhoeae* to azithromycin, significantly reduce the activity of erythromycin versus azithromycin against *N. gonorrhoeae*. Limited data showing the efficacy of erythromycin against ophthalmia neonatorum further accentuate concerns regarding the appropriateness of ocular prophylaxis with 0.5% erythromycin ophthalmic ointment.[12]

Efficacy of Neonatal Ocular Prophylaxis for Prevention of Neonatal Gonococcal Conjunctivitis

Despite its widespread use in the United States and continued recommendations for use from the CDC and the USPSTF,[7,8] data on the actual efficacy of neonatal prophylaxis with erythromycin ointment for the prevention of gonococcal ophthalmia are very limited. Major confounding variables are prenatal screening and treatment of pregnant women for *N. gonorrhoeae*.

Credé's original data from 1881 found that 2% silver nitrate reduced the incidence of gonococcal conjunctivitis from 7.6% to 0.5%.[1] In the following years, neonatal ocular prophylaxis with silver nitrate was implemented and required either by law or public health regulations in many countries globally. Use of 2% silver nitrate was associated with severe chemical conjunctivitis in many infants.[10,34] The concentration was reduced to 1% in most of the United States during the 1900s. After the introduction of neonatal ocular prophylaxis with silver nitrate in Europe and the United States, the incidence of gonococcal ophthalmia steadily declined.[35] However, as the use of 1% silver nitrate was still associated with chemical conjunctivitis in many infants, many jurisdictions switched to antibiotics, including penicillin, erythromycin, tetracycline, sulfonamides, and chloramphenicol, as they became available in the 1950s and later. Clinical data on the efficacy of these regimens for the prevention of gonococcal ophthalmia were limited. However, screening and treatment of pregnant women for gonococcal infection were being implemented around the same time.[4]

Kapoor et al.[36] conducted an extensive review of intervention for preventing ophthalmia neonatorum for the *Cochrane Database of Systematic Reviews* in 2020. They included 30 trials with a total of 79,198 neonates conducted from 1951 to 2015. All of the studies were randomized or quasi-randomized. Over half of the studies (18) were conducted in high-income settings in the United States, Europe, Israel, and Canada; 15 were conducted in low- and middle-income settings in Africa, Iran, China, Indonesia, and Mexico. Tetracycline 1%, erythromycin 0.5%, povidone–iodine 2.5%, and silver nitrate 1% were the most frequently used preparations. Most of the studies from low- and middle-income countries did not test women prenatally for either *N. gonorrhoeae* or *C. trachomatis*; thus, the actual prevalence of these infections in these populations was not known. In several studies, only those infants who presented with conjunctivitis were seen and evaluated, and no infants were followed up prospectively. Several studies from high-income countries did not report any cases of gonococcal conjunctivitis, even in the no-prophylaxis groups. Screening pregnant women for *N. gonorrhoeae* was part of routine prenatal care in those countries. None of the studies reported any data on the development of serious sequelae including corneal perforation or blindness. Kapoor et al.[36] concluded that there were no data on whether neonatal prophylaxis for ophthalmia neonatorum prevents any serious adverse outcomes.[36] The authors also felt that, although neonatal ocular prophylaxis may lead to a reduction in acute conjunctivitis of any etiology, the evidence for an effect on gonococcal and chlamydial conjunctivitis was less certain.

From 1985 to 1987, Hammerschlag et al.[37] conducted a prospective study of neonatal ocular prophylaxis, comparing 1% silver nitrate drops and erythromycin and tetracycline ophthalmic ointments for the prevention of neonatal chlamydial conjunctivitis in an inner-city population in Brooklyn, NY. Although the study was not initially planned to evaluate the efficacy of these preparations to prevent gonococcal ophthalmia, the researchers were able to examine the impact on gonococcal ophthalmia as the three preparations were rotated monthly and given to all infants born at Kings County Hospital during the study period. Gonococcal ophthalmia occurred in eight of the 12,431 infants (0.06%) who were delivered during this period. One infant in the silver nitrate group (0.03%), four in the erythromycin group (0.1%), and three in the tetracycline group (0.07%) developed gonococcal ophthalmia ($P > 0.05$).

In 2017, Kreisel et al.[38] examined the national rates of reported *C. trachomatis* and *N. gonorrhoeae* conjunctivitis among infants less than 1 year of age in the United States from 2010 to 2015. It was assumed that most of these cases were perinatal. There were 563 cases with a specimen source of either eye or conjunctiva. *N. gonorrhoeae* accounted for 42 cases (7.5%) compared to 521 cases of *C. trachomatis* infection (92.5%). The rate of gonococcal conjunctivitis was 0.2 cases per 100,000 live births/year during the period studied. There were no data on whether the mothers had prenatal care or were screened for gonorrhea or chlamydia. The USPSTF, in a position document published in 2019,[8] continued to recommend ocular prophylaxis for all newborns to prevent gonococcal ophthalmia, despite the absence of any new data. They did not specify which preparation to use. Currently, erythromycin ophthalmic ointment is the only preparation available for neonatal prophylaxis in the United States. There is only one manufacturer in the United States, and there have been interruptions in the supply. In 2009, the CDC informed physicians of a shortage of 0.5% erythromycin ointment due to changes in the manufacturers, and a set of interim guidelines was provided to clinicians regarding alternative agents (i.e., azithromycin drops, gentamicin ophthalmic preparations).[39] However, there are no data on these alternatives for this indication, and the use of gentamicin ophthalmic ointment has been associated with severe ocular reactions in infants.[39,40] There were subsequent shortages of erythromycin ointment in the United States from 2019 through May of 2021.

Impact of Prenatal Screening and Treatment on the Incidence of Neonatal Gonococcal Ophthalmia

The incidence of neonatal gonococcal ophthalmia is related to the prevalence of gonococcal infection in women of child-bearing age. Treatment of sexually active women and their sex partners has been recommended since the 1970s, and the first CDC treatment recommendations for gonorrhea were published in 1972, 1974, and 1979.[41] The recommendations specifically state that, "All pregnant women should have endocervical cultures examined for gonococci as an integral part of prenatal care." The treatment regimen recommended at that time was a single dose of aqueous procaine penicillin IM plus oral probenecid as the drug regimen of choice for uncomplicated gonorrhea in men and women, including pregnant women.[42] Erythromycin was only recommended for use in pregnant women who were allergic to penicillin; intramuscular cefazolin and spectinomycin were alternatives. Due to increasing resistance, penicillin and tetracycline were no longer recommended for treatment of gonorrhea in 1989. Single-dose IM ceftriaxone became the treatment of choice for treatment of uncomplicated gonorrhea in adolescents and adults, including pregnant women, in 1989.[43]

In 2015, the Canadian Pediatric Society (CPS) recommended discontinuing ocular prophylaxis to prevent gonococcal ophthalmia.[12] The rationales for this change were that silver nitrate was no longer available, erythromycin ophthalmic ointment was the only currently available antibiotic eye ointment, and that neither prevented chlamydial ophthalmia. The CPS recommended placing an emphasis on enhanced prenatal screening. The recommendations were similar to those currently recommended in the 2021 CDC Sexually Transmitted Infections Treatment Guidelines.[7] All pregnant women should be screened for gonorrhea and chlamydial infection at the first prenatal visit and treated. Those who were infected and treated should be tested again to confirm microbiologic cure and tested again in the third trimester or, if not then, at delivery. The mother's sexual partners should also be treated. In addition, women who initially tested negative but were at risk for acquiring gonococcal infection later in pregnancy should be tested again in the third trimester. Mothers who were not screened should be tested at delivery, and their infants should be treated with one dose of IM ceftriaxone. The CPS referred to the 2010 CDC Sexually Transmitted Diseases Treatment Guidelines,[44] which contained similar screening recommendations. In addition to recommending ocular prophylaxis with erythromycin, the CDC also recommended that infants born to mothers with untreated gonorrhea receive prophylactic treatment with a single dose of IM ceftriaxone, regardless of whether they received neonatal ocular prophylaxis. This recommendation has been dropped from subsequent editions of the CDC Guidelines but is still recommended in the current *Red Book*,[45] which states that, because gonococcal ophthalmia, infection at other anatomic sites, or disseminated infection can develop in infants who have received ocular prophylaxis, infants born to mothers with untreated gonorrhea should receive a single dose of ceftriaxone, as described previously, even if they received ocular prophylaxis. Single-dose ceftriaxone (20–50 mg/kg, maximum dose 125 mg) is also the recommended therapy for gonococcal ophthalmia in infants.

Data on infant outcomes after implementation of the CPS recommendations are very limited. Ivensky et al.[46] assessed prenatal screening rates for *N. gonorrhoeae* and *C. trachomatis* in a birthing and tertiary care center in Montréal, Quebec. They retrospectively reviewed a list of all women who delivered at the facility between April 2015 and March 2016. Of the 2688 women who delivered during this period, 2245 were screened at least once (83.5%); only two of 2206 (0.09%) had gonococcal infection. No data were provided on whether these women were treated prenatally or the outcomes of the infants born to mothers who were not screened, including gonococcal ophthalmia. The investigators concluded that the screening rates were suboptimal and that universal ocular prophylaxis cannot be discontinued. Ocular prophylaxis was in effect during this period, although there were shortages of erythromycin ophthalmic ointments in Canada. Gonococcal infection, including perinatal infection defined as occurring in infants <4 weeks of age, is a reportable disease in Canada. Rates of reported cases in children <1 year of age from 2016, when ocular prophylaxis was discontinued, to 2019 increased from 0.52 to 2.15 cases/per 100,000.[47] No data were presented on how many of these cases were neonatal conjunctivitis. Kreisel et al.[38] reported that the rate of gonococcal conjunctivitis in infants in the United States was 0.2 cases per 100,000 live births/year from 2010 to 2015, despite the use of ocular prophylaxis with erythromycin ophthalmic ointment.

In 2018, Comunián-Carrrasco et al.[48] reviewed published studies on the treatment of gonorrhea in pregnancy which included multiple regimens (IM ceftriaxone, oral cefixime, oral amoxicillin plus probenecid, and IM spectinomycin). Although they found high levels of cure of gonococcal infections, none of the trials included in the review followed the infants after delivery. However, the results of the ocular prophylaxis trial by Hammerschlag et al.[37] in 1989, which was discussed earlier, supports the efficacy of prenatal screening and treatment of gonorrhea for the prevention of gonococcal ophthalmia. During the study period, 248 of 9128 women (2.7%) who were registered in the prenatal clinic at Kings County Hospital had positive cultures for *N. gonorrhoeae*. All of these women were treated after the diagnosis in the prenatal clinic, and none of their infants developed gonococcal ophthalmia. However, gonococcal ophthalmia occurred in eight of 3303 infants whose mothers were not registered in the prenatal clinic (0.24%); seven of the eight infants (87.5%) were born to women who had received no prenatal care. One mother received prenatal care at another institution. These results suggest that prenatal screening and treatment of pregnant women had a greater impact on the subsequent development of gonococcal ophthalmia than neonatal ocular prophylaxis. Banniettis et al.,[49] in a subsequent study in the same population, audited the records of women registered for prenatal care in the prenatal clinic at University Hospital of Brooklyn over a 2-year period from 2016 through 2017. A total of 608 women were enrolled; the prevalence of gonococcal infection was 1% overall and 2% in women under 25 years of age. Over 60% of the women were screened more than once. All of the women with gonococcal infection were treated with a single 250-mg IM ceftriaxone dose. In contrast, the prevalence of chlamydial infection was 5.6% overall, and 11.8% in women less than 25 years of age. All of the women with chlamydial infection were treated with a single dose of 1 g of azithromycin orally. There were no cases of gonococcal or chlamydial conjunctivitis in any of the infants born to these women during the study period.

The CDC continues to recommend routine ocular prophylaxis in their 2021 Sexually Transmitted Infections Treatment Guidelines,[8] referring to the USPSTF recommendations. No new data have been provided; however, the CDC recommended focusing on prenatal screening for *N. gonorrhoeae*. The CDC recommended screening all pregnant women at risk, defined as women <25 years of age and those >25 years who have a new sex partner, more than one sex partner, a sex partner with concurrent partners, or a sex partner with an STI or who lives in a community with high rates of gonorrhea at the first prenatal visit. Infected women should be treated and retested in 3 months and in the third trimester or at time of delivery; sex partners should also be tested and treated. Most importantly, the CDC now recommends retesting those pregnant women considered at high risk in the third trimester and screening at delivery for women at high risk who were not tested during pregnancy, specifically those who did not have prenatal care. If erythromycin ointment is unavailable, infants at high risk for exposure to *N. gonorrhoeae*, such as those born to mothers with no prenatal care or untreated gonorrhea, should be administered one dose of ceftriaxone IM. In a notice from the CDC on the shortage of erythromycin ophthalmic ointment last reviewed May 24, 2021, the agency stated: "It is important to remember that prenatal screening is the best method of preventing gonococcal ophthalmia neonatorum among newborns."

Conclusions

Implementation of screening and treatment of pregnant women for gonococcal infection is the most effective way to prevent neonatal gonococcal infection. There are no data that confirm that neonatal ocular prophylaxis with 0.5% erythromycin is effective, especially in populations where prenatal screening and treatment are routine. Increasing macrolide resistance in *N. gonorrhoeae* will very likely have a negative effect on efficacy. Shortages of erythromycin ophthalmic ointment are inevitable, as there is currently only one manufacturer in the United States, and, as seen with other generic antibiotics including cefotaxime, it may be dropped from production as being unprofitable.[50] Continuation of neonatal ocular prophylaxis in resource-poor settings such as Africa, has been recommended, as there is no maternal screening for *N. gonorrhoeae* and *C. trachomatis*.[51,52] Currently all newborn infants in Ghana receive 1% tetracycline ointment as neonatal ocular prophylaxis; however, the rate of tetracycline resistance of *N. gonorrhoeae* in this population is 73%.[53]

Gonococcal infection during pregnancy can be associated with significant morbidities. Infants may also become infected at sites other than the conjunctivae, leading to disseminated infection. These infections would not be prevented by neonatal ocular prophylaxis. Preliminary data on the use of emerging testing technologies based on DNA and RNA amplification for *N. gonorrhoeae* and *C. trachomatis* suggest that etiologic testing and treatment of pregnant women in low-resource settings, rather than the implementation of neonatal ocular prophylaxis, are feasible and will improve maternal and neonatal health outcomes globally.[52,54] Legislative and regulatory mandates for universal neonatal ophthalmia prophylaxis in countries with organized healthcare systems are no longer evidence based and should be withdrawn.

REFERENCES

1. Credé CSF. Die Verhuetung der Augenentzundung der Neugeborenen [Prevention of inflammatory eye disease in the newborn]. *Arch Gynaekol*. 1881;18:367-370.
2. Thygeson P, Stone Jr W. Epidemiology of inclusion conjunctivitis. *Arch Ophthalmol*. 1942;27(1):91-122.
3. Kardos N, Demain AL. Penicillin: the medicine with the greatest impact on therapeutic outcomes. *Appl Microbiol Biotechnol*. 2011;92(4):677-687.
4. Brockelhurst P. Antibiotics for gonorrhoeae in pregnancy. *Cochrane Database Syst Rev*. 2002;(2):CD000098.
5. Centers for Disease Control and Prevention. Recommendations for the prevention and management of *Chlamydia trachomatis* infections, 1993. *MMWR Recomm Rep*. 1993;42(RR-12):1-39.
6. Smith-Norowitz T, Ukaegbu C, Kohlhoff S, Hammerschlag MR. Neonatal prophylaxis with antibiotic containing ointments does not reduce incidence of chlamydial conjunctivitis in newborns. *BMC Infect Dis*. 2021;21(1):270.
7. Centers for Disease Control and Prevention. Sexually transmitted infections treatment guidelines 2021. *MMWR Recomm Rep*. 2021;70(RR-4):1-192.
8. US Preventative Services Task Force, Curry SJ, Krist AH, et al. Ocular prophylaxis for gonococcal ophthalmia neonatorum: US Preventative Services Task Force reaffirmation recommendation statement. *JAMA*. 2019;321(4):394-398.
9. Laga M, Meheus A, Piot P. Epidemiology and control of ophthalmia neonatorum. *Bull WHO*. 1989;67(5):471-477.
10. Walhberg V. Reconsideration of Credé prophylaxis. A study of maternity and neonatal care. *Acta Paediatr Scand Suppl*. 1982; 295:1-73.
11. WHO. *WHO Guidelines for the Treatment of Neisseria Gonorrhoeae*. Geneva: World Health Organization; 2016.
12. Moore DL, MacDonald NE, Canadian Paediatric Society, Infectious Diseases and Immunization Committee. Preventing ophthalmia neonatorum. *Paediatr Child Health*. 2015;20(2): 93-96.
13. Derbie A, Mekonnen D, Woldeamanuel Y, Abebe T. Azithromycin resistant gonococci: a literature review. *Antimicrob Resist Infect Control*. 2020;9(1):138.
14. Bremond-Gignac D, Chiambaretta F, Milazzo S. A European perspective on topical ophthalmic antibiotics: current and evolving options. *Ophthalmol Eye Dis*. 2011;3:29-43.
15. Unemo M, Shafer WM. Antimicrobial resistance in *Neisseria gonorrhoeae* in the 21st century: past, evolution, and future. *Clin Microbiol Rev*. 2014;27(3):587-613.
16. Slaney L, Chubb H, Ronald A, Brunham R. In-vitro activity of azithromycin, erythromycin, ciprofloxacin and norfloxacin against *Neisseria gonorrhoeae*, *Haemophilus ducreyi*, and *Chlamydia trachomatis*. *J Antimicrob Chemother*. 1990;25(suppl A):1-5.
17. Holderman JL, Thomas JC, Schlanger K, et al. Sustained transmission of *Neisseria gonorrhoeae* with high-level resistance to azithromycin, in Indianapolis, Indiana, 2017–2018. *Clin Infect Dis*. 2021;73(5):808-815.
18. Government of Canada. *National Surveillance of Antimicrobial Susceptibilities of Neisseria gonorrhoeae - 2015*. Available at: https://www.canada.ca/en/public-health/services/publications/drugs-health-products/national-surveillance-antimicrobial-susceptibilities-neisseria-gonorrhoeae-annual-summary-2015.html. Accessed December 12, 2021.
19. Workowski KA, Bolan GA, Centers for Disease Control and Prevention. Sexually transmitted diseases treatment guidelines, 2015. *MMWR Recomm Rep*. 2015;64(RR-03):1-137. Erratum in *MMWR Recomm Rep*. 2015;64(33):924.
20. St Cyr S, Barbee L, Workowski KA, et al. Update to CDC's treatment guidelines for gonococcal infection, 2020. *MMWR Morb Mortal Wkly Rep*. 2020;69(50):1911-1916.
21. Zar HJ. Neonatal chlamydial infections prevention and treatment. *Pediatr Drugs*. 2005;7(2):103-110.
22. Moran JS, Levine WC. Drugs of choice for the treatment of uncomplicated gonococcal infections. *Clin Infect Dis*. 1995; 20(suppl 1):S47-S65.
23. Lahra MM, Shoushtari M, George CRR, Armstrong BH, Hogan TR, National Neisseria Network, Australia. Australian Gonococcal Surveillance Programme Annual Report, 2019. *Commun Dis Intell (2018)*. 2020;15:44.

24. Young H, Moyes A, McMillan A. Azithromycin and erythromycin resistant *Neisseria gonorrhoeae* following treatment with azithromycin. *Int J STD AIDS*. 1997;8(5):299-302.
25. Kirkcaldy RD, Harvey A, Papp JR, et al. *Neisseria gonorrhoeae* antimicrobial susceptibility surveillance - The Gonococcal Isolate Surveillance Project, 27 Sites, United States, 2014. *MMWR Surveill Summ*. 2016;65(7):1-19.
26. Selb R, Buder S, Dudareva S, et al. Markedly decreasing azithromycin susceptibility of *Neisseria gonorrhoeae*, Germany, 2014 to 2021. *Euro Surveill*. 2021;26(31):2100616.
27. Gieseker KE, Learner ER, Mauk K, et al. Demographic and epidemiological characteristics associated with reduced antimicrobial susceptibility to *Neisseria gonorrhoeae* in the United States, strengthening the US response to resistant gonorrhea, 2018 to 2019. *Sex Transm Dis*. 2021;48(12S suppl 2):S118-S123.
28. Kong FYS, Horner P, Unemo M, et al. Pharmacokinetic considerations regarding the treatment of bacterial sexually transmitted infections with azithromycin: a review. *J Antimicrob Chemother*. 2019;74(5):1157-1166.
29. Suzuki T, Kitagawa Y, Maruyama Y, et al. Conjunctivitis caused by *Neisseria gonorrhoeae* isolates with reduced cephalosporin susceptibility and multidrug resistance. *J Clin Microbiol*. 2013;51(12):4246-4248.
30. Agrahari V, Mandal A, Agrahari V, et al. A comprehensive insight on ocular pharmacokinetics. *Drug Deliv Transl Res*. 2016;6(6):735-754.
31. Isenberg SJ, Apt L, McCarty J, et al. Development of tearing in preterm and term neonates. *Arch Ophthalmol*. 1998;116(6):773-776.
32. del Amo EM, Rimpela AK, Heikkinen E, et al. Pharmacokinetic aspects of retinal drug delivery. *Prog Retinal Eye Res*. 2017;57:134-185.
33. Lim LT, Ah-kee EY, Collins CE. Common eye drops and their implications for pH measurements in the management of chemical eye injuries. *Int J Ophthalmol*. 2014;7(6):1067-1068.
34. Wahlberg V, Moberg Kallings I, Winberg J. Reconsideration of Credé's prophylaxis. I. Epidemiologic aspects of gonorrheal and chlamydial infection. Local effects of sliver nitrate and hexarginum. *Acta Paediatr Scand*. 1982;71(s295):27-36.
35. Fitzgerald HE, McCreal CE. Reconsideration of Credé's prophylaxis. Introduction. *Acta Paediatr Scand*. 1982;71(s295):9-21.
36. Kapoor VS, Evans JR, Vedula SS. Interventions for preventing ophthalmia neonatorum. *Cochrane Database Syst Rev*. 2020;9(9):CD001862.
37. Hammerschlag MR, Cummings CC, Roblin PM, Williams TH, Delke I. Efficacy of neonatal ocular prophylaxis for the prevention of chlamydial and gonococcal conjunctivitis. *New Engl J Med*. 1989;320(120):769-772.
38. Kreisel K, Weston E, Braxton J, Llata E, Torrone E. Keeping an eye on chlamydia and gonorrhea conjunctivitis in infants in the United States, 2010–2015. *Sex Transm Dis*. 2017;44(6):356-358.
39. Erythromycin opthalmic ointment shortage. https://www.cdc.gov/std/treatment/drugnotices/FDA-Statement-Erythromycin-Ophthalmic-Ointment-7-8-2022-Final.pdf. Accessed April 4, 2023.
40. Nathawad R, Mendez H, Ahmad A, et al. Severe ocular reactions after neonatal ocular prophylaxis with gentamicin ophthalmic ointment. *Pediatr Infect Dis J*. 2011;30(2):175-176.
41. Centers for Disease Control and Prevention. *CDC's STI Treatment Guidelines Timeline: The Evolution of Sexual Healthcare*. Available at: https://www.cdc.gov/std/treatment-guidelines/timeline.htm. Accessed December 27, 2021.
42. Gonorrhea. Recommended treatment schedules—1974. *J Pediatr*. 1975;86(5):794-798.
43. Centers for Disease Control (CDC). 1989 CDC sexually transmitted diseases treatment guidelines. *MMWR Suppl*. 1989;38:(8):1-43.
44. Centers for Disease Control and Prevention. Sexually Transmitted Diseases Treatment Guidelines, 2010. *MMWR Recomm Rep*. 2010;59(RR-12):1-110.
45. Kimberlin DW, Barnett ED, Lynfield R, Sawyer, MH, eds. *Red Book: 2021 Report of the Committee on Infectious Diseases*. 32nd ed. Itasca, IL: American Academy of Pediatrics; 2021.
46. Ivensky V, Mandel R, Boulay AC, Lavallée C, Benoît J, Labbé AC. Suboptimal prenatal screening of *Chlamydia trachomatis* and *Neisseria gonorrhoeae* infections in a Montréal birthing and tertiary care centre: a retrospective cohort study. *Can Commun Dis Rep*. 2021;47(4):209-215.
47. Government of Canada. *Notifiable Diseases Online*. Available at: https://diseases.canada.ca/notifiable/. Accessed January 26, 2023.
48. Comunián-Carrasco G, Peña-Martí GE, Martí-Carvajal AJ. Antibiotics for treating gonorrhea in pregnancy. *Cochrane Database Syst Rev*. 2018;2(2):CD011167.
49. Banniettis N, Wisecup K, Byland L, Watanabe I, Hammerschlag MR, Kohlhoff S. Association of routine *Chlamydia trachomatis* screening during pregnancy and seroprevalence of chlamydial infection in children, 1991–2015. *J Pediatr Infect Dis Soc*. 2021;10(2):172-174.
50. U.S. Food and Drug Administration. *Current and Resolved Drug Shortages and Discontinuations Reported to FDA: Cefotaxime Sodium Injection*. Available at: https://www.accessdata.fda.gov/scripts/drugshortages/dsp_ActiveIngredientDetails.cfm?AI=Cefotaxime%20Sodium%20Injection&st=c&tab=tabs-1#:~:text=(Reverified%2010%2F14%2F2021)&text=SteriMax%20in%20conjunction%20with%20FDA,%2D877%2D404%2D3338. Accessed February 4, 2022.
51. Galega FP, Heymann DL, Nasah BT. Gonococcal ophthalmia neonatorum: the case for prophylaxis in tropical Africa. *Bull World Health Org*. 1984;62(1):95-98.
52. Medline A, Davey DV, Klausner JD. Lost opportunity to save newborn lives: variable national antenatal screening policies for *Neisseria gonorrhoeae* and *Chlamydia trachomatis*. *Int J STD AIDS*. 2017;28:660-666.
53. Boadi-Kusi SB, Kyei S, Holdbrook S, Abu EK, Ntow J, Ateko AM. A study of ophthalmia neonatorum in the central region of Ghana: causative agents and antibiotic susceptibility patterns. *Glob Pediatr Health*. 2021;8:2333794X211019700.
54. Grant JS, Chico RM, Lee ACC, et al. Sexually transmitted infections in pregnancy: a narrative review of the global research gaps, challenges, and opportunities. *Sex Transm Dis*. 2020;47(12):779-789.

Chapter 11

Organ Dysfunction in Sepsis and Necrotizing Enterocolitis

Brynne Archer Sullivan, MD, MSCR; Zachary Andrew Vesoulis, MD, MSCI

Key Points

- Sepsis and necrotizing enterocolitis are common sources of morbidity and mortality in the premature infant population.
- There is a lack of consensus on the definition of neonatal sepsis, confounded by the overlap between pathologic and non-pathologic variability in vital signs, physiology, and exam findings.
- Improved outcomes in neonatal sepsis and sepsis-like illness will require prompt intervention guided by sensitive, multimodal detection of end-organ dysfunction.

Sepsis and sepsis-like illnesses, including necrotizing enterocolitis (NEC), remain among the most common causes of mortality in premature infants.[1] Neonatal sepsis kills thousands of newborns every year, and survivors commonly suffer serious morbidities.[2,3] The risk of sepsis and NEC is not evenly distributed across the population of all infants, with incidences increasing as gestational age decreases. Among those born before 28 weeks' gestation, the rate of sepsis can be as high as 30% to 40%.[4] The host response to infection is designed to fight off pathogens but often does so at the expense of normal organ function.[5] The immune response signals inflammatory cascades with checks and balances from anti-inflammatory pathways, mediated by the autonomic nervous system.[6] Much, if not all, of the morbidity and mortality associated with sepsis is the result of organ dysfunction; thus, the diagnosis and treatment of neonatal sepsis must be calibrated to the presence and severity of organ dysfunction.[7]

Despite this need, definitions of sepsis based on organ dysfunction, originally developed for adult and older pediatric patients, perform poorly in preterm neonates, confounded by the generally unstable physiology of prematurity. As a result, most clinical trials have relied on the blood culture result alone as an unequivocal, albeit limited, definition of neonatal sepsis.[8] Currently, experts are working to develop a core outcome set for clinical trials of neonatal sepsis.[9] In 2005, the International Pediatric Sepsis Consensus Conference defined sepsis syndromes and organ failure for pediatric patients.[10] These definitions modified those for adult patients with systemic inflammatory response syndrome (SIRS), sepsis, severe sepsis, septic shock, and organ dysfunction for children in six age groups, including term neonates, but notably not including premature infants. Some have suggested modifications to the pediatric SIRS criteria for application to premature infants,[11,12] but one study evaluating the accuracy of the modified SIRS criteria for premature infants found them to only modestly improve sensitivity from about 40% to 50%.[12] More work is needed to develop consensus definitions for sepsis to operationalize organ dysfunction[13] in premature infants with immature organ systems. The Pediatric Organ Dysfunction Information Update Mandate (PODIUM) Collaborative was founded to better define organ dysfunction in pediatric sepsis, yet their work excludes premature infants.[14] Recognizing and treating organ dysfunction early in the course of neonatal sepsis is an important yet challenging goal, especially in premature infants.[7] Therefore, this review will focus on the pathophysiology of organ dysfunction in neonatal sepsis and NEC, with an emphasis on questions and controversies yet to be answered.

Organ Dysfunction Severity

End-organ dysfunction occurs when homeostasis is disrupted and the organ is no longer able to adequately support the body. Dysfunction may arise from many sources, including hypoxia, ischemia, destruction of tissue by infectious organisms, or altered function induced by local or systemic inflammation. Although organized as distinct units of the body, organs function as a network, and the physiology of one system reflects and adapts to changes in others.[15,16] Although organ dysfunction is the proximal cause of sepsis-related mortality, early signs may be subtle and the time course of progression to overt failure depends on complex interactions between the pathogen, the host, and the treatment.

The Pathogen

The causative organism plays an important role in modulating the severity of illness during a bloodstream infection. Our understanding of the pathophysiology of neonatal sepsis is limited by blood cultures with a substantial number of false-negative and false-positive results.[17,18] Studies of neonatal sepsis with bacteremia show that Gram-negative organisms cause mortality and serious organ dysfunction more often than sepsis caused by Gram-positive bacteria.[19–21] Different pathogens trigger different immune responses because of their unique virulence factors, referred to as pathogen-associated molecular patterns (PAMPs). For example, lipopolysaccharide (LPS), an integral component of the cell membrane in Gram-negative bacteria, activates immune cells via host receptors, such as Toll-like receptors. There is significant variability in PAMPs and their interaction with human receptors,[22] underlining the complex, diverse, and unique inter-individual differences in the clinical manifestation of sepsis episodes.[11]

Furthermore, the chronologic age of the preterm infant at the time of infection impacts the profile of the most likely organism; Gram-negative organisms are more common in early-onset sepsis (within the first 3 days after birth) and Gram-positive organisms are more common in premature infants with late-onset sepsis.[1,23] Sepsis caused by fungus[24,25] and viruses[26–28] can also lead to organ dysfunction and serious illness but compose a minority of infections.

Although we often focus on bloodstream infections as the cause of the sepsis syndrome in neonates, NEC presents with a similar but subtly distinct course of illness. The systemic inflammatory syndrome that frequently accompanies NEC in premature infants develops in part due to disruption of the normal interface between enterocytes and the microbial flora of the intestinal tract.[29,30] Toll-like receptors of the innate immune system mediate the initial inflammatory response to pathogenic intestinal microbes,[31] and the disease progresses with an inflammatory cascade leading to sepsis and shock just as a bloodstream infection would. These two processes are not always distinct, as many bloodstream infections in premature infants probably arise from the translocation of intestinal bacteria into the bloodstream.[32–34] Similarly, pneumonia, urinary tract infection, focal intestinal perforation, and other localized infections may also lead to a sepsis-like illness with organ dysfunction in premature infants.[11,35,36]

The Host

Virulence factors of the pathogen play a major part in the severity of illness, but host factors influence the sepsis trajectory, as well. The immune response depends on many variables, including the infant's gestational and postnatal age.[37,38] Fatal or severe sepsis occurs in some cases because the neonatal immune response is less robust than that of an adult or child,[38] leaving them more susceptible to systemic infection and organ dysfunction.[39,40] Sex is a biological risk factor with a slightly higher incidence of sepsis in males.[41–43] Black or non-White race has been associated with higher neonatal sepsis risk,[44,45] likely due to the complex influence of socioeconomic and maternal health factors. Molecular studies have identified genetic polymorphisms associated with a higher risk of sepsis.[46–48] Studies in adults have shown a specific tumor necrosis factor polymorphism to be a risk marker for worse outcomes in severe sepsis,[49] but a small study was unable to confirm the association in neonates with sepsis.[50]

The Treatment

Although recent studies have identified promising areas for therapies targeting specific aspects of the immature immune system,[51–53] supportive care and antibiotics remain the primary treatment options for bacterial sepsis. Early goal-directed treatment of sepsis became a focus of adult sepsis guidelines and outcome metrics after evidence of mortality reduction,[54] although several subsequent clinical trials have failed to show an impact on outcomes with specific or bundled interventions.[55–57] In neonatology, delivery room protocols for the extremely premature infant[58] are analogous to early goal-directed therapy bundles for shock in adults and pediatric patients,[59] but no clinical trials have studied this in the setting of neonatal septic shock. Before this can happen, clinicians and scientists must establish consensus on how to define neonatal sepsis and related outcomes in translational research, clinical trials, and routine clinical care. Only then will assessments of novel biomarkers and monitoring technologies as targets of goal-directed therapy in neonates provide the evidence necessary.[60] Antibiotic prescribing practices differ widely among neonatal intensive care units (NICUs), particularly for choices in empiric coverage while awaiting the blood culture result.[61,62] Prolonged antibiotic treatment for clinical signs of sepsis or shock despite a negative blood culture occurs often but with center variability in the frequency and duration.[63,64]

Until improved treatment and prevention strategies become available for clinical use, efforts should focus on timely identification of sepsis or NEC, with the aim of avoiding irreversible damage or dysfunction. Although careful clinical observation and laboratory monitoring, including blood cultures, remain the mainstay of evaluation, promising new technologies are beginning to emerge that utilize physiological biomarkers to identify at-risk infants. Predictive monitoring technology has been shown to augment traditional clinical measures, reducing sepsis-associated mortality[65] in very-low-birth-weight (VLBW) infants and improving neurodevelopmental outcomes for survivors.[66]

Organ Dysfunction in Sepsis and NEC by System

The significant inter-individual variation in pathogen, host, and treatment factors combine to create a unique sepsis course for each neonate. This variability is primarily expressed through diversity of end-organ dysfunction and failure which can be attributed in part to a dysregulated immune response to infection. Although immune activation is essential for effective eradication of invading microorganisms, excessive inflammation can precipitate a metabolic or immune dysfunction cascade that can be difficult to treat or reverse and may lead to late mortality.[67] The primary goal of timely diagnosis and treatment of sepsis is to protect or restore the perfusion of organs so they will maintain their function. Understanding the progression of organ dysfunction during sepsis allows clinicians to anticipate future problems and to provide targeted supportive treatment.

NERVOUS SYSTEM

The sepsis syndrome alters nervous system function in a way that can be leveraged for the identification of sepsis and as a target for treatment efficacy in order to maximize injury reduction. The autonomic nervous system (ANS) mediates a large part of the immune response to sepsis and septic shock.[68] Sensory nerves and receptors in every organ carry signals triggered by PAMPs, cytokines, or immune cells to the brainstem, where an efferent signal is transmitted via sympathetic or parasympathetic nerve fibers. Sepsis generally induces a stress response, consisting of simultaneous activation of sympathetic nerve signals and inhibition of vagal nerve signaling, recognized as the "fight or flight" response; however, there is also evidence of direct firing of the vagus nerve triggered by LPS and cytokines.[69,70] This sepsis-induced vagal stimulation generates abnormal heart rate patterns in premature infants[71,72] that can be detected using special monitors. Furthermore, the cholinergic anti-inflammatory response generates secondary vagal nerve activation, with downstream effects of suppressing immune cells, such as macrophages, and the release of inflammatory molecules, such as tumor necrosis factor.[73–75] Given the extensive involvement in the response to sepsis, vagal nerve stimulation or ANS modulation may have a role in the treatment of septic shock.[76]

The central nervous system may also be affected by sepsis through dysfunction and injury. Hypoperfusion of the brain typically occurs during the decompensated phase of shock, which usually occurs later in the course of the illness. Low blood pressure, hypoxia, and impaired autoregulation have been associated with brain injury, including intraventricular and cerebellar hemorrhage.[77–79] Seizures due to sepsis are uncommon and occur more often with gram-negative sepsis and meningitis[80,81] and frequently end with death.

The inflammatory reaction of sepsis and NEC, even without hemorrhage, has also been linked to the development of white matter injury. The periventricular white matter is incompletely vascularized in preterm infants and is highly vulnerable to perfusion deficits.[82,83] Some cytokines may damage white matter directly.

Infants may have encephalopathy without overt injury in the setting of sepsis. Lethargy or decreased activity is a commonly cited indication for sepsis evaluation and may have a higher positive predictive value than other early clinical signs.[84–86] These findings are often subjective and difficult to assess in a non-verbal patient bundled in an incubator for most of the day. One group has successfully developed an algorithm to quantify activity levels using electrocardiogram waveform data to detect decreased infant movement.[87,88] This technology is promising for use in predictive monitoring to alert clinicians to early, objective changes in activity that indicate an imminent deterioration due to infection.

CARDIOVASCULAR SYSTEM

The heart and blood vessels function together to perfuse organs with vital nutrients, facilitate gas exchange, and carry molecules throughout the body. We measure the function of the cardiovascular system primarily using heart rate and blood pressure. Normal heart rate and blood pressure ranges vary with gestational age and postnatal age.[89,90] However, the numerous physiologic and iatrogenic influences on the cardiovascular system in the preterm neonate make it difficult to define normal ranges.[91] With immature organ systems and transitional physiology, extremely premature infants frequently have symptoms such as hypotension and respiratory failure in the absence of infection. Additionally, the mode of respiratory support, common medications, bleeding, and painful procedures all affect heart rate and blood pressure throughout an infant's course in the NICU. As clinical practice and monitoring equipment vary among centers, small differences in heart rate and oxygen saturation exist among VLBW infants cared for in different NICUs.[92] Cardiovascular dysfunction must be recognized and treated early in the course of illness. Resuscitation guidelines for the management of septic shock focus on supporting cardiovascular function to perfuse vital organs. In patients with shock, we presume that timely restoration of tissue perfusion improves outcomes, although supportive data are lacking.[11,93]

Signs of cardiovascular dysfunction include hypotension, decreased capillary refill time, metabolic acidosis, and decreased urine output. Transitional physiology may confound accurate assessment of the impact of individual findings in the extremely premature infant. For example, all neonates have a period of relative oliguria for the first 24 hours after birth. During this period, it is difficult to distinguish normal urine output from acute kidney injury or developing shock. Very premature infants or term infants with respiratory illnesses may have invasive, continuous blood pressure monitoring using an arterial line in the first few days after birth. Outside of this period, non-invasive cuff pressures are typically used for routine monitoring, although there have been a number of reports of significant discrepancy between invasive and non-invasive blood pressure measurements.[94,95] Although it is generally recognized that systolic, mean, and diastolic blood pressure increases by approximately 1 mmHg per day for the first few days following birth, there is significant disagreement over the definition of "hypotension." One definition, first made by Zubrow et al.,[96] suggests that the lower limit of the mean arterial blood pressure should be equal to the gestational age in weeks. This target may be too low in extremely preterm infants, and an alternative lower limit of 30 mmHg for the avoidance of brain injury has been suggested.[97] That cutoff value has not been validated.

In healthy term infants, blood pressure might be measured one or two times (or possibly not at all) during the birth hospitalization. Signs of hypoperfusion might first be detected with changes in skin color, activity, or feeding. Peripheral vasoconstriction often precedes hypotension in an attempt to maintain central perfusion; therefore, measuring the difference between core temperature and peripheral temperature might detect early cardiovascular dysfunction.[98] An ongoing clinical trial is studying continuous core-to-peripheral temperature difference measurement to predict sepsis and improve outcomes.[99]

Prompt and effective treatment of hypotension should be a clinical priority. In a study of organ dysfunction in cases of fatal sepsis, the percentage of patients receiving vasopressor medications increased more for cases where mortality occurred closer to the diagnosis of sepsis. About half of all patients with fatal sepsis were receiving pressors at the time of death.[19] Once diagnosed, the treatment of hypotension typically starts with fluid resuscitation. As extremely premature infants are more sensitive to rapid volume expansion, with an increased risk of adverse pulmonary and neurologic outcomes,[100] resuscitation is most often focused on administration of small volumes of fluid and early transition to vasopressors. In the immature heart, stroke volume is essentially fixed, and changes in cardiac output are driven entirely by increases in heart rate, a tenuous relationship with a fixed upper limit.[11] Dopamine is the most widely used anti-hypotensive drug, without supportive clinical evidence.[101,102] Historically, dobutamine was used as an alternative first-line agent; however, a number of direct comparison studies have demonstrated superior benefit for dopamine.[103–105] Not surprisingly, the use of dobutamine has decreased.[93,106]

Various secondary treatment options have been utilized. Hydrocortisone use has increased over time because of the high incidence of relative adrenal insufficiency.[107] Several studies have shown that the use of hydrocortisone in neonates with shock can reduce fluid and pressor requirements.[108] Caution should be urged when using hydrocortisone concurrently with indomethacin, as this combination has been associated with the complication of spontaneous intestinal perforation.[109,110] Vasopressin and epinephrine may be effective in early treatment of hypotension, as well,[111,112] although these medications remain less well studied. More recently, favorable evidence has emerged to support the use of norepinephrine as a second-line treatment with a more favorable side effect profile.[113]

Monitoring the response to treatment of cardiovascular dysfunction includes continuous blood pressure monitoring when available, measuring urine output, and normalizing acidosis or serum lactate. Functional echocardiography is gaining attention and evidence as a valuable tool for assessing the response to volume and pressors using serial measurements of cardiac output, myocardial function, and other parameters.[114–116]

The hallmarks of the sympathetic response triggered by sepsis include tachycardia[117] and hypotension. Due to their parasympathetic dominance, sepsis-related cardiovascular dysfunction in preterm infants presents equally or more often as episodes of bradycardia rather than tachycardia. Bradycardic episodes commonly occur in conjunction with apnea and desaturation[118] but may also occur as a result of firing of the vagus nerve in response to PAMPs or cytokines.[69] Although the vagus nerve may be stimulated by sepsis-related inflammation, the primary impact is globally impaired autonomic function, which can be detected as decreased heart rate variability, or the standard deviation of the length of time between successive heartbeats. The signature of depressed variability punctuated by heart rate decelerations is a well-studied physiomarker of neonatal sepsis,[119–123] representing the effects of inflammation on autonomic control of heart rate.[70] This distinct pattern can be leveraged to provide a sepsis early-warning system. Tachycardia and abnormal heart rate characteristics often improve with the treatment of sepsis but may remain elevated due to ongoing ANS signaling.

RESPIRATORY SYSTEM

Changes in the respiratory status, including the need for, or escalation of, support and supplemental oxygen, often raise concerns for neonatal sepsis and present early in the course of infection.[85,86,124,125] Cytokines and prostaglandins mediate sepsis-associated apnea.[126,127] Prostaglandin E_2 (PGE_2) production is upregulated by the proinflammatory cytokine interleukin 1B, and PGE_2 levels correlate with the number of apnea and desaturation events in infants with bacteremia or meningitis.[126,128,129]

Characteristically, a term infant is more likely to present with tachypnea and a preterm infant is more likely to have apnea or recurrent episodes of hypoxia.[85,130] As with other organ systems, it can be difficult to differentiate the influence of developmentally expected conditions such as surfactant deficiency, apnea of prematurity, atelectasis, and evolving chronic lung disease from new manifestations of illness in preterm infants. For these reasons, respiratory dysfunction is a sensitive yet non-specific sign of neonatal sepsis. In an analysis of apnea events with bradycardia and oxygen desaturation using a quantitative apnea detection algorithm, the number and duration of events correlated with decreasing maturity and increased preceding many but not all cases of sepsis and NEC.[118]

An increase in supplemental oxygen requirement for a premature infant could indicate inadequate respiratory support or inadequate tissue perfusion due to worsening sepsis. It may also indicate surfactant inactivation. For this reason, exogenous surfactant administration could be considered for some infants, even late preterm or term, with respiratory failure due to pneumonia.[131] The hypoxia and acidosis triggered by sepsis can lead to secondary concerns including pulmonary hypertension, either as persistent pulmonary hypertension of the newborn in recently delivered infants, or acquired pulmonary hypertension for infants with chronic lung disease later in the hospital course. Oxygen and inhaled nitric oxide are the first-line treatments for pulmonary hypertension. In more mature infants with respiratory failure that does not respond to medical treatment and advanced mechanical ventilation, extracorporeal membrane oxygenation may be indicated for supportive treatment. In one study, among infants who died during sepsis, most were on a ventilator and received supplemental oxygen for several days preceding sepsis diagnosis; all of the infants had a significant rise in mean FiO_2 between sepsis diagnosis and death.[19]

HEMATOLOGIC SYSTEM

Pro-inflammatory cytokines and chemokines trigger immune cell production, activation, and release, including neutrophils and other white blood cells. Neutrophils represent an important component of the innate immune response to bacterial infection. Mature and immature neutrophils are stored in the bone marrow for ready release. In neonates, these stores are depleted quickly, resulting in neutropenia[132] rather than neutrophilia, as seen in older children and adults who have a greater capacity to ramp up production. Severe neutropenia is more common in severe or fatal sepsis, which has prompted the study of exogenous immune stimulants such as granulocyte colony-stimulating factor for its potential to prevent infection or reduce the severity of illness during infection.[133] Although early studies showed that this treatment increased neutrophil counts and stores, no studies have shown an impact on survival or outcomes.

Laboratory studies provide an important adjunctive component to the blood culture and physiologic assessment during sepsis evaluation. Two commonly used tests, the complete blood count (CBC) and the C-reactive protein (CRP), provide markers of inflammation and the immune response. Although characteristic changes occur during sepsis, both tests lack specificity. Although CRP was initially cited as a highly sensitive marker for sepsis, with high positive and negative predictive values,[124,134,135] subsequent evaluation has demonstrated significantly lower performance than initially proposed.[136–138] CRP production falls downstream of several steps in the inflammatory response to pathogens, causing a delay in the time from the stimulation of production to a measurable rise in CRP. Therefore, sepsis is often suspected before CRP rises, which limits its predictive and diagnostic utility. CRP-guided protocols for duration of antibiotic therapy can be effective,[139] but their use may result in the unnecessary extension of antibiotic treatment and impede antibiotic stewardship efforts.[140] The components of a complete blood count with differential are often used to screen for infection. However, the variable response and timing of the production of white blood cells by the immature immune system result in poor sensitivity and specificity for prediction of a positive blood culture or adverse sepsis outcomes.[141–143] Large studies show high specificity and negative predictive value for EOS diagnosis but poor sensitivity of all CBC components.[23,142,144] Notably, multiple studies have shown that hematologic markers have significantly greater performance in combination and when performed serially, rather than individually at a single time point.[144–146] Although the clinical practicability of repeated laboratory measures is unclear, this finding underscores the importance of multimodal evaluation to better capture the diverse expression of sepsis in individual patients.

Analogous to the inflammatory response, pathogen invasion activates a pro-coagulatory response as a mechanism to trap and contain organisms in the vasculature. If this response progresses unchecked, disseminated intravascular coagulopathy (DIC) may develop and cause significant hematologic dysfunction.[147] DIC is a consumptive coagulopathy that occurs following excessive formation of microthrombi, resulting in a state where both bleeding and clotting can occur.[148] This process is mediated in part by inflammatory cytokines. Levels of specific cytokines measured at the time of sepsis diagnosis may predict the risk of DIC during that sepsis episode.[149]

RENAL SYSTEM

As cardiac output and vascular integrity worsen with progression of the sepsis syndrome, perfusion to the neonatal kidneys decreases, and the risk of acute kidney injury (AKI) and renal dysfunction increases. As with hypotension, clear diagnostic criteria for AKI are lacking due to differences in definitions, creatinine sampling, and timing.[150] Nevertheless, preterm neonates are uniquely at risk for AKI due to a confluence of developmental and iatrogenic risk factors, compounded by sepsis-related dysfunction.[151]

As with most organs, the preterm kidney is not completely developed, a process that continues even past term gestation, with a doubling of the number of nephrons between 20 and 35 weeks' gestation.[152] Renal blood flow rapidly changes, with a doubling or even tripling of the fraction of the cardiac output reaching the kidneys over the course of the first week, and the changes continue until maximal consumption of cardiac output at 2 years of age.[152] The relatively low perfusion and oliguria early in the neonatal course leave infants with a unique risk of kidney injury compared with older children and adults.[153]

The mechanisms of renal injury during sepsis include oxidative stress and direct parenchyma or tubule damage (as in acute tubular necrosis). PAMPs, such as LPS, mediate this injury in conjunction with systemic cardiovascular compromise and impaired perfusion.[154] In one study, 20% of late-onset sepsis cases had AKI within 7 days of a positive blood culture. AKI also occurred in infants with a sepsis syndrome without a positive blood culture but with lower frequency and severity.[155] Other studies report a high incidence of AKI in sepsis and NEC,[150,156] and a large, epidemiological study of late-onset AKI in neonates identified sepsis and NEC as major risk factors.[151] Iatrogenic factors may further exacerbate AKI; nephrotoxic medications such as vancomycin and gentamicin are common first-line drugs for the treatment of Gram-positive infections (where methicillin resistance is a concern) and Gram-negative infections, respectively. In one study, 74% of infants identified in a multi-hospital database received at least one nephrotoxic drug, and their use was associated with an adjusted relative risk of AKI of 3.68.[157]

Although neonatal AKI is frequently reversible, it can have long-term consequences[158] and presents challenges to the acute management of the patient, particularly in the setting of concurrent sepsis. Decreased urine output leads to the retention of excessive free water, potentially causing electrolyte disturbances such as hyponatremia. Although fluid resuscitation is the mainstay of treatment for the distributive shock that often accompanies sepsis, significant consideration must be given to the total volume administered if it will not be excreted at expected rates. Care should be taken to dose renally cleared medications and supplemental electrolytes such as potassium appropriately to prevent toxicity.

GASTROINTESTINAL SYSTEM

The intestinal tract of the preterm infant has dual vulnerabilities in the setting of sepsis. First, the low perfusion priority and impaired splanchnic autoregulation[159,160] make it vulnerable to ischemic injury during periods of poor perfusion. Second, there has been extensive study of the preterm microbiome, finding that altered microbiomes containing pathogenic bacteria are commonly observed preceding the development of NEC[161] and that common NICU interventions such as antibiotic use contribute to this alteration.

As with dysfunction in other organ systems, the clinical manifestation of intestinal injury is variable and ranges from no abnormality to transmural necrosis of the large and small bowel. The connection between a positive blood culture and gastrointestinal dysfunction remains tenuous at best and requires careful monitoring to initiate timely supportive treatment. Most of what we know about organ dysfunction, sepsis, and NEC has come from observational studies, which inform clinical care and future study design.[162] Feeding intolerance may be considered a harbinger of intestinal pathology, but repeated analyses of gastric residuals demonstrate that this common practice does not predict or reduce rates of NEC,[163,164] but it does impact the nutrition and growth potential of infants.[165,166] Transfusion of red blood cells has also been implicated in the development of NEC,[167] a critical concern as blood transfusions are frequently given to improve the oxygen-carrying capacity of infected infants with cardiorespiratory failure. A number of theories for this finding have been proposed, including the immunogenicity of prepared red blood cell products, which contain increased levels of cytokines, free hemoglobin, and red blood cell fragments.[167] Subsequent detailed examination has revealed that the preceding anemia may be the proximal cause of transfusion-associated NEC rather than the transfusion itself.[168,169] This finding further underlines the mechanism by which sepsis-related perfusion defects exacerbate common NICU morbidities.

Many questions and controversies remain regarding intestinal dysfunction in neonatal sepsis and NEC. Several clinical trials have studied interventions for neonatal sepsis and NEC, but with variable definitions of sepsis and outcomes and unclear generalizability.[8,9] Sepsis and shock occur in neonates even when the blood culture is negative and no focal infection is diagnosed. In research and clinical care, these "clinical sepsis" events are frequently treated as falsely negative blood cultures, and infants receive antibiotic treatment as if the culture had been positive. In reality, the sensitivity of a culture of at least 1 mL of blood, using modern methods in upper-income countries, is about 99%.[17,170,171]

Guidelines and Monitoring

The diverse and idiosyncratic clinical expressions of sepsis in preterm neonates has led to the current, highly fragmented approach to monitoring, diagnosis, and treatment. As has been demonstrated, comprehensive assessment of sepsis impact and treatment response requires integration of information from multiple organ systems. Inclusion of infants with and without positive blood cultures and infants with and without organ dysfunction, as well as a lack of a more universal measure of illness severity, hampers forward progress. Therefore, experts have called for a working group to review the evidence and develop definitions and guidelines.[13]

Guidelines for adult sepsis use the sequential organ failure assessment (SOFA) score and culture results to define sepsis and septic shock.[172] SOFA assigns points for increasing measures of dysfunction in each of six organ systems, and the score is calculated by adding the points. Recently, a neonatal SOFA score was developed[173] using data from an observational study of fatal sepsis[19] to guide thresholds for assigning points to calculate the score. The score performed well for predicting mortality during sepsis in a single-center, external validation study[174] and a large, multicenter cohort of preterm infants.[175] An alternative score, neonatal multiple organ dysfunction, utilizes a similar strategy of assigning increasing point values to worsening function across a range of organ systems and is strongly predictive of mortality.[176]

Physiologic monitoring can also be leveraged to capture a cross-sectional overview of organ dysfunction early in the sepsis course. Algorithms utilizing computational assessment of heart rate characteristics can identify preclinical signs of sepsis and NEC and lead to improved outcomes for patients.[71,86,122,177] Alternative technology, such as near-infrared spectroscopy, can be used to detect changes in organ function including alterations in the splanchnic–cerebral oxygenation ratio for infants with significant anemia.[178,179]

Conclusion

Sepsis and NEC remain significant problems for infants admitted to the NICU, including the potential for significant morbidity and mortality. The neonatal sepsis syndrome, influenced by the unstable physiology of transition and overlap with common non-sepsis conditions, not only is unique to this patient population but is also highly variable between neonates. Future lines of investigation should focus on defining organ dysfunction and sepsis and advancing care of the infant with sepsis through development of multimodal, cross-organ evaluation. Providing clinicians with the earliest possible warning of sepsis and the tools necessary to track the response to treatment will save lives and improve outcomes for survivors.

REFERENCES

1. Shane AL, Stoll BJ. Neonatal sepsis: progress towards improved outcomes. *J Infect*. 2014;68(suppl 1):S24-S32.
2. Shane AL, Sánchez PJ, Stoll BJ. Neonatal sepsis. *Lancet*. 2017; 390(10104):1770-1780.
3. Liu L, Oza S, Hogan D, et al. Global, regional, and national causes of under-5 mortality in 2000–15: an updated systematic analysis with implications for the Sustainable Development Goals. *Lancet*. 2016;388(10063):3027-3035.
4. Greenberg RG, Kandefer S, Do BT, et al. Late-onset sepsis in extremely premature infants: 2000–2011. *Pediatr Infect Dis J*. 2017; 36(8):774-779.
5. Hasday JD, Fairchild KD, Shanholtz C. The role of fever in the infected host. *Microbes Infect*. 2000;2(15):1891-1904.
6. Tracey KJ. Reflex control of immunity. *Nat Rev Immunol*. 2009;9(6): 418-428.

7. Wynn JL, Polin RA. Progress in the management of neonatal sepsis: the importance of a consensus definition. *Pediatr Res.* 2018;83(1-1):13-15.
8. Hayes R, Hartnett J, Semova G, et al. Neonatal sepsis definitions from randomised clinical trials [published online ahead of print November 6, 2021]. *Pediatr Res.* Available at: https://doi.org/10.1038/s41390-021-01749-3.
9. Henry CJ, Semova G, Barnes E, et al. Neonatal sepsis: a systematic review of core outcomes from randomised clinical trials. *Pediatr Res.* 2022;91(4):735-742.
10. Goldstein B, Giroir B, Randolph A, International Consensus Conference on Pediatric Sepsis. International Pediatric Sepsis Consensus Conference: definitions for sepsis and organ dysfunction in pediatrics. *Pediatr Crit Care Med.* 2005;6(1):2-8.
11. Wynn JL, Wong HR. Pathophysiology and treatment of septic shock in neonates. *Clin Perinatol.* 2010;37(2):439-479.
12. Coggins S, Harris MC, Grundmeier R, Kalb E, Nawab U, Srinivasan L. Performance of pediatric systemic inflammatory response syndrome and organ dysfunction criteria in late-onset sepsis in a quaternary neonatal intensive care unit: a case-control study. *J Pediatr.* 2020;219:133-139.e1.
13. Molloy EJ, Wynn JL, Bliss J, et al. Neonatal sepsis: need for consensus definition, collaboration and core outcomes. *Pediatr Res.* 2020;88(1):2-4.
14. Bembea MM, Agus M, Akcan-Arikan A, et al. Pediatric Organ Dysfunction Information Update Mandate (PODIUM) contemporary organ dysfunction criteria: executive summary. *Pediatrics.* 2022;149(1 suppl 1):S1-S12.
15. Moorman JR, Lake DE, Ivanov PC. Early detection of sepsis—a role for network physiology? *Crit Care Med.* 2016;44(5):e312-e313.
16. Shashikumar SP, Li Q, Clifford GD, Nemati S. Multiscale network representation of physiological time series for early prediction of sepsis. *Physiol Meas.* 2017;38(12):2235-2248.
17. Connell TG, Rele M, Cowley D, Buttery JP, Curtis N. How reliable is a negative blood culture result? Volume of blood submitted for culture in routine practice in a children's hospital. *Pediatrics.* 2007;119(5):891-896.
18. Jawaheer G, Neal TJ, Shaw NJ. Blood culture volume and detection of coagulase negative staphylococcal septicaemia in neonates. *Arch Dis Child Fetal Neonatal Ed.* 1997;76(1):F57-F58.
19. Wynn JL, Kelly MS, Benjamin DK, et al. Timing of multiorgan dysfunction among hospitalized infants with fatal fulminant sepsis. *Am J Perinatol.* 2017;34(7):633-639.
20. Shah J, Jefferies AL, Yoon EW, Lee SK, Shah PS, Canadian Neonatal Network. Risk factors and outcomes of late-onset bacterial sepsis in preterm neonates born at < 32 weeks' gestation. *Am J Perinatol.* 2015;32(7):675-682.
21. Goh GL, Lim CSE, Sultana R, De La Puerta R, Rajadurai VS, Yeo KT. Risk factors for mortality from late-onset sepsis among preterm very-low-birthweight infants: a single-center cohort study from Singapore. *Front Pediatr.* 2021;9:801955.
22. Kumar S, Ingle H, Prasad DVR, Kumar H. Recognition of bacterial infection by innate immune sensors. *Crit Rev Microbiol.* 2013;39(3):229-246.
23. Hornik CP, Fort P, Clark RH, et al. Early and late onset sepsis in very-low-birth-weight infants from a large group of neonatal intensive care units. *Early Hum Dev.* 2012;88(suppl 2):S69-S74.
24. Kaufman D, Fairchild KD. Clinical microbiology of bacterial and fungal sepsis in very-low-birth-weight infants. *Clin Microbiol Rev.* 2004;17(3):638-680.
25. Manzoni P, Farina D, Leonessa M, et al. Risk factors for progression to invasive fungal infection in preterm neonates with fungal colonization. *Pediatrics.* 2006;118(6):2359-2364.
26. Ronchi A, Michelow IC, Chapin KC, et al. Viral respiratory tract infections in the neonatal intensive care unit: the VIRIoN-I study. *J Pediatr.* 2014;165(4):690-696.
27. Verboon-Maciolek MA, Krediet TG, Gerards LJ, Fleer A, van Loon TM. Clinical and epidemiologic characteristics of viral infections in a neonatal intensive care unit during a 12-year period. *Pediatr Infect Dis J.* 2005;24(10):901-904.
28. Kidszun A, Klein L, Winter J, et al. Viral infections in neonates with suspected late-onset bacterial sepsis–a prospective cohort study. *Am J Perinatol.* 2017;34(1):1-7.
29. Pammi M, Cope J, Tarr PI, et al. Intestinal dysbiosis in preterm infants preceding necrotizing enterocolitis: a systematic review and meta-analysis. *Microbiome.* 2017;5(1):31.
30. Rusconi B, Good M, Warner BB. The microbiome and biomarkers for necrotizing enterocolitis: are we any closer to prediction? *J Pediatr.* 2017;189:40-47.e2.
31. Afrazi A, Sodhi CP, Richardson W, et al. New insights into the pathogenesis and treatment of necrotizing enterocolitis: toll-like receptors and beyond. *Pediatr Res.* 2011;69(3):183-188.
32. Van Camp JM, Tomaselli V, Drongowski R, Coran AG. Bacterial translocation in the newborn rabbit: effect of age on frequency of translocation. *Pediatr Surg Int.* 1995;10(2-3):134-137.
33. Sherman MP. New concepts of microbial translocation in the neonatal intestine: mechanisms and prevention. *Clin Perinatol.* 2010;37(3):565-579.
34. Masi AC, Stewart CJ. The role of the preterm intestinal microbiome in sepsis and necrotising enterocolitis. *Early Hum Dev.* 2019;138:104854.
35. Stoll BJ, Hansen N. Infections in VLBW infants: studies from the NICHD Neonatal Research Network. *Semin Perinatol.* 2003;27(4):293-301.
36. Sullivan BA, Grice SM, Lake DE, Moorman JR, Fairchild KD. Infection and other clinical correlates of abnormal heart rate characteristics in preterm infants. *J Pediatr.* 2014;164(4):775-780.
37. Sangild PT, Strunk T, Currie AJ, Nguyen DN. Editorial: immunity in compromised newborns. *Front Immunol.* 2021;12:732332.
38. Wynn J, Cornell TT, Wong HR, Shanley TP, Wheeler DS. The host response to sepsis and developmental impact. *Pediatrics.* 2010;125(5):1031-1041.
39. Raymond SL, Stortz JA, Mira JC, Larson SD, Wynn JL, Moldawer LL. Immunological defects in neonatal sepsis and potential therapeutic approaches. *Front Pediatr.* 2017;5:14.
40. Luce WA, Hoffman TM, Bauer JA. Bench-to-bedside review: developmental influences on the mechanisms, treatment and outcomes of cardiovascular dysfunction in neonatal versus adult sepsis. *Crit Care.* 2007;11(5):228.
41. Klein SL, Flanagan KL. Sex differences in immune responses. *Nat Rev Immunol.* 2016;16(10):626-638.
42. Stevenson DK, Verter J, Fanaroff AA, et al. Sex differences in outcomes of very low birthweight infants: the newborn male disadvantage. *Arch Dis Child Fetal Neonatal Ed.* 2000;83(3):F182-F185.
43. Boghossian NS, Geraci M, Edwards EM, Horbar JD. Sex differences in mortality and morbidity of infants born at less than 30 weeks' gestation. *Pediatrics.* 2018;142(6):e20182352.
44. Wallace ME, Mendola P, Kim SS, et al. Racial/ethnic differences in preterm perinatal outcomes. *Am J Obstet Gynecol.* 2017;216(3):306.e1-306.e12.
45. Travers CP, Carlo WA, McDonald SA, et al. Racial/ethnic disparities among extremely preterm infants in the united states from 2002 to 2016. *JAMA Netw Open.* 2020;3(6):e206757.

46. Esposito S, Zampiero A, Pugni L, et al. Genetic polymorphisms and sepsis in premature neonates. *PLoS ONE*. 2014;9(7): e101248.
47. Dahmer MK, Randolph A, Vitali S, Quasney MW. Genetic polymorphisms in sepsis. *Pediatr Crit Care Med*. 2005;6(suppl 3): S61-S73.
48. Abu-Maziad A, Schaa K, Bell EF, et al. Role of polymorphic variants as genetic modulators of infection in neonatal sepsis. *Pediatr Res*. 2010;68(4):323-329.
49. Majetschak M, Flohé S, Obertacke U, et al. Relation of a TNF gene polymorphism to severe sepsis in trauma patients. *Ann Surg*. 1999;230(2):207-214.
50. Weitkamp JH, Stüber F, Bartmann P. Pilot study assessing TNF gene polymorphism as a prognostic marker for disease progression in neonates with sepsis. *Infection*. 2000;28(2):92-96.
51. Wynn JL, Wilson CS, Hawiger J, et al. Targeting IL-17A attenuates neonatal sepsis mortality induced by IL-18. *Proc Natl Acad Sci U S A*. 2016;113(19):E2627-E2635.
52. Schüller SS, Kramer BW, Villamor E, Spittler A, Berger A, Levy O. Immunomodulation to prevent or treat neonatal sepsis: past, present, and future. *Front Pediatr*. 2018;6:199.
53. Wynn JL, Neu J, Moldawer LL, Levy O. Potential of immunomodulatory agents for prevention and treatment of neonatal sepsis. *J Perinatol*. 2009;29(2):79-88.
54. Rivers E, Nguyen B, Havstad S, et al. Early goal-directed therapy in the treatment of severe sepsis and septic shock. *N Engl J Med*. 2001;345(19):1368-1377.
55. Caironi P, Tognoni G, Masson S, et al. Albumin replacement in patients with severe sepsis or septic shock. *N Engl J Med*. 2014; 370(15):1412-1421.
56. Asfar P, Meziani F, Hamel JF, et al. High versus low blood-pressure target in patients with septic shock. *N Engl J Med*. 2014; 370(17):1583-1593.
57. Yealy DM, Kellum JA, Huang DT, et al. A randomized trial of protocol-based care for early septic shock. *N Engl J Med*. 2014; 370(18):1683-1693.
58. Wyckoff MH. Initial resuscitation and stabilization of the periviable neonate: the Golden-Hour approach. *Semin Perinatol*. 2014;38(1):12-16.
59. Carcillo JA, Han K, Lin J, Orr R. Goal-directed management of pediatric shock in the emergency department. *Clin Pediatr Emerg Med*. 2007;8(3):165-175.
60. Finer NN, Kinsella JP. Neonatal intensive care perspective. *Pediatr Crit Care Med*. 2011;12:S62-S65.
61. Sullivan BA, Panda A, Wallman-Stokes A, et al. Antibiotic spectrum index: a new tool comparing antibiotic use in three NICUs. *Infect Control Hosp Epidemiol*. 2022;43(11):1553-1557.
62. Rubin LG, Sánchez PJ, Siegel J, et al. Evaluation and treatment of neonates with suspected late-onset sepsis: a survey of neonatologists' practices. *Pediatrics*. 2002;110(4):e42.
63. Cotten CM, Taylor S, Stoll B, et al. Prolonged duration of initial empirical antibiotic treatment is associated with increased rates of necrotizing enterocolitis and death for extremely low birth weight infants. *Pediatrics*. 2009;123(1):58-66.
64. Greenberg RG, Chowdhury D, Hansen NI, et al. Prolonged duration of early antibiotic therapy in extremely premature infants. *Pediatr Res*. 2019;85(7):994-1000.
65. Fairchild KD, Schelonka RL, Kaufman DA, et al. Septicemia mortality reduction in neonates in a heart rate characteristics monitoring trial. *Pediatr Res*. 2013;74(5):570-575.
66. King WE, Carlo WA, O'Shea TM, Schelonka RL, HRC Neurodevelopmental Follow-Up Investigators. Multivariable predictive models of death or neurodevelopmental impairment among extremely low birth weight infants using heart rate characteristics. *J Pediatr*. 2022;242:137-144.e4.
67. Appiah MG, Park EJ, Akama Y, et al. Cellular and exosomal regulations of sepsis-induced metabolic alterations. *Int J Mol Sci*. 2021;22(15):8295.
68. Carrara M, Ferrario M, Bollen Pinto B, Herpain A. The autonomic nervous system in septic shock and its role as a future therapeutic target: a narrative review. *Ann Intensive Care*. 2021;11(1):80.
69. Fairchild KD, Srinivasan V, Moorman JR, Gaykema RPA, Goehler LE. Pathogen-induced heart rate changes associated with cholinergic nervous system activation. *Am J Physiol Regul Integr Comp Physiol*. 2011;300(2):R330-R339.
70. Fairchild KD, Saucerman JJ, Raynor LL, et al. Endotoxin depresses heart rate variability in mice: cytokine and steroid effects. *Am J Physiol Regul Integr Comp Physiol*. 2009;297(4): R1019-R1027.
71. Griffin MP, O'Shea TM, Bissonette EA, Harrell FE, Lake DE, Moorman JR. Abnormal heart rate characteristics preceding neonatal sepsis and sepsis-like illness. *Pediatr Res*. 2003;53(6):920-926.
72. Fairchild KD, O'Shea TM. Heart rate characteristics: physiomarkers for detection of late-onset neonatal sepsis. *Clin Perinatol*. 2010;37(3):581-598.
73. Tracey KJ. Reflexes in immunity. *Cell*. 2016;164(3):343-344.
74. Borovikova LV, Ivanova S, Zhang M, et al. Vagus nerve stimulation attenuates the systemic inflammatory response to endotoxin. *Nature*. 2000;405(6785):458-462.
75. Andersson U, Tracey KJ. Neural reflexes in inflammation and immunity. *J Exp Med*. 2012;209(6):1057-1068.
76. Tracey KJ. Physiology and immunology of the cholinergic anti-inflammatory pathway. *J Clin Invest*. 2007;117(2):289-296.
77. Vesoulis ZA, Bank RL, Lake D, et al. Early hypoxemia burden is strongly associated with severe intracranial hemorrhage in preterm infants. *J Perinatol*. 2019;39(1):48-53.
78. Ng IHX, da Costa CS, Zeiler FA, et al. Burden of hypoxia and intraventricular haemorrhage in extremely preterm infants. *Arch Dis Child Fetal Neonatal Ed*. 2020;105(3):242-247.
79. Villamor-Martinez E, Fumagalli M, Alomar YI, et al. Cerebellar hemorrhage in preterm infants: a meta-analysis on risk factors and neurodevelopmental outcome. *Front Physiol*. 2019;10:800.
80. Ter Horst HJ, van Olffen M, Remmelts HJ, de Vries H, Bos AF. The prognostic value of amplitude integrated EEG in neonatal sepsis and/or meningitis. *Acta Paediatr*. 2010;99(2):194-200.
81. Prieto CL, Colomer BF, Sastre JBL. Prognostic factors of mortality in very low-birth-weight infants with neonatal sepsis of nosocomial origin. *Am J Perinatol*. 2013;30(5):353-358.
82. Volpe JJ. Postnatal sepsis, necrotizing entercolitis, and the critical role of systemic inflammation in white matter injury in premature infants. *J Pediatr*. 2008;153(2):160-163.
83. Khwaja O, Volpe JJ. Pathogenesis of cerebral white matter injury of prematurity. *Arch Dis Child Fetal Neonatal Ed*. 2008;93(2): F153-F161.
84. Verstraete EH, Blot K, Mahieu L, Vogelaers D, Blot S. Prediction models for neonatal health care-associated sepsis: a meta-analysis. *Pediatrics*. 2015;135(4):e1002-e1014.
85. Fanaroff AA, Korones SB, Wright LL, et al. Incidence, presenting features, risk factors and significance of late onset septicemia in very low birth weight infants. The National Institute of Child Health and Human Development Neonatal Research Network. *Pediatr Infect Dis J*. 1998;17(7):593-598.
86. Sullivan BA, Nagraj VP, Berry KL, et al. Clinical and vital sign changes associated with late-onset sepsis in very low birth weight infants at 3 NICUs. *J Neonatal Perinatal Med*. 2021;14(4): 553-561.

87. Joshi R, Bierling BL, Long X, et al. A ballistographic approach for continuous and non-obtrusive monitoring of movement in neonates. *IEEE J Transl Eng Health Med*. 2018;6:2700809.
88. Joshi R, Kommers D, Oosterwijk L, Feijs L, van Pul C, Andriessen P. Predicting neonatal sepsis using features of heart rate variability, respiratory characteristics, and ECG-derived estimates of infant motion. *IEEE J Biomed Health Inform*. 2020;24(3):681-692.
89. Alonzo CJ, Nagraj VP, Zschaebitz JV, Lake DE, Moorman JR, Spaeder MC. Blood pressure ranges via non-invasive and invasive monitoring techniques in premature neonates using high resolution physiologic data. *J Neonatal Perinatal Med*. 2020;13(3):351-358.
90. Alonzo CJ, Nagraj VP, Zschaebitz JV, Lake DE, Moorman JR, Spaeder MC. Heart rate ranges in premature neonates using high resolution physiologic data. *J Perinatol*. 2018;38(9):1242-1245.
91. Hegyi T, Carbone MT, Anwar M, et al. Blood pressure ranges in premature infants. I. The first hours of life. *J Pediatr*. 1994;124(4):627-633.
92. Zimmet AM, Sullivan BA, Fairchild KD, et al. Vital sign metrics of VLBW infants in three NICUs: implications for predictive algorithms. *Pediatr Res*. 2021;90(1):125-130.
93. Seri I, Noori S. Diagnosis and treatment of neonatal hypotension outside the transitional period. *Early Hum Dev*. 2005;81(5):405-411.
94. Werther T, Aichhorn L, Baumgartner S, Berger A, Klebermass-Schrehof K, Salzer-Muhar U. Discrepancy between invasive and non-invasive blood pressure readings in extremely preterm infants in the first four weeks of life. *PLoS ONE*. 2018;13(12):e0209831.
95. Troy R, Doron M, Laughon M, Tolleson-Rinehart S, Price W. Comparison of noninvasive and central arterial blood pressure measurements in ELBW infants. *J Perinatol*. 2009;29(11):744-749.
96. Zubrow AB, Hulman S, Kushner H, Falkner B. Determinants of blood pressure in infants admitted to neonatal intensive care units: a prospective multicenter study. Philadelphia Neonatal Blood Pressure Study Group. *J Perinatol*. 1995;15(6):470-479.
97. Miall-Allen VM, de Vries LS, Whitelaw AG. Mean arterial blood pressure and neonatal cerebral lesions. *Arch Dis Child*. 1987;62(10):1068-1069.
98. Knobel-Dail RB, Sloane R, Holditch-Davis D, Tanaka DT. Negative temperature differential in preterm infants less than 29 weeks gestational age: associations with infection and maternal smoking. *Nurs Res*. 2017;66(6):442-453.
99. Dail RB, Everhart KC, Hardin JW, et al. Predicting infection in very preterm infants: a study protocol. *Nurs Res*. 2021;70(2):142-149.
100. Bakshi S, Koerner T, Knee A, Singh R, Vaidya R. Effect of fluid bolus on clinical outcomes in very low birth weight infants. *J Pediatr Pharmacol Ther*. 2020;25(5):437-444.
101. Seri I, Rudas G, Bors Z, Kanyicska B, Tulassay T. Effects of low-dose dopamine infusion on cardiovascular and renal functions, cerebral blood flow, and plasma catecholamine levels in sick preterm neonates. *Pediatr Res*. 1993;34(6):742-749.
102. Barrington K, Brion LP. Dopamine versus no treatment to prevent renal dysfunction in indomethacin-treated preterm newborn infants. *Cochrane Database Syst Rev*. 2002;(3):CD003213.
103. Filippi L, Pezzati M, Poggi C, Rossi S, Cecchi A, Santoro C. Dopamine versus dobutamine in very low birthweight infants: endocrine effects. *Arch Dis Child Fetal Neonatal Ed*. 2007;92(5):F367-F371.
104. Greenough A, Emery EF. Randomized trial comparing dopamine and dobutamine in preterm infants. *Eur J Pediatr*. 1993;152(11):925-927.
105. Klarr JM, Faix RG, Pryce CJ, Bhatt-Mehta V. Randomized, blind trial of dopamine versus dobutamine for treatment of hypotension in preterm infants with respiratory distress syndrome. *J Pediatr*. 1994;125(1):117-122.
106. Rios DR, Moffett BS, Kaiser JR. Trends in pharmacotherapy for neonatal hypotension. *J Pediatr*. 2014;165(4):697-701.e1.
107. Watterberg KL. Adrenal insufficiency and cardiac dysfunction in the preterm infant. *Pediatr Res*. 2002;51(4):422-424.
108. Seri I, Tan R, Evans J. Cardiovascular effects of hydrocortisone in preterm infants with pressor-resistant hypotension. *Pediatrics*. 2001;107(5):1070-1074.
109. Attridge JT, Clark R, Walker MW, Gordon PV. New insights into spontaneous intestinal perforation using a national data set: (1) SIP is associated with early indomethacin exposure. *J Perinatol*. 2006;26(2):93-99.
110. Paquette L, Friedlich P, Ramanathan R, Seri I. Concurrent use of indomethacin and dexamethasone increases the risk of spontaneous intestinal perforation in very low birth weight neonates. *J Perinatol*. 2006;26(8):486-492.
111. Rios DR, Kaiser JR. Vasopressin versus dopamine for treatment of hypotension in extremely low birth weight infants: a randomized, blinded pilot study. *J Pediatr*. 2015;166(4):850-855.
112. Lee G, Kaiser JR, Moffett BS, Rodman E, Toy C, Rios DR. Efficacy of low-dose epinephrine continuous infusion in neonatal intensive care unit patients. *J Pediatr Pharmacol Ther*. 20214;26(1):51-55.
113. Rizk MY, Lapointe A, Lefebvre F, Barrington KJ. Norepinephrine infusion improves haemodynamics in the preterm infants during septic shock. *Acta Paediatr*. 2018;107(3):408-413.
114. Sehgal A, McNamara PJ. Does point-of-care functional echocardiography enhance cardiovascular care in the NICU? *J Perinatol*. 2008;28(11):729-735.
115. El-Khuffash AF, McNamara PJ. Neonatologist-performed functional echocardiography in the neonatal intensive care unit. *Semin Fetal Neonatal Med*. 2011;16(1):50-60.
116. Kluckow M, Seri I, Evans N. Functional echocardiography: an emerging clinical tool for the neonatologist. *J Pediatr*. 2007;150(2):125-130.
117. Kingwell BA, Thompson JM, Kaye DM, McPherson GA, Jennings GL, Esler MD. Heart rate spectral analysis, cardiac norepinephrine spillover, and muscle sympathetic nerve activity during human sympathetic nervous activation and failure. *Circulation*. 1994;90(1):234-240.
118. Fairchild K, Mohr M, Paget-Brown A, et al. Clinical associations of immature breathing in preterm infants: part 1–central apnea. *Pediatr Res*. 2016;80(1):21-27.
119. Griffin MP, Scollan DF, Moorman JR. The dynamic range of neonatal heart rate variability. *J Cardiovasc Electrophysiol*. 1994;5(2):112-124.
120. Griffin MP, Lake DE, Bissonette EA, Harrell FE, O'Shea TM, Moorman JR. Heart rate characteristics: novel physiomarkers to predict neonatal infection and death. *Pediatrics*. 2005;116(5):1070-1074.
121. Lake DE, Fairchild KD, Moorman JR. Complex signals bioinformatics: evaluation of heart rate characteristics monitoring as a novel risk marker for neonatal sepsis. *J Clin Monit Comput*. 2014;28(4):329-339.
122. Kovatchev BP, Farhy LS, Cao H, Griffin MP, Lake DE, Moorman JR. Sample asymmetry analysis of heart rate characteristics

with application to neonatal sepsis and systemic inflammatory response syndrome. *Pediatr Res*. 2003;54(6):892-898.

123. Griffin MP, Moorman JR. Toward the early diagnosis of neonatal sepsis and sepsis-like illness using novel heart rate analysis. *Pediatrics*. 2001;107(1):97-104.
124. Ohlin A, Björkqvist M, Montgomery SM, Schollin J. Clinical signs and CRP values associated with blood culture results in neonates evaluated for suspected sepsis. *Acta Paediatr*. 2010;99(11):1635-1640.
125. Kumar RS, Otero NA, Abubakar MO, et al. Framework for considering abnormal heart rate characteristics and other signs of sepsis in very low birth weight infants [published online ahead of print December 7, 2021]. *Am J Perinatol*. Available at: https://doi.org/10.1055/a-1715-3727.
126. Siljehav V, Hofstetter AM, Leifsdottir K, Herlenius E. Prostaglandin E2 mediates cardiorespiratory disturbances during infection in neonates. *J Pediatr*. 2015;167(6):1207-1213.e3.
127. Balan KV, Kc P, Hoxha Z, Mayer CA, Wilson CG, Martin RJ. Vagal afferents modulate cytokine-mediated respiratory control at the neonatal medulla oblongata. *Respir Physiol Neurobiol*. 2011;178(3):458-464.
128. Hofstetter AO, Saha S, Siljehav V, Jakobsson PJ, Herlenius E. The induced prostaglandin E2 pathway is a key regulator of the respiratory response to infection and hypoxia in neonates. *Proc Natl Acad Sci U S A*. 2007;104(23):9894-9899.
129. Herlenius E. An inflammatory pathway to apnea and autonomic dysregulation. *Respir Physiol Neurobiol*. 2011;178(3):449-457.
130. Gonzalez BE, Mercado CK, Johnson L, Brodsky NL, Bhandari V. Early markers of late-onset sepsis in premature neonates: clinical, hematological and cytokine profile. *J Perinat Med*. 2003;31(1):60-68.
131. Tan K, Lai NM, Sharma A. Surfactant for bacterial pneumonia in late preterm and term infants. *Cochrane Database Syst Rev*. 2012;(2):CD008155.
132. Christensen RD, Rothstein G, Anstall HB, Bybee B. Granulocyte transfusions in neonates with bacterial infection, neutropenia, and depletion of mature marrow neutrophils. *Pediatrics*. 1982;70(1):1-6.
133. Gillan ER, Christensen RD, Suen Y, Ellis R, van de Ven C, Cairo MS. A randomized, placebo-controlled trial of recombinant human granulocyte colony-stimulating factor administration in newborn infants with presumed sepsis: significant induction of peripheral and bone marrow neutrophilia. *Blood*. 1994;84(5):1427-1433.
134. Kawamura M, Nishida H. The usefulness of serial C-reactive protein measurement in managing neonatal infection. *Acta Paediatr*. 1995;84(1):10-13.
135. Benitz WE, Han MY, Madan A, Ramachandra P. Serial serum C-reactive protein levels in the diagnosis of neonatal infection. *Pediatrics*. 1998;102(4):E41.
136. Nuntnarumit P, Pinkaew O, Kitiwanwanich S. Predictive values of serial C-reactive protein in neonatal sepsis. *J Med Assoc Thai*. 2002;85(suppl 4):S1151-S1158.
137. Hisamuddin E, Hisam A, Wahid S, Raza G. Validity of C-reactive protein (CRP) for diagnosis of neonatal sepsis. *Pak J Med Sci*. 2015;31(3):527-531.
138. Cantey JB, Bultmann CR. C-reactive protein testing in late-onset neonatal sepsis: hazardous waste. *JAMA Pediatr*. 2020;174(3):235-236.
139. Coggins SA, Wynn JL, Hill ML, et al. Use of a computerized C-reactive protein (CRP) based sepsis evaluation in very low birth weight (VLBW) infants: a five-year experience. *PLoS ONE*. 2013;8(11):e78602.
140. Singh N, Gray JE. Antibiotic stewardship in NICU: de-implementing routine CRP to reduce antibiotic usage in neonates at risk for early-onset sepsis. *J Perinatol*. 2021;41(10):2488-2494.
141. Ottolini MC, Lundgren K, Mirkinson LJ, Cason S, Ottolini MG. Utility of complete blood count and blood culture screening to diagnose neonatal sepsis in the asymptomatic at risk newborn. *Pediatr Infect Dis J*. 2003;22(5):430-434.
142. Hornik CP, Benjamin DK, Becker KC, et al. Use of the complete blood cell count in early-onset neonatal sepsis. *Pediatr Infect Dis J*. 2012;31(8):799-802.
143. Blommendahl J, Janas M, Laine S, Miettinen A, Ashorn P. Comparison of procalcitonin with CRP and differential white blood cell count for diagnosis of culture-proven neonatal sepsis. *Scand J Infect Dis*. 2002;34(8):620-622.
144. Shaaban HA, Safwat N. Mean platelet volume in preterm: a predictor of early onset neonatal sepsis. *J Matern Fetal Neonatal Med*. 2020;33(2):206-211.
145. Aydın B, Dilli D, Zenciroğlu A, Karadağ N, Beken S, Okumuş N. Mean platelet volume and uric acid levels in neonatal sepsis. *Indian J Pediatr*. 2014;81(12):1342-1346.
146. Bomela HN, Ballot DE, Cory BJ, Cooper PA. Use of C-reactive protein to guide duration of empiric antibiotic therapy in suspected early neonatal sepsis. *Pediatr Infect Dis J*. 2000;19(6):531-535.
147. Hathaway WE, Mull MM, Pechet GS. Disseminated intravascular coagulation in the newborn. *Pediatrics*. 1969;43(2):233-240.
148. Roman J, Velasco F, Fernandez F, et al. Coagulation, fibrinolytic and kallikrein systems in neonates with uncomplicated sepsis and septic shock. *Haemostasis*. 1993;23(3):142-148.
149. Ng PC, Li K, Leung TF, et al. Early prediction of sepsis-induced disseminated intravascular coagulation with interleukin-10, interleukin-6, and RANTES in preterm infants. *Clin Chem*. 2006;52(6):1181-1189.
150. Starr MC, Charlton JR, Guillet R, et al. Advances in neonatal acute kidney injury. *Pediatrics*. 2021;148(5):e2021051220.
151. Charlton JR, Boohaker L, Askenazi D, et al. Late onset neonatal acute kidney injury: results from the AWAKEN Study. *Pediatr Res*. 2019;85(3):339-348.
152. Botwinski CA, Falco GA. Transition to postnatal renal function. *J Perinat Neonatal Nurs*. 2014;28(2):150-154; E3-E4.
153. Selewski DT, Charlton JR, Jetton JG, et al. Neonatal acute kidney injury. *Pediatrics*. 2015;136(2):e463-e473.
154. Plotnikov EY, Brezgunova AA, Pevzner IB, et al. Mechanisms of LPS-induced acute kidney injury in neonatal and adult rats. *Antioxidants (Basel)*. 2018;7(8):105.
155. Coggins SA, Laskin B, Harris MC, et al. Acute kidney injury associated with late-onset neonatal sepsis: a matched cohort study. *J Pediatr*. 2021;231:185-192.e4.
156. Garg PM, Britt AB, Ansari MAY, et al. Severe acute kidney injury in neonates with necrotizing enterocolitis: risk factors and outcomes. *Pediatr Res*. 2021;90(3):642-649.
157. Mohamed TH, Abdi HH, Magers J, Prusakov P, Slaughter JL. Nephrotoxic medications and associated acute kidney injury in hospitalized neonates. *J Nephrol*. 2022;35(6):1679-1687.
158. Harer MW, Charlton JR, Tipple TE, Reidy KJ. Preterm birth and neonatal acute kidney injury: implications on adolescent and adult outcomes. *J Perinatol*. 2020;40(9):1286-1295.
159. Fortune PM, Wagstaff M, Petros AJ. Cerebro-splanchnic oxygenation ratio (CSOR) using near infrared spectroscopy may

be able to predict splanchnic ischaemia in neonates. *Intensive Care Med*. 2001;27(8):1401-1407.
160. Bozzetti V, Paterlini G, Meroni V, et al. Evaluation of splanchnic oximetry, Doppler flow velocimetry in the superior mesenteric artery and feeding tolerance in very low birth weight IUGR and non-IUGR infants receiving bolus versus continuous enteral nutrition. *BMC Pediatr*. 2012;12:106.
161. Neu J, Pammi M. Pathogenesis of NEC: impact of an altered intestinal microbiome. *Semin Perinatol*. 2017;41(1):29-35.
162. Escobar GJ. What have we learned from observational studies on neonatal sepsis? *Pediatr Crit Care Med*. 2005;6(suppl 3): S138-S145.
163. Abiramalatha T, Thanigainathan S, Ninan B. Routine monitoring of gastric residual for prevention of necrotising enterocolitis in preterm infants. *Cochrane Database Syst Rev*. 2019;7: CD012937.
164. Cobb BA, Carlo WA, Ambalavanan N. Gastric residuals and their relationship to necrotizing enterocolitis in very low birth weight infants. *Pediatrics*. 2004;113(1 Pt 1):50-53.
165. Elia S, Ciarcià M, Miselli F, Bertini G, Dani C. Effect of selective gastric residual monitoring on enteral intake in preterm infants. *Ital J Pediatr*. 2022;48(1):30.
166. Parker LA, Weaver M, Murgas Torrazza RJ, et al. Effect of gastric residual evaluation on enteral intake in extremely preterm infants: a randomized clinical trial. *JAMA Pediatr*. 2019;173(6):534-543.
167. Mohamed A, Shah PS. Transfusion associated necrotizing enterocolitis: a meta-analysis of observational data. *Pediatrics*. 2012;129(3):529-540.
168. Ozcan B, Aydemir O, Isik DU, Bas AY, Demirel N. Severe anemia is associated with intestinal injury in preterm neonates. *Am J Perinatol*. 2020;37(6):603-606.
169. Patel RM, Knezevic A, Shenvi N, et al. Association of red blood cell transfusion, anemia, and necrotizing enterocolitis in very low-birth-weight infants. *JAMA*. 2016;315(9):889-897.
170. Schelonka RL, Chai MK, Yoder BA, Hensley D, Brockett RM, Ascher DP. Volume of blood required to detect common neonatal pathogens. *J Pediatr*. 1996;129(2):275-278.
171. Cantey JB, Prusakov P. A proposed framework for the clinical management of neonatal "culture-negative" sepsis. *J Pediatr*. 2022;244:203-211.
172. Seymour CW, Liu VX, Iwashyna TJ, et al. Assessment of clinical criteria for sepsis: for the Third International Consensus Definitions for Sepsis and Septic Shock (Sepsis-3). *JAMA*. 2016;315(8):762-774.
173. Wynn JL, Polin RA. A neonatal sequential organ failure assessment score predicts mortality to late-onset sepsis in preterm very low birth weight infants. *Pediatr Res*. 2020;88(1): 85-90.
174. Zeigler AC, Ainsworth JE, Fairchild KD, Wynn JL, Sullivan BA. Sepsis and mortality prediction in very low birth weight infants: analysis of HeRO and nSOFA [published online ahead of print May 10, 2021]. *Am J Perinatol*. Available at: https://doi.org/10.1055/s-0041-1728829.
175. Fleiss N, Coggins SA, Lewis AN, et al. Evaluation of the neonatal sequential organ failure assessment and mortality risk in preterm infants with late-onset infection. *JAMA Netw Open*. 2021;4(2):e2036518.
176. Janota J, Simak J, Stranak Z, Matthews T, Clarke T, Corcoran D. Critically ill newborns with multiple organ dysfunction: assessment by NEOMOD score in a tertiary NICU. *Ir J Med Sci*. 2008;177(1):11-17.
177. Churpek MM, Adhikari R, Edelson DP. The value of vital sign trends for detecting clinical deterioration on the wards. *Resuscitation*. 2016;102:1-5.
178. Braski K, Weaver-Lewis K, Loertscher M, Ding Q, Sheng X, Baserga M. Splanchnic–cerebral oxygenation ratio decreases during enteral feedings in anemic preterm infants: observations under near-infrared spectroscopy. *Neonatology*. 2018;113(1): 75-80.
179. Howarth CN, Leung TS, Banerjee J, Eaton S, Morris JK, Aladangady N. Regional cerebral and splanchnic tissue oxygen saturation in preterm infants – longitudinal normative measurements. *Early Hum Dev*. 2022;165:105540.

SECTION 2

Pharmacology

Chapter 12

Antibiotic Considerations for Necrotizing Enterocolitis

Julie Autmizguine, MD, MHS; Ahmed Moussa, MD, MMed; Joseph Y. Ting, MBBS, MPH

Key Points

- Necrotizing enterocolitis (NEC) results in an intra-abdominal infection, and treatment includes antimicrobial therapy, bowel rest, parenteral nutrition, and surgery, if clinically or radiologically indicated.
- In the absence of evidence-based guidelines, many antibiotic combinations are used for NEC treatment in the current practice.
- Ampicillin and gentamicin are probably adequate for the treatment of stage I or IIA NEC.
- For proven stage IIB or III NEC, antimicrobial treatment may include anaerobic coverage.

Necrotizing enterocolitis (NEC) is a common and devastating disease in infants with an incidence of approximately 1 per 1000 live births.[1] Prematurity is an important risk factor with up to 9% of preterm infants ≤28 weeks' gestational age affected.[2–4] Despite treatment, mortality remains high following NEC.[5] Surviving infants face complications such as failure to thrive, gastrointestinal problems including strictures and adhesions, cholestasis, short bowel syndrome with or without intestinal failure, and neurodevelopmental impairment.[6–9] Spontaneous intestinal bowel perforation, sometimes confused with NEC, is a different clinical entity occurring in the first week of life in preterm infants[10,11] and is not discussed in this chapter. The etiology of NEC is multifactorial, and its treatment includes bowel rest, antibiotics, parenteral nutrition, and, in specific situations, surgery. In this chapter, we discuss the different options for antimicrobial therapy of NEC.

Pathogenesis of NEC

Current evidence suggests that tissue injury results from intestinal inflammation caused by disruption of the gut microbiome and an altered immune response.[12–15] Preterm infants are especially at high risk of dysbiosis given their exposure to antibiotics and their prolonged hospitalization.[13,16,17] Prolonged antibiotic exposure in uninfected preterm infants has been associated with an increased risk of NEC.[18–20] NEC ultimately results in bacterial overgrowth, mimicking a complicated intra-abdominal infection characterized by bowel inflammation with mucosal edema, ulcerations, hemorrhages and coagulation necrosis, localized or diffused peritonitis, and, in some cases, sepsis and bowel perforation.

Clinical Presentation and Diagnosis of NEC

Age of onset is typically inversely proportional to gestational age.[21] Although relatively rare, term and near-term infants usually develop NEC in the first week of life and very preterm infants after the third week of life.[22,23] NEC presents with both digestive and systemic manifestations. Infants generally have abdominal distention and/or tenderness, feeding intolerance, and occult or grossly bloody stools. Nonspecific systemic symptoms include apnea and bradycardia, lethargy, poor perfusion, and respiratory distress. Disease can be mild with only feeding intolerance or sudden and fulminant with multiple organ failure.

Laboratory studies supporting the diagnosis of NEC include abnormal complete blood count with neutropenia or thrombocytopenia, hyponatremia, high C-reactive protein, and metabolic acidosis. Radiological studies are used to confirm the diagnosis of NEC and determine the stage of disease severity according to Bell's criteria (Table 12.1).[24] Plain abdominal radiography may reveal distended, fixed bowel loops, air fluid levels, pneumatosis intestinalis (intramural gas), portal venous gas, or pneumoperitoneum in the case of intestinal perforation. In recent years, data have accumulated regarding the potential benefits of using abdominal ultrasound in the diagnosis and management of NEC.[25]

Although many pathogens have been associated with NEC, no specific microorganism has consistently been linked to this condition. Blood culture is positive in 7% to 30% of cases, and ≤1% of infants with NEC present with an associated meningitis.[28–31] More rarely, *Candida* spp. and viruses (e.g., cytomegalovirus, rotavirus, and norovirus) have also been associated with NEC.[32–34] For most infants with NEC, however, no microorganism is identified, and a polymicrobial infection with endogenous intestinal flora may be assumed. Therefore, antibiotic empirical therapy should be active against enteric Gram-negative aerobic and facultative anaerobic bacilli such as Enterobacteriaceae (e.g., *Escherichia coli*, *Klebsiella* spp.); enteric Gram-positive streptococci (e.g., *Streptococcus anginosus*); and, in some situations, obligate anaerobic bacilli (e.g., *Clostridium perfringens*, *Bacteroides fragilis*).[28–30] *C. perfringens* seems to be associated with more severe and fulminant NEC presentations.[35] However, it is still unclear whether, in general, anaerobic bacteria play a

TABLE 12.1 Modified Bell Staging for Nec

Bell's Stages	Abdominal Signs and Symptoms	Systemic Signs and Symptoms	Radiological Features	Treatment
Stage I, Suspected NEC				
IA	Feeding intolerance, mild abdominal distention, occult blood in stools	Mild systemic symptoms (apnea and bradycardia, temperature instability)	Nonspecific, normal or signs of ileus, mild intestinal dilatation	Close clinical observation NPO Consider antibiotics without anaerobic coverage
IB	Stage IA plus grossly bloody stools			
Stage II, Proven NEC				
IIA, mild IIB, moderate	Prominent abdominal distension, abdominal tenderness and wall edema, grossly bloody stools	Mild systemic symptoms (as stage I) Moderate systemic symptoms (stage I plus thrombocytopenia, metabolic acidosis)	Intestinal dilatation, pneumatosis intestinalis, portal venous gas	Close clinical, laboratory and radiological observation NPO, gastric decompression, intravenous fluids and antibiotics with or without anaerobic coverage
Stage III, Advanced NEC				
IIIA	As for stage II plus signs of peritonitis	Severe systemic symptoms (stage II plus need for mechanical ventilation, hypotension and shock, severe metabolic and respiratory acidosis, disseminated intravascular coagulation)	Stage II plus fixed bowel loops, severe ascites	Same as stage II, including anaerobic coverage Consider surgical intervention
IIIB			Stage IIIB plus pneumoperitoneum	Same as stage III plus exploratory laparotomy and resection of necrotic bowel or peritoneal drainage

NPO, nil per os (nothing by mouth). Adapted from Walsh and Kliegman[26] and Hall et al.[27]

pathogenic or a protective role in the pathogenesis of NEC. Disruption of the intestinal mucosa with subsequent intramural invasion by anaerobic bacteria causes pneumatosis intestinalis.[36] But, anaerobic bacteria are also known to produce short-chain fatty acids potentially regulating the intestinal inflammatory response.[37] Moreover, Gram-negative rods, as opposed to anaerobic bacteria, are predominant in stools of very-low-birth-weight (VLBW) infants (birth weight <1500 g) who have developed NEC compared to those who have not.[17]

Antimicrobial Therapy in the Management of NEC

Infants with NEC should be given bowel rest, medical supportive care with parenteral nutrition, volume expansion, vasopressors, ventilation, and blood product transfusions if needed. The clinical and radiological evolution will determine the need for surgery for the most severe cases.[13] Given the local bacterial overgrowth from the endogenous intestinal flora, management typically includes broad-spectrum antibiotics.

ANTIBIOTIC REGIMENS

To date, studies have failed to demonstrate the optimal antimicrobial treatment for NEC.[31,38,39] The only guideline addressing this issue was published by the Surgical Infection Society and the Infectious Diseases Society of America in 2010. Even though these guidelines mainly discuss the treatment of complicated intra-abdominal infections in adults and older children, they recommend broad-spectrum antibiotics, including ampicillin, gentamicin, and metronidazole, as well as ampicillin, cefotaxime, and metronidazole or meropenem for NEC.[40] They also specify that clindamycin should not be routinely used in older children and adults because of resistance of *Bacteroides fragilis*, but the data in infants with NEC are not sufficient to make similar recommendations. Finally, antifungal therapy should only be added if clinical history is consistent with fungal infection.[40] Due to the lack of an evidence-based guidelines, multiple empiric antibiotic combinations are used for the treatment of NEC in current practice.[31,41,42]

Observational Studies

Several observational retrospective studies comparing antibiotic regimens have been published.[31,41–44] The combination of ampicillin, gentamicin, and metronidazole is the most frequently used regimen.[31,42] Most of the observational studies report similar outcomes regardless of antibiotic regimens, but the majority are single-center studies with limited sample size. Two retrospective studies have observed differences in outcomes. In a comparison of cefotaxime–vancomycin with ampicillin–gentamicin in 90 infants (<2500 g birth weight) with NEC,[44] the cefotaxime–vancomycin regimen was associated with lower mortality and less peritoneal-positive bacterial culture in the more premature infants. This study was limited by its observational design and small sample size. Furthermore, some pathogens isolated were *Staphylococcus* spp., which are not typically involved in the pathogenesis of NEC and are not covered by ampicillin or gentamicin.

The largest study involved a retrospective cohort of 2780 VLBW infants with NEC in which outcomes were compared between those with and without anaerobic antimicrobial therapy on the first day of NEC.[41] Results suggest that, for infants with medical NEC, anaerobic coverage is not associated with lower mortality but is associated with a small increased risk of intestinal strictures (odds ratio [OR] = 1.73; 95% confidence interval [CI], 1.11–2.72; $P = 0.02$). However, among infants with surgical NEC, anaerobic antimicrobial therapy was associated with lower mortality (OR = 0.71; 95% CI, 0.52–0.95; $P = 0.02$). These results suggest that anaerobic coverage is beneficial in cases of severe and perforated (stage III) NEC. Given the retrospective design of this study, the use of anaerobic antimicrobial therapy may have been confounded with symptom severity. Therefore, the higher incidence of strictures observed in infants treated with anaerobic antimicrobial therapy could be explained by more severe disease rather than as a consequence of the antimicrobial treatment.

Randomized Controlled Trials

One randomized controlled trial (RCT) assessed the addition of oral gentamicin to parenteral ampicillin and gentamicin. In this small cohort ($N = 20$), the clinical courses and outcomes were comparable.[45]

A second RCT compared ampicillin–gentamicin to ampicillin–gentamicin–clindamycin for the treatment of NEC in 42 premature infants.[46] This study showed no beneficial effect on mortality or intestinal perforation with the addition of clindamycin to the initial regimen, but it did observe a significantly longer time to successful reinstitution of enteral feeding and a higher incidence of late stricture formation in the clindamycin group (5/15 with clindamycin vs. 1/18 without; $P = 0.02$). Of note, infants were excluded if intestinal perforation occurred <12 hours after randomization, and therefore the results are most comparable to the medical NEC subgroup of infants from the observational study described above.

The largest and most recent randomized controlled trial compared three antibiotic regimens given for ≤10 days: (1) ampicillin–gentamicin–metronidazole, (2) ampicillin–gentamicin–clindamycin, and (3) piperacillin–tazobactam–gentamicin.[38] Randomization occurred within 48 hours after initiation of therapy. The study population ($N = 180$; ≤33 weeks' gestational age at birth) was broader than previous studies, as it included different types of complicated intra-abdominal infections in preterm infants. Stage II or III NEC was the most common diagnosis (59%), but infants with spontaneous intestinal perforation or perforation associated with other intestinal diseases were also included. Due to slow enrollment, eligible infants already receiving study regimens were enrolled without randomization (29% of the cohort). Safety was similar in all treatment groups. More specifically, mortality rates up to 90 days after treatment were 4.22% (95% CI, 1.39–12.13) in the ampicillin–gentamicin–metronidazole group; 4.53% (95% CI, 1.21–15.50) in the ampicillin–gentamicin–clindamycin group; and 4.07 (95% CI, 1.22–12.70) in the piperacillin–tazobactam–gentamicin group, after adjusting for treatment group and gestational age. Intestinal strictures were uncommon, with no difference between treatment groups (5%, 4%, and 6% in the ampicillin–gentamicin–metronidazole, ampicillin–gentamicin–clindamycin, and piperacillin–tazobactam–gentamicin groups, respectively; $P = 0.99$). Although not powered for efficacy, investigators also reported no differences in therapeutic success. Despite some limitations related to the challenges inherent in conducting trials in critically ill premature infants, this important study demonstrated that all three regimens are safe in premature infants with complicated intra-abdominal infection. Unfortunately, this trial did not close the debate over the need to include anaerobic antimicrobial therapy for NEC because all three regimens provided anaerobic coverage.

DURATION OF ANTIBIOTIC TREATMENT

There is no evidence supporting the optimal duration of antimicrobial therapy for NEC. In a single-center retrospective study, infants with medical NEC receiving ampicillin, gentamicin, and metronidazole for ≤10 days versus >10 days had similar outcomes.[31] For a complicated intra-abdominal infection in children and adults, antimicrobial therapy is limited to 4 to 7 days unless there are signs of an uncontrolled infection.[40] As sometimes seen in clinical practice, antimicrobial therapy may be discontinued after 5 to 7 days in stage I or IIA NEC, if symptoms are resolved.[40] If stage II NEC is confirmed, some experts recommend treatment for 7 to 14 days.[13,27] For infants presenting with bacteremia or sepsis, duration of the antimicrobial therapy may be extended to 10 to 14 days. In summary, even in the absence of evidence-based guidelines, experts agree that antimicrobial therapy should last between 5 and 14 days, depending on the evolution.[13,40,27] If an intra-abdominal abscess has been identified, antibiotics should be continued until a clinical and radiological response is established.

Conclusion

In summary, there is insufficient evidence to support one antibiotic regimen over another for the treatment of NEC. Given that broad-spectrum antibiotics (including third-generation cephalosporins and carbapenems) increase the risk for adverse outcomes (invasive candidiasis, increased risk of colonization with antimicrobial-resistant organisms, and microbiota alterations), narrow-spectrum regimens and short-therapy durations are encouraged. Empirical antimicrobial treatment of NEC should be effective against most pathogenic bacteria usually present in the intestinal flora for all infants. For medical NEC, the data are insufficient to recommend anaerobic coverage for all infants because studies have not shown any benefit regarding survival or other clinical outcomes. In infants with Bell stage I, consider parenteral antibiotics such as ampicillin and gentamicin pending cultures and evolution. Weak evidence from one large multicenter retrospective study suggests that anaerobic coverage could reduce mortality in preterm infants with NEC who require surgical treatment (stage III).[41] Although no evidence supports anaerobic coverage for infants with stage II NEC, it may be considered in infants with the most severe forms (stage IIB) who present with moderate systemic symptoms or thrombocytopenia, or metabolic acidosis. Therefore, in infants with Bell stage IIB or III NEC, therapy may include anaerobic coverage with metronidazole or clindamycin in addition to ampicillin–gentamicin or piperacillin–tazobactam as a single agent. Additional coverage with vancomycin or antifungals should only be added based on the patient's microbiologic results and clinical evolution. Clinicians should also consider local resistance rates to guide their antibiotic choice.

REFERENCES

1. Holman RC, Stoll BJ, Curns AT, Yorita KL, Steiner CA, Schonberger LB. Necrotising enterocolitis hospitalisations among neonates in the United States. *Paediatr Perinat Epidemiol*. 2006;20(6):498-506.
2. Bell EF, Hintz SR, Hansen NI, et al. Mortality, in-hospital morbidity, care practices, and 2-year outcomes for extremely preterm infants in the US, 2013–2018. *JAMA*. 2022;327(3):248-263.
3. Qian T, Zhang R, Zhu L, et al. Necrotizing enterocolitis in low birth weight infants in China: mortality risk factors expressed by birth weight categories. *Pediatr Neonatol*. 2017;58(6):509-515.
4. Stoll BJ, Hansen NI, Bell EF, et al. Trends in care practices, morbidity, and mortality of extremely preterm neonates, 1993–2012. *JAMA*. 2015;314(10):1039-1051.
5. Horbar JD, Edwards EM, Greenberg LT, et al. Variation in performance of neonatal intensive care units in the United States. *JAMA Pediatr*. 2017;171(3):e164396.
6. Mondal A, Misra D, Al-Jabir A, Hubail D, Ward T, Patel B. Necrotizing enterocolitis in neonates: has the brain taken a hit 10 years later? *J Pediatr Neurosci*. 2021;16(1):30-34.
7. Humberg A, Spiegler J, Fortmann MI, et al. Surgical necrotizing enterocolitis but not spontaneous intestinal perforation is associated with adverse neurological outcome at school age. *Sci Rep*. 2020;10(1):2373.
8. Matei A, Montalva L, Goodbaum A, Lauriti G, Zani A. Neurodevelopmental impairment in necrotising enterocolitis survivors: systematic review and meta-analysis. *Arch Dis Child Fetal Neonatal Ed*. 2020;105(4):432-439.
9. Federici S, De Biagi L. Long term outcome of infants with NEC. *Curr Pediatr Rev*. 2019;15(2):111-114.
10. Vongbhavit K, Underwood MA. Intestinal perforation in the premature infant. *J Neonatal Perinatal Med*. 2017;10(3):281-289.
11. Meyer CL, Payne NR, Roback SA. Spontaneous, isolated intestinal perforations in neonates with birth weight less than 1,000 g not associated with necrotizing enterocolitis. *J Pediatr Surg*. 1991;26(6):714-717.
12. Bazacliu C, Neu J. Pathophysiology of necrotizing enterocolitis: an update. *Curr Pediatr Rev*. 2019;15(2):68-87.
13. Lin PW, Stoll BJ. Necrotising enterocolitis. *Lancet*. 2006;368(9543):1271-1283.
14. Schnabl KL, Van Aerde JE, Thomson AB, Clandinin MT. Necrotizing enterocolitis: a multifactorial disease with no cure. *World J Gastroenterol*. 2008;14(14):2142-2161.
15. Itani T, Ayoub Moubareck C, Mangin I, Butel MJ, Karam Sarkis D. Individual variations in intestinal microbiota were higher in preterm infants with necrotising enterocolitis than healthy controls. *Acta Paediatr*. 2019;108(12):2294-2295.
16. Torrazza RM, Neu J. The altered gut microbiome and necrotizing enterocolitis. *Clin Perinatol*. 2013;40(1):93-108.
17. Warner BB, Deych E, Zhou Y, et al. Gut bacteria dysbiosis and necrotising enterocolitis in very low birthweight infants: a prospective case-control study. *Lancet*. 2016;387(10031):1928-1936.
18. Kuppala VS, Meinzen-Derr J, Morrow AL, Schibler KR. Prolonged initial empirical antibiotic treatment is associated with adverse outcomes in premature infants. *J Pediatr*. 2011;159(5):720-725.
19. Ting JY, Roberts A, Sherlock R, et al. Duration of initial empirical antibiotic therapy and outcomes in very low birth weight infants. *Pediatrics*. 2019;143(3):e20182286.
20. Esaiassen E, Fjalstad JW, Juvet LK, van den Anker JN, Klingenberg C. Antibiotic exposure in neonates and early adverse outcomes: a systematic review and meta-analysis. *J Antimicrob Chemother*. 2017;72(7):1858-1870.
21. González-Rivera R, Culverhouse RC, Hamvas A, Tarr PI, Warner BB. The age of necrotizing enterocolitis onset: an application of Sartwell's incubation period model. *J Perinatol*. 2011;31(8):519-523.
22. Yee WH, Soraisham AS, Shah VS, Aziz K, Yoon W, Lee SK. Incidence and timing of presentation of necrotizing enterocolitis in preterm infants. *Pediatrics*. 2012;129(2):e298-e304.
23. Gordon PV, Clark R, Swanson JR, Spitzer A. Can a national dataset generate a nomogram for necrotizing enterocolitis onset? *J Perinatol*. 2014;34(10):732-735.
24. Bell MJ, Ternberg JL, Feigin RD, et al. Neonatal necrotizing enterocolitis. Therapeutic decisions based upon clinical staging. *Ann Surg*. 1978;187(1):1-7.
25. Alexander KM, Chan SS, Opfer E, et al. Implementation of bowel ultrasound practice for the diagnosis and management of necrotising enterocolitis. *Arch Dis Child Fetal Neonatal Ed*. 2021;106(1):96-103.
26. Walsh MC, Kliegman RM. Necrotizing enterocolitis: treatment based on staging criteria. *Pediatr Clin North Am*. 1986;33(1):179-201.
27. Hall NJ, Eaton S, Pierro A. Royal Australasia of Surgeons Guest Lecture. Necrotizing enterocolitis: prevention, treatment, and outcome. *J Pediatr Surg*. 2013;48(12):2359-2367.
28. Kliegman RM, Walsh MC. The incidence of meningitis in neonates with necrotizing enterocolitis. *Am J Perinatol*. 1987;4(3):245-248.
29. Chan KL, Saing H, Yung RW, Yeung YP, Tsoi NS. A study of pre-antibiotic bacteriology in 125 patients with necrotizing enterocolitis. *Acta Paediatr Suppl*. 1994;396:45-48.

30. Uauy RD, Fanaroff AA, Korones SB, Phillips EA, Phillips JB, Wright LL. Necrotizing enterocolitis in very low birth weight infants: biodemographic and clinical correlates. National Institute of Child Health and Human Development Neonatal Research Network. *J Pediatr*. 1991;119(4):630-638.
31. Murphy C, Nair J, Wrotniak B, Polischuk E, Islam S. Antibiotic treatments and patient outcomes in necrotizing enterocolitis. *Am J Perinatol*. 2020;37(12):1250-1257.
32. Brook I. Microbiology and management of neonatal necrotizing enterocolitis. *Am J Perinatol*. 2008;25(2):111-118.
33. Parra-Herran CE, Pelaez L, Sola JE, Urbiztondo AK, Rodriguez MM. Intestinal candidiasis: an uncommon cause of necrotizing enterocolitis (NEC) in neonates. *Fetal Pediatr Pathol*. 2010;29(3): 172-180.
34. Rotbart HA, Levin MJ, Yolken RH, Manchester DK, Jantzen J. An outbreak of rotavirus-associated neonatal necrotizing enterocolitis. *J Pediatr*. 1983;103(3):454-459.
35. Dittmar E, Beyer P, Fischer D, et al. Necrotizing enterocolitis of the neonate with *Clostridium perfringens*: diagnosis, clinical course, and role of alpha toxin. *Eur J Pediatr*. 2008;167(8):891-895.
36. Pear BL. Pneumatosis intestinalis: a review. *Radiology*. 1998;207(1): 13-19.
37. Smith PM, Howitt MR, Panikov N, et al. The microbial metabolites, short-chain fatty acids, regulate colonic Treg cell homeostasis. *Science*. 2013;341(6145):569-573.
38. Smith MJ, Boutzoukas A, Autmizguine J, et al. Antibiotic safety and effectiveness in premature infants with complicated intraabdominal infections. *Pediatr Infect Dis J*. 2021;40(6):550-555.
39. Shah D, Sinn JK. Antibiotic regimens for the empirical treatment of newborn infants with necrotising enterocolitis. *Cochrane Database Syst Rev*. 2012;(8):CD007448.
40. Solomkin JS, Mazuski JE, Bradley JS, et al. Diagnosis and management of complicated intra-abdominal infection in adults and children: guidelines by the Surgical Infection Society and the Infectious Diseases Society of America. *Clin Infect Dis*. 2010;50(2):133-164.
41. Autmizguine J, Hornik CP, Benjamin Jr DK, et al. Anaerobic antimicrobial therapy after necrotizing enterocolitis in VLBW infants. *Pediatrics*. 2015;135(1):e117-e125.
42. Blackwood BP, Hunter CJ, Grabowski J. Variability in antibiotic regimens for surgical necrotizing enterocolitis highlights the need for new guidelines. *Surg Infect (Larchmt)*. 2017;18(2):215-220.
43. Luo LJ, Li X, Yang KD, Lu JY, Li LQ. Broad-spectrum antibiotic plus metronidazole may not prevent the deterioration of necrotizing enterocolitis from stage II to III in full-term and near-term infants: a propensity score-matched cohort study. *Medicine (Baltimore)*. 2015;94(42):e1862.
44. Scheifele DW, Ginter GL, Olsen E, Fussell S, Pendray M. Comparison of two antibiotic regimens for neonatal necrotizing enterocolitis. *J Antimicrob Chemother*. 1987;20(3):421-429.
45. Hansen TN, Ritter DA, Speer ME, Kenny JD, Rudolph AJ. A randomized, controlled study of oral gentamicin in the treatment of neonatal necrotizing enterocolitis. *J Pediatr*. 1980;97(5): 836-839.
46. Faix RG, Polley TZ, Grasela TH. A randomized, controlled trial of parenteral clindamycin in neonatal necrotizing enterocolitis. *J Pediatr*. 1988;112(2):271-277.

Chapter 13

Antiseizure Medications and Treatments in Neonates

Amanda G. Sandoval Karamian, MD; Courtney J. Wusthoff, MD, MS

Key Points

- Initial/emergent management of neonatal seizures includes stabilization of the neonate, assessment and correction of reversible causes of seizures, and evaluation for sepsis/meningitis at the same time as antiseizure medications (ASMs) are initiated.
- Despite limited efficacy data and concern for adverse effects, phenobarbital remains the first-line treatment for most neonatal seizures.
- Limited evidence supports phenytoin, benzodiazepines, lidocaine, and levetiracetam as second- or third-line agents.
- Other third-line agents may also be used for refractory seizures, but there is limited evidence regarding their safety and efficacy.
- Empiric pyridoxine, pyridoxal 5′-phosphate (PLP), and folinic acid trials should be considered in neonates with seizures refractory to therapy with multiple ASMs while diagnostic biochemical and genetic testing is performed.

Introduction

GOALS OF THERAPY

Untreated neonatal seizures have been shown to cause neuronal apoptosis and are associated with poor neurodevelopmental outcomes in both animal and human studies.[1–5] Although controversy remains regarding the degree to which seizure treatment might affect outcomes, most providers attempt to control neonatal seizures with the use of antiseizure medications (ASMs). As such, the overarching goal of treatment is usually to minimize the acute seizure burden for the neonate. At the same time, different providers and specific clinical scenarios may warrant a distinct consideration of the potential benefits of seizure treatment against the potential risks. When selecting ASMs, it is helpful to be explicit about the goals of therapy for each individual case.

The majority of neonatal seizures are acute symptomatic seizures.[1] That is, they are symptomatic of acute brain injury such as hypoxic–ischemic encephalopathy (HIE) or stroke. Animal models and observational studies suggest that increased seizure burden in the setting of acute neonatal brain injury is associated with worsened outcomes.[2–4] For this reason, when treating acute symptomatic seizures, the initial goal of treatment is typically resolution of all seizures. Of note, this includes both clinical seizures and subclinical (electrographic-only) seizures. Over 85% of neonatal seizures are subclinical, with no outward clinical signs visible.[6] Subclinical seizures can only be identified through the use of electroencephalography (EEG). As such, continuous electroencephalography (cEEG) is required for accurate diagnosis of neonatal seizures.[6–8] The updated neonatal seizure classification from the International League Against Epilepsy (ILAE) emphasizes the key role of EEG in the diagnosis of neonatal seizures and recommends EEG as the first step in the evaluation of a critically ill neonate at risk for or with clinically suspected seizures.[9] If cEEG is not available, amplitude-integrated electroencephalography (aEEG) may be used, although aEEG is known to have lower sensitivity and specificity compared with cEEG. With treatment for neonatal seizures, about half of neonates will have electroclinical dissociation, meaning outward signs might resolve even as EEG seizures continue.[10] cEEG monitoring is therefore particularly important after initiating treatment to accurately evaluate response as treatment is continued and to target complete resolution of seizures.

In contrast, approximately 20% of neonatal seizures are symptomatic of underlying brain malformation or neonatal-onset epilepsy, meaning ongoing seizures are expected. In these cases, the goal of treatment is more likely to reduce the seizure burden as much as possible using oral agents, but with the knowledge that some breakthrough seizures may continue. cEEG may be useful in these cases to clarify which clinical events are true seizures with an electrographic correlate.

In rare cases, such as when palliative care has been selected, the goal of treatment might be only suppression of clinical seizures to maximize patient and parental comfort. In these cases, EEG is not necessary. The main consideration is efficacy of the ASM for the outward control of symptoms.

Regardless, it is essential to establish and communicate the goals of treatment for each neonate with seizures when initiating therapy. Treatment choices are heavily influenced by a shared understanding of the goal of treatment (e.g., complete resolution of seizures, seizure control as best as possible with oral agents, suppression of clinical seizures). These goals may be revisited throughout the course of treatment, and, as goals are revised, good communication is essential.

OVERVIEW OF THERAPY

In any case of suspected neonatal seizures, the first steps in management are securing and maintaining the infant's airway, confirming adequate ventilation, and ensuring adequate circulation and perfusion. cEEG should be placed as soon as possible after the infant is stabilized and can be placed concurrently with subsequent steps in evaluation and treatment. Interventions should not be delayed for EEG placement. The next step in acute management is to assess for reversible causes of seizure, including hypocalcemia, hypoglycemia, and hypomagnesemia. Serum concentrations of electrolytes and glucose should be rapidly obtained and any electrolyte abnormalities or hypoglycemia corrected. Infants should also be evaluated for infectious causes of seizures, such as meningitis and sepsis, with appropriate antimicrobial therapy initiated. If seizures are highly suspected clinically or are confirmed on EEG, a loading dose of an ASM should be given as soon as possible. See Table 13.1 for dosing guidelines and Figure 13.1 for a suggested treatment algorithm.

TABLE 13.1 Antiseizure Medication Dosing and Serum Levels

ASM	Loading Dose	Maintenance Dosing	Target Serum Level
Phenobarbital	20 mg/kg IV; may give additional doses of 10 mg/kg up to 40 mg/kg total	5 mg/kg/day divided into one to two doses	Obtain level 1–2 hr after loading dose; target range 20–40 µg/mL
Phenytoin/ fosphenytoin	15–20 mg PE/kg IV; may give additional 10 mg PE/kg once	3–5 mg/kg/day divided into two to four doses	Obtain level 1 hr after loading dose; target level 10–20 µg/mL total or 1–2 µg/mL free phenytoin
Midazolam	0.05 mg/kg IV over 10 min	Continuous infusion of 0.15 mg/kg/hr; may increase stepwise by 0.05 mg/kg/hr up to maximum of 0.5 mg/kg/hr	No established drug-level monitoring
Lorazepam	0.05–0.1 mg/kg IV given over 2–5 min; may repeat up to total dose of 0.15 mg/kg	—	—
Clonazepam	0.01 mg/kg IV	0.01 mg/kg/dose for 3–5 doses	—
Levetiracetam	20–50 mg/kg IV	30–50 mg/kg/day divided into two doses	No established drug-level monitoring
Topiramate	5–10 mg/kg enteral	1–5 mg/kg/day	5–20 µg/mL in adults; not established in neonates

Please see Table 13.2 for lidocaine dosing.

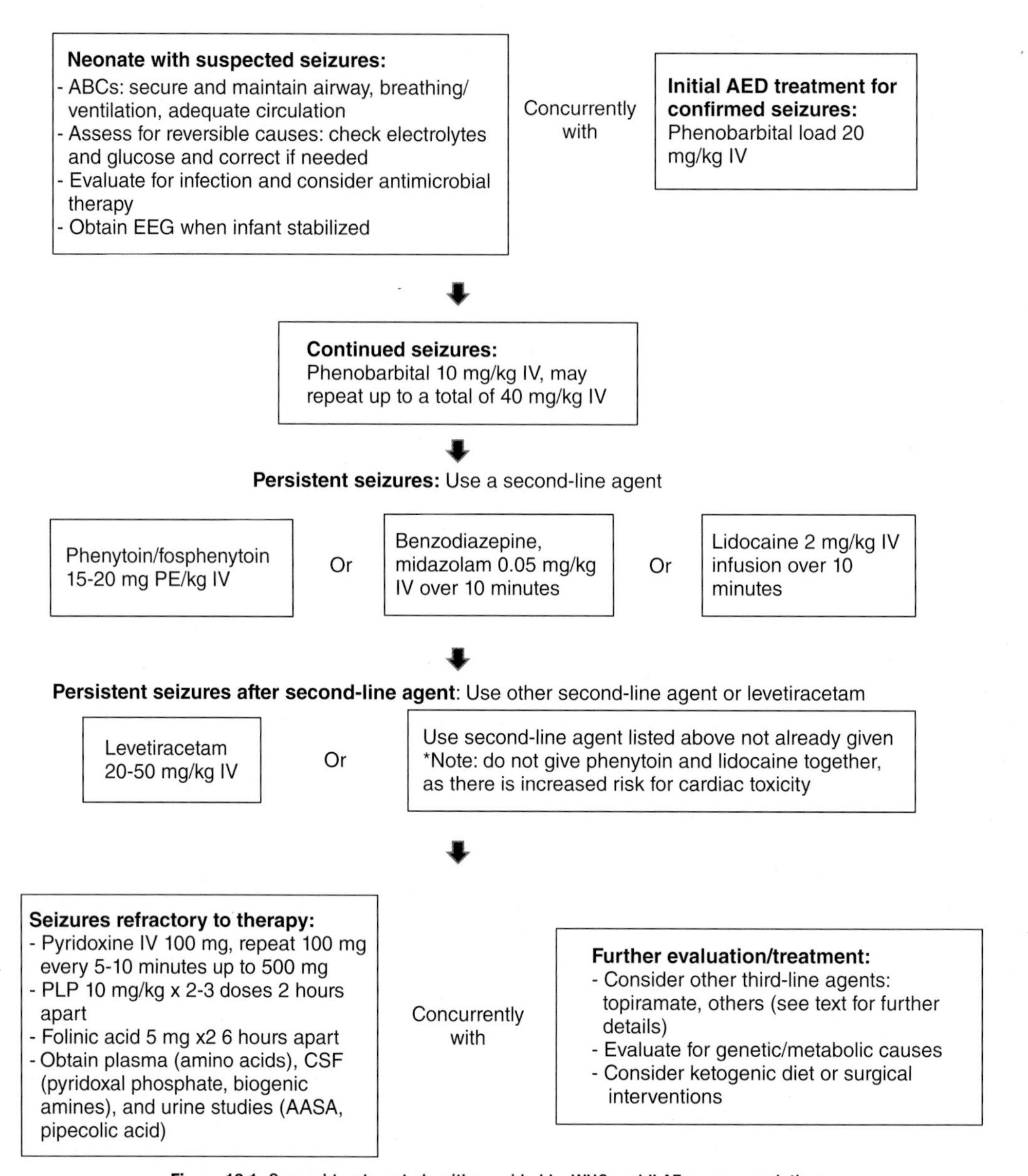

Figure 13.1 General treatment algorithm guided by WHO and ILAE recommendations.

Current ILAE and World Health Organization (WHO) recommendations and expert consensus support phenobarbital as the first-line agent for the treatment of neonatal seizures.[8] Seizures unresponsive or only partially responsive to phenobarbital should be treated with an additional second-line agent: phenytoin, benzodiazepines, or lidocaine.[8] Although not yet included in official guidelines, levetiracetam is increasingly popular as a second-line agent, as well. No clear guidelines exist for third-line treatment, other than use of second-line agents already noted. Choice of a third-line agent is largely dependent on clinician and institutional preference. In neonates with seizures refractory to adequate doses of multiple ASMs and when there is no clear etiology for seizures identified, vitamin-responsive epileptic encephalopathies should be considered. Trials of pyridoxine, pyridoxal 5′-phosphate (PLP), and folinic acid should be performed. Evaluation for specific genetic and metabolic causes of neonatal seizures should also be performed, with consideration of the ketogenic diet in select cases. Neuroimaging should be obtained to evaluate for acute causes of seizure and structural abnormalities as soon as possible; magnetic resonance imaging is the preferred imaging modality.[11,12] Identification of the underlying cause of seizures can be helpful in guiding the choice of treatment and informing the duration of anticipated treatment.

Antiseizure Medications

PHENOBARBITAL

Phenobarbital, although an older ASM, remains the mainstay of treatment for neonatal seizures. The 2011 WHO guidelines on neonatal seizures designate phenobarbital as a first-line treatment.[8] Similarly, surveys of child neurologists and neonatologists confirm that phenobarbital remains the first-choice medication for most physicians treating neonatal seizures.[13–16] This is largely because phenobarbital has the largest evidence base, with the most animal model data and greatest clinical experience.[17–22]

Mechanism of Action

Phenobarbital is a barbiturate, which acts as an agonist at the gamma-aminobutyric acid type A (GABA-A) receptor to enhance inhibitory neurotransmission. Phenobarbital binding to the GABA-A receptor triggers opening of the postsynaptic chloride ion channel, which in mature neurons results in chloride entering the cell, hyperpolarizing the cell, and thus reducing excitability (see Figure 13.2A). In immature neurons, however, there is age-specific increased expression of a specific sodium–potassium–chloride cotransporter, NKCC1, that causes immature neurons to have much higher intracellular chloride levels than exist in mature neurons. Due to this high intracellular concentration of chloride in an immature neuron, when the GABA-A receptor is activated to open the chloride ion channel, there is not an influx of chloride. There may be little change, or even an outflow of chloride, with resulting depolarization (excitation). This correlates with the clinical finding that phenobarbital is incompletely effective for controlling neonatal seizures.[23] Ongoing research investigates whether adjunctive agents might enhance the efficacy of phenobarbital by manipulating chloride concentrations (see later discussion of bumetanide). It has also been proposed that phenobarbital reduces excitatory neurotransmission

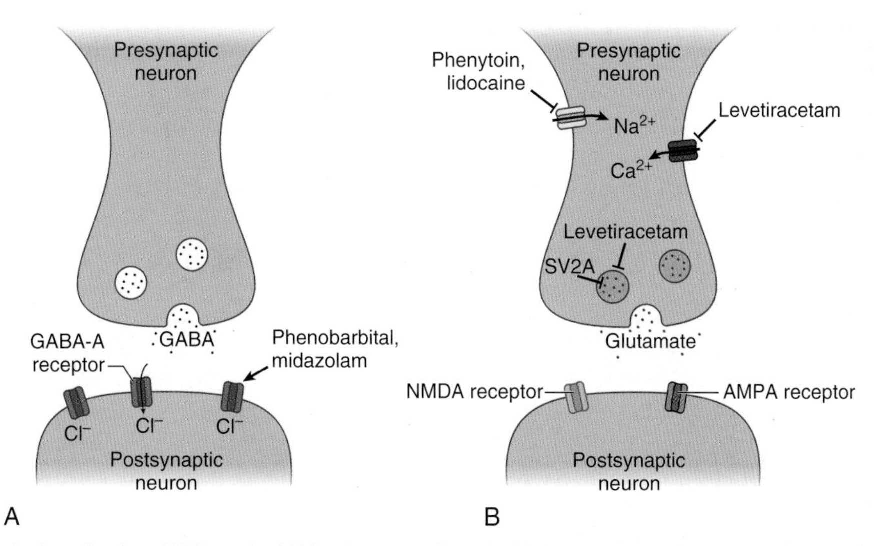

Figure 13.2 (A) Mechanism of action of ASMs at the GABAergic synapse. Phenobarbital and midazolam both act via the GABA-A receptor to open postsynaptic chloride channels. (B) Mechanism of action of ASMs at the glutamatergic synapse. Phenytoin/fosphenytoin and lidocaine both inhibit presynaptic voltage-gated sodium channels. Levetiracetam blocks presynaptic glutamate release via synaptic vesicle protein 2A and inhibits presynaptic calcium channels to prevent calcium influx into the neuron.

across the glutamatergic synapse through action on the alpha-amino-3-hydroxy-5-methyl-4-isoxazolepropionic acid (AMPA)/kainite glutamate receptor (see Figure 13.2B).[20]

Efficacy

Despite extensive clinical use, there is a paucity of high-grade clinical evidence supporting the efficacy of phenobarbital. The first published randomized trial of phenobarbital for the treatment of neonatal seizures was conducted by Painter and colleagues in 1999.[24] This study included 59 neonates with acute seizures confirmed on EEG. The majority had identified acute causes of seizure, such as HIE or stroke. Subjects were randomized to receive either phenobarbital first or phenytoin first. If seizures continued, the other drug was added. Among neonates receiving phenobarbital first, only 43% had control of seizures (vs. 45% response rate with phenytoin). With the addition of phenytoin, this increased to 57%. Subsequent retrospective and small prospective studies have similarly reported that phenobarbital monotherapy provides seizure control rates of 43% to 63%.[25–27] Consistent across these studies has been lower efficacy in neonates with significantly abnormal background EEG[25,28] or with worse initial seizure burden.[24] A second randomized trial was published in 2020 comparing levetiracetam to phenobarbital for neonatal seizure treatment.[29] Eighty-three neonates with seizures were randomized and received either levetiracetam 40 mg/kg or phenobarbital 20 mg/kg as first-line therapy, with an additional 20 mg/kg of levetiracetam or 20 mg/kg of phenobarbital if seizures continued. The other medication was given as second-line therapy if seizures were not controlled. After the first dose, seizures stopped in 70% of those treated with phenobarbital versus 21% in the levetiracetam group. This increased to 80% for phenobarbital and 28% for levetiracetam after the second dose. The efficacy of phenobarbital as the second-line medication was 54%, and the efficacy of levetiracetam was 17%. Phenobarbital (20–40 mg/kg) was significantly more efficacious than levetiracetam (40–60 mg/kg) in this study.[29]

Of note, evidence suggests that phenobarbital should only be used for treatment of existing seizures and not for prophylaxis before seizures in neonates with encephalopathy.[30] A *Cochrane Review* found that, although prophylactic phenobarbital did reduce the risk of seizures for neonates with perinatal asphyxia, there was no reduction in mortality and no data to suggest improved long-term outcomes.[31] Similarly, prophylactic phenobarbital does not enhance the efficacy of hypothermia in limiting brain injury from HIE.[32]

Dosing

Initial phenobarbital treatment for confirmed seizures is a loading dose of 20 mg/kg intravenous (IV). After the initial load, neonates are typically started on short-term maintenance therapy of 5 mg/kg/day, divided into either twice-daily doses or as one daily dose.[17,18,20,33] The recommended loading dose is the same in the setting of therapeutic hypothermia.[33] If seizures do not subside on EEG after the initial 20-mg/kg loading dose, additional doses of 10 mg/kg can be given up to a total load of 40 mg/kg.[17,27] A phenobarbital level should be checked 1 to 2 hours after the loading dose is given, with a target level of 20 to 40 μg/mL.[17,18,24] Some patients may require levels up to 60 μg/mL to achieve seizure control,[34] although increased sedation is noted with levels >50 μg/mL.[18]

The half-life of phenobarbital varies widely with postnatal age, especially when given orally. In the first 10 days of life, there is delayed and incomplete absorption of phenobarbital from the gastrointestinal tract and the half-life is typically long, with increasing clearance in days 11 to 30 and 31 to 70.[34,35] Therefore, neonates may require increasing doses to achieve the same therapeutic effect after the first few weeks of life.

Metabolism of phenobarbital is inhibited by several drugs, including phenytoin. These medications may increase serum phenobarbital concentrations.[35] There are conflicting reports in the current literature regarding the effect of hypothermia on phenobarbital clearance. Shellhaas et al.[36] found that therapeutic hypothermia did not influence clearance of phenobarbital in a study of 39 infants with seizures undergoing cooling for hypoxic ischemic encephalopathy. A small single-center study of 19 neonates, however,[33] found that hypothermic infants had higher plasma concentrations and longer half-lives of phenobarbital compared with their normothermic counterparts.

Adverse Effects, Contraindications, and Monitoring

The most commonly encountered side effects with phenobarbital use are sedation and respiratory depression.[18,34,35] Other potential adverse effects include hypotension, skin rash, hepatotoxicity, and blood dyscrasia.[34] A large retrospective study showed an association between increased neonatal exposure to phenobarbital and worse neurodevelopmental outcomes. This included cognitive and motor scores on the Bayley Scales of Infant and Toddler Development (8- and 9-point decrease per 100 mg/kg cumulative dose) and increased rates of cerebral palsy (2.3-fold increase per 100 mg/kg phenobarbital).[4] This is in keeping with the body of animal evidence demonstrating increased neuronal apoptosis, altered synaptic development, and long-term behavioral changes with early phenobarbital use.[2,37,38] Thus, although phenobarbital remains commonly used, there are concerns regarding overuse and adverse neurodevelopmental effects and an urgent need for alternative drugs.

PHENYTOIN/FOSPHENYTOIN

Phenytoin/fosphenytoin is a common second-line agent for the treatment of neonatal seizures.[14,39] A recent systematic review demonstrated that there is no strong evidence that phenytoin is superior or inferior to the alternative second-line ASMs levetiracetam or lidocaine.[17] WHO guidelines on the treatment of neonatal seizures also recommend phenytoin as a second-line treatment after phenobarbital, along with consideration of a benzodiazepine or lidocaine.[8] A 2009 survey of European neonatologists found that phenytoin was most commonly used as a third-line treatment after benzodiazepines.[15]

Mechanism of Action

Phenytoin primarily acts at the glutamatergic synapse by inhibiting voltage-gated sodium channels (see Figure 13.2B). In doing so, phenytoin prevents depolarization of the presynaptic neuron, which in turn inhibits excitatory neurotransmission at the glutamatergic synapse.[20] Fosphenytoin is a phosphate ester prodrug of phenytoin that can be given parenterally and is associated with fewer infusion-related adverse effects, but it is more expensive.[15]

Efficacy

In the only randomized controlled trial of phenytoin versus phenobarbital for first-line treatment of neonatal seizures, phenytoin had a response rate of 45% with complete seizure cessation, similar to phenobarbital.[24] In a later study, among neonates with seizures refractory to phenobarbital, phenytoin achieved seizure control in 16%.[40] There have been specific reports of the efficacy of phenytoin in treating neonatal-onset encephalopathies, including *SCN2A* and *KCNQ2* encephalopathy.[41,42] Further work is needed to clarify whether phenytoin has superior efficacy compared with other agents for these diseases.

Dosing

The typical loading dose of phenytoin is 15 to 20 mg/kg IV.[17,22] Of note, fosphenytoin is typically dosed in phenytoin equivalents (PEs); thus, a dose of 20 mg/kg phenytoin is equivalent to fosphenytoin 20 mg PE/kg. Neonates receiving phenytoin must have cardiac monitoring during infusion therapy per current WHO guidelines, and the infusion rates should not exceed 1 to 3 mg/kg/min for phenytoin or 2 mg/kg/min for fosphenytoin, given the risk for arrhythmia and/or bradycardia, especially with rapid infusions of phenytoin.[8] An additional 10-mg/kg load may be considered if seizures persist.[22] Further repeat doses are to be avoided due to the risks of toxicity with higher serum levels. Phenytoin levels should be obtained 1 hour after the loading dose is given,[17] with the goal range being 10 to 20 μg/mL.[35] Increasing adverse effects are seen at concentrations >30 μg/mL.[35] Because phenytoin is albumin bound, in patients with abnormal albumin levels a free phenytoin level may be more reliable. A therapeutic range for free phenytoin is typically 1 to 2 μg/mL.

Maintenance dosing is typically 3 to 5 mg/kg/day divided two to four times daily.[17,22] However, because of rapid hepatic metabolism in the neonate, it can be challenging to maintain therapeutic phenytoin levels even with four-times-daily dosing. Thus, dosing is frequently adjusted to target a blood level in the goal range and is rarely continued beyond the acute period.

Adverse Effects, Contraindications, and Monitoring

There are several drug–drug interactions to consider when using phenytoin. Acutely, the most important is avoidance of phenytoin when lidocaine has recently been given, as these drugs have a similar mechanism of action and combined have a much increased risk for cardiovascular effects. When considering chronic use, aluminum-, magnesium-, or calcium-containing antacids reduce the absorption of phenytoin, and valproic acid displaces phenytoin from albumin-binding sites and inhibits its metabolism.[35] Phenobarbital and carbamazepine may also have variable effects on the serum concentration of phenytoin.[35]

Several adverse effects have been seen with phenytoin use in neonates and older children. In the trial by Painter and colleagues,[24] there were no significant adverse effects, and no changes in heart rate, heart rhythm, or respiratory status were observed. However, phenytoin has been described as causing arrhythmias, hypotension, and hepatotoxicity.[34,43,44] Soft-tissue injury from extravasation of phenytoin has also been described, with the development of blue discoloration and blistering noted.[34,45,46] All of these effects are less severe with fosphenytoin versus phenytoin.[22,34,46] One case report in a 1-month-old infant described ileus at toxic phenytoin levels (serum concentration 91.8 μg/mL).[47]

The long-term risks of phenytoin administration are less clear. Similar to effects seen with phenobarbital, phenytoin has been demonstrated to cause neuronal apoptosis in the developing white matter of rat pups.[2] Widespread dose-dependent neurodegeneration has been demonstrated in rat pups, with a threshold dose of 20 mg/kg.[38] Specific effects on the cerebellum have also been studied, with cerebellar cells and motor coordination deficits seen in rat pups exposed to phenytoin.[48] Further study is needed to determine whether these animal studies translate to clinical deficits in humans.

LIDOCAINE

Lidocaine is widely used as a second- or third-line agent for neonatal seizures in Europe, though it is less often used in North America. In a survey of European neonatologists, providers from all hospitals except one reported using lidocaine as the third-line treatment for refractory neonatal seizures, after phenobarbital and benzodiazepines.[15] The 2011 WHO guidelines include lidocaine as a second-line agent, along with phenytoin or benzodiazepines, for neonatal seizures that do not respond to initial treatment with phenobarbital.[8] There is no high-quality evidence to clearly support the efficacy of any one of the second-line therapies over the others.[17]

Mechanism of Action

An amine derivative of cocaine, lidocaine has many applications, including use as an anesthetic, sedative, antiarrhythmic, and anticonvulsant.[49] As an ASM, lidocaine reduces excitatory neurotransmission at the glutamatergic synapse (see Figure 13.2B). It does so by inhibiting voltage-gated sodium channels, in turn preventing depolarization of the presynaptic neuron.[20]

Efficacy

There have been no randomized, controlled trials to demonstrate the efficacy of lidocaine, although other evidence supports its use. Variable response rates have been reported for lidocaine, ranging from 53% to 76%,[26,50–52] with a particularly high seizure control rate of 91% reported in one small series of hypothermic infants receiving lidocaine as add-on therapy.[53] In a large retrospective study of 413 term and preterm infants, 71% had "good" (no seizures for >4 hours, no need for rescue medication) or "intermediate" (no seizures for 0–2 hours, but rescue medication needed after 2–4 hours) response to lidocaine.[54] Lidocaine response rates may vary based on gestational age, as one study reported seizure control in 76% of full-term neonates versus only 55% of preterm neonates.[55] Limited evidence suggests that lidocaine may be more efficacious than midazolam, but larger prospective studies are needed to confirm these findings.[51,55]

Dosing

Lidocaine is primarily metabolized by hepatic cytochrome P450 into two bioactive anticonvulsant metabolites that are renally excreted; thus, lidocaine elimination involves both hepatic and renal clearance.[49,56] It has a short half-life of 90 to 100 minutes and therefore is typically given as a continuous infusion.[56] Acceptable dosing regimens vary. Most begin with a loading dose of 2 mg/kg IV over 10 minutes, followed by a maintenance infusion of 2 to 6 mg/kg/hr titrated to seizure control; it is then typically continued for 12 to 24 hours and then rapidly weaned off for a total infusion duration of <48 hours.[15] A loading dose of 2 mg/kg IV over 10 minutes is used for neonates regardless of gestational age, birth weight, or cooling status.[19] The most commonly used maintenance regimen consists of an infusion over a total of 30 hours, with an initial infusion rate of 6 mg/kg/hr for 6 hours, followed by a reduction to 4 mg/kg/hr for 12 hours, and then another reduction to 2 mg/kg/hr for 12 hours, for a total dosage of 110 mg/kg.[52,55]

TABLE 13.2 **Lidocaine Dosing**

	Loading Dose	First Infusion	Second Infusion	Third Infusion
General dosing[54]	2 mg/kg IV, given over 10 min	6 mg/kg/hr for 6 hr	4 mg/kg/hr for 12 hr	2 mg/kg/hr for 12 hr
Birth weights 0.8–1.5 kg[48]		5 mg/kg/hr for 4 hr	2.5 mg/kg/hr for 6 hr	1.25 mg/kg/hr for 12 hr
Birth weights 1.6–2.5 kg[48]		6 mg/kg/hr for 4 hr	3 mg/kg/hr for 6 hr	1.5 mg/kg/hr for 12 hr
Birth weights 2.6–4.5 kg[48]		7 mg/kg/hr for 4 hr	3.5 mg/kg/hr for 6 hr	1.75 mg/kg/hr for 12 hr
Hypothermia, birth weights 2.0–2.5 kg[52]		6 mg/kg/hr for 3.5 hr	3 mg/kg/hr for 12 hr	1.5 mg/kg/hr for 12 hr
Hypothermia, birth weights 2.5–4.5 kg[52]		7 mg/kg/hr for 3.5 hr	3.5 mg/kg/hr for 12 hr	1.75 mg/kg/hr for 12 hr

Care must be used when setting or adjusting lidocaine infusion rates, as some protocols list rates as mg/min, whereas others list them as mg/kg/hr or mg/hr.

Preterm neonates have a lower clearance of lidocaine.[49,57] A proposed weight-adjusted regimen for low-birth-weight and very-low-birth-weight neonates was developed to avoid supratherapeutic lidocaine levels in these patients; several variations of this regimen have been described.[19] In one pharmacokinetic study, therapeutic hypothermia reduced the clearance of lidocaine in neonates by 24% compared with historic normothermic controls; therefore, a decreased dosing regimen was proposed for this population, as well.[53] See Table 13.2 for further details.

Adverse Effects, Contraindications, and Monitoring

Lidocaine levels can be checked after completion of the initial infusion dose, with a goal concentration of 6 to 7 μg/mL.[49] A practical limitation of this is that lidocaine is typically used for <48 hours, so results of level checks may not return in sufficient time to be relevant for treatment decisions. When levels are rapidly available, plasma concentrations of >9 μg/mL should be avoided, given the increased risk for adverse effects. Because of the risk for arrhythmias, neonates treated with lidocaine require continuous cardiac monitoring throughout infusion.[8,58]

The adverse effect of most concern with lidocaine is cardiac toxicity, including bradycardia, ventricular tachycardia, prolonged QRS complex, and irregular heart rate.[20,52,58] There is increased risk of cardiac effects with plasma concentrations of >9 μg/mL and after use of other cardiotoxic agents, including phenytoin.[20] For this reason, lidocaine should be avoided in neonates with congenital heart disease and infants who have received phenytoin in the preceding 24 hours.[19,34] Rates of cardiotoxicity range from 0% to 5% across multiple studies.[50,53,58] A large retrospective study reported a cardiac event rate of 1.3% to 1.9% in term and preterm neonates due to lidocaine; however, this rate was only 0.4% with appropriately dosed regimens.[55] The common practice of limiting lidocaine use to <48 hours is based on hopes of limiting the accumulation of lidocaine and its metabolites to limit the risk for cardiotoxicity.[52]

Paradoxically, lidocaine has proconvulsant activity at higher concentrations, although this mechanism is not well understood.[52,56] Several case reports describe seizure after lidocaine administration for circumcision in otherwise healthy neonates.[59,60] It has been speculated that these cases may reflect inadvertent intravenous administration instead of local administration of lidocaine at anesthetic doses. At the doses used for neonatal seizure treatment, however, there is no evidence of a proconvulsant effect. When appropriately dosed and monitored, lidocaine can provide good efficacy for treatment of seizures in cases where phenobarbital has failed to provide complete seizure control.

BENZODIAZEPINES

Benzodiazepines, including midazolam, lorazepam, and clonazepam, are a second- or third-line treatment option for neonatal seizures. In a survey of European neonatologists, 85% reported use of midazolam as their second-line treatment for neonatal seizures after phenobarbital.[15] In an international survey of primarily American neurologists and neonatologists, lorazepam was the first treatment choice of 22% for preterm neonates and 23% for term neonates.[16] When asked about using lorazepam as a second- or third-line treatment, 27% endorsed use in preterm neonates and 26% endorsed use in term neonates.[16] Midazolam was used as a first-line therapy by 3% of providers in term or preterm infants and was used as a second- or third-line treatment by 24% for preterm and 25% for term infants.[16] The 2011 WHO guidelines include benzodiazepines as second-line agents, along with phenytoin or lidocaine, for neonatal seizures that do not respond to initial treatment with phenobarbital.[8] Given the potential effects of sedation and respiratory depression, some authors recommend this class of medications as second- or third-line therapy and use it primarily in already-intubated neonates.[17]

Mechanism of Action

Benzodiazepines act on the postsynaptic side of the GABAergic synapse, modulating the chloride channel in the GABA-A receptor to increase inhibitory neurotransmission (see Figure 13.2A).[20] It has been proposed that, because midazolam is more lipophilic than lorazepam, midazolam crosses the blood–brain barrier more easily and has a more rapid onset of action.[18]

Efficacy

As with many other ASMs discussed here, a variable response to treatment has been observed with benzodiazepines, and high-quality evidence for efficacy is lacking. A very small study randomized neonates to benzodiazepines or lidocaine as second-line treatment after phenobarbital failure; this study found no effect on seizure burden with midazolam (three neonates) or clonazepam (three neonates).[26] In contrast, in a study with eight neonates receiving midazolam, 50% had a partial response.[51] Other series have reported higher rates of seizure control ranging from 67% to 100%.[27,61–63] In two small studies of lorazepam, there was good to immediate response in 86% to 100% after treatment; however, both studies suffered from small sample size, with only seven patients each, and inconsistent use of EEG to confirm electrographic seizure activity.[64,65]

Dosing

Midazolam is primarily metabolized by cytochrome P450 enzymes in the liver, relying on hepatic clearance.[61] Typical midazolam dosing is a load of 0.05 mg/kg given intravenously over 10 minutes, followed by a continuous infusion of 0.15 mg/kg/hr to a maximum of 0.5 mg/kg/hr, increasing stepwise by 0.05 mg/kg/hr as needed for seizure control.[18,19,61,66] Clonazepam may be given as a 0.01-mg/kg intravenous loading dose followed by a 0.01-mg/kg/dose for an additional three to five doses if needed.[18] Lorazepam is typically given only as a loading dose of 0.05 to 0.1 mg/kg IV over 2 to 5 minutes, with no maintenance regimen.[18,19,22,64,65] The loading dose may be repeated up to a total dose 0.15 mg/kg if needed.[18,19,65] Therapeutic hypothermia does not appear to affect the pharmacokinetics of midazolam; however, concomitant use of inotropes decreases midazolam clearance by 33%.[66]

Adverse Effects, Contraindications, and Monitoring

Potential adverse effects with benzodiazepines include hypotension, sedation, and respiratory depression, although some studies report no significant adverse effects within their cohorts.[27,64,65] Reported rates of hypotension vary widely, with as many as 33% to 38% of neonates treated with midazolam requiring inotropic support for hypotension in two small studies.[63,67] An inverse relationship between midazolam plasma concentration and mean arterial blood pressure was described in a prospective pharmacokinetic study of midazolam.[66] Lower rates were reported in a review of midazolam and lorazepam for both sedation and seizure control in neonates, with hypotension in only 8% and respiratory depression in 5%.[68] Midazolam may cause less respiratory depression and sedation than lorazepam because it is relatively faster acting.[22] The potential for adverse effects is greater when benzodiazepines are used in combination or when benzodiazepines are used in combination with barbiturates.

Of note, a retrospective study reported better neurodevelopmental outcomes at 1 year of life in infants treated with midazolam compared with infants who did not respond to treatment with phenobarbital/

phenytoin.[27] This, however, may be more reflective of the damage caused by untreated seizures in neonates with improved neurodevelopmental outcomes in infants with better seizure control, rather than a specific benefit of midazolam. Of the benzodiazepines used for neonatal seizures, the largest body of evidence exists for midazolam; however, more studies are needed to evaluate its safety and efficacy in this population.

LEVETIRACETAM

Levetiracetam is an increasingly common second- or third-line treatment for neonatal seizures. It has been approved by the U.S. Food and Drug Administration for children as young as 1 month.[17] Its use for treating seizures of various etiologies has been described in term and preterm infants, including some as immature as 23 weeks' gestational age, without significant adverse effects.[69–71] Because of this lack of significant adverse effects, levetiracetam is increasingly popular. In a 2007 survey of child neurologists, 47% reported using levetiracetam as second- or third-line treatment for neonatal seizures.[72] Though there is no evidence-based recommendation by the ILAE regarding use of any current agent used to treat neonatal seizures, they acknowledge that there is evidence to support levetiracetam as a therapy for seizures in older infants.[73] Levetiracetam is not, however, currently included in the WHO guidelines for treatment of neonatal seizures.[8,74]

Mechanism of Action

Levetiracetam inhibits excitatory neurotransmission at the glutamatergic synapse through inhibition of N-type calcium channels on the presynaptic neuron (see Figure 13.2B). This prevents the influx of calcium into the cell, which in turn blocks exocytosis of intracellular vesicles containing glutamate.[20] Levetiracetam additionally prevents the release of glutamate from intracellular vesicles through modulation of synaptic vesicle protein 2A.[20,56,74,75]

Efficacy

One randomized trial has compared levetiracetam to phenobarbital for neonatal seizure treatment.[29] In this trial, published in 2020, Sharpe et al.[29] demonstrated seizure cessation in 21% of neonates treated with 40 mg/kg of levetiracetam as first-line therapy, increasing to 28% after an additional 20 mg/kg. The efficacy of levetiracetam for seizure cessation as a second-line medication after phenobarbital was 17%. Although phenobarbital (20–40 mg/kg) was significantly more efficacious than levetiracetam (40–60 mg/kg) in this study, there were more adverse events in the phenobarbital group in the short term.[29]

Additional limited evidence for the efficacy of levetiracetam is available from other types of studies. In one retrospective cohort of 23 neonates treated with levetiracetam, 35% had a reduction in seizures of >50% within 24 hours, with an additional 17% of neonates showing improvement within 24 to 72 hours.[76] In another retrospective study of 22 neonates, 32% had complete cessation of seizures on EEG after a loading dose of levetiracetam, 64% had seizure cessation within 24 hours, and up to 86% were seizure free by 48 hours.[77] In a separate retrospective study of 12 preterm neonates, 82% had complete cessation of seizures on EEG within 24 hours.[69] A prospective study of levetiracetam pharmacokinetics in 18 neonates showed similar results, with a cessation of seizures in 33% of neonates treated with lower doses (20-mg/kg load) versus 42% at higher doses (40-mg/kg load).[78] In a prospective feasibility study of levetiracetam administered as the first-line antiepileptic agent to 38 neonates, 79% were seizure free by the end of the first week of treatment. However, >50% of the study population required loading doses of 20 to 40 mg/kg phenobarbital as adjunctive therapy.[71] It is difficult to draw definitive conclusions about the efficacy of levetiracetam as monotherapy for neonatal seizures, given the limitations of studies to date, but the available data suggest that levetiracetam may be less effective than phenobarbital.[29]

Dosing

Most authors recommend a loading dose of 40 to 50 mg/kg IV levetiracetam,[17,77,78] although some extend this range to 20 to 50 mg/kg.[18,77] Maintenance dosing ranges from 20 to 25 mg/kg every 12 hours[77] or 30 mg/kg/day divided into twice- or three-times-daily dosing.[56] A small prospective pharmacokinetic study of levetiracetam concluded that the best levels were achieved using a loading dose of 40 mg/kg IV, followed by maintenance dosing of 10 mg/kg every 8 hours to keep trough levels at >20 μg/mL in the first 3 days, then to keep trough levels at >10 μg/mL in the rest of the first week, although goal levels are unclear in neonates.[78] A different prospective pharmacokinetic modeling study suggested that higher loading doses are needed for neonates compared with older children and adults, due to the higher volume of distribution in neonates. These authors also recommended only twice-daily dosing in the first few weeks of life, even with a levetiracetam half-life of 8.9 hours, due to immature renal function in neonates.[79] Other authors have similarly advised higher-loading doses for this reason.[56] Similarly, because preterm neonates have less-mature renal function, longer half-lives may be seen in preterm compared with term newborns.[56]

Adverse Effects, Contraindications, and Monitoring

Levetiracetam does not require routine drug-level monitoring,[17,74] as there is a limited side-effect profile and no well-established reference ranges for neonates.[74] Metabolism does not involve the cytochrome P450 system, and it is primarily renally excreted. There are no known clinically relevant drug–drug interactions with levetiracetam.[18]

Unlike many other ASMs, levetiracetam is not thought to cause neuronal apoptosis or disrupt synaptic development.[80–82] Some animal data suggest that levetiracetam may exert neuroprotective effects after hypoxic injury, with reduced neuronal apoptosis noted in rat pups treated with levetiracetam.[83]

Levetiracetam has been well tolerated in several study populations, with no acute adverse effects reported in term and preterm neonates,[69,76–78] although some infants were noted to be somnolent in the first 24 hours after the loading dose was given.[79] Temporary irritability reported in one patient improved with pyridoxine supplementation.[77] There is one case report of a neonate developing anaphylactic shock after 10 mg/kg of IV levetiracetam.[84]

In one follow-up study, levetiracetam use correlated with decreased cognitive and motor scores on the Bayley Scales of Infant and Toddler Development at 24-month follow-up; however, this was to a much-lesser degree than was associated with phenobarbital use (2- vs. 8-point cognitive score and 3- vs. 9-point motor score decreases with levetiracetam vs. phenobarbital, respectively). No association was found between levetiracetam exposure and development of cerebral palsy.[4] Although further research is needed to fully understand long-term outcomes after levetiracetam use, the adverse-effect profile demonstrated to date makes this an attractive treatment option for neonatal seizures.

EMERGING THERAPIES

Topiramate

Topiramate is a second-generation ASM sometimes used to treat refractory neonatal seizures, despite a lack of data in neonates.[17,18] In a 2007 survey of pediatric neurologists, 54% recommended treatment of neonatal seizures with topiramate in at least some circumstances, either alone or with other agents.[72] This drug is not included in the current WHO guidelines for treatment of neonatal seizures.

Topiramate is thought to have multiple mechanisms of action, the most well characterized being inhibition of voltage-gated sodium channels on the presynaptic glutamatergic neuron to prevent depolarization.[20] It is also thought to act as a GABA-A receptor agonist, as well as an AMPA/kainite glutamate receptor antagonist.[85,86]

Small case series have reported efficacy in neonatal seizures. One retrospective cohort of six term newborns reported seizure reduction in 67%,[87] and 100% seizure control was achieved in a case series of three neonates with refractory seizures.[88] There is one reported ongoing trial of topiramate therapy in the setting of therapeutic hypothermia for HIE. This study is investigating the primary outcome of clinical or EEG seizures before hospital discharge.[89]

No intravenous formulation of topiramate is currently available commercially, limiting its use for acute seizures.[72] Topiramate is given to neonates as crushed tablets or extemporaneous liquid suspension, either orally or via nasogastric tube. Different doses have been reported, with loading doses typically 5 to 10 mg/kg and a maintenance dose of 1 to 5 mg/kg/day.[87,90] The therapeutic range for blood levels in adults is 5 to 20 μg/mL, but no therapeutic range of levels has been established for neonates.[18,90] Clearance may be prolonged in hypothermia, meaning that doses may have to be administered less often.[91]

No adverse effects have been noted in the published case series of topiramate in neonates, though necrotizing enterocolitis has been rarely reported in preterm neonates.[87,90,91] Due to its inhibition of carbonic anhydrase in the renal tubules, topiramate can cause metabolic acidosis. However, no clinically significant decreases in serum bicarbonate were noted in a study of neonates receiving topiramate and undergoing hypothermia, a population already at risk for metabolic acidosis due to asphyxia and renal impairment.[91] Anecdotal reports of metabolic acidosis, transient hyperammonemia, and irritability or feeding problems were reported in a survey of pediatric neurologists.[72]

Given the well-described cognitive effects of topiramate in older children and adults, there has been concern for neurodevelopmental consequences of chronic administration early in life.[92–95] However, animal studies suggest that topiramate may have neuroprotective effects and does not increase apoptosis.[96,97] Some animal studies even demonstrate improved cognitive function after treatment with topiramate, although this may be reflective of the detrimental effects of uncontrolled seizures on the developing brain rather than a specific benefit of topiramate.[98,99]

Carbamazepine/Oxcarbazepine

Carbamazepine and its structural derivative oxcarbazepine are less frequently used for neonatal seizures, although they may have a role in specific neonatal-onset epilepsies. Mutations in the *KCNQ2* gene affect voltage-gated potassium channels and cause 10% of early infantile epileptic encephalopathies associated with intractable seizures and developmental delay.[42] Carbamazepine and oxcarbazepine block voltage-gated sodium channels that colocalize with KCNQ potassium channels, which is hypothesized to affect the function of the potassium channel complex. As such, carbamazepine and oxcarbazepine, along with other sodium channel blockers including phenytoin, may be a preferred therapy for seizures in neonates with *KCNQ2* encephalopathy.[42,100]

A small study of preterm infants with refractory seizures reported that 90% achieved good clinical seizure control with carbamazepine. The true efficacy is unknown, however, as this study did not use EEG monitoring to assess response.[101] A small case series of patients with benign familial neonatal epilepsy primarily due to mutations in *KCNQ2* or *KCNQ3* also reported high rates of seizure freedom (88%) after carbamazepine administration; however, this was often after receiving other first-line ASMs.[102] Carbamazepine has been given as an initial dose of 10 mg/kg, followed by maintenance therapy of 5 to 7 mg/kg every 8 hours starting 24 hours after the loading dose.[103] A drop in serum concentrations between days 8 and 15 of life has been observed due to increased capacity of liver cytochrome CYP3A4 to metabolize the drug.[56] Of note, enzyme induction by phenobarbital and phenytoin may cause increased elimination of carbamazepine.[56] In the few studies of carbamazepine in neonates, no significant adverse effects were reported.[101,103] Generally, this agent is used only when other treatments have failed or when a specific neonatal-onset epilepsy diagnosis suggests potential efficacy.

Valproic Acid

Little literature exists to support the use of valproic acid in neonates. There is generally reluctance to use valproic acid due to the known risk of (and black box warning for) hepatic failure with this drug in young children. In particular, valproate should not be used when there is the possibility of a metabolic or mitochondrial disorder. At the same time, some providers do still use valproic acid for refractory seizures with a clearly identified cause that is not metabolic or mitochondrial. In a survey of Israeli neurologists and neonatologists, neurologists were more likely to recommend valproic acid and topiramate for the treatment of intractable neonatal seizures versus lidocaine and benzodiazepines recommended by neonatologists.[104] The mechanism of action of valproic acid is not completely understood; its multiple targets include inhibition of sodium channels and increased GABA function.[56] A loading dose of 20 to 30 mg/kg of rectal valproic acid in two neonates followed by maintenance therapy in one patient of 30 mg/kg/day rectally divided twice daily achieved good seizure control in a case report of two neonates who failed phenobarbital and phenytoin.[105] If valproic acid is used in a neonate, it should be in close consultation with a child neurologist.

Lacosamide

Lacosamide is rarely used in the treatment of neonatal seizures, and data in this population are currently limited. Lacosamide acts on sodium channels; however, it has a unique mechanism of selectively enhancing slow sodium channel inactivation.[106] Current evidence is limited to small case reports, with seizure cessation in the three neonates described.[107,108] Given the mechanism of action at the sodium channels, there may be a role in neonatal-onset epilepsies due to channelopathies. One of the case reports described two cases of *SCN2A* associated neonatal epilepsy with seizures responsive to lacosamide.[107] There is an ongoing trial assessing the efficacy, safety, and pharmacokinetics of lacosamide in neonates with refractory neonatal seizures.[109]

Bumetanide

Although phenobarbital is currently used as a monotherapy for first-line treatment of neonatal seizures, there is some evidence for a potential role for chloride cotransporters as adjunctive therapies with phenobarbital to reduce phenobarbital resistance. However, recent safety concerns have tempered early enthusiasm for these agents.

Bumetanide is a loop diuretic that inhibits the sodium–potassium–chloride cotransporters NKCC1 and NKCC2, both of which move chloride into cells. NKCC2 is expressed in renal tubular cells, whereas neurons express NKCC1 with increased expression in immature neurons, making this a potential target for ASMs in neonates. As mentioned previously (see the earlier discussion of phenobarbital), GABA may be excitatory in immature neurons with higher intracellular levels of chloride, due to high NKCC1 expression with low KCC2 potassium chloride cotransporter expression. By blocking NKCC1, bumetanide may prevent intracellular chloride accumulation, which may then allow GABA agonists to have greater effect.[18,20,34,86]

In two recent studies of neonatal rat pups, one demonstrated increased efficacy of phenobarbital with bumetanide versus phenobarbital alone.[110] However, the other demonstrated no difference between phenobarbital plus adjunctive therapy with bumetanide versus phenobarbital alone.[111] Unfortunately, a large phase I/II trial assessing use of bumetanide was stopped early due to hearing loss and poor efficacy. A review of this study emphasized that there was a reduced seizure burden seen with bumetanide use and argued that hearing loss may not be entirely attributable to the study drug.[112,113] An additional pilot randomized controlled trial of bumetanide was recently completed and demonstrated greater seizure reduction in neonates treated with bumetanide in combination with phenobarbital over phenobarbital alone.[114] Hearing impairment occurred in 8% (2/26) of surviving neonates treated with bumetanide, lower than the 27% in the prior phase I/II trial and not significantly different from the control group.[114] With the evidence currently available, the use of bumetanide for the treatment of neonatal seizures cannot be recommended at this time pending further study.

Other Therapies

KETOGENIC DIET

The ketogenic diet is a dietary therapy in which the majority of caloric intake is fat to put the body in a state of chronic ketosis, in turn altering energy supply to the brain. The ketogenic diet is used in children with intractable epilepsy with good evidence, although it is used less commonly in neonates and there is less published evidence for its use in this population.[115,116] There may be a role for the ketogenic diet in certain cases of inborn errors of metabolism, and it is the treatment of choice in patients with pyruvate dehydrogenase complex deficiency or glucose transporter 1 (GLUT-1) deficiency.[73,117] A case series of three neonates with early myoclonic epilepsy and nonketotic hyperglycinemia demonstrated good seizure response to the ketogenic diet after failure of multiple ASMs.[118] More high-quality evidence is needed to determine the safety and efficacy of the ketogenic diet in neonates.

SURGERY

With technologic advances enhancing the precision of epilepsy surgery, more options are now available for neonates with intractable seizures. Current ILAE recommendations state that standard care for infants with seizures should include identifying patients who are potential candidates for epilepsy surgery.[73] Although not common among neonates, surgery may be considered as an option in select cases of refractory seizures.

VITAMIN SUPPLEMENTATION

A minority of neonates with seizures have underlying disorders of metabolism that respond to specific vitamin supplementation. These conditions are sometimes described as *vitamin-responsive epilepsies*. In addition, there are reports of vitamin supplementation reducing neonatal seizures due to other causes, although these are less consistent. For neonates with seizures of unknown etiology that remain refractory to conventional ASMs, an empiric trial of vitamin supplementation is warranted. After an empiric vitamin treatment has been started, it should be continued until confirmatory testing returns, unless another clear etiology for seizures is found. This may be up to several weeks, depending on laboratory capabilities.

PYRIDOXINE

Pyridoxine-dependent epilepsy (PDE) is a rare cause of intractable seizures in neonates due to a deficiency of alpha-aminoadipic semialdehyde dehydrogenase (antiquitin).[119] Neonates with intractable seizures not responsive to therapy with ASMs should receive an empiric trial of pyridoxine (vitamin B_6) therapy.[18,19,34] Patients should be monitored with cEEG and given 100 mg of pyridoxine intravenously, watching for response on EEG. In some regimens, it is proposed that doses of 100 mg may be repeated every 5 to 10 minutes up to a cumulative dose of 500 mg, at which point no further pyridoxine should be given.[119] This should be done only in an intensive care unit setting with respiratory support resources readily available, as first administration of pyridoxine may result in respiratory arrest in neonates responsive to treatment.[120,121] Patients with a positive response to intravenous pyridoxine should be maintained on enteral pyridoxine 15 to 18 mg/kg/day divided into twice-daily doses,[119] although ranges up to 15 to 30 mg/kg/day divided into two or three doses up to a maximum of 200 mg/day have been reported in neonates.[122] Lifelong therapy with pyridoxine is required in patients with PDE.[119] Adjuvant therapy with folinic acid 3 to 5 mg/kg/day has been suggested for infants with PDE.[122]

The diagnosis of pyridoxine-dependent seizures is typically made by clinical and electrographic response to intravenous pyridoxine, although biochemical tests (elevated serum pipecolic acid levels and elevated serum, cerebrospinal fluid [CSF], or urine levels of alpha-aminoadipic semialdehyde [AASA]) and testing of the *ALDH7A1* gene are becoming available.[119,123-125] It is important to note that pipecolic acid and AASA levels cannot be followed as a measure of treatment response, as these will remain elevated with treatment.[123,124] Conversely, these markers may remain abnormal and may be useful for identifying affected patients even if drawn after a trial of pyridoxine has been initiated. Pyridoxine therapy is known to cause dorsal root ganglionopathy and sensory neuropathy at high doses; therefore, the maximum dose of 30 mg/kg/day should be observed.[119,121,122]

PYRIDOXAL 5′-PHOSPHATE

PLP-dependent seizures are caused by a deficiency of pyridox(am)ine 5′-phosphate oxidase (PNPO) encoded by the *PNPO* gene.[119,126] Similar to PDE, PNPO deficiency should be suspected in neonates with intractable seizures unresponsive to ASM treatment, and empiric PLP therapy should be trialed.[18,19,34] Because PLP is less readily available than pyridoxine, in practice many neonates have completed a pyridoxine trial before a PLP trial is initiated. However, if PLP is available, this can be given as empiric therapy for both PDE and PLP-dependent seizures.

PLP is given enterally, with a recommended dose of 30 mg/kg/day divided into three or four doses, given for at least 3 to 5 days to observe for clinical and EEG response.[119,121] Acutely, a trial of 10 mg/kg/dose for two doses given 2 hours apart can be considered.[126] If the diagnosis is confirmed, maintenance therapy of 30 to 50 mg/kg/day divided in four to six doses should be continued.[119,126] As with PDE, lifelong therapy is required, and hepatic function should be monitored, given reports of cirrhosis with treatment.[122,127]

A diagnosis of PLP can be confirmed by serum, urine, and CSF metabolic studies. Increased CSF L-DOPA, 3-methoxytyrosine, threonine, and glycine with decreased CSF homovanillic acid and 5-hydroxyindoleacetic acid, increased urine vanillactic acid, and increased plasma levels of threonine and glycine are characteristic of PNPO deficiency.[128,129] This may be more directly tested with demonstration of decreased levels of PLP in the CSF or *PNPO* gene sequencing.[130]

FOLINIC ACID

First described in 1995, folinic acid–responsive seizures are another cause of vitamin-responsive epileptic encephalopathy.[131] Treatment with folinic acid should be considered in neonates with intractable seizures not responsive to pyridoxine or with a transient response to pyridoxine.[132] There is some crossover between patients who respond to pyridoxine and those who respond to folinic acid, as patients with a yet-to-be-identified folinic acid–responsive CSF marker (termed *peak X*)[121] also have antiquin mutations, and patients with PDE also often have the same elevated peak in their CSF.[119,133] Patients should be treated with enteral folinic acid (5-formyltetrahydrofolate) 3 to 5 mg/kg/day for 3 to 5 days to evaluate for response to treatment, followed by maintenance therapy of 3 to 5 mg/kg/day divided into three doses.[119] A trial of 5 mg for two doses given 6 hours apart in the acute period can be considered.[126] Care must be used to avoid confusion with folic acid, a common mistake when folinic acid is prescribed.

BIOTIN

Biotinidase deficiency is another rare cause of intractable epilepsy in neonates caused by mutations of the biotinidase *BTD* gene.[134] It is associated with optic atrophy with visual loss, sensorineural hearing loss, conjunctivitis, cheilosis, and alopecia.[122] Testing for this disorder is included in most newborn screening programs. Profound or severe deficiency is characterized by <10% enzymatic activity, whereas 10% to 30% of activity is retained in cases of partial deficiency. Neonates with both partial and severe deficiency should be treated with 5 to 20 mg of biotin daily, and patients must continue lifelong therapy.[122,134,135]

Discontinuation of Therapy

After acute seizures resolve, the duration of ongoing ASM treatment required is largely dependent on the cause of the seizures. In cases of neonatal-onset epilepsy, ASMs will likely be required in the long term and thus should be continued at the time of hospital discharge. For neonates with acute symptomatic seizures or seizures of unknown cause, however, ongoing ASM treatment beyond hospital discharge is not always necessary. The 2015 ILAE Task Force Report does not include recommendations for how long neonates with seizures should be treated, given there was no clear evidence available at that time.[73] The 2011 WHO guidelines on this topic, based on expert opinion in the absence of supporting data, state that medication may be discontinued abruptly before hospital discharge without tapering in neonates who achieve seizure control on a single ASM. However, if more than one ASM is required for seizure control, the expert consensus recommends discontinuing medications one by one, with phenobarbital being the final medication to discontinue.[8]

Historically, providers had recommended continuation of ASM therapy for several months before tapering medications.[136] More recent practice is trending toward discontinuation of ASM therapy during the neonatal period to avoid the potential neurodevelopmental problems linked to chronic ASM administration. In a large multicenter prospective cohort study, practices varied widely, with timing of medication discontinuation largely dependent on the institution, etiology of seizures, and EEG and examination findings.[137] There was large variability in practice among hospitals; some sites sent the vast majority of neonates home on ASMs (>85%), whereas others discontinued medication in almost all patients before discharge. An older retrospective study demonstrated no significant correlation between seizure etiology or initial examination with recurrence of seizures during the tapering of ASMs. The presence of normal background on EEG and normal computed tomography findings were correlated with successful tapering of ASMs.[138]

A more recent large multicenter comparative effectiveness study examined outcomes of 270 neonates with acute symptomatic seizures who were continued on ASMs at hospital discharge versus those for whom ASMs were discontinued prior to hospital discharge. This study showed no significant difference in either the rates of post-neonatal epilepsy or neurodevelopmental outcomes at 24 months between the groups.[139] Given the lack of benefit with prolonged ASM use, the authors suggest that, if neonatal seizures are known to be due to an acute, symptomatic cause, then ASM may usually be discontinued prior to hospital discharge.

Given the concerns for long-term adverse effects with chronic ASM administration, we recommend early discontinuation of ASMs for neonates with acute symptomatic seizures. Our own practice is to continue maintenance ASM dosing until seizures are totally controlled for at least 48 hours. Subsequently, for neonates with seizures due to ischemic injury or with no cause identified, ASMs are stopped before hospital discharge. If multiple ASMs were required in the acute period, it may be that one or more ASMs are stopped before discharge, with the last ASM continued until follow-up with a neurologist a few weeks after discharge. In acute symptomatic seizures with a higher risk for recurrence (e.g., hemorrhage), we do consider a longer initial treatment period.

Ideally, medication tapering and discontinuation are performed in the neonatal intensive care unit, where the infant can be closely monitored for seizure recurrence. In neonates with neonatal-onset epilepsy, ASMs most often should be continued at hospital discharge. Discontinuation of therapy, however, is ultimately provider and institution dependent.

Conclusion

Current recommendations for the treatment of neonatal seizures are largely based on historical experience, with a dearth of high-quality evidence to support the use of the aforementioned therapies. Currently available ASMs have been demonstrated to achieve only a partial response, and further research into optimal treatment regimens for this population is needed. The suggested treatments in this chapter are based on the recommendations of ILAE and WHO guidelines, experts in the field, and the evidence available in the literature, but they should be tailored and adjusted for each individual patient.

REFERENCES

1. Glass HC, Shellhaas RA, Wusthoff CJ, et al. Contemporary profile of seizures in neonates: a prospective cohort study. *J Pediatr*. 2016;174:98-103.e1.
2. Kaushal S, Tamer Z, Opoku F, Forcelli PA. Anticonvulsant drug-induced cell death in the developing white matter of the rodent brain. *Epilepsia*. 2016;57(5):727-734.
3. Kang SK, Kadam SD. Neonatal seizures: impact on neurodevelopmental outcomes. *Front Pediatr*. 2015;3:101.
4. Maitre NL, Smolinsky C, Slaughter JC, Stark AR. Adverse neurodevelopmental outcomes after exposure to phenobarbital and levetiracetam for the treatment of neonatal seizures. *J Perinatol*. 2013;33(11):841-846.
5. van Rooij LGM, Toet MC, van Huffelen AC, et al. Effect of treatment of subclinical neonatal seizures detected with aEEG: randomized, controlled trial. *Pediatrics*. 2010;125(2):e358-e366.
6. Shellhaas RA, Chang T, Tsuchida T, et al. The American Clinical Neurophysiology Society's Guideline on continuous electroencephalography monitoring in neonates. *J Clin Neurophysiol*. 2011;28(6):611-617.
7. Boylan GB, Stevenson NJ, Vanhatalo S. Monitoring neonatal seizures. *Semin Fetal Neonatal Med*. 2013;18(4):202-208.
8. World Health Organization. *Guidelines on Neonatal Seizures*. Available at: https://apps.who.int/iris/bitstream/handle/10665/77756/9789241548304_eng.pdf;sequence=1. Accessed January 30, 2023.
9. Pressler RM, Cilio MR, Mizrahi EM, et al. The ILAE classification of seizures and the epilepsies: modification for seizures in the neonate. Position paper by the ILAE Task Force on Neonatal Seizures. *Epilepsia*. 2021;62(3):615-628.
10. Scher MS, Alvin J, Gaus L, Minnigh B, Painter MJ. Uncoupling of EEG-clinical neonatal seizures after antiepileptic drug use. *Pediatr Neurol*. 2003;28(4):277-280.
11. Weeke LC, Groenendaal F, Toet MC, et al. The aetiology of neonatal seizures and the diagnostic contribution of neonatal cerebral magnetic resonance imaging. *Dev Med Child Neurol*. 2015;57(3):248-256.
12. Osmond E, Billetop A, Jary S, Likeman M, Thoresen M, Luyt K. Neonatal seizures: magnetic resonance imaging adds value in the diagnosis and prediction of neurodisability. *Acta Paediatr*. 2014;103(8):820-826.
13. Wickström R, Hallberg B, Bartocci M. Differing attitudes toward phenobarbital use in the neonatal period among neonatologists and child neurologists in Sweden. *Eur J Paediatr Neurol*. 2013; 17(1):55-63.
14. Hellström-Westas L, Boylan G, Ågren J. Systematic review of neonatal seizure management strategies provides guidance on anti-epileptic treatment. *Acta Paediatr*. 2015;104(2):123-129.
15. Vento M, De Vries L, Alberola A, et al. Approach to seizures in the neonatal period: a European perspective. *Acta Paediatr*. 2010;99(4):497-501.
16. Glass HC, Kan J, Bonifacio SL, Ferriero DM. Neonatal seizures: treatment practices among term and preterm infants. *Pediatr Neurol*. 2012;46(2):111-115.
17. Slaughter LA, Patel AD, Slaughter JL. Pharmacological treatment of neonatal seizures: a systematic review. *J Child Neurol*. 2013;28(3):351-364.
18. van Rooij LGM, van den Broek MPH, Rademaker CMA, de Vries LS. Clinical management of seizures in newborns : diagnosis and treatment. *Paediatr Drugs*. 2013;15(1):9-18.
19. van Rooij LGM, Hellström-Westas L, de Vries LS. Treatment of neonatal seizures. *Semin Fetal Neonatal Med*. 2013;18(4): 209-215.
20. Donovan MD, Griffin BT, Kharoshankaya L, Cryan JF, Boylan GB. Pharmacotherapy for neonatal seizures: current knowledge and future perspectives. *Drugs*. 2016;76(6):647-661.
21. Brodie MJ, Kwan P. Current position of phenobarbital in epilepsy and its future. *Epilepsia*. 2012;53(suppl 8):40-46.
22. Sankar JM, Agarwal R, Deorari A, Paul VK. Management of neonatal seizures. *Indian J Pediatr*. 2010;77(10):1129-1135.
23. Booth D, Evans DJ. Anticonvulsants for neonates with seizures. *Cochrane Database Syst Rev*. 2004;(4):CD004218.
24. Painter MJ, Scher MS, Stein AD, et al. Phenobarbital compared with phenytoin for the treatment of neonatal seizures. *N Engl J Med*. 1999;341(7):485-489.
25. Spagnoli C, Seri S, Pavlidis E, Mazzotta S, Pelosi A, Pisani F. Phenobarbital for neonatal seizures: response rate and predictors of refractoriness. *Neuropediatrics*. 2016;47(5):318-326.
26. Boylan GB, Rennie JM, Chorley G, et al. Second-line anticonvulsant treatment of neonatal seizures: a video-EEG monitoring study. *Neurology*. 2004;62(3):486-488.
27. Castro Conde JR, Hernández Borges AA, Doménech Martínez E, González Campo C, Perera Soler R. Midazolam in neonatal seizures with no response to phenobarbital. *Neurology*. 2005;64(5): 876-879.

28. Boylan GB, Rennie JM, Pressler RM, Wilson G, Morton M, Binnie CD. Phenobarbitone, neonatal seizures, and video-EEG. *Arch Dis Child Fetal Neonatal Ed*. 2002;86(3):F165-F170.
29. Sharpe C, Reiner GE, Davis SL, et al. Levetiracetam versus phenobarbital for neonatal seizures: a randomized controlled trial. *Pediatrics*. 2020;145(6):e20193182.
30. Evans DJ, Levene MI, Tsakmakis M. Anticonvulsants for preventing mortality and morbidity in full term newborns with perinatal asphyxia. *Cochrane Database Syst Rev*. 2007;(3): CD001240.
31. Young L, Berg M, Soll R. Prophylactic barbiturate use for the prevention of morbidity and mortality following perinatal asphyxia. *Cochrane Database Syst Rev*. 2016;(5):CD001240.
32. Sarkar S, Barks JD, Bapuraj JR, et al. Does phenobarbital improve the effectiveness of therapeutic hypothermia in infants with hypoxic-ischemic encephalopathy? *J Perinatol*. 2012;32(1):15-20.
33. Filippi L, la Marca G, Cavallaro G, et al. Phenobarbital for neonatal seizures in hypoxic ischemic encephalopathy: a pharmacokinetic study during whole body hypothermia. *Epilepsia*. 2011;52(4):794-801.
34. Glass HC. Neonatal seizures: advances in mechanisms and management. *Clin Perinatol*. 2014;41(1):177-190.
35. Patsalos PN, Berry DJ, Bourgeois BFD, et al. Antiepileptic drugs—best practice guidelines for therapeutic drug monitoring: a position paper by the subcommission on therapeutic drug monitoring, ILAE Commission on Therapeutic Strategies. *Epilepsia*. 2008;49(7):1239-1276.
36. Shellhaas RA, Ng CM, Dillon CH, Barks JDE, Bhatt-Mehta V. Population pharmacokinetics of phenobarbital in infants with neonatal encephalopathy treated with therapeutic hypothermia. *Pediatr Crit Care Med*. 2013;14(2):194-202.
37. Gutherz SB, Kulick CV, Soper C, Kondratyev A, Gale K, Forcelli PA. Brief postnatal exposure to phenobarbital impairs passive avoidance learning and sensorimotor gating in rats. *Epilepsy Behav*. 2014;37:265-269.
38. Bittigau P, Sifringer M, Ikonomidou C. Antiepileptic drugs and apoptosis in the developing brain. *Ann N Y Acad Sci*. 2003;993:103-114; discussion 123-124.
39. Shetty J. Neonatal seizures in hypoxic–ischaemic encephalopathy – risks and benefits of anticonvulsant therapy. *Dev Med Child Neurol*. 2015;57(suppl 3):40-43.
40. Bye A, Flanagan D. Electroencephalograms, clinical observations and the monitoring of neonatal seizures. *J Paediatr Child Health*. 1995;31(6):503-507.
41. Howell KB, McMahon JM, Carvill GL, et al. SCN2A encephalopathy: a major cause of epilepsy of infancy with migrating focal seizures. *Neurology*. 2015;85(11):958-966.
42. Pisano T, Numis AL, Heavin SB, et al. Early and effective treatment of KCNQ2 encephalopathy. *Epilepsia*. 2015;56(5):685-691.
43. Pathak G, Upadhyay A, Pathak U, Chawla D, Goel SP. Phenobarbitone versus phenytoin for treatment of neonatal seizures: an open-label randomized controlled trial. *Indian Pediatr*. 2013;50(8):753-757.
44. Appleton RE, Gill A. Adverse events associated with intravenous phenytoin in children: a prospective study. *Seizure*. 2003;12(6):369-372.
45. Sharief N, Goonasekera C. Soft tissue injury associated with intravenous phenytoin in a neonate. *Acta Paediatr*. 1994;83(11): 1218-1219.
46. Mueller EW, Boucher BA. Fosphenytoin: current place in therapy. *J Pediatr Pharmacol Ther*. 2004;9(4):265-273.
47. Lowry JA, Vandover JC, DeGreeff J, Scalzo AJ. Unusual presentation of iatrogenic phenytoin toxicity in a newborn. *J Med Toxicol*. 2005;1(1):26-29.
48. Ohmori H, Ogura H, Yasuda M et al. Developmental neurotoxicity of phenytoin on granule cells and Purkinje cells in mouse cerebellum. *J Neurochem*. 1999;72(4):1497-1506.
49. van den Broek MPH, Huitema ADR, van Hasselt JGC, et al. Lidocaine (lignocaine) dosing regimen based upon a population pharmacokinetic model for preterm and term neonates with seizures. *Clin Pharmacokinet*. 2011;50(7):461-469.
50. Lundqvist M, Ågren J, Hellström-Westas L, Flink R, Wickström R. Efficacy and safety of lidocaine for treatment of neonatal seizures. *Acta Paediatr*. 2013;102(9):863-867.
51. Shany E, Benzaqen O, Watemberg N. Comparison of continuous drip of midazolam or lidocaine in the treatment of intractable neonatal seizures. *J Child Neurol*. 2007;22(3):255-259.
52. Malingré MM, Van Rooij LGM, Rademaker CMA, et al. Development of an optimal lidocaine infusion strategy for neonatal seizures. *Eur J Pediatr*. 2006;165(9):598-604.
53. van den Broek MPH, Rademaker CMA, van Straaten HLM, et al. Anticonvulsant treatment of asphyxiated newborns under hypothermia with lidocaine: efficacy, safety and dosing. *Arch Dis Child Fetal Neonatal Ed*. 2013;98(4):F341-F345.
54. Weeke LC, Toet MC, van Rooij LGM, et al. Lidocaine response rate in aEEG-confirmed neonatal seizures: retrospective study of 413 full-term and preterm infants. *Epilepsia*. 2016;57(2):233-242.
55. Weeke LC, Schalkwijk S, Toet MC, van Rooij LGM, de Vries LS, van den Broek MPH. Lidocaine-associated cardiac events in newborns with seizures: incidence, symptoms and contributing factors. *Neonatology*. 2015;108(2):130-136.
56. Tulloch JK, Carr RR, Ensom MHH. A systematic review of the pharmacokinetics of antiepileptic drugs in neonates with refractory seizures. *J Pediatr Pharmacol Ther*. 2012;17(1):31-44.
57. Rey E, Radvanyi-Bouvet MF, Bodiou C, et al. Intravenous lidocaine in the treatment of convulsions in the neonatal period: monitoring plasma levels. *Ther Drug Monit*. 1990;12(4):316-320.
58. van Rooij LGM, Toet MC, Rademaker KMA, Groenendaal F, de Vries LS. Cardiac arrhythmias in neonates receiving lidocaine as anticonvulsive treatment. *Eur J Pediatr*. 2004;163(11):637-641.
59. Rezvani M, Finkelstein Y, Verjee Z, Railton C, Koren G. Generalized seizures following topical lidocaine administration during circumcision: establishing causation. *Paediatr Drugs*. 2007; 9(2):125-127.
60. Moran LR, Hossain T, Insoft RM. Neonatal seizures following lidocaine administration for elective circumcision. *J Perinatol*. 2004;24(6):395-396.
61. van Leuven K, Groenendaal F, Toet MC, et al. Midazolam and amplitude-integrated EEG in asphyxiated full-term neonates. *Acta Paediatr*. 2004;93(9):1221-1227.
62. Sheth RD, Buckley DJ, Gutierrez AR, Gingold M, Bodensteiner JB, Penney S. Midazolam in the treatment of refractory neonatal seizures. *Clin Neuropharmacol*. 1996;19(2):165-170.
63. Sirsi D, Nangia S, LaMothe J, Kosofsky BE, Solomon GE. Successful management of refractory neonatal seizures with midazolam. *J Child Neurol*. 2008;23(6):706-709.
64. Deshmukh A, Wittert W, Schnitzler E, Mangurten HH. Lorazepam in the treatment of refractory neonatal seizures. A pilot study. *Am J Dis Child*. 1986;140(10):1042-1044.
65. Maytal J, Novak GP, King KC. Lorazepam in the treatment of refractory neonatal seizures. *J Child Neurol*. 1991;6(4):319-323.
66. van den Broek MPH, van Straaten HLM, Huitema ADR, et al. Anticonvulsant effectiveness and hemodynamic safety of midazolam in

full-term infants treated with hypothermia. *Neonatology*. 2015; 107(2):150-156.
67. Hu KC, Chiu NC, Ho CS, Lee ST, Shen EY. Continuous midazolam infusion in the treatment of uncontrollable neonatal seizures. *Acta Paediatr Taiwan*. 2003;44(5):279-281.
68. Ng E, Klinger G, Shah V, Taddio A. Safety of benzodiazepines in newborns. *Ann Pharmacother*. 2002;36(7-8):1150-1155.
69. Khan O, Cipriani C, Wright C, Crisp E, Kirmani B. Role of intravenous levetiracetam for acute seizure management in preterm neonates. *Pediatr Neurol*. 2013;49(5):340-343.
70. Shoemaker MT, Rotenberg JS. Levetiracetam for the treatment of neonatal seizures. *J Child Neurol*. 2007;22(1):95-98.
71. Ramantani G, Ikonomidou C, Walter B, Rating D, Dinger J. Levetiracetam: safety and efficacy in neonatal seizures. *Eur J Paediatr Neurol*. 2011;15(1):1-7.
72. Silverstein FS, Ferriero DM. Off-label use of antiepileptic drugs for the treatment of neonatal seizures. *Pediatr Neurol*. 2008;39(2): 77-79.
73. Wilmshurst JM, Gaillard WD, Vinayan KP, et al. Summary of recommendations for the management of infantile seizures: Task Force Report for the ILAE Commission of Pediatrics. *Epilepsia*. 2015;56(8):1185-1197.
74. Mruk AL, Garlitz KL, Leung NR. Levetiracetam in neonatal seizures: a review. *J Pediatr Pharmacol Ther*. 2015;20(2):76-89.
75. Lynch BA, Lambeng N, Nocka K, et al. The synaptic vesicle protein SV2A is the binding site for the antiepileptic drug levetiracetam. *Proc Natl Acad Sci U S A*. 2004;101(26): 9861-9866.
76. Abend NS, Gutierrez-Colina AM, Monk HM, Dlugos DJ, Clancy RR. Levetiracetam for treatment of neonatal seizures. *J Child Neurol*. 2011;26(4):465-470.
77. Khan O, Chang E, Cipriani C, Wright C, Crisp E, Kirmani B. Use of intravenous levetiracetam for management of acute seizures in neonates. *Pediatr Neurol*. 2011;44(4):265-269.
78. Sharpe CM, Capparelli EV, Mower A, Farrell MJ, Soldin SJ, Haas RH. A seven-day study of the pharmacokinetics of intravenous levetiracetam in neonates: marked changes in pharmacokinetics occur during the first week of life. *Pediatr Res*. 2012; 72(1):43-49.
79. Merhar SL, Schibler KR, Sherwin CM, et al. Pharmacokinetics of levetiracetam in neonates with seizures. *J Pediatr*. 2011;159(1):152-154.e3.
80. Forcelli PA, Janssen MJ, Vicini S, Gale K. Neonatal exposure to antiepileptic drugs disrupts striatal synaptic development. *Ann Neurol*. 2012;72(3):363-372.
81. Kim JS, Kondratyev A, Tomita Y, Gale K. Neurodevelopmental impact of antiepileptic drugs and seizures in the immature brain. *Epilepsia*. 2007;48(suppl 5):19-26.
82. Manthey D, Asimiadou S, Stefovska V, et al. Sulthiame but not levetiracetam exerts neurotoxic effect in the developing rat brain. *Exp Neurol*. 2005;193(2):497-503.
83. Kilicdag H, Daglıoglu K, Erdogan S, et al. The effect of levetiracetam on neuronal apoptosis in neonatal rat model of hypoxic ischemic brain injury. *Early Hum Dev*. 2013;89(5):355-360.
84. Koklu E, Ariguloglu EA, Koklu S. Levetiracetam-induced anaphylaxis in a neonate. *Pediatr Neurol*. 2014;50(2):192-194.
85. Vesoulis ZA, Mathur AM. Advances in management of neonatal seizures. *Indian J Pediatr*. 2014;81(6):592-598.
86. Pressler RM, Mangum B. Newly emerging therapies for neonatal seizures. *Semin Fetal Neonatal Med*. 2013;18(4):216-223.
87. Glass HC, Poulin C, Shevell MI. Topiramate for the treatment of neonatal seizures. *Pediatr Neurol*. 2011;44(6):439-442.
88. Riesgo R, Winckler MI, Ohlweiler L, et al. Treatment of refractory neonatal seizures with topiramate. *Neuropediatrics*. 2012; 43(6):353-356.
89. Hoffman KR. *Topiramate in Neonates Receiving Whole Body Cooling for Hypoxic Ischemic Encephalopathy*. Available at: https://clinicaltrials.gov/ct2/show/NCT01765218. Accessed January 30, 2023.
90. Filippi L, la Marca G, Fiorini P, et al. Topiramate concentrations in neonates treated with prolonged whole body hypothermia for hypoxic ischemic encephalopathy. *Epilepsia*. 2009;50(11):2355-2361.
91. Filippi L, Poggi C, la Marca G, et al. Oral topiramate in neonates with hypoxic ischemic encephalopathy treated with hypothermia: a safety study. *J Pediatr*. 2010;157(3):361-366.
92. Ortinski P, Meador KJ. Cognitive side effects of antiepileptic drugs. *Epilepsy Behav*. 2004;5(suppl 1):S60-S65.
93. Thompson PJ, Baxendale SA, Duncan JS, Sander JW. Effects of topiramate on cognitive function. *J Neurol Neurosurg Psychiatry*. 2000;69(5):636-641.
94. Lee S, Sziklas V, Andermann F, et al. The effects of adjunctive topiramate on cognitive function in patients with epilepsy. *Epilepsia*. 2003;44(3):339-347.
95. Meador KJ, Loring DW, Hulihan JF, Kamin M, Karim R, CAPSS-027 Study Group. Differential cognitive and behavioral effects of topiramate and valproate. *Neurology*. 2003;60(9): 1483-1488.
96. Schubert S, Brandl U, Brodhun M, et al. Neuroprotective effects of topiramate after hypoxia–ischemia in newborn piglets. *Brain Res*. 2005;1058(1-2):129-136.
97. Glier C, Dzietko M, Bittigau P, Jarosz B, Korobowicz E, Ikonomidou C. Therapeutic doses of topiramate are not toxic to the developing rat brain. *Exp Neurol*. 2004;187(2):403-409.
98. Zhao Q, Hu Y, Holmes GL. Effect of topiramate on cognitive function and activity level following neonatal seizures. *Epilepsy Behav*. 2005;6(4):529-536.
99. Cha BH, Silveira DC, Liu X, Hu Y, Holmes GL. Effect of topiramate following recurrent and prolonged seizures during early development. *Epilepsy Res*. 2002;51(3):217-232.
100. Kato M, Yamagata T, Kubota M, et al. Clinical spectrum of early onset epileptic encephalopathies caused by KCNQ2 mutation. *Epilepsia*. 2013;54(7):1282-1287.
101. Hoppen T, Elger CE, Bartmann P. Carbamazepine in phenobarbital-nonresponders: experience with ten preterm infants. *Eur J Pediatr*. 2001;160(7):444-447.
102. Sands TT, Balestri M, Bellini G, et al. Rapid and safe response to low-dose carbamazepine in neonatal epilepsy. *Epilepsia*. 2016;57(12):2019-2030.
103. Singh B, Singh P, al Hifzi I, Khan M, Majeed-Saidan M. Treatment of neonatal seizures with carbamazepine. *J Child Neurol*. 1996;11(5):378-382.
104. Bassan H, Bental Y, Shany E, et al. Neonatal seizures: dilemmas in workup and management. *Pediatr Neurol*. 2008;38(6): 415-421.
105. Steinberg A, Shalev RS, Amir N. Valproic acid in neonatal status convulsivus. *Brain Dev*. 1986;8(3):278-279.
106. Rogawski MA, Tofighy A, White HS, Matagne A, Wolff C. Current understanding of the mechanism of action of the antiepileptic drug lacosamide. *Epilepsy Res*. 2015;110:189-205.
107. Hadar FH, Eli H, Ayelet L, et al. Lacosamide for SCN2A-related intractable neonatal and infantile seizures. *Epileptic Disord*. 2018;20(5):440-446.
108. Bertozzi V, Bonardi CM, Biscalchin G, Tona C, Amigoni A, Sartori S. Efficacy of lacosamide in neonatal-onset super-refractory

status epilepticus: a case report. *Epileptic Disord.* 2021;23(4):655-660.

109. UCB Biopharma SRL. *A Study to Evaluate the Efficacy, Safety, and Pharmacokinetics of Lacosamide in Neonates with Repeated Electroencephalographic Neonatal Seizures (LENS)*. Available at: https://clinicaltrials.gov/ct2/show/study/NCT04519645. Accessed January 30, 2023.
110. Cleary RT, Sun H, Huynh T, et al. Bumetanide enhances phenobarbital efficacy in a rat model of hypoxic neonatal seizures. *PLoS ONE.* 2013;8(3):e57148.
111. Kang SK, Markowitz GJ, Kim ST, Johnston MV, Kadam SD. Age- and sex-dependent susceptibility to phenobarbital-resistant neonatal seizures: role of chloride co-transporters. *Front Cell Neurosci.* 2015;9:173.
112. Pressler RM, Boylan GB, Marlow N, et al. Bumetanide for the treatment of seizures in newborn babies with hypoxic ischaemic encephalopathy (NEMO): an open-label, dose finding, and feasibility phase 1/2 trial. *Lancet Neurol.* 2015;14(5):469-477.
113. Thoresen M, Sabir H. Epilepsy: neonatal seizures still lack safe and effective treatment. *Nat Rev Neurol.* 2015;11(6):311-312.
114. Soul JS, Bergin AM, Stopp C, et al. A pilot randomized, controlled, double-blind trial of bumetanide to treat neonatal seizures. *Ann Neurol.* 2021;89(2):327-340.
115. Freeman JM, Kossoff EH. Ketosis and the ketogenic diet, 2010: advances in treating epilepsy and other disorders. *Adv Pediatr.* 2010;57(1):315-329.
116. Martin K, Jackson CF, Levy RG, Cooper PN. Ketogenic diet and other dietary treatments for epilepsy. *Cochrane Database Syst Rev.* 2016;2:CD001903.
117. Rubenstein JE. Use of the ketogenic diet in neonates and infants. *Epilepsia.* 2008;49(suppl 8):30-32.
118. Cusmai R, Martinelli D, Moavero R, et al. Ketogenic diet in early myoclonic encephalopathy due to non ketotic hyperglycinemia. *Eur J Paediatr Neurol.* 2012;16(5):509-513.
119. Gospe SM. Neonatal vitamin-responsive epileptic encephalopathies. *Chang Gung Med J.* 2010;33(1):1-12.
120. Bass NE, Wyllie E, Cohen B, Joseph SA. Pyridoxine-dependent epilepsy: the need for repeated pyridoxine trials and the risk of severe electrocerebral suppression with intravenous pyridoxine infusion. *J Child Neurol.* 1996;11(5):422-424.
121. Stockler S, Plecko B, Gospe SM, et al. Pyridoxine dependent epilepsy and antiquitin deficiency: clinical and molecular characteristics and recommendations for diagnosis, treatment and follow-up. *Mol Genet Metab.* 2011;104(1-2):48-60.
122. Pearl PL. Amenable treatable severe pediatric epilepsies. *Semin Pediatr Neurol.* 2016;23(2):158-166.
123. Plecko B, Paul K, Paschke E, et al. Biochemical and molecular characterization of 18 patients with pyridoxine-dependent epilepsy and mutations of the antiquitin (ALDH7A1) gene. *Hum Mutat.* 2007;28(1):19-26.
124. Bok LA, Struys E, Willemsen MAAP, Been JV, Jakobs C. Pyridoxine-dependent seizures in Dutch patients: diagnosis by elevated urinary alpha-aminoadipic semialdehyde levels. *Arch Dis Child.* 2007;92(8):687-689.
125. Baxter P. Pyridoxine-dependent seizures: a clinical and biochemical conundrum. *Biochim Biophys Acta.* 2003;1647(1-2):36-41.
126. Pearl PL. New treatment paradigms in neonatal metabolic epilepsies. *J Inherit Metab Dis.* 2009;32(2):204-213.
127. Sudarsanam A, Singh H, Wilcken B, et al. Cirrhosis associated with pyridoxal 5′-phosphate treatment of pyridoxamine 5′-phosphate oxidase deficiency. *JIMD Rep.* 2014;17:67-70.
128. Bräutigam C, Hyland K, Wevers R, et al. Clinical and laboratory findings in twins with neonatal epileptic encephalopathy mimicking aromatic L-amino acid decarboxylase deficiency. *Neuropediatrics.* 2002;33(3):113-117.
129. Clayton PT, Surtees RA, DeVile C, Hyland K, Heales SJR. Neonatal epileptic encephalopathy. *Lancet.* 2003;361(9369):1614.
130. Van Hove JLK, Lohr NJ. Metabolic and monogenic causes of seizures in neonates and young infants. *Mol Genet Metab.* 2011;104(3):214-230.
131. Hyland K, Buist NR, Powell BR, et al. Folinic acid responsive seizures: a new syndrome? *J Inherit Metab Dis.* 1995;18(2):177-181.
132. Nicolai J, van Kranen-Mastenbroek VHJM, Wevers RA, Hurkx WAPT, Vles JSH. Folinic acid-responsive seizures initially responsive to pyridoxine. *Pediatr Neurol.* 2006;34(2):164-167.
133. Gallagher RC, Van Hove JLK, Scharer G, et al. Folinic acid-responsive seizures are identical to pyridoxine-dependent epilepsy. *Ann Neurol.* 2009;65(5):550-556.
134. Zempleni J, Hassan YI, Wijeratne SS. Biotin and biotinidase deficiency. *Expert Rev Endocrinol Metab.* 2008;3(6):715-724.
135. Wolf B. Clinical issues and frequent questions about biotinidase deficiency. *Mol Genet Metab.* 2010;100(1):6-13.
136. Volpe JJ. Neonatal seizures: current concepts and revised classification. *Pediatrics.* 1989;84(3):422-428.
137. Shellhaas RA, Chang T, Wusthoff CJ, et al. Treatment duration after acute symptomatic seizures in neonates: a multicenter cohort study. *J Pediatr.* 2017;181:298-301.e1.
138. Brod SA, Ment LR, Ehrenkranz RA, Bridgers S. Predictors of success for drug discontinuation following neonatal seizures. *Pediatr Neurol.* 1988;4(1):13-17.
139. Glass HC, Soul JS, Chang T, et al. Safety of early discontinuation of antiseizure medication after acute symptomatic neonatal seizures. *JAMA Neurol.* 2021;78(7):817-825.

Chapter 14

Neuroprotective Therapies in Newborns

Sonia L. Bonifacio, MD; Krisa P. Van Meurs, MD

Key Points

- Preterm and term infants are at risk of acquiring brain injury with lasting neurodevelopmental sequelae.
- Mechanisms of brain injury in the developing brain are related to unique vulnerabilities due to the maturational stage of the various types of cells in the brain.
- The pathogenesis of brain injury in both preterm and term infants provides multiple opportunities for therapeutic intervention, such as addressing excitotoxicity, inflammation, oxidative stress, cytokines, and mechanisms of repair and regeneration.
- In the future, it is plausible that a cocktail of medications may be prescribed to address the mechanisms of brain injury at different time points during the injury and repair process.
- Antenatal steroids and magnesium sulfate should be administered to women at risk of delivering a premature infant, as they have been proven to reduce the risk of developing intraventricular hemorrhage.
- Therapeutic hypothermia is the standard of care for term and near-term infants with moderate to severe hypoxic–ischemic encephalopathy, but its use in infants with mild HIE or in infants at 33 to 35 weeks' gestation requires further study. Additional drugs such as erythropoiesis-stimulating agents, xenon, melatonin, and allopurinol are being studied as single-agent therapies or as adjunctive treatments to further reduce the risk of death or disability in these infants.

Introduction

Sick infants are at significant risk for the acquisition of perinatal brain injury. Concerns about long-term neurologic sequelae have increased along with improved survival of extremely premature infants, movement of the limits of viability toward earlier gestational ages, and increased survival among infants with complex medical and surgical conditions. According to the Centers for Disease Control and Prevention, one in 10 infants born in the United States in 2020 was premature. Mortality is highest among the smallest and youngest premature infants, and 40% of survivors have cognitive or physical disabilities. The lifetime cost associated with cognitive and physical disabilities is >$1,000,000 per family, without accounting for parental loss of work to care for a disabled child or family emotional burdens.

Major advances in respiratory and cardiovascular care have not been matched by advances in prevention or treatment of brain injury in premature infants. The best protective strategy remains prevention of preterm birth. Neuroprotective strategies for premature infants focus on antenatal management and postnatal strategies such as providing thermoregulation and maintenance of hemodynamic and respiratory stability, particularly in the first 3 to 7 days after birth. Current regimens thought to further improve neurologic outcomes in preterm infants include antenatal administration of betamethasone or magnesium sulfate, delivery in an appropriate center with a well-trained and experienced resuscitation team, use of delayed cord clamping at birth, postnatal treatment with indomethacin or caffeine, and use of neuroprotective bundles aimed at reducing intraventricular hemorrhage (IVH).

For term infants, there has been significant progress over the last 15 years for those with neonatal encephalopathy due to presumed perinatal asphyxia, also known as hypoxic–ischemic encephalopathy (HIE). Eleven randomized controlled trials (RCTs) that enrolled >1500 infants demonstrated the efficacy of therapeutic hypothermia in reducing the risks of death and neurodevelopmental impairment in infants with HIE.[1] Therapeutic hypothermia is the only clinically available treatment for moderate to severe HIE and is considered the standard of care for this patient population.[2] Several medications, including erythropoietin (EPO), darbepoetin, xenon, topiramate, melatonin, magnesium sulfate, and stem cells are under evaluation to determine if they provide neuroprotection in addition to that of hypothermia. Other agents have been evaluated in animals but are not yet ready for clinical trials. In this chapter, we review neuroprotective strategies and therapies currently in use or being evaluated for use in preterm or term infants.

Neuroprotective Therapies and Strategies for Premature Infants

The pathophysiology of brain injury in premature infants is complex, reflecting developmental susceptibility of the immature and rapidly changing preterm brain,[3,4] fragility of the vascular germinal matrix (where IVHs originate),[5] and the impacts of various measures needed to sustain life outside of the womb.[6,7] The chronic inflammatory state often associated with life-sustaining intensive care is postulated to interfere with normal brain development and may account for the focal injuries to and abnormal maturation of white matter detected using advanced magnetic resonance and diffusion tensor imaging techniques.[8–14] Chronic mechanical ventilation, oxygen exposure, sepsis, necrotizing enterocolitis, surgery (e.g., ligation of a patent ductus arteriosus), and suboptimal nutrition all likely contribute to the brain pathology observed in this population. At 24 weeks' gestation, the white matter is populated predominantly by immature oligodendrocytes and lacks myelination, and the cortex is undergoing development and reorganization via neuronal migration and synaptogenesis. Over the next 12 to 16 weeks, while the extremely premature infant is cared for in the neonatal intensive care unit (NICU), the brain undergoes tremendous growth and development (Figure 14.1). Abnormal development of the brain may be caused by direct damage to the brain tissue (as occurs in periventricular hemorrhagic infarction, or PVHI, previously known as grade 4 IVH) or by interruption of normal development without tissue disruption.[15] Between 24 and 32 weeks' postmenstrual age, preoligodendrocytes and the subplate neurons are highly vulnerable to oxidative injury, hypoxia, and excitotoxicity.[15] Impaired maturation of preoligodendrocytes leads to abnormalities of the white matter on ultrasound and magnetic resonance imaging (MRI), and later poor head growth, motor abnormalities such as cerebral palsy, and other neurodevelopmental disabilities.

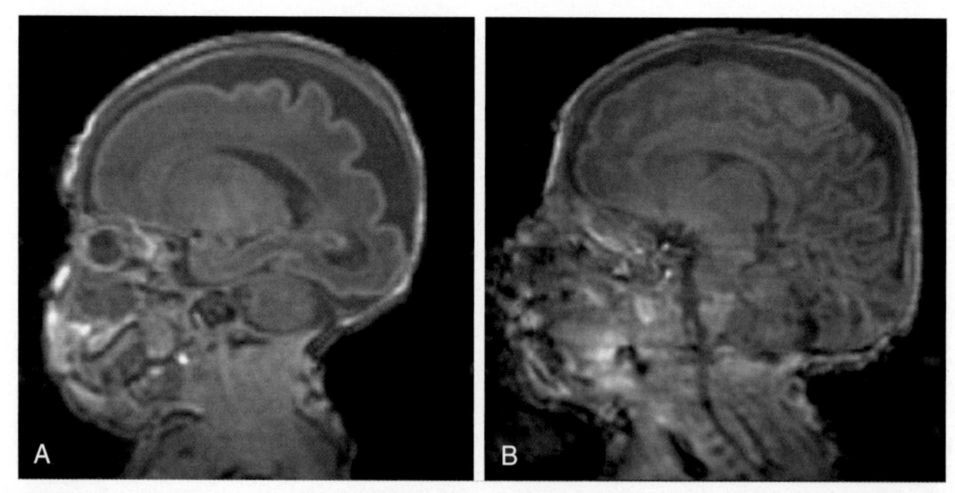

Figure 14.1 MRI images of a preterm infant born at 26 weeks gestation. (A) Midline sagittal image acquired between 26 and 27 weeks. (B) The same infant imaged 7 weeks later. Note the growth and development of complexity during the interval while the infant was cared for in the intensive care nursery.

Care Bundles to Reduce IVH and Improve Neurodevelopmental Outcome

Care practices during the antenatal and perinatal period may affect the pathogenesis of brain injury. Due to the complex pathophysiology that leads to the development of IVH, care bundles based on avoidance of abnormal physiologic or coagulopathic states have been used in quality improvement studies to attempt to reduce IVH and ultimately improve neurodevelopmental outcome.[16] Antenatal steroids and magnesium sulfate are both associated with lower rates of IVH. Management at the time of delivery, including delayed cord clamping,[17] resuscitation by an experienced team, and practices such as early continuous positive airway pressure,[18] slow rates of volume administration of infusion, and gentle or noninvasive ventilation strategies may also reduce brain injury.[18] Midline head positioning, minimal handling, reduction of stress and painful procedures, and addressing nutritional deficiencies have been identified as potentially helpful.[16,19] Given the premature infant's limited ability to autoregulate cerebral blood flow, measures should be taken to avoid hypotension, hypertension, and hypocarbia or hypercarbia. Hyperoxia is also toxic to the developing brain by promoting production of oxygen free radicals.[20] Targeted oxygen saturation goals may help prevent exposure to high oxygen levels. Early introduction of breast milk (mother's own or donor milk) may improve immune status and early gut function and thus reduce the risk of developing necrotizing enterocolitis.[21] Developmental care practices such as containment devices, protection from noise and light, and kangaroo or skin-to-skin care are also frequently included in care bundles.[22] However, evidence that demonstrates the efficacy of these methods to prevent high-grade IVH, PVHI, periventricular leukomalacia, or long-term motor or cognitive impairment remains limited.

Antenatal Betamethasone

Among very-low-birth-weight infants (<1500 g), the incidence of IVH is about 20%.[23] In extremely low-birth-weight infants (<1000 g), the incidence of IVH is 45%.[23] Increasing use of antenatal betamethasone since the 1980s has been associated with a commensurate reduction in the rate of IVH.[24] The initial studies of antenatal steroids in the 1970s and 1980s, including the landmark study of Liggins and Howie in 1972,[25] had the primary goal of improving respiratory outcomes. The most recent *Cochrane Review*, which includes data on >8000 infants, shows that antenatal steroid treatment is also associated with decreased risk of perinatal death (relative risk [RR] = 0.72; 95% confidence interval [CI], 0.58–0.89), neonatal death (RR = 0.69; 95% CI, 0.59–0.81), any grade of IVH (RR = 0.55; 95% CI, 0.40–0.76), and severe (grade 3 or 4) IVH (RR = 0.26; 95% CI, 0.11–0.60).[26] Despite these and other benefits, meta-analyses have not shown an improvement in long-term developmental outcomes.

The mechanisms by which antenatal steroid treatment reduces IVH are thought to be similar to those of indomethacin, including structural stabilization and reduced permeability of the basement membrane of the germinal matrix vasculature. In theory, these changes should make the fragile germinal matrix more tolerant to changes in cerebral blood flow caused by episodes of hypoxia, hypercarbia, or hypocarbia or unstable blood pressure.

Recent work has focused on the relationships between the risk of IVH and the proximity of antenatal betamethasone exposure to delivery or repeated courses of antenatal steroids. A recent study of 429 infants <28 weeks at birth evaluated the impact of proximity of steroid exposure and severe IVH (grade 3 or 4).[27] In premature infants born ≥10 days after a course of maternal betamethasone, the rate of severe IVH was 17% compared with 7% for those born <10 days after steroid exposure (adjusted odds ratio [aOR] = 4.16; 95% CI, 1.59–10.87; *P* = 0.004). This higher risk of IVH potentially may be reversed by a repeat course of steroids, because infants who received a second course had a rate of IVH of 8%, similar to that for infants born <10 days after the first course. Investigators examined the dose-dependent effect of antenatal corticosteroids (ANS) on neonatal mortality, morbidities, and neurodevelopmental outcome by comparing cohorts 401 to 1000 g or 22 to 27 weeks' gestation with no ANS, partial ANS, and complete ANS. This observational study found significant differences in death (43%, 29.6%, and 25.2%, respectively), severe IVH (23.3%, 19.1, and 11.7%, respectively), death or necrotizing enterocolitis

(48.1%, 37.1%, and 32.5%, respectively), death or bronchopulmonary dysplasia (74.9%, 68.9%, and 65.5%, respectively), and the primary outcome of death or neurodevelopmental impairment (68.1%, 54.4%, and 48.1%, respectively). These results emphasize the importance of prompt administration of ANS to women with threatened preterm delivery with a goal of providing a complete course prior to delivery.[28] A recent RCT performed by the National Institute of Child Health and Human Development Maternal–Fetal Medicine Units Network in women at 34 to 36 weeks 5 days of gestation at high risk for delivery found a significantly reduced risk of neonatal respiratory complications in the betamethasone-treated group but no difference in IVH.[29] Given the beneficial impact of antenatal steroids on both respiratory and neurologic outcomes, it should be the goal to administer betamethasone to all women at risk of delivery at <37 weeks' gestation.

Magnesium Sulfate

Magnesium sulfate was introduced to prevent maternal eclampsia and was then used as a tocolytic agent. It was later recognized in the late 1980s and early 1990s to have neuroprotective effects, with a reduction in the rate of IVH after treatment of mothers with preeclampsia. Concurrently, animal evidence of neuroprotection in age-appropriate models suggested benefit for human fetuses in the range of 26 to 34 weeks' gestational age.[30] Several subsequent controlled trials, including four in which the primary outcome was neuroprotection of the fetus, have confirmed this effect. Meta-analyses demonstrate a clear reduction in the risk of cerebral palsy at 18 to 24 months of corrected age, but data on whether this benefit is sustained at early childhood are conflicting.[31] Antenatal administration to mothers at risk of preterm delivery reduces the risk of cerebral palsy (RR = 0.68; 95% CI, 0.54–0.97) and the rate of substantial gross motor dysfunction (unable to walk without assistance at age 2 years) (RR = 0.61; 95% CI, 0.44–0.85).[31] Antenatal magnesium sulfate administration is considered standard of care by the American College of Obstetricians and Gynecologists for women presenting with preterm labor at <32 weeks' gestation and expected to deliver within 7 days. Dosing regimens vary, in the range of a 4- to 6-g loading dose followed by 1 to 2 g/hr by continuous infusion for 12 to 24 hours.

The mechanism of neuroprotective action of magnesium sulfate is not well understood. Magnesium is important for key cellular processes such as glycolysis, oxidative phosphorylation, protein synthesis, DNA and RNA aggregation, and maintenance of cell membrane integrity. Magnesium is also involved in mechanisms of cell death and dysfunction, modulating inflammatory cytokines and free radicals, and preventing excitotoxic calcium injury by reducing calcium entry into cells. Finally, magnesium may have important hemodynamic effects that stabilize cerebral blood flow and thus reduce the risk of IVH.[30]

Caffeine

Apnea, defined as cessation of breathing for more than 15 seconds, occurs in at least 85% of infants born at <34 weeks' gestation and is frequently accompanied by bradycardia and desaturation. Caffeine, a methylxanthine respiratory stimulant, is one of the most commonly used medications in premature infants.[32] Methylxanthines reduce both apnea and the need for mechanical ventilation. However, methylxanthines inhibit adenosine receptors, and adenosine preserves brain adenosine triphosphate (ATP) levels during experimental hypoxia and ischemia.[33] They also increase oxygen consumption and may diminish growth.[34] Accordingly, there was uncertainty about short- and long-term benefits or risks of methylxanthine treatment.[35]

This uncertainty was addressed by the Caffeine for Apnea of Prematurity (CAP) trial, an RCT in infants with birth weights of 500 to 1250 g (N = 2006).[36] The primary outcome was a composite outcome of death, cerebral palsy or cognitive delay, deafness, or blindness assessed at 18 to 21 months of age.[37] Caffeine decreased death or survival with neurodevelopmental disability (40.2% vs. 46.2%; aOR = 0.77; 95% CI, 0.64–0.93; P = 0.008). Significant reductions in cerebral palsy and cognitive delay were observed without any difference in the rates of death, deafness, or blindness. The number of infants needed to prevent one adverse outcome was 16 (95% CI, 9–56).

When the CAP trial participants were seen at 5 years of age, caffeine therapy was no longer associated with a significantly lower risk of death or disability (21.1% vs. 24.8%; aOR = 0.82; 95% CI, 0.65–1.03; P = 0.09).[38] Interestingly, the incidence of cognitive impairment at 5 years was similar in the placebo- and caffeine-treated groups and was lower than at 18 months, but gross motor impairment was less severe in the caffeine-treated infants, who had better motor coordination and visual perception. The rate of developmental coordination disorder (a form of motor dysfunction not associated with cerebral palsy or cognitive dysfunction, defined as motor performance less than the fifth percentile on the Movement Assessment Battery for Children) was lower in the caffeine-treated group (11.3% vs. 15.2%; OR = 0.71; 95% CI, 0.52–0.97; P = 0.032).[39] This was felt to be an important finding, because developmental coordination disorder is associated with learning disabilities, poor school performance, behavioral problems, poor social skills, and low self-esteem. The CAP trial has now followed 76% of the original cohort to 11 years of age, when the primary outcome was functional impairment defined as a composite of poor academic performance, motor impairment, and behavior problems. Rates of functional impairment were not significantly different between the groups, but caffeine therapy was associated with a reduced risk of motor impairment (19.7% vs. 27.5%; OR = 0.66; 95% CI, 0.48–0.90; P = 0.009).[40]

Caffeine has been called a silver bullet in neonatology because of its wide therapeutic index, tolerability, and efficacy in reducing bronchopulmonary dysplasia, patent ductus arteriosus, severe retinopathy of prematurity, and neurodevelopmental disability. Few drugs used in the neonatal period have been tested in RCTs with follow-up out to 11 years with continued evidence of benefit. The exact mechanisms responsible for neuroprotection remain incompletely elucidated. Brain microstructural changes consisting of improved myelination have been seen in the caffeine-treated group, and larger MRI studies are underway to better understand this finding.[41]

Indomethacin

Indomethacin, a nonsteroidal anti-inflammatory drug, diminishes prostaglandin production by inhibiting the activity of cyclooxygenase. Indomethacin was initially used in neonatology to promote closure of the ductus arteriosus, but administration within hours after birth also has independent effects that reduce early IVH. Meta-analyses show that indomethacin administered prophylactically (within 24 hours of birth) can reduce the risk of grade III or IV IVH (RR = 0.66; 95% CI, 0.53–0.82; number needed to treat, 20). Despite a reduction in severe IVH, prophylactic indomethacin has not been shown to improve longer-term neurodevelopment in very-low-birth-weight infants.[42] The mechanisms of IVH prevention are thought to include promotion of vascular stability during episodes of hypoxia or hypercapnia, preventing ischemia-related hyperperfusion. Indomethacin is also thought to promote maturation of the germinal matrix.[43,44]

Erythropoiesis-Stimulating Agents: Erythropoietin/Darbepoetin

Preclinical studies have found neuronal repair, regeneration, antioxidant, anti-inflammatory, and antiapoptotic effects of erythropoiesis-stimulating agents (ESAs).[45] EPO is an endogenous cytokine produced by the liver in the fetus and in the kidney postnatally. Although primarily known for its effects on erythropoiesis, EPO is also produced in the brain, where it acts as a growth factor and neuroprotectant for the developing brain.[46] Several cell types in the brain, including neurons, oligodendrocytes, astrocytes, and microglia, produce EPO. Neuroprotective properties include promoting transcription of antiapoptotic genes, reduction of inflammation and oxidation, and long-term effects that promote healing, such as angiogenesis, neurogenesis, and olidendrogenesis. EPO production is stimulated by hypoxia, although prolonged periods of hypoxia are thought to be required to upregulate production. In rodent and nonhuman primate models of hypoxia–ischemia, EPO has demonstrated both histologic and functional benefit. A surprising and clinically appealing property identified in a rodent model of hypoxia–ischemia is that EPO could provide functional and histologic neuroprotection even if administered 7 days after the insult.[47] These characteristics make ESAs promising therapeutic agents for brain injury in preterm infants and for term infants with HIE.

ESAs appear to be ideal neuroprotectants to combat brain injury in premature infants. As reviewed earlier, inflammation and arrest of cellular development are characteristics of brain injury in preterm infants. EPO combats inflammation and promotes neurogenesis. It has been widely used to stimulate erythropoiesis in preterm infants, who often are exposed to EPO for several weeks during their hospital course, providing ample data on safety and tolerability. Neuroprotective doses are higher than those needed to stimulate red blood cell production. Animal and human studies have been performed to elucidate appropriate dosing strategies.[48] Darbepoetin alfa (Darbe) is a long-acting form of EPO. An RCT comparing Darbe (10 µg/kg/wk), EPO (400 U/kg three times per week), and placebo, with dosing starting at <48 hours after birth and continuing through 35 weeks' postmenstrual age, was performed to evaluate if Darbe and EPO would reduce transfusion needs in premature infants born weighing 500 to 1250 g.[49] At follow-up of 80 of the 102 randomized infants at 18 to 22 months of age, infants in the Darbe and EPO groups had significantly higher cognitive scores than those in the placebo group.[50] In addition, none of the ESA-treated patients developed cerebral palsy, compared with five in the placebo group, and the odds of neurodevelopmental impairment were lower in the ESA-treated group (OR = 0.18; 95% CI, 0.05–0.63). This benefit of ESAs persisted at 3.5 to 4 years of age, with higher full-scale and performance IQ in treated infants compared with those who received placebo.[51] A large phase III trial of darbepoetin to improve red cell mass and provide neuroprotection has completed enrollment and is in the follow-up phase. This trial recruited 650 infants born at 23 to 28 weeks' gestation for enrollment within 24 hours after birth. Darbe or placebo was administered weekly at a dose of 10 µg/kg weekly. The primary outcome is the composite cognitive score on the Bayley III examination at a corrected gestational age of 26 months (NCT03169881).

Neuroprotective effects of EPO have also been directly studied in premature infants. The Swiss EPO Neuroprotection Trial Group recently reported neurodevelopmental outcomes for preterm infants (26–32 weeks' gestation at birth; mean, 29 weeks) who were randomized to receive high-dose EPO (3000 U/kg) or placebo at 3, 12 to 18, and 36 to 42 hours after birth. There were no differences in the primary outcome between the study groups. The mean mental developmental index (MDI) of the Bayley II at 2 years of age was 93.5 (95% CI, 91.2–95.8) in the EPO group and 94.5 (95% CI, 90.8–98.5) in the placebo group.[52] Compared with other trials of ESAs, which showed benefit in this population, this trial enrolled slightly older infants, the control group had a higher than expected MDI score, and the duration of the EPO dosing regimen was much shorter. The latter may not adequately address the mechanism of brain injury in premature infants. A U.S. trial of EPO in preterm infants (Preterm Erythropoietin Neuroprotection Trial [PENUT]; NCT01378273) was recently completed. This is a multicenter, placebo-controlled, randomized trial of 941 preterm infants (24–28 weeks) randomized to placebo or high-dose EPO (1000 U/kg intravenous [IV] every 48 hours for 6 doses for the first 2 weeks after birth) followed by low-dose EPO (400 U/kg subcutaneous three times per week until 32-6/7 weeks) with neurodevelopmental outcome determined at 24 to 26 months of age. The trial failed to demonstrate a benefit of EPO with equal rates of death or severe neurodevelopmental impairment at 2 years of age.[53]

Management of Pain Versus Impact of Analgesics and Sedatives on the Developing Brain

The impact of pain on the developing brain and neurodevelopmental outcome is a recent area of focus in neonatal care. Measures to provide comfort and developmentally appropriate care are emphasized to support the developing brain. The NICU in no way resembles the relatively quiet, dark, and insulated environment in which the fetus develops in utero. Premature infants in the NICU are constantly stimulated and have interrupted sleep–wake cycles. The optimal balance between overstimulation and understimulation is uncertain, as leaving a developing infant in a dark incubator without interaction is also unlikely to promote healthy development. Recent studies have addressed the importance of the NICU environment and parental interaction on neurodevelopment.[54,55] Exposure to maternal voice improves infant physiologic stability and reduces pain.[56,57] In contrast, a growing body of literature describes ill effects of painful procedures on brain development, as measured by MRI or by neurodevelopment at school age. Routine procedures in the NICU, such as heel sticks for laboratory monitoring or placement of intravenous lines, are painful. Many infants experience more than 100 of these procedures while under our care. Recent investigations have identified that the number of painful procedures affects white matter development and is associated with lower IQ at age 7.[58] Some painful procedures cannot be avoided, so treatment with analgesics and sedatives may be warranted. However, there is also a growing body of evidence demonstrating adverse impacts of some of these medications on the developing brain. Fentanyl and morphine have been associated with both injury to and abnormal growth of the cerebellum,[59,60] and midazolam has been associated with abnormalities of the hippocampus.[61] Although not frequently used in the NICU environment, animal data suggest that inhaled anesthetics may trigger neuronal apoptosis (programmed cell death).[62] Best practices to better balance the need for painful procedures and sedation or analgesia need to be developed to minimize the risk of iatrogenic neurodevelopmental harm.

Neuroprotective Strategies for Term Infants

Brain injury due to hypoxia–ischemia is an important cause of death or significant neurodevelopmental disability. HIE is a major cause of neonatal death across the globe, with an incidence ranging from one to six per 1000 live births. Hypoxic or ischemic insults may trigger multiple pathways that result in cell death. The initial event can result in immediate cell death (cellular necrosis) or trigger processes that evolve over a period of hours to days or weeks post-insult (Figure 14.2).[63] These pathways include oxidative stress, inflammation, and excitatory pathways, which lead to both early and late cellular dysfunction and may trigger programmed cell death (apoptosis). A hypoxic–ischemic insult immediately leads to

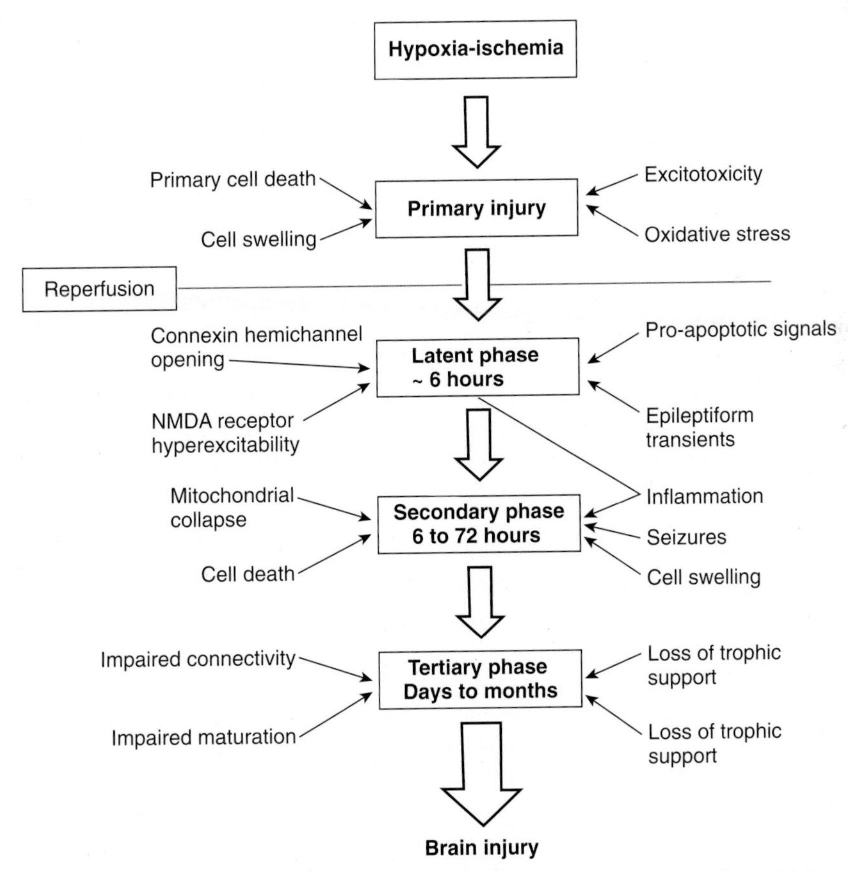

Figure 14.2 **Mechanisms of evolving neuronal injury cascade after an hypoxic–ischemic insult during the primary, latent, secondary, and tertiary phases of injury that occur over hours, days, weeks, and months, highlighting potential therapeutic targets for prevention and repair.** (Image from Davidson JO, et al. Therapeutic hypothermia for neonatal hypoxic–ischemic encephalopathy—where to go from here? *Front Neurol.* 2015;6:198.)

cellular depolarization, release of excitotoxins, calcium entry into cells, and cell lysis. After the insult there is a period of reperfusion, which may correlate with clinical resuscitation, during which aerobic metabolism recovers but the earlier mentioned deleterious pathways have been triggered. The insult itself is a trigger that causes downstream cascades that are thought to occur in a latent phase (6–15 hours after the insult) and a secondary phase (6 hours to 3 days after the insult), during which secondary energy failure may occur (see Figure 14.2). Drugs that may ameliorate or block these pathways, thus reducing apoptosis and neuronal injury and thereby preventing neurodevelopmental impairments, are discussed later.

Clinically Available Treatments: Therapeutic Hypothermia

Therapeutic hypothermia was first identified in the mid-1900s to provide neuroprotection after hypoxic–ischemic insults in animal studies. As early as the 1950s, improved outcomes were reported in small studies of immersing apneic infants in water baths until the onset of spontaneous respiration.[64] Hypothermia was not tested again in large RCTs until the late 1990s. In 2013, a meta-analysis of 11 RCTs including >1500 infants found that therapeutic hypothermia significantly decreased the rate of death or moderate to severe neurodisability.[1] Treatment with hypothermia resulted in a significant reduction in the risk of death or disability (RR = 0.75; 95% CI, 0.68–0.83; number needed to treat, 7; 95% CI, 5–10). Therapeutic hypothermia appears to be most beneficial when initiated within 6 hours after birth. Although not yet proven, some data suggest that initiating treatment within 4 hours after birth may optimize efficacy.[65,66] Infants are cooled to 33.5°C ± 0.5°C for 72 hours, then rewarmed slowly over 6 hours. Most centers use servo-regulated cooling devices that circulate cold water through a blanket that is either placed underneath or wrapped around the infant, although cooling caps with moderate body hypothermia have also been used. Overall, the treatment is safe, with few adverse effects. Some adverse effects, including persistent pulmonary hypertension (about 25% of infants), coagulopathy, and thrombocytopenia, may be related directly to perinatal asphyxia itself.

The mechanisms by which hypothermia provides neuroprotection are not completely understood. Hypothermia likely affects many of the pathways triggered by hypoxic–ischemic insults.[67] One primary effect is a reduction in the metabolic rate. The metabolic rate decreases by 5% with each reduction in body temperature of 1°C, resulting in decreased energy consumption and delay of anoxic cell depolarization. The neonatal brain is one of the most metabolically active organs, with the neurons in the cortex and the deep gray structures being much more metabolically active than the white matter. Reducing the metabolic rate in these areas of the brain may impede the injurious cellular cascades that are triggered after a hypoxic–ischemic insult.

Recent trials of longer and deeper hypothermia and late-onset hypothermia (onset between >6 and <24 hours after birth) have been completed. The longer and deeper cooling trial was terminated early due to safety concerns in the deeper and longer arms of the study, with increased mortality compared with the standard cooling (33.5°C for 72 hours) arm, although death in all arms was lower than in the initial trials of hypothermia.[68] Using Bayesian statistics, the late hypothermia trial demonstrated a 77% chance of some benefit but only a 58% chance that late hypothermia would result in a 10% or greater reduction in the risk of death or disability.[69] Treatment of premature infants (33–35 weeks' gestation) is being studied in an RCT (NCT01793129) that has completed enrollment of 168 newborns; analysis will again use Bayesian statistics due to the limited sample size. A trial of therapeutic hypothermia performed in India, Sri Lanka, and Bangladesh to determine the efficacy and safety in low- and middle-income countries (LMICs) found that cooling did not reduce death or disability.[70] The primary outcome occurred in 42.2% in the hypothermia group compared to 31.3% in the control group ($P = 0.02$). The authors concluded that therapeutic hypothermia should not be offered in LMICs even when tertiary NICU care is available. Around 80% of the infants in this trial had white-matter injury, suggesting a subacute or partial prolonged hypoxia that may explain the absence of neuroprotection.

Therapies Under Study

ERYTHROPOIESIS-STIMULATING AGENTS

An appealing aspect of ESAs is that they are thought to promote neurogenesis and repair post-injury and have efficacy even when administered 24 hours or more after an insult.[47,71] Several human studies have evaluated ESAs, either alone or in combination with hypothermia, as a treatment for infants with HIE. A phase I dose escalation safety and pharmacokinetics study identified an EPO dose of 1000 U/kg intravenously every 48 hours as providing serum concentrations equivalent to the neuroprotective ranges identified in animal studies (NCT00719407).[72] The phase I/II Neonatal Erythropoietin and Therapeutic Hypothermia Outcomes in Newborn Brain Injury (NEATO) trial aimed at determining safety and feasibility of enrolling infants with HIE treated with hypothermia into an RCT of EPO or placebo within 24 hours of delivery. The dosing regimen was 1000 U/kg at 1, 2, 3, 5, and 7 days of age. Secondary outcomes included brain injury on MRI within the first week after birth and motor and developmental testing at 1 year of age. EPO was associated with decreased brain injury and improved motor performance.[73] A large phase III trial (High-Dose Erythropoietin for Asphyxia and Encephalopathy [HEAL]; NCT02811263) was recently completed. There was no significant difference in the rate of death or neurodevelopmental impairment between those treated with high-dose EPO in addition to hypothermia versus hypothermia alone (53% vs. 50%; RR = 1.03; 95% CI, 0.86–1.24), and there was a concern for harm, as EPO-treated infants suffered a higher burden of serious adverse events.[74]

ESAs are also being studied in infants with stroke, a focal hypoxic–ischemic injury. A double-blinded, placebo-controlled, randomized trial of darbepoetin for perinatal arterial ischemic stroke is being planned. Infants will be eligible if they are identified to have a middle cerebral artery stroke within 1 week of birth and will receive two doses of darbepoetin 10 μg/kg IV or placebo. The study will include 80 patients to be enrolled at two centers in Canada and one in the Netherlands (NCT03171818). The primary outcome is stroke tissue volume loss at 6 to 8 weeks after birth, and secondary outcomes include neurodevelopment at 18 months of age.

TOPIRAMATE

Topiramate, an anticonvulsant, is thought to act by inhibiting activation of glutamate receptors, thus preventing programmed cell death. Topiramate also blocks sodium and calcium channels, inhibits carbonic anhydrase, and affects mitochondrial permeability. In vitro and in vivo animal data suggest a beneficial effect of topiramate. A safety and feasibility study in 44 infants with HIE, comparing topiramate 10 mg/kg for 3 days with placebo, was recently completed (NCT01241019).[75] There were no differences in safety or other outcome measures, but epilepsy was less frequent in treated infants. Larger trials are needed to determine if adding topiramate to hypothermia further improves outcomes.

XENON

Xenon is a rare and inert noble gas known for its anesthetic and neuroprotective properties. Neuroprotective effects of xenon are likely mediated by inhibition of the *N*-methyl-D-aspartate glutamate receptor, dampening the excitotoxic phase of acute neurologic injury. Other neuroprotective actions of xenon may include activation of two-pore potassium channels, modulation of neuroapoptosis and inflammation, induction of hypoxia-inducible factor alpha, and activation of ATP-sensitive potassium channels. Xenon crosses the blood–brain barrier rapidly as a result of a low blood/gas partition coefficient. Xenon is used in Europe as an anesthetic but is not U.S. Food and Drug Administration (FDA)-approved in the United States. Its high cost makes its use as an anesthetic difficult to justify; however, it may have a role in pediatric anesthesia where anesthetic-induced neurotoxicity is a concern. Xenon is attractive for use in critically ill infants due to cardiovascular stability and myocardial protective properties.

In both in vitro and in vivo animal models, xenon and hypothermia together provide greater neuroprotection after hypoxic–ischemic injury than either treatment alone.[76,77] In an animal model of hypoxia–ischemia, dramatic improvements in function and histology were observed after administration of xenon.[77] The combination of xenon with therapeutic hypothermia is effective even when xenon administration is delayed.[78,79] However, a recent study cautioned that animals subjected to severe hypoxia–ischemia and either hypothermia alone or hypothermia plus 50% xenon did not demonstrate a benefit as measured by hemispheric brain area or subventricular zone neuronal cell counts.[80]

Clinical data on xenon use in human newborns with HIE are limited. A feasibility study in 14 infants with moderate to severe HIE who were receiving <35% oxygen increased xenon treatment time stepwise from 3 to 18 hours.[81] Xenon was delivered using a closed-circuit delivery system utilizing a modified standard anesthesia workstation with modified breathing hoses.[82] Xenon caused sedation and attenuated background amplitude integrated electroencephalogram. Seizures occurred with rapid xenon tapering but not with slow weaning. There were no adverse cardiovascular or respiratory effects. Mortality in this small study was 20%; 64% of survivors had Bayley II mental and motor scores >70.

A recently published trial randomized 92 infants with HIE to either 30% xenon for 24 hours along with cooling or to cooling alone at a median age of 11 hours.[83] There were no significant differences in the primary MRI outcomes of the reduced lactate to *N*-acetylaspartate ratio in the thalamus and preserved fractional anisotropy in the posterior limb of the internal capsule. The authors concluded that treatment with 30% xenon for 24 hours started more than 6 hours after birth did not have additional neuroprotective benefits when compared with cooling alone. The study was adequately powered to detect changes in fractional anisotropy but not for the other MRI outcome measure. The timing, dose, or duration of xenon use may not have been optimal. Another trial currently enrolling is the CoolXenon3 trial (NCT02071394). Newborns are randomized to 50% xenon for 18 hours or hypothermia alone. The primary outcome is survival without moderate or severe disability, defined as a Bayley III composite score of <85. A transport device to deliver xenon in an ambulance to allow earlier initiation of treatment has been developed.[84]

Xenon has potent anticonvulsant effects that are likely due to glutamate receptor blockade. In five infants treated with 30% xenon, seizures stopped during xenon therapy but recurred within minutes after xenon was stopped.[85] Suppression of seizures may contribute to the neuroprotective effect of xenon. Further clinical trial results with long-term outcome measures in humans are needed to determine if the neuroprotective benefits seen in animal models will be confirmed in humans.

MELATONIN

Melatonin, a low-molecular-weight hormone secreted by the pineal gland, is best known for its role in regulation of circadian rhythm but it also has important roles in normal neurodevelopment. Because melatonin readily crosses the placenta and the blood–brain barrier, it has drawn interest as a candidate treatment to reduce the risk of hypoxic–ischemic injury in high-risk deliveries. The role of its antioxidative, antiapoptotic, and anti-inflammatory activities in protecting the developing brain has been studied in animal models of both premature and term brain injury.[86] In rodent models of HIE, melatonin is neuroprotective when given either prophylactically or immediately after an hypoxic–ischemic insult. In sheep models of both term and preterm brain injury, prophylactic melatonin was neuroprotective, with effects that were specific for gestational age, such as preservation of mature oligodendrocytes in the preterm model and reduced neuronal death and astrogliosis in the term model. In a piglet model of HIE, animals treated with melatonin (5 mg/kg/hr for 5 hours starting 10 minutes after resuscitation and repeated at 24 hours) in conjunction with therapeutic hypothermia for 24 hours had decreased histologic damage in both gray- and white-matter regions, and magnetic resonance spectroscopy demonstrated decreased lactate with preservation of cerebral ATP.[87]

One small trial randomized 15 infants to treatment with melatonin (10 mg/kg orally for 5 days) with hypothermia and 15 to hypothermia alone.[88] Melatonin was well tolerated without adverse effects and was associated with decreased white-matter injury on MRI and increased survival with a normal neurologic examination at 6 months of age. The sample size was small, and long-term neurodevelopmental follow-up is not available. The optimal neuroprotective dose of melatonin is not yet known. An ongoing dose-escalation study in infants with moderate to severe HIE receiving therapeutic hypothermia will randomize 30 infants and increase the dose from 0.5 to 5 mg/kg (NCT02621944).

ALLOPURINOL

Allopurinol, a xanthine oxidase inhibitor, acts as a neuroprotectant by preventing the formation of free radicals that trigger programmed cell death. Free-radical production occurs after reperfusion and reoxygenation after a hypoxic–ischemic insult. Allopurinol was neuroprotective in a rodent model of hypoxic–ischemic injury but did not improve neurodevelopmental outcome in a small human study of neonatal HIE.[89] A study enrolled only 32 of a planned 100 infants; all had severe HIE, and none was cotreated with hypothermia. The dose of allopurinol was 40 mg/kg within 4 hours after birth and then repeated at 12 hours of age. The study was stopped early due to the likelihood of not finding a difference in outcome between the groups. It is not known whether allopurinol may be more effective in moderate HIE, in conjunction with hypothermia, or with earlier initiation. One small RCT ($N = 53$) gave antenatal allopurinol to mothers with nonreassuring fetal heart rate patterns or fetal acidemia.[90] Cord blood was obtained and evaluated for lactate and S-100B, a marker of brain injury. Infants with measurable levels of allopurinol or its metabolite had lower S-100B levels, suggesting that early treatment with allopurinol should be further investigated. A proposed placebo-controlled, double-blinded trial of early allopurinol (20 mg/kg within 30 minutes of birth followed by a second dose at 12 hours of age) along with hypothermia, the Effect of Allopurinol for Hypoxic-Ischemic Brain Injury on Neurocognitive Outcome (ALBINO) trial (NCT03162653), is currently enrolling patients.

MAGNESIUM SULFATE

The neuroprotective effects of magnesium sulfate are reviewed in the preterm section. Evidence regarding neuroprotective effects of magnesium sulfate in term infants with HIE is inconsistent.[91] In animal models, there appears to be some additive neuroprotection by combining magnesium with hypothermia. The results of the one small RCT to evaluate safety of magnesium sulfate plus hypothermia for HIE (MagCool Study; NCT01646619) have not yet been published. Magnesium in addition to melatonin and/or EPO is being investigated in some low-income countries where hypothermia therapy is not readily available.

SILDENAFIL

Sildenafil, a selective phosphodiesterase type 5 (PDE5) inhibitor is also being studied in animal models and clinical trials of hypoxic–ischemic brain injury. Its mechanism of action is regulation of the second messenger cyclic guanosine monophosphate (cGMP) by inhibiting the effect of PDE5 that breaks down the phosphodiesteric bond of cGMP and hydrolyzes cGMP into GMP. It was first studied in adults and used to treat erectile dysfunction.[92] Since then, it has also been studied and approved for the treatment of pulmonary arterial hypertension in adults, and its use has been extrapolated to treat newborns with persistent pulmonary hypertension. Sildenafil is known to cross the blood–brain barrier and has been studied in animal models of adult neurological disorders, such as Alzheimer's disease, stroke, and multiple sclerosis, among others.[92] There are now animal studies of neonatal brain injury that explore the effect of sildenafil. The neuroprotective effects of sildenafil include neurogenesis, synaptoplasticity, modulation of microglial activation, inhibition of death of oligodendrocytes, and inhibition of inflammation. These actions are similar to those of other neuroprotective treatments. In rodent models, histological benefits include both reduced apoptosis and increased neurogenesis, as well as functional improvements compared to untreated animals.[92] There are now two clinical trials of sildenafil in neonates with HIE (NCT02812433 and NCT04169191).

STEM CELL THERAPY

Stem cell–based therapy to prevent or repair perinatal brain injury is an area of active investigation.[93–96] Stem cell therapies may act by diverse mechanisms at different phases of brain injury. Early studies focused on the ability of stem cells to engraft and replace dying cells. In general, the net increase in cell numbers in the brain was negligible, despite significant functional improvements. This suggests that the key mechanism is the release of neurotropic and immunomodulatory factors. This is an attractive neuroprotectant for term infants with HIE, as often the etiology and precise timing of the brain injury are unclear.

Umbilical cord blood (UCB) contains a rich and diverse mixture of stem and progenitor cells with the potential to generate a variety of cell types. UCB is one of the most abundant sources of nonembryonic stem cells and has high engraftment rates when used for transplantation with low rates of graft-versus-host disease. UCB also contains a population of mesenchymal stem cells, which have a high potential for neural differentiation.[97] In animal models of stroke and hypoxia–ischemia, UCB decreases clinical sequelae and neuroimaging abnormalities.[98,99]

Investigators studied the feasibility and safety of autologous cord blood in 23 infants with moderate to severe HIE (NCT00593242).[100] Infants were eligible if they were ≥35 weeks and met the National Institute of Child Health and Human Development criteria for therapeutic hypothermia. Cord blood was collected in deliveries of mothers who had previously consented for public banking or in deliveries where obstetric staff thought the infant might meet cooling criteria. The cord blood was volume and red blood cell reduced and divided into aliquots containing 1 to 5 × 10^7 nucleated cells. All infants were treated with therapeutic hypothermia and, after pretreatment with hydrocortisone, were given up to four UCB infusions. The first dose was given as soon as possible after birth and subsequent doses at 24, 48, and 72 hours of age.

In 2011, the FDA began regulation of UCB, and the investigational new drug protocol was modified to administer only two doses in the first 48 hours. The volume of UCB collected varied, but even the lowest collected volumes provided cell numbers adequate for at least one dose containing the target cell number. No significant adverse events occurred, but oxygen saturation decreased by 1% to 2% after the third and fourth infusions ($P < 0.05$). One-year outcomes were compared with a cohort of 82 infants who did not have UCB available and were cooled. All infants treated with autologous UCB and 87% in the comparison group survived to 1 year ($P = 0.12$). Bayley III testing was available for 18 treated infants (78%) and 46 in the comparison group (56%); in these subgroups, 74% of the UCB group and 41% of the comparison group had Bayley III scores ≥ 85 in all three testing domains (cognitive, language, and motor development). Stem cell therapy remains an intriguing possibility for newborns identified to be at risk of brain injury. Additional research is needed to determine the most appropriate cell type, dose, timing, and mode of administration, as well as to provide sufficient data on safety and outcome.

REFERENCES

1. Jacobs SE, Berg M, Hunt R, Tarnow-Mordi WO, Inder TE, Davis PG. Cooling for newborns with hypoxic ischaemic encephalopathy. *Cochrane Database Syst Rev*. 2013;(1):CD003311.
2. Papile LA, Baley JE, Benitz W, et al. Hypothermia and neonatal encephalopathy. *Pediatrics*. 2014;133(6):1146-1150.
3. Ferriero DM, Miller SP. Imaging selective vulnerability in the developing nervous system. *J Anat*. 2010;217(4):429-435.
4. Lynn S, Huang EJ, Elchuri S, et al. Selective neuronal vulnerability and inadequate stress response in superoxide dismutase mutant mice. *Free Radic Biol Med*. 2005;38(6):817-828.
5. Volpe JJ. Intraventricular hemorrhage and brain injury in the premature infant. Neuropathology and pathogenesis. *Clin Perinatol*. 1989;16(2):361-386.
6. Glass HC, Bonifacio SL, Chau V, et al. Recurrent postnatal infections are associated with progressive white matter injury in premature infants. *Pediatrics*. 2008;122(2):299-305.
7. Bonifacio SL, Glass HC, Chau V, et al. Extreme premature birth is not associated with impaired development of brain microstructure. *J Pediatr*. 2010;157(5):726-732.e1.
8. Back SA, Luo NL, Borenstein NS, Levine JM, Volpe JJ, Kinney HC. Late oligodendrocyte progenitors coincide with the developmental window of vulnerability for human perinatal white matter injury. *J Neurosci*. 2001;21(4):1302-1312.
9. Back SA, Luo NL, Borenstein NS, Volpe JJ, Kinney HC. Arrested oligodendrocyte lineage progression during human cerebral white matter development: dissociation between the timing of progenitor differentiation and myelinogenesis. *J Neuropathol Exp Neurol*. 2002;61(2):197-211.
10. Haynes RL, Xu G, Folkerth RD, Trachtenberg FL, Volpe JJ, Kinney HC. Potential neuronal repair in cerebral white matter injury in the human neonate. *Pediatr Res*. 2011;69(1):62-67.
11. Kinney HC, Haynes RL, Xu G, et al. Neuron deficit in the white matter and subplate in periventricular leukomalacia. *Ann Neurol*. 2012;71(3):397-406.
12. Back SA, Rivkees SA. Emerging concepts in periventricular white matter injury. *Semin Perinatol*. 2004;28(6):405-414.
13. Chau V, McFadden DE, Poskitt KJ, Miller SP. Chorioamnionitis in the pathogenesis of brain injury in preterm infants. *Clin Perinatol*. 2014;41(1):83-103.
14. Hagberg H, Mallard C, Ferriero DM, et al. The role of inflammation in perinatal brain injury. *Nat Rev Neurol*. 2015;11(4):192-208.
15. Back SA. Brain injury in the preterm infant: new horizons for pathogenesis and prevention. *Pediatr Neurol*. 2015;53(3):185-192.
16. McLendon D, Check J, Carteaux P, et al. Implementation of potentially better practices for the prevention of brain hemorrhage and ischemic brain injury in very low birth weight infants. *Pediatrics*. 2003;111(4 Pt 2):e497-e503.
17. Mercer JS, Vohr BR, McGrath MM, Padbury JF, Wallach M, Oh W. Delayed cord clamping in very preterm infants reduces the incidence of intraventricular hemorrhage and late-onset sepsis: a randomized, controlled trial. *Pediatrics*. 2006;117(4):1235-1242.
18. Barton SK, Tolcos M, Miller SL, et al. Unraveling the links between the initiation of ventilation and brain injury in preterm infants. *Front Pediatr*. 2015;3:97.

19. Schmid MB, Reister F, Mayer B, Hopfner RJ, Fuchs H, Hummler HD. Prospective risk factor monitoring reduces intracranial hemorrhage rates in preterm infants. *Dtsch Arztebl Int*. 2013; 110(29-30):489-496.
20. Sabir H, Jary S, Tooley J, Liu X, Thoresen M. Increased inspired oxygen in the first hours of life is associated with adverse outcome in newborns treated for perinatal asphyxia with therapeutic hypothermia. *J Pediatr*. 2012;161(3):409-416.
21. Meinzen-Derr J, Poindexter B, Wrage L, Morrow AL, Stoll B, Donovan EF. Role of human milk in extremely low birth weight infants' risk of necrotizing enterocolitis or death. *J Perinatol*. 2009;29(1):57-62.
22. Als H, McAnulty GB. The Newborn Individualized Developmental Care and Assessment Program (NIDCAP) with Kangaroo Mother Care (KMC): comprehensive care for preterm infants. *Curr Womens Health Rev*. 2011;7(3):288-301.
23. Ballabh P. Intraventricular hemorrhage in premature infants: mechanism of disease. *Pediatr Res*. 2010;67(1):1-8.
24. Wei JC, Catalano R, Profit J, Gould JB, Lee HC. Impact of antenatal steroids on intraventricular hemorrhage in very-low-birth weight infants. *J Perinatol*. 2016;36(5):352-356.
25. Liggins GC, Howie RN. A controlled trial of antepartum glucocorticoid treatment for prevention of the respiratory distress syndrome in premature infants. *Pediatrics*. 1972;50(4):515-525.
26. Roberts D, Brown J, Medley N, Dalziel SR. Antenatal corticosteroids for accelerating fetal lung maturation for women at risk of preterm birth. *Cochrane Database Syst Rev*. 2017;3:CD004454.
27. Liebowitz M, Clyman RI. Antenatal betamethasone: a prolonged time interval from administration to delivery is associated with an increased incidence of severe intraventricular hemorrhage in infants born before 28 weeks gestation. *J Pediatr*. 2016;177:114-120.e1.
28. Chawla S, Natarajan G, Shankaran S, et al. Association of neurodevelopmental outcomes and neonatal morbidities of extremely premature infants with differential exposure to antenatal steroids. *JAMA Pediatr*. 2016;170(12):1164-1172.
29. Gyamfi-Bannerman C, Thom EA, Blackwell SC, et al. Antenatal betamethasone for women at risk for late preterm delivery. *N Engl J Med*. 2016;374(14):1311-1320.
30. Marret S, Doyle LW, Crowther CA, Middleton P. Antenatal magnesium sulphate neuroprotection in the preterm infant. *Semin Fetal Neonatal Med*. 2007;12(4):311-317.
31. Bain E, Middleton P, Crowther CA. Different magnesium sulphate regimens for neuroprotection of the fetus for women at risk of preterm birth. *Cochrane Database Syst Rev*. 2012;(2):CD009302.
32. Hsieh EM, Hornik CP, Clark RH, Laughon MM, Benjamin Jr DK, Smith PB. Medication use in the neonatal intensive care unit. *Am J Perinatol*. 2014;31(9):811-821.
33. Fredholm BB. Astra Award Lecture. Adenosine, adenosine receptors and the actions of caffeine. *Pharmacol Toxicol*. 1995; 76(2):93-101.
34. Thurston JH, Hauhard RE, Dirgo JA. Aminophylline increases cerebral metabolic rate and decreases anoxic survival in young mice. *Science*. 1978;201(4356):649-651.
35. Henderson-Smart DJ, Steer P. Methylxanthine treatment for apnea in preterm infants. *Cochrane Database Syst Rev*. 2001;(3): CD000140.
36. Schmidt B, Roberts RS, Davis P, et al. Caffeine therapy for apnea of prematurity. *N Engl J Med*. 2006;354(20):2112-2121.
37. Schmidt B, Roberts RS, Davis P, et al. Long-term effects of caffeine therapy for apnea of prematurity. *N Engl J Med*. 2007; 357(19):1893-1902.
38. Schmidt B, Anderson PJ, Doyle LW, et al. Survival without disability to age 5 years after neonatal caffeine therapy for apnea of prematurity. *JAMA*. 2012;307(3):275-282.
39. Doyle LW, Schmidt B, Anderson PJ, et al. Reduction in developmental coordination disorder with neonatal caffeine therapy. *J Pediatr*. 2014;165(2):356-359.e2.
40. Schmidt B, Roberts RS, Anderson PJ, et al. Academic performance, motor function, and behavior 11 years after neonatal caffeine citrate therapy for apnea of prematurity: an 11-year follow-up of the CAP randomized clinical trial. *JAMA Pediatr*. 2017;171(6):564-572.
41. Doyle LW, Cheong J, Hunt RW, et al. Caffeine and brain development in very preterm infants. *Ann Neurol*. 2010;68(5):734-742.
42. Fowlie PW, Davis PG, McGuire W. Prophylactic intravenous indomethacin for preventing mortality and morbidity in preterm infants. *Cochrane Database Syst Rev*. 2010;(7):CD000174.
43. Coyle MG, Oh W, Petersson KH, Stonestreet BS. Effects of indomethacin on brain blood flow, cerebral metabolism, and sagittal sinus prostanoids after hypoxia. *Am J Physiol*. 1995;269 (4 Pt 2):H1450-H1459.
44. Ment LR, Stewart WB, Ardito TA, Huang E, Madri JA. Indomethacin promotes germinal matrix microvessel maturation in the newborn beagle pup. *Stroke*. 1992;23(8):1132-1137.
45. Gonzalez FF, Ferriero DM. Neuroprotection in the newborn infant. *Clin Perinatol*. 2009;36(4):859-880, vii.
46. Juul SE, Pet GC. Erythropoietin and neonatal neuroprotection. *Clin Perinatol*. 2015;42(3):469-481.
47. Larpthaveesarp A, Georgevits M, Ferriero DM, Gonzalez FF. Delayed erythropoietin therapy improves histological and behavioral outcomes after transient neonatal stroke. *Neurobiol Dis*. 2016;93:57-63.
48. Patel S, Ohls RK. Darbepoetin administration in term and preterm neonates. *Clin Perinatol*. 2015;42(3):557-566.
49. Ohls RK, Christensen RD, Kamath-Rayne BD, et al. A randomized, masked, placebo-controlled study of darbepoetin alfa in preterm infants. *Pediatrics*. 2013;132(1):e119-e127.
50. Ohls RK, Kamath-Rayne BD, Christensen RD, et al. Cognitive outcomes of preterm infants randomized to darbepoetin, erythropoietin, or placebo. *Pediatrics*. 2014;133(6):1023-1030.
51. Ohls RK, Cannon DC, Phillips J, et al. Preschool assessment of preterm infants treated with darbepoetin and erythropoietin. *Pediatrics*. 2016;137(3):e20153859.
52. Natalucci G, Latal B, Koller B, et al. Effect of early prophylactic high-dose recombinant human erythropoietin in very preterm infants on neurodevelopmental outcome at 2 years: a randomized clinical trial. *JAMA*. 2016;315(19):2079-2085.
53. Juul SE, Comstock BA, Wadhawan R, et al. A randomized trial of erythropoietin for neuroprotection in preterm infants. *N Engl J Med*. 2020;382(3):233-243.
54. Reynolds LC, Duncan MM, Smith GC, et al. Parental presence and holding in the neonatal intensive care unit and associations with early neurobehavior. *J Perinatol*. 2013;33(8):636-641.
55. Pineda RG, Neil J, Dierker D, et al. Alterations in brain structure and neurodevelopmental outcome in preterm infants hospitalized in different neonatal intensive care unit environments. *J Pediatr*. 2014;164(1):52-60.e2.
56. Filippa M, Panza C, Ferrari F, et al. Systematic review of maternal voice interventions demonstrates increased stability in preterm infants. *Acta Paediatr*. 2017;106(8):1220-1229.
57. Chirico G, Cabano R, Villa G, Bigogno A, Ardesi M, Dioni E. Randomised study showed that recorded maternal voices reduced pain in preterm infants undergoing heel lance procedures

in a neonatal intensive care unit. *Acta Paediatr*. 2017;106(10): 1564-1568.
58. Vinall J, Miller SP, Bjornson BH, et al. Invasive procedures in preterm children: brain and cognitive development at school age. *Pediatrics*. 2014;133(3):412-421.
59. Zwicker JG, Miller SP, Grunau RE, et al. Smaller cerebellar growth and poorer neurodevelopmental outcomes in very preterm infants exposed to neonatal morphine. *J Pediatr*. 2016;172: 81-87.e2.
60. McPherson C, Haslam M, Pineda R, Rogers C, Neil JJ, Inder TE. Brain injury and development in preterm infants exposed to fentanyl. *Ann Pharmacother*. 2015;49(12):1291-1297.
61. Duerden EG, Guo T, Dodbiba L, et al. Midazolam dose correlates with abnormal hippocampal growth and neurodevelopmental outcome in preterm infants. *Ann Neurol*. 2016;79(4):548-559.
62. Creeley CE. From drug-induced developmental neuroapoptosis to pediatric anesthetic neurotoxicity—where are we now? *Brain Sci*. 2016;6(3):32.
63. Davidson JO, Wassink G, van den Heuij LG, Bennet L, Gunn AJ. Therapeutic hypothermia for neonatal hypoxic-ischemic encephalopathy—where to from here? *Front Neurol*. 2015;6:198.
64. Westin B, Miller Jr JA, Nyberg R, Wedenberg E. Neonatal asphyxia pallida treated with hypothermia alone or with hypothermia and transfusion of oxygenated blood. *Surgery*. 1959;45(5): 868-879.
65. Azzopardi DV, Strohm B, Edwards AD, et al. Moderate hypothermia to treat perinatal asphyxial encephalopathy. *N Engl J Med*. 2009;361(14):1349-1358.
66. Thoresen M, Tooley J, Liu X, et al. Time is brain: starting therapeutic hypothermia within three hours after birth improves motor outcome in asphyxiated newborns. *Neonatology*. 2013;104(3): 228-233.
67. Gunn AJ, Laptook AR, Robertson NJ, et al. Therapeutic hypothermia translates from ancient history in to practice. *Pediatr Res*. 2017;81(1-2):202-209.
68. Shankaran S, Laptook AR, Pappas A, et al. Effect of depth and duration of cooling on deaths in the NICU among neonates with hypoxic ischemic encephalopathy: a randomized clinical trial. *JAMA*. 2014;312(24):2629-2639.
69. Laptook AR, Shankaran S, Tyson JE, et al. Effect of therapeutic hypothermia initiated after 6 hours of age on death or disability among newborns with hypoxic-ischemic encephalopathy: a randomized clinical trial. *JAMA*. 2017;318(16):1550-1560.
70. Thayyil S, Pant S, Montaldo P, et al. Hypothermia for moderate or severe neonatal encephalopathy in low-income and middle-income countries (HELIX): a randomised controlled trial in India, Sri Lanka, and Bangladesh. *Lancet Glob Health*. 2021;9(9): e1273-e1285.
71. Sun Y, Zhang L, Chen Y, Zhan L, Gao Z. Therapeutic targets for cerebral ischemia based on the signaling pathways of the GluN2B C terminus. *Stroke*. 2015;46(8):2347-2353.
72. Wu YW, Bauer LA, Ballard RA, et al. Erythropoietin for neuroprotection in neonatal encephalopathy: safety and pharmacokinetics. *Pediatrics*. 2012;130(4):683-691.
73. Wu YW, Mathur AM, Chang T, et al. High-dose erythropoietin and hypothermia for hypoxic-ischemic encephalopathy: a phase II trial. *Pediatrics*. 2016;137(6):e20160191.
74. Wu YW. Randomized controlled trial of erythropoietin for neonatal hypoxic–ischemic encephalopathy. Paper presented at PAS 2022, Denver, CO, April 21–25, 2022.
75. Filippi L, Fiorini P, Catarzi S, et al. Safety and efficacy of topiramate in neonates with hypoxic ischemic encephalopathy treated with hypothermia (NeoNATI): a feasibility study. *J Matern Fetal Neonatal Med*. 2018;31(8):973-980.
76. Hobbs C, Thoresen M, Tucker A, Aquilina K, Chakkarapani E, Dingley J. Xenon and hypothermia combine additively, offering long-term functional and histopathologic neuroprotection after neonatal hypoxia/ischemia. *Stroke*. 2008;39(4):1307-1313.
77. Ma D, Hossain M, Chow A, et al. Xenon and hypothermia combine to provide neuroprotection from neonatal asphyxia. *Ann Neurol*. 2005;58(2):182-193.
78. Martin JL, Ma D, Hossain M, et al. Asynchronous administration of xenon and hypothermia significantly reduces brain infarction in the neonatal rat. *Br J Anaesth*. 2007;98(2):236-240.
79. Thoresen M, Hobbs CE, Wood T, Chakkarapani E, Dingley J. Cooling combined with immediate or delayed xenon inhalation provides equivalent long-term neuroprotection after neonatal hypoxia-ischemia. *J Cereb Blood Flow Metab*. 2009;29(4):707-714.
80. Sabir H, Osredkar D, Maes E, Wood T, Thoresen M. Xenon combined with therapeutic hypothermia is not neuroprotective after severe hypoxia–ischemia in neonatal rats. *PLoS One*. 2016;11(6):e0156759.
81. Dingley J, Tooley J, Liu X, et al. Xenon ventilation during therapeutic hypothermia in neonatal encephalopathy: a feasibility study. *Pediatrics*. 2014;133(5):809-818.
82. Rawat S, Dingley J. Closed-circuit xenon delivery using a standard anesthesia workstation. *Anesth Analg*. 2010;110(1):101-109.
83. Azzopardi D, Robertson NJ, Bainbridge A, et al. Moderate hypothermia within 6 h of birth plus inhaled xenon versus moderate hypothermia alone after birth asphyxia (TOBY-Xe): a proof-of-concept, open-label, randomised controlled trial. *Lancet Neurol*. 2016;15(2):145-153.
84. Dingley J, Liu X, Gill H, et al. The feasibility of using a portable xenon delivery device to permit earlier xenon ventilation with therapeutic cooling of neonates during ambulance retrieval. *Anesth Analg*. 2015;120(6):1331-1336.
85. Azzopardi D, Robertson NJ, Kapetanakis A, et al. Anticonvulsant effect of xenon on neonatal asphyxial seizures. *Arch Dis Child Fetal Neonatal Ed*. 2013;98(5):F437-F439.
86. Alonso-Alconada D, Alvarez A, Arteaga O, Martinez-Ibarguen A, Hilario E. Neuroprotective effect of melatonin: a novel therapy against perinatal hypoxia-ischemia. *Int J Mol Sci*. 2013; 14(5):9379-9395.
87. Robertson NJ, Faulkner S, Fleiss B, et al. Melatonin augments hypothermic neuroprotection in a perinatal asphyxia model. *Brain*. 2013;136(Pt 1):90-105.
88. Aly H, Elmahdy H, El-Dib M, et al. Melatonin use for neuroprotection in perinatal asphyxia: a randomized controlled pilot study. *J Perinatol*. 2015;35(3):186-191.
89. Benders MJ, Bos AF, Rademaker CM, et al. Early postnatal allopurinol does not improve short term outcome after severe birth asphyxia. *Arch Dis Child Fetal Neonatal Ed*. 2006;91(3):F163-F165.
90. Torrance HL, Benders MJ, Derks JB, et al. Maternal allopurinol during fetal hypoxia lowers cord blood levels of the brain injury marker S-100B. *Pediatrics*. 2009;124(1):350-357.
91. Galinsky R, Bennet L, Groenendaal F, et al. Magnesium is not consistently neuroprotective for perinatal hypoxia-ischemia in term-equivalent models in preclinical studies: a systematic review. *Dev Neurosci*. 2014;36(2):73-82.
92. Xiong Y, Wintermark P. The role of sildenafil in treating brain injuries in adults and neonates. *Front Cell Neurosci*. 2022;16:879649.
93. Bennet L, Tan S, Van den Heuij L, et al. Cell therapy for neonatal hypoxia-ischemia and cerebral palsy. *Ann Neurol*. 2012;71(5): 589-600.

94. Liao Y, Cotten M, Tan S, Kurtzberg J, Cairo MS. Rescuing the neonatal brain from hypoxic injury with autologous cord blood. *Bone Marrow Transplant*. 2013;48(7):890-900.
95. Sun JM, Kurtzberg J. Cord blood for brain injury. *Cytotherapy*. 2015;17(6):775-785.
96. Castillo-Melendez M, Yawno T, Jenkin G, Miller SL. Stem cell therapy to protect and repair the developing brain: a review of mechanisms of action of cord blood and amnion epithelial derived cells. *Front Neurosci*. 2013;7:194.
97. Lim JY, Park SI, Oh JH, et al. Brain-derived neurotrophic factor stimulates the neural differentiation of human umbilical cord blood-derived mesenchymal stem cells and survival of differentiated cells through MAPK/ERK and PI3K/Akt-dependent signaling pathways. *J Neurosci Res*. 2008;86(10):2168-2178.
98. Pimentel-Coelho PM, Magalhaes ES, Lopes LM, deAzevedo LC, Santiago MF, Mendez-Otero R. Human cord blood transplantation in a neonatal rat model of hypoxic-ischemic brain damage: functional outcome related to neuroprotection in the striatum. *Stem Cells Dev*. 2010;19(3):351-358.
99. van Velthoven CT, Dzietko M, Wendland MF, et al. Mesenchymal stem cells attenuate MRI-identifiable injury, protect white matter, and improve long-term functional outcomes after neonatal focal stroke in rats. *J Neurosci Res*. 2017;95(5):1225-1236.
100. Cotten CM, Murtha AP, Goldberg RN, et al. Feasibility of autologous cord blood cells for infants with hypoxic-ischemic encephalopathy. *J Pediatr*. 2014;164(5):973-979.e1.

Chapter 15

Pharmacological Therapy of Neonatal Abstinence Syndrome

Prabhakar Kocherlakota, MD; Edmund F. La Gamma, MD

Key Points

- Neonatal abstinence syndrome (NAS) secondary to maternal use of opioids during pregnancy continues to remain a major problem in neonates.
- Nonpharmacological measures are the first-line treatment in the management of NAS.
- Morphine remains the most popular medication in the treatment of NAS, although methadone and buprenorphine are also effective.
- Adjunct medications (e.g., phenobarbital, clonidine) are not without adverse effects and may be necessary when NAS is not controllable with primary medications.

Neonatal abstinence syndrome (NAS) is a constellation of clinical signs that are a consequence of the abrupt discontinuation of chronic fetal exposure to substances used, misused, or abused by the mother during pregnancy.[1] As the opioid crisis expanded across the United States, the incidence of NAS grew in parallel. The incidence of NAS increased from 1.6 per 1000 in-hospital births in 2004 to 8.8 per 1000 in-hospital births in 2016,[2] increasing by 83% from 2010 to 2017.[3] The incidence differs among countries, regions, and states; within states, counties, and county areas; and between rural and urban areas. In 2016, approximately 31,765 infants with NAS were cared for in hospitals across the United States.[2] The incidence of NAS in the southern United States was nearly twice as high as that in the Northeast or Midwest and almost three times as high as that in the West.[2] Another study showed that 42% of infants with NAS were born in the southern United States in 2016.[4] In 2016, the rate of NAS in West Virginia was the highest for any state (53 per 1000 live births).[3] NAS has become more common in rural counties than in urban counties.[5] Among rural infants, the incidence of NAS increased from 1.2 to 7.5 per 1000 hospital births from 2004 to 2014 and from 1.4 to 4.8 per 1000 hospital births among urban infants.[6] The incidence of NAS was higher in areas with higher long-term unemployment and greater shortages of mental health clinicians.[7] Regional variations in the incidence of NAS have led to a disproportionate burden in highly affected areas within the country.

The incidence of opioid use disorder (OUD) in pregnancy increased from 3.5 to 8.2 per 1000 delivery hospitalizations in the United States between 2010 and 2017.[3] In a study of 10,741 mothers with OUD, 58% of infants developed NAS.[8] In a study of 8059 mothers that was conducted from 2012 to 2018, 41% of infants exposed to opioids in utero required neonatal intensive care unit (NICU) admission, compared to 14% of infants not exposed to opioids.[9] The prevalence of polysubstance use increased from 60.5% in 2007 to 64.1% in 2017. It has increased more rapidly in rural areas than in urban areas in recent years.[10] Polysubstance use is associated with more severe and increased incidence of withdrawal in infants born to mothers with OUD.[1] Medication use for OUD during pregnancy is associated with decreased fetal death, preterm birth, growth restriction, and reduced maternal overdose.[8,11] It has been reported that, for each week of medication for OUD during pregnancy, the odds of preterm births decreased by 1%, the odds of overdose decreased by 2%, and the odds of NAS increased by 41%.[8] The COVID-19 pandemic has worsened the opioid problem among pregnant women due to social distancing, "stay-home" limitations, and lack of access to resources, among other pandemic-related issues.[12]

NAS is more common among Caucasians and in the population using Medicaid. In a study of 32,128 pediatric NAS admissions in 4200 hospitals across the United States in 2016, 80% were Caucasians and 84% were on Medicaid.[5] The majority of infants were born in low-income ZIP Code areas.[3] Opioid-exposed infants had lower birth weights, shorter birth lengths, smaller head circumferences, and lower gestational ages than unexposed infants.[13] Male gender, maternal smoking, and high methadone doses are other risk factors for NAS.[1] NAS is less common and less severe in preterm infants compared to term infants.[14] The signs of withdrawal are usually seen within 2 to 3 days of birth. The risk of NAS also depends on the dose, duration, and timing of the prenatal opioid exposure.[15] The average length of hospital stay (LOS) for pharmacological treatment is 16 to 18 days.[5] There is a higher chance of readmission among infants with NAS after discharge from the hospital, and 9.1% of NAS infants compared to 6.2% of non-NAS infants needed readmission within a year of discharge in a study of 10,087 readmissions.[16] Similar observations were reported in another study of 3842 infants with NAS.[17] The pathophysiology and clinical presentation of these infants were described in the previous edition of this text.[18]

Terminology

The National Institutes of Health uses the term neonatal opioid withdrawal syndrome (NOWS) because NAS is often a result of opioid use during pregnancy by the mother.[19] However, the term NOWS is restricted to opioid withdrawal and excludes other illegal substances such as amphetamines, cocaine, and marijuana, as well as medications such as selective serotonin reuptake inhibitors, benzodiazepines, or tricyclic antidepressants, which can also cause withdrawal in infants.[1] In addition, the use of combinations of opioids and nonopioids, prescribed and unprescribed drugs, or legal and illicit substances has become common. In a study of 659 cases of NAS, one-third of the infants did not have evidence of exposure to opioids.[20] In a recent observation from Japan, 54% of infants born to mothers on oral psychotropic or anticonvulsant drugs during pregnancy developed withdrawal symptoms (32.4% of those born to mothers taking a single drug and 62.9% of those born to mothers taking two or more drugs).[21] There have been instances where the term NOWS has been used for opioid-exposed infants, and the term NAS has been used for polysubstance-exposed infants. Inconsistent terminology may further complicate this complex problem. We believe the term NAS is more encompassing, and NOWS is more limiting. Hence, NAS is used in this chapter.

Problems in the Management of NAS

The major problems hindering progress in NAS management are related to the limited ability to diagnose, assess severity, include nonpharmacological measures, and apply evidence-based guidelines for pharmacological treatment.

Clinical Definition

Every disease requires a simple, reliable, and acceptable diagnosis. A definitive diagnosis is necessary for proper clinical management, future research, public health surveillance, and implementation of control measures. Moreover, a standardized case definition can contribute to a better understanding of the exact incidence of disease, disease spectrum, disease burden, and effects of individual substance exposure. Currently, the diagnosis of NAS is clinical, with most reports being based on clinical diagnosis by physicians. Most of the scientific literature is based on the International Classification of Diseases (ICD) codes. The diagnosis differs among providers and hospitals, and this may cause underreporting or overreporting. Opioid exposure does not imply opioid withdrawal. States across the United States use a variety of different definitions. Some states require toxicology confirmation, clinical withdrawal signs, Finnegan scores, and/or >2 days of hospitalization.[22] The Council of State and Territorial Epidemiologists published a position statement in 2019 recommending standardized surveillance definitions for use across the United States.[23] However, the definition was soon found to have issues with its applicability. In a retrospective analysis of 863 cases of confirmed NAS identified by ICD codes, 66% received pharmacotherapy, 23% did not require pharmacotherapy, and 9% did not meet the criteria for

NAS.[24] In January 2022, the U.S. Department of Health and Human Services announced criteria for the clinical definition of NAS that include (1) in utero exposure to opioids with or without other psychotropic substances (recommended to be collected via confidential maternal self-report; toxicology testing also acceptable with maternal informed consent), and (2) two of the five signs: excessive crying, fragmented sleep, tremors (disturbed or undisturbed), hypertonia, and gastrointestinal disturbances.[25] This definition may improve diagnosis, but it requires clarification regarding timing, mothers' refusal of toxicological screening, and definitions for some of the clinical signs.

Clinical Assessment

A fundamental problem in the management of NAS is the lack of an ideal instrument to assess the severity of withdrawal in infants. The Modified Finnegan Neonatal Abstinence Scoring Tool (M-FNAST) is the most commonly used scoring system for NAS assessment.[26] However, the M-FNAST is complex and lengthy, and the items included in the M-FNAST are based on subjective criteria, with arbitrary item weighting.[27,28] In addition, it lacks precise definitions for some items and includes some signs unrelated to NAS severity.[29] Several other scoring systems have been proposed, but many have not achieved widespread adoption for several reasons, including uncertainty about their reliability, validity, and utility.[30,31] Scoring systems that shortened or simplified the M-FNAST were mostly statistical models and were never used in clinical settings.[32,33] In addition, different studies used different criteria for initiating pharmacotherapy, further complicating the management of NAS.[34,35] Grossman et al.[36] included the infant's ability to successfully breastfeed, sleep, and be consoled in their Eat, Sleep, and Console (ESC) system. However, such an assessment does not quantify withdrawal, lacks objectivity, and may not be appropriate for all infants with NAS. In addition, the ESC system did not change the length of hospitalization or treatment (LOT) when nonpharmacological measures were not included.[35] Clinicians have been looking for a better system for the assessment of NAS in infants.[37] Hence, we have proposed a new scoring system, NAS SCORES, a 10-item, user-friendly scale instrument. NAS SCORES is a physiology-based assessment of withdrawal, with equal emphasis on the infant's central nervous system, autonomic nervous system, and neurobehavior.[38] A prospective randomized study to determine the benefits of NAS SCORES in managing infants with NAS is still needed.

Management of NAS

NONPHARMACOLOGICAL CARE

The management of NAS includes both pharmacological and nonpharmacological measures. Nonpharmacological measures often suffice for mild withdrawal and are crucial for the success of pharmacological treatment. These measures are safe, less costly, and easy to implement, and they can be considered in all infants with NAS.[39] Nonpharmacological measures can also be continued after hospital discharge. These interventions have been used more frequently in the last 10 years. The goal of nonpharmacological interventions is to reduce the need for pharmacotherapy. These interventions[40,41] consist of the following: (1) soothing support measures, such as swaddling, pacifier use, prone positioning, holding, skin-to-skin contact, volunteers or cuddlers to hold the baby, and skin-care bundle to prevent skin irritation; (2) environmental support measures, including a low-noise and low-stimulation environment, rocking, massage therapy, musical therapy, and rooming-in; (3) nutritional support measures, such as frequent small feeds, demand feeds, high-calorie feeds, and breastfeeding; (4) social support measures, including a compassionate and nonjudgmental approach and consolation therapy; and (5) family support measures, such as partner support and parental participation. Rooming-in of the mother and infant also encourages active parental participation in infant care,[42] and parental presence has been reported to decrease Finnegan scores and delay the need for pharmacological therapy.[43]

The mother is central to all nonpharmacological supportive measures because the success of nonpharmacological support depends on active maternal participation.[44] The mother is the best treatment for the infant (Figure 15.1). Breastfeeding has been explicitly shown to decrease the need for initiating pharmacological treatment, the amount of morphine needed for treatment, LOT, and LOS.[45–47] Although specific

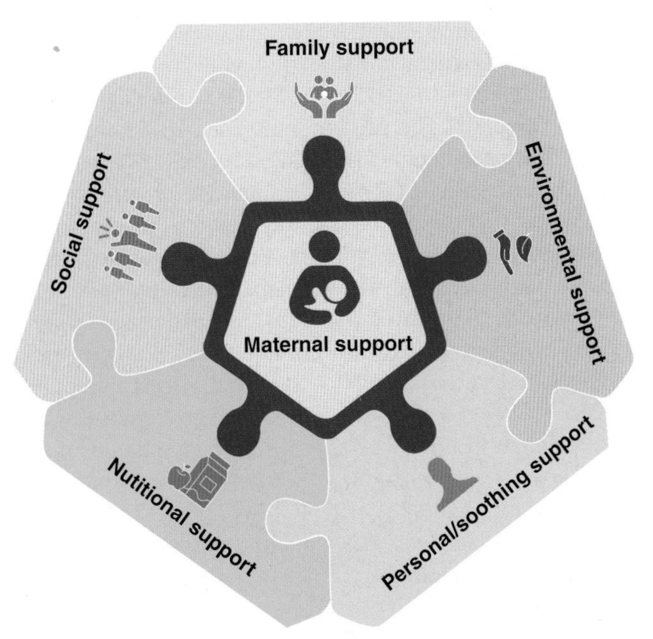

Figure 15.1 Nonpharmacological supports: mother is the center of supports. Mother is the best medicine for the infant. Mother can integrate and augment all other support measures.

interventions vary by location, ~95% of NICUs offered some form of nonpharmacological care as the initial management.[48] The nonpharmacological interventions can be individualized based on the behavioral patterns of each infant

However, there are multiple barriers to the implementation of nonpharmacological measures, including (1) absent, minimal, or inadequate maternal participation; (2) inability to breastfeed; (3) lack of structural capacity to offer rooming-in facilities; (4) lack of financial or organizational support for prolonged parental stay; (5) inadequate staff or volunteers; (6) lack of parental education and understanding; (7) complex and challenging patient populations; and (8) lack of training for clinical staff to manage the mother–infant dyad.[49] The COVID-19 pandemic has complicated NAS management in many ways, including prolonging the hospital stay for infants, impeding parental presence and volunteer participation, loss of access to rooming-in facilities, and other social and family support issues.[50] A recent meta-analysis was uncertain whether nonpharmacological care for opioid withdrawal in newborns decreased the length of hospitalization or the use of pharmacological treatment, as the analysis was restricted by heterogeneity of the studies, lack of definitions for interventions, and scarcity of outcome data.[51] We believe that larger, well-designed studies will help determine the effect of nonpharmacological care on opioid withdrawal in newborns.

PHARMACOLOGICAL MANAGEMENT

NAS is a multisystemic but treatable disease. However, there are wide variations in NAS management, and no evidence-based treatment guidelines are available. Management of NAS is symptomatic and depends on the severity of substance withdrawal signs. NAS rarely causes death, but it is associated with severe morbidity and prolonged LOS.[52]

All infants with NAS need nonpharmacological treatment measures initially. Pharmacological interventions are replacement therapeutics to minimize the effects of abrupt termination of opioid exposure in utero. Pharmacological measures are indicated in the following scenarios: (1) withdrawal not controlled by nonpharmacological measures; (2) serious complications, such as seizures; (3) severe diarrhoea leading to dehydration; (4) feeding difficulties leading to failure to thrive; and (5) severe comorbidities requiring immediate attention. In a study of 3264 infants with NAS from 2013 to 2016, 70% needed treatment.[53] In another study of 1377 infants from 2016 to 2017, 48% received pharmacological treatment.[54] The proportion of infants requiring pharmacotherapy is decreasing. In a quality improvement study of 275 infants from 2015 to 2017, the proportion of pharmacologically treated infants decreased from 87% to 40%.[35] The proportion of infants with NAS who receive medication differs from institution to institution. In another recent study, the proportion of infants receiving pharmacological therapy across various hospitals ranged from 6% to 100%.[54] Pharmacological treatment may be necessary more often in infants exposed to concomitant antenatal opioids and benzodiazepines. In a study of 822 infants with NAS, 41% of those who required pharmacotherapy had been exposed to antenatal benzodiazepines, compared to 31% of those not requiring pharmacotherapy.[55]

To date, no universally accepted standardized pharmacotherapy for NAS treatment has been established,[56] nor has a drug been approved by the U.S. Food and Drug Administration (FDA) for NAS. The first-line treatments include morphine, methadone, or buprenorphine, and second-line therapies include clonidine and phenobarbital. Opioid treatment, which is recommended by the American Academy of Pediatrics (AAP), is superior to other medications, as it is associated with less treatment failure.[57] However, opioid therapy may prolong hospital stays.[53] Due to the lack of adequately powered randomized controlled trials comparing opioids, heterogeneity in methods and reporting, and lack of long-term outcome data (including adverse events), no one opioid can be recommended over another.[58] Pharmacotherapy cannot eliminate all signs of withdrawal. Also, complete withdrawal in an infant exposed to opioids throughout pregnancy is a lengthy process.[59] Withdrawal in the infant can have an initial acute course followed by a subacute or chronic and relapsing process. When the initial acute symptoms subside, infants can be weaned rapidly or managed with nonpharmacological measures, and the infant can be discharged and managed at home. Home therapy may be associated with prolonged LOT and require frequent emergency room visits.[60] Pharmacotherapy is often predicated on the center's or practitioner's preference, irrespective of the specific opioid exposure for the fetus. Current dosing protocols are often empirically conceived and generally lack pharmacokinetics and pharmacodynamic rationale. The complex nature of withdrawal, polysubstance use by pregnant women, and multiple substantiated or unsubstantiated nonpharmacological interventions may complicate the determination of the advantages or disadvantages of the pharmacological management of NAS. Delays in pharmacological therapy are associated with higher morbidity and extended LOS.[61] Pharmacotherapy with an opioid is the standard of care, although NAS is also a self-limiting disorder, treatment can be continued in or out of the hospital, and there is no single criterion for the effectiveness of any protocol.

Two recent reports suggested that Caucasian infants were more likely than African-American infants to be treated with pharmacological measures; however, it is unclear whether these patients required treatment or received the treatment.[62,63] There is no known metabolic or genetic evidence of different treatments based on race or sex. The pharmacological properties, doses, and other details of opioids are summarized in Table 15.1.

Medications

MORPHINE

Morphine, a natural μ-opioid receptor agonist, is the most-used medication in the treatment of NAS. Of infants receiving pharmacotherapy for NAS, 80% to 90% are being treated with oral morphine. In a recent study of 1377 infants given medications for NAS from July 2016 to June 2017, 86% were treated with morphine as the primary pharmacological medication.[54] Oral morphine can decrease agitation, improve feeding, and control severe withdrawal symptoms. Older opioid preparations such as paregoric and tincture of opium are no longer used. Paregoric includes multiple toxic ingredients, including papaverine, noscapine, and camphor, as well as other substances, and tincture of opium contains ethanol and codeine, and its alkaloid content of morphine is not standardized.[69] Oral morphine solution is stable and free of alcohol; because it has a short serum half-life, it requires frequent administration.[70,71] There is a wide variation in the initiation, escalating dose, and weaning process for

TABLE 15.1 Pharmacology of Opioids in the Management of NAS[1,64–68]

Property	Morphine	Methadone	Buprenorphine
Mechanism of action	μ receptor agonist Partial δ receptor agonist κ receptor agonist	μ receptor agonist Partial δ receptor agonist κ receptor agonist *N*-methyl-D aspartate antagonist	Partial μ receptor agonist δ receptor antagonist κ receptor antagonist
Origin of opioid	Natural	Synthetic	Semi-synthetic
Route of administration	Oral; can be given intravenously	Oral	Sublingual
Half-life	4.1–7.6 hr	19.4–41 hr	11 hr
Bioavailability	48%	85% (41%–95%)	51% sublingual 15% oral
Protein binding	20%	85%–90%	96%
Solubility	Hydrophilic	Lipophilic	Lipophilic
Initial dose	0.05–0.1 mg/kg/dose	0.05–0.1 mg/kg/dose	5.3 μg/kg/dose
Maximum dose	1.3 mg/kg/d	1 mg/kg/d	60 μg/kg/d
Frequency	Q 3–4 hr	Q 6–12 hr	Q 8 hr
Alcohol content	0%	8%–15%	30%
Weaning	10% every 24–48 hr	10% every 24–48 hr	10% every 24 hr
Metabolism	Metabolized in liver Glucuronidation by UGT 2B7 Excreted through bile and kidney (5%–10% unchanged)	Metabolized in liver demethylation by CYP2B6 Excreted through kidney (15%–60% unchanged)	Metabolized in liver dealkylation by CYP3A4 Excreted through bile and kidney (10–30% unchanged)
Metabolites	Morphine-6-glucoronide (active) (10%–15%) Morphine-3-glucoronide (inactive) (45%–55%)	2-Ethylidene-1,5-dimethyl-3,3-diphenylpyrrolidine (inactive) 2-Ethyl-5-methyl-3,3-diphenyl-1-pyrroline hydrochloride (inactive)	Norbuprenorphine (active) Buprenorphine-3-glucuronide (inactive)
Elimination	Active and inactive products Elimination changes with age	Inactive products Elimination changes with age	Active and inactive products Elimination changes with age
Adverse effects	Respiratory depression Apnea Constipation Sedation Vomiting	Sedation Prolonged QTc interval Respiratory depression	Hyperthermia Tachycardia Sedation

morphine. The initial dose varies from 0.03 to 0.1 mg/kg/dose, and the escalating dose varies from 0.025 to 0.1 mg/kg/dose. Changing the initial dosage or frequency does not appear to yield significant improvement.[72] There is no consensus about the maximum dose of morphine for controlling the signs of NAS in infants. Additional medications may be considered when the maximal dose does not decrease the withdrawal scores significantly.

Oral morphine is prepared in a concentration of 0.4 or 0.5 mg/mL; hence, it must be used with caution, lest errors happen during administration. Home treatment with morphine is not an option.[73] Morphine remains popular, as its safety is well established, and dose adjustments can be easily managed. Wide variability in the dose regimen of morphine may be due to the duration and timing of fetal exposure, elimination and metabolism of drugs in the mother and fetus, and simultaneous exposure to different substances.[74]

METHADONE

Methadone, a synthetic complete μ-opioid receptor agonist, is the second most commonly used medication in NAS treatment.[54] A recent multicenter study reported that 13.4% of infants who received pharmacologic therapy for NOWS were treated with methadone.[54] Methadone is a lipid-soluble and highly protein-bound drug. There is no clearance maturation with age, unlike morphine.[75] It is commercially prepared and may not require dilution. The long half-life of methadone facilitates reduced inter-dose variation in serum concentrations. The longer interval needed to achieve steady state allows less-frequent dose adjustments and permits less interruption of feeding and sleeping. However, the long half-life may also make dose adjustment difficult. Caution should be exercised when methadone is used along with other medications; phenobarbital and omeprazole may decrease or increase methadone levels, respectively.[76] Infants can be discharged home on methadone,[77] although pediatricians have concerns regarding out-of-hospital methadone treatment.[78] Methadone labeling by the FDA has a Black Box Warning of a prolonged QTc interval. An earlier study demonstrated that maternal methadone causes a transient but clinically insignificant prolongation of QTc in infants[79]. However, a recent study confirmed that methadone did not prolong QTc interval in infants.[80]

BUPRENORPHINE

Buprenorphine, a semi-synthetic derivative of thebaine with partial μ-receptor agonist action, is increasingly being utilized to treat NAS. It has a long half-life.[81] There are no sedative and respiratory depression effects, as seen with morphine, or cardiovascular toxicities, as seen with methadone. Because of its ceiling effect, buprenorphine has a wider safety margin than full agonists such as morphine or methadone.[82] Phenobarbital has minimal impact on buprenorphine clearance.[83] Because of extensive first-pass metabolism, buprenorphine is administered sublingually rather than orally. The bioavailability of sublingually administered buprenorphine in neonates is unknown. The pharmacokinetic and pharmacodynamic profiles are well documented in the literature.[84] Buprenorphine clearance increases with age. Buprenorphine must be compounded, and the solution can be stable for 30 days when stored at room temperature.[85] However, the average concentration of alcohol in buprenorphine solution is 30%. The exposure–response relationship of buprenorphine was recently established to verify the efficacy and safety of buprenorphine in the treatment of neonates with NAS using pharmacokinetic and pharmacodynamic models.[86] Some recent reports suggest that buprenorphine may be more appropriate than other opiates for reducing LOT and LOS.[87]

MORPHINE VERSUS METHADONE

Several studies have compared the effectiveness of morphine to methadone. The description of the studies, number of infants enrolled, outcomes, and the authors' comments are included in Table 15.2. Eleven studies that included 10,450 infants were part of this analysis. It is difficult to draw conclusions from these studies, as nine were retrospective and eight were not protocolized. Six of the nine retrospective studies showed no difference between morphine and methadone in NAS management, and the other three drew contrasting conclusions. One study discontinued methadone treatment outside the hospital,[78] and two other studies continued home treatment.[89,91] Both prospective studies observed decreased LOS and LOT with methadone; however, the number of subjects enrolled in these studies was small.[94,96] Brown et al.,[94] in a single-center randomized study, found that methadone was associated with decreased LOT; however, mothers in the morphine group had received much higher doses of methadone antenatally. In their multicenter randomized controlled trial, Davis et al.[96] did not find any differences in unadjusted results between the morphine and methadone groups, but there was a 14% reduction in LOS and 16% reduction in LOT after adjustment for study site and maternal opioid used. There were no differences in neurobehavioral outcomes when infants were followed up at 18 months of age.[98] Systematic reviews and meta-analyses have shown no significant differences between methadone and morphine regarding LOT or LOS.[99–103] There was no difference in treatment failure between these medications. It should be recalled that both morphine and methadone are associated with short-term side-effects and long-term adverse neurological effects. In the absence of evidence-based superiority of morphine or methadone, the choice for either drug is at the discretion of the medical provider, depending on one's experience and preference.

TABLE 15.2 **Studies Comparing Morphine to Methadone in the Treatment of NAS**

Study	Number of Patients	Study Design	Results (days) (Morphine vs. Methadone)	Comments
Lainwala et al.[88]	Morphine: 17 Methadone: 29	Retrospective chart review Two hospitals	LOS (median): 36 vs. 40	No statistical significance Deodorized tincture of opium and morphine solution were grouped together Not adequately powered
Napolitano et al.[78]	Morphine: 139 Methadone: 154	Retrospective single-center	LOS (mean): 20 vs. 13	No statistical inference 89% discharged home on methadone
Hall et al.[89]	Morphine: 232 Methadone: 151	Retrospective	LOT (mean): 15.6 vs. 16.2 LOS (mean): 21.6 vs. 21.5	Protocol-driven cohort study No statistical significance Phenobarbital use: 23% vs. 37% Number of days on phenobarbital: 12 vs. 20*
Patrick et al.[90]	Morphine: 6 hospitals Methadone: 6 hospitals (total = 1424)	Retrospective cohort, multicenter	LOT (mean): 22.2 vs. 17.4* LOS (mean): 25.0 vs. 21*	Wide variation in protocols Methadone use decreased from 44% to 11% Nonpharmacological measures not provided Stand-alone children's hospital data (mostly) Individual group statistics not provided
Lee et al.[91]	Morphine: 48 Methadone: 41	Retrospective cohort	LOS (mean): 21.6 vs. 11.4	Methadone had the lowest LOS of all medications Wide variation of LOS within individual hospitals Inpatient treatment for morphine and combined inpatient and home treatment with methadone
Karna[92]	Morphine: 254 Methadone: 88	Retrospective cohort	LOT (mean): 16 vs. 19	State-quality collaborative study No statistical significance Adjunct medicine required more with morphine
Young et al.[93]	Morphine: 13 Methadone: 13	Retrospective chart review, single-center	LOS (mean): 12.08 vs. 44.23* LOT (mean): 7.46 vs. 38.08*	Morphine: Score-based protocol Methadone: Weight-based protocol Morphine: Finnegan scores Methadone: Neonatal withdrawal inventory scores No difference in average score No difference in the need for adjunct therapy
Brown et al.[94]	Morphine: 16 Methadone: 15	Prospective, randomized, double-blind, single-center	LOT (median): 21 vs. 14*	Median maternal methadone dose of 160 mg in morphine group and 72 mg in methadone group LOS not provided Nonpharmacological measures not included
Burke et al.[95]	Morphine: 16 Methadone: 15	Retrospective chart review	LOT (mean): 45 vs. 42 LOS (mean): 21 vs. 22	Single-center study Developmental outcomes were compared Finnegan scores were much higher with morphine Newborns treated with morphine had higher scores in cognitive and gross motor domains
Davis et al.[96]	Morphine: 59 Methadone: 59	Prospective, randomized, blinded multicenter	LOT (mean): 14.7 vs. 16.6* LOS (mean): 18.9 vs. 21.1*	Hybrid dosing regimen Delay to procure preservative-free methadone No significant difference in unadjusted analysis Recruitment did not meet the sample size target Lack of power analysis
Tolia et al.[97]	Morphine: 6480 Methadone: 1187	Retrospective cohort	LOS (median): 21 vs.17*	Multivariable Cox proportional hazard model No standardized protocol across the study Assessments and threshold not included Nonpharmacological measures not included Adjunct medications use: 26 vs. 17* Feeding problems: 20 vs. 15*

$^{*}P < 0.05$.

LOT, length of hospitalization or treatment; *LOS,* length of hospital stay.

BUPRENORPHINE VERSUS MORPHINE OR METHADONE

Buprenorphine is the newest opioid in the management of NAS. The description of the studies, number of infants enrolled, outcomes, and these authors' comments are included in Table 15.3. Eight studies consisting of 979 infants were analyzed to determine the effectiveness of buprenorphine over morphine or methadone.[104–111] Among eight studies comparing buprenorphine with morphine or methadone, three were prospective,[104–106] three were retrospective,[107–109] and two were for quality improvement.[110,111] In a small prospective randomized study, Kraft et al.[104,105]

TABLE 15.3 Comparison of Buprenorphine to Morphine or Methadone in the Treatment of NAS

Study	Number of Patients	Study Design	Dose of Buprenorphine (μg/kg/d)	Buprenorphine vs. Morphine or Methadone Results (Days)	Comments
Kraft et al.[104]	Morphine: 12 Buprenorphine: 13	Prospective, randomized, open-label, phase I trial	13.2	LOT (mean): 22 vs. 32 LOS (mean): 27 vs. 38	Pilot study Mothers were on buprenorphine Single-center study Adjunct treatment: buprenorphine (25%) vs. morphine (8%) One patient in the buprenorphine group had a seizure (withdrawn from the study)
Kraft et al.[105]	Morphine: 12 Buprenorphine: 12	Prospective, randomized open-label	15.9	LOT (mean): 23 vs. 38* LOS (mean): 32 vs. 42	Single-center, open-label study Treatment based on MOTHER NAS scores Adjunct treatment: buprenorphine (25%) vs. morphine (8%) One patient in buprenorphine group developed abnormal liver function tests
Kraft et al.[106]	Morphine: 30 Buprenorphine: 33	Prospective, randomized double-blind	15.9	LOT (median): 15 vs. 28* LOS (median): 21 vs. 33*	Randomized single-center study Study period: 5 years Gestation: >37 weeks Treatment based on MOTHER NAS scores Infants exposed to benzodiazepines excluded Adjunct treatment (no difference): buprenorphine (15%) vs. morphine (23%) Adverse events (no difference): buprenorphine (39%) vs. morphine (33%)
Hall et al.[107]	Methadone: 163 Buprenorphine: 38	Retrospective Buprenorphine: 1 hospital Methadone: 5 hospitals	13.2	LOT (mean): 9.4 vs. 14.0* LOS (mean): 16.3 vs. 20.7*	Cohort study Gestation: >34 weeks Treatment based on Finnegan scores Adjunct treatment (no difference): buprenorphine (24%) vs. methadone (25%)
Hall et al.[108]	Morphine: 110 Methadone: 76 Buprenorphine: 174	Retrospective	13.5	LOS (mean): 7.4 vs. 10.4* LOT (mean): 12.4 vs. 15.2*	Cohort Single-center study Adjunct therapy (46 % vs. 52%) Methadone-group infants were smaller Polysubstance abuse excluded

TABLE 15.3 Comparison of Buprenorphine to Morphine or Methadone in the Treatment of NAS—cont'd

Study	Number of Patients	Study Design	Dose of Buprenorphine (μg/kg/d)	Buprenorphine vs. Morphine or Methadone Results (Days)	Comments
Taleghani et al.[109]	Methadone: 108 Buprenorphine: 48	Retrospective	NA	LOT (median): 8 vs. 15* LOS (median): 13 vs. 20*	Multicenter cohort study Gestation age: >35 weeks Median cumulative morphine dose equivalent less in buprenorphine group Adjunct treatment: buprenorphine (71%) vs. methadone (32%)*
Bhandary et al.[110]	Morphine: 64 Buprenorphine: 37	Plan–Do–Study–Act (PDSA)	15.9	LOT (mean): 14.5 vs. 8.5 LOS (mean): 18.5 vs. 13	Single-center study 50% of mothers on buprenorphine Buprenorphine solution contained 30% alcohol No statistical inference included
Hein et al.[111]	Morphine: 17 Buprenorphine: 32	PDSA	15.9	LOT (mean): 6.5 vs. 10	Single-center study Phenobarbital was first tried for 2 days No statistical inference included Modified ESC used Buprenorphine or morphine used as adjunct medication

*$P < 0.05$.
LOT, length of hospitalization or treatment; *LOS*, length of hospital stay; *ESC*, eat, sleep and console system.

observed shorter LOT and LOS with a relatively high dose of buprenorphine. Another randomized, double-blind study demonstrated decreased LOS and LOT in infants treated with buprenorphine compared to those treated with morphine.[106] However, there was no difference regarding the percentage of infants requiring adjuncts, and infants of mothers taking benzodiazepines were excluded. All three retrospective studies concluded in favor of buprenorphine over morphine or methadone.[107–109] However, two of three studies used a dose of buprenorphine that was considered by Kraft et al.[105] to be too low to be effective in infants. Both quality-improvement studies also favored buprenorphine, although statistical conclusions were missing.[110,111] Multiple reviews, systematic analyses, and meta-analyses observed moderate evidence with regard to LOS and LOT in favor of buprenorphine compared to morphine or methadone.[103,112–115] However, most of the systematic reviews and meta-analyses had significant limitations, with the majority of studies being single-center or non-blinded or using nonpharmacological therapies. In addition, buprenorphine has a high alcohol content, and adjunct medications are often needed. Large multicenter randomized controlled trials considering both pharmacologic and nonpharmacological factors are warranted before definitive recommendations are developed for the role of buprenorphine in the management of NAS.

Weaning Process

Any infant stable on opioid replacement treatment needs to be weaned off the medications as soon as possible for the following reasons: (1) to decrease exposure to opioids, as none of the opioids is entirely safe; (2) to decrease the LOT and LOS, as the weaning process dictates these measures; (3) to decrease opioid-induced dependence, as prolonged exposure can lead to drug tolerance; and (4) maturation of clearance of medications can modify the opioid levels in infants. The longer the weaning process, the higher the cost of health care. A treatment reduction of 2 days may reduce healthcare costs by more than $15 million per year in the present time.[116] Structured protocols decreased LOT and LOS compared to unstructured protocols.[117] Lack of a proper weaning protocol can lead to overtreatment or undertreatment of withdrawal. In the absence of a standardized approach, patients are frequently treated at the provider's discretion. Currently, significant practice variation exists within and among institutions concerning the weaning of infants off opioids. Weaning may be done after a desired time or when a desired response is obtained; the actual dose can be calculated using current weight or birth weight, the medication may be weaned by a fixed amount or a fixed percentage, and the response to weaning can be measured by a scoring system or by the level of medication in the blood. The fixed-dose reduction has been the standard practice for many years. Most clinicians wean opioids by 10% every 2 to 3 days, provided that the infant does not show any relapse.[96] There are studies underway with increasing the dose-weaning steps from 10% to 15% or 20% or decreasing the frequency of weaning from 48 hours to 24 hours.[116]

Opioid medication doses are usually administered in a weight-based manner, but some caregivers employ dosing based on symptoms, as measured by the Finnegan score.[118] A recent retrospective observational study failed to show any benefit with score-based weaning; in a study of 146 infants, score-based protocol infants had longer LOS and required a higher total amount of morphine than weight-based infants.[34] Rescue-dose protocols (dosage increase in response to increased withdrawal scores during weaning) were associated with decreased LOT and LOS.[119] Standard weaning protocols involve the management of methadone doses based on clinical response and the amount of medication used. In a nonrandomized quality-improvement study of methadone weaning, a symptom-triggered approach decreased LOT and LOS and lowered the amount of methadone required compared to a fixed-schedule tapering protocol.[120] In a study of 93 infants treated with a pharmacokinetic-based weaning protocol compared to 267 infants on a standard weaning protocol, Hall et al.[121] found decreased LOS and LOT, but neither the amount of methadone required for treating NAS nor the need for adjunct therapy was reduced. A similar evaluation of buprenorphine weaning is also underway.[122] The wide pharmacokinetic variabilities seen with medications in infants may inhibit the broader application of such dosing regimen.[123]

Although different approaches have been developed to decrease LOT and LOS, most studies were restricted to single centers, retrospective observations, nonrandomized designs, and insufficient infant recruitment. More research is required to further support the weaning process in NAS through clinical trials or prospective observational studies, preferably in a multicenter setting.

Adjunct Medications

Adjunct medications are nonopioid substances that are often used in addition to opioids in NAS treatment. The indications for adjunct medications may include the following: (1) infant shows a failure to respond to a single opioid; (2) the maximum dose of opioid has been reached; (3) side-effects prohibit continued use of opioids; (4) there is a desire to decrease the exposure to opioids; (5) infant relapses after adequate treatment of withdrawal; or (6) a reduction of LOT is required. In a multicenter cross-sectional study of 1377 infants, 32% of infants with NAS received adjunct medications.[46] In a quality-improvement study from 2015 to 2017, the use of adjunct medications decreased from 34% to 2%.[35] Phenobarbital and clonidine are the commonly used adjunct medications. The pharmacological properties, doses, and side-effects of phenobarbital and clonidine are shown in Table 15.4.

PHENOBARBITAL

Phenobarbital is a long-acting barbiturate that reduces neuronal activity by blocking glutamatergic neurotransmission.[126] The half-life of phenobarbital in a term infant is 103 hours at birth; it decreases as clearance matures and is 67 hours at 4 weeks of age.[124] Phenobarbital has been used both as a first-line and as an adjunct medication in NAS treatment. However, it does not prevent seizures at the doses administered for withdrawal nor does it improve the gastrointestinal manifestation of NAS.[127] Phenobarbital is more often used to manage nonopioid NAS and polydrug abuse.[128] The limitations for the use of phenobarbital include sedative effects, a long half-life, rapid development of tolerance, alcohol content of 15%, and

TABLE 15.4 Pharmacology, Doses, and Side-Effects of Adjunct Medications[64–66, 124,125]

	Phenobarbital	Clonidine
Mechanism of action	Gamma-aminobutyric acid (GABA) receptor agonist	Centrally acting alpha-adrenergic receptor agonist
Route of administration	Oral, intravenous, intramuscular	Oral, intravenous, epidural, transdermal
Half-life	82–148 hr	14 hr
Bioavailability	49%	75%–90%
Protein binding	35%	20%–40%
Solubility	Hydrophilic	Lipophilic
Loading dose	16–20 mg/kg	0.5–1 μg/kg
Maintenance dose	2–4 mg/kg/day	1–1.5 μg/kg/dose
Frequency	Q 12 hr	Q 3–4 hr
Alcohol content	15%	None
Metabolism	Metabolized in liver by *N*-glucosidation Phenobarbital and metabolites excreted through the kidney (80%)	Excreted through kidney (60%) Rest metabolized in the liver
Elimination	Kidney (20%–40%)	Kidney (40%–60%)
Adverse effects	Respiratory depression Apnea Sedation Vomiting	Hypotension Bradycardia Rebound hypertension Sedation

long-term neurocognitive sequelae.[129] A recent meta-analysis did not favor using phenobarbital as the primary mode of treatment for NAS.[138] The AAP also favors opiates over phenobarbital in the treatment of opiate-induced NAS.[57]

CLONIDINE

Clonidine prevents noradrenaline surge, which is a hallmark of opioid withdrawal.[29,131] Clonidine has no respiratory depression effect; however, the theoretical risk of hypotension, bradycardia, and other cardiovascular effects may prohibit increased use of this drug.[132] Clonidine can counteract noradrenaline excess but has no impact on other consequences of withdrawal. The half-life of clonidine decreases with increasing age.[133] Clonidine can be used as a single-replacement therapy or as an adjunct medication in NAS treatment.[130] In a prospective randomized double-blind study, clonidine use decreased LOT but there were no differences in LOS or motor, cognitive, or language scores between the clonidine and morphine groups.[134]

PHENOBARBITAL VERSUS CLONIDINE

Several studies were done to study the effectiveness of phenobarbital or clonidine as adjunct medication to opioids. Phenobarbital has significant neurological adverse effects, and clonidine has substantial cardiovascular effects. Phenobarbital solution is commercially available, whereas clonidine must be compounded. However, infants can be discharged home with either medication. The phenobarbital dose can be easily titrated at home, whereas the clonidine dose must be carefully monitored because of cardiovascular effects. Phenobarbital clearance depends on hepatic maturation, and clonidine clearance depends upon renal maturation. Drug interactions with opioids are a concern with phenobarbital but not with clonidine. In addition, the combination of phenobarbital with an opioid may cause respiratory depression in neonates. The effects of exposure on the developing brain are a concern with phenobarbital, whether during short-term or long-term use.[144] In contrast, no such adverse long-term neurological outcomes have been reported with clonidine. The levels of both medications can be monitored.

Eleven studies, seven retrospective and four prospective, that involved 1148 infants were analyzed. In three studies, opioid and phenobarbital combination was compared to opioid alone; in four studies, opioid and clonidine combination was compared to opioid; and, in four studies, phenobarbital and opioid combination was compared to clonidine and opioid combination. This analysis was made much more difficult by heterogeneity in the study designs, as in some studies adjunct medication was used along with opioids from the initiation of treatment, whereas in other studies adjunct medication was used only in infants who did not respond adequately to opioids. Historically, phenobarbital had been used more often when a second-line medication was required, but a recent study reported that clonidine was used in 54% of infants and phenobarbital was used in 37% of infants who received secondary medication.[54] The description of the studies, number of infants enrolled, outcomes, and these authors' comments are included in Table 15.5.

Coyle et al.[135] decreased LOS with phenobarbital, and Agthe et al.[136] reduced LOT with clonidine as adjunct medications to tincture of opium. A phenobarbital and morphine combination increased LOS compared to a phenobarbital and methadone combination in one study, but conflicting results were obtained in another.[89,92] Four studies directly compared phenobarbital to clonidine as an adjunct to morphine; in both prospective studies, phenobarbital decreased LOT, LOS, and duration of opioid therapy or total morphine dose.[140,142.] In a large retrospective multicenter study of 180 infants, phenobarbital

TABLE 15.5 Studies with Adjunct Medication Use in the Treatment of Neonatal Abstinence Syndrome

Study	Primary Medication	Adjunct Medication	Results	Comments
Studies comparing phenobarbital and opioid to opioids alone				
Coyle et al.[135]	Deodorized tincture of opium (DTO)	Phenobarbital: 10 Placebo: 10	LOS (mean days): 38 vs. 79* Maximum DTO dose (mL): 4.7 vs. 16.8*	Partial randomized study Duration of phenobarbital treatment: 3.5 months
Hall et al.[89]	Morphine: 86 Methadone: 34	Phenobarbital	LOT (mean): morphine (19.6 days) vs. methadone: (12.0 days)*	Retrospective Weaning protocol Multi-hospital study
Karna[92]	Morphine: 99 Methadone:15	Phenobarbital	LOT (mean): morphine (24 days) vs. methadone (37 days)*	Retrospective State Quality Collaborative study Polydrug-exposed neonates
Studies comparing morphine alone to clonidine and morphine				
Agthe et al.[136]	Deodorized DTO	Clonidine: 40 Placebo: 40	LOS (median days): 11 vs. 15* Morphine (total dose): 7.7 mg vs. 19.2 mg*	Prospective, randomized, double-blinded, placebo-controlled study Seven infants rebounded in the clonidine group Increased amount of DTO in the placebo
Esmelli et al.[137]	Morphine: 64 Clonidine: 29	Phenobarbital Chloral hydrate	LOT (mean days): 35 vs. 14* LOS (mean days): 44 vs. 32*	Retrospective Clonidine given as IV infusion No follow-up done Adjunct medication added after maximum dose of primary medication No comparison between subgroups
Bader et al.[138]	Morphine: 72	Morphine + clonidine: 65	LOS (mean days): 30 vs. 20* LOT (mean days): 28 vs. 18* Morphine dose (mg/kg): 6.9 vs. 3.4*	Retrospective Different time periods Days on morphine: 26.1 vs. 14.7* Phenobarbital required 5% vs. 3%
Gullickson et al.[139]	Morphine: 22	Morphine + clonidine: 100	LOT with morphine (mean days): 11.3 vs. 17.8* Peak morphine dose (mg/kg q3h): 0.1 vs. 0.14*	Retrospective cohort study Period of study: 9 years Detailed information missing

TABLE 15.5 Studies with Adjunct Medication Use in the Treatment of Neonatal Abstinence Syndrome—cont'd

Study	Primary Medication	Adjunct Medication	Results	Comments
Studies comparing phenobarbital vs. clonidine as adjunct medications to morphine				
Surran et al.[140]	Morphine	Phenobarbital: 34 Clonidine: 32	LOT with morphine (mean days): 12.4 vs. 19.5* Total morphine dose (mg/kg/d): 3.8 vs. 6.7	Prospective, randomized, single-center study Discharged home on phenobarbital No difference in total morphine dose No long-term follow-up Two failures in clonidine group Discontinued after an interim analysis
Devlin et al.[141]	Morphine	Phenobarbital: 146 Clonidine: 44	LOT with morphine (mean days): 35 vs. 26.5* LOS (mean days): 42 vs. 33*	Retrospective cohort study Historical controls Different time periods (2005–2014 vs. 2014–2017) Different regimens of morphine treatment (q3h vs. q4h) Adjunct treatment 63% vs. 39%*
Brusseau et al [142]	Morphine	Phenobarbital: 11 Clonidine: 14	LOT with morphine (mean days): 25.5 vs. 34.4* LOT with adjunct meds (mean days): 22 vs. 33* LOS (mean days): 31 vs. 41*	Prospective, randomized study Small in numbers, single-center clonidine group Hypotension: 3 infants Rebound hypertension: 2 infants
Merhar et al.[143]	Morphine	Phenobarbital: 72 Clonidine: 108	LOS (mean days): 26.4 vs. 36.5* LOT with morphine (mean days): 20.8 vs. 28.1* Peak morphine dose (mg/kg): 0.08 vs. 0.07*	Retrospective, cohort study Large, multicenter, contemporary observational study After adjusting covariable, LOS was lower with phenobarbital Out-of-hospital treatment: 78% vs. 29%*

*$P < 0.05$.

reduced LOS, LOT, and morphine dose,[143] but the other retrospective study reached opposite conclusions.[141] A recent meta-analysis concluded that the current data are insufficient to determine the safety and incidence of adverse events in infants treated with phenobarbital or clonidine combined with opioids.[130] However, in a recent policy statement, AAP advised clinicians to consider the use of clonidine as a second-line drug over phenobarbital, mainly out of concern for the adverse neurological outcomes associated with phenobarbital.[56] But, we advise readers to await confirmation from further studies to favor clonidine over phenobarbital as an adjunct medication in NAS treatment.

Conclusions

NAS is a major public health crisis in the United States and other countries. NAS is a complex disease, and there is a need for a practical clinical definition of NAS. There are no biological markers to assess the severity of NAS; hence, it is necessary to have a simple, reliable, and valid scoring system for the assessment of NAS. Moreover, nonpharmacological interventions must be utilized before initiating pharmacological measures, and having a practical, structured protocol for NAS management is essential. Evidence-based pharmacological interventions are the need of the day. Studies suggest there may or may not be benefits of one opioid over another opioid at this point, but the weaning process must be rapid, as long as there are no relapses. This is because none of the medications used in the treatment of NAS is entirely safe, either in the short or long term, so treatment must be restricted to as short a duration as possible. All NAS infants need to be carefully followed up, as they may experience short- and long-term adverse effects. The optimal growth and development of infants in a safe environment are the goals.

REFERENCES

1. Kocherlakota P. Neonatal abstinence syndrome. *Pediatrics*. 2014;134:e547-e561.
2. Leech AA, Cooper WO, McNeer E, Scott TA, Patrick SW. Neonatal abstinence syndrome in the United States, 2004–16. *Health Aff (Millwood)*. 2020;39:764-767.
3. Hirai AH, Ko JY, Owens PL, Stocks C, Patrick SW. Neonatal abstinence syndrome and maternal opioid-related diagnoses in the US, 2010–2017. *JAMA*. 2021;325:146-155.
4. Strahan AE, Guy Jr GP, Bohm M, Frey M, Ko JY. Neonatal abstinence syndrome incidence and health care costs in the United States, 2016. *JAMA Pediatr*. 2020;174:200-202.
5. Ramphul K, Mejias SG, Joynauth J. An update on the burden of neonatal abstinence syndrome in the United States. *Hosp Pediatr*. 2020;10:181-184.
6. Villapiano NL, Winkelman TN, Kozhimannil KB, Davis MM, Patrick SW. Rural and urban differences in neonatal abstinence syndrome and maternal opioid use, 2004 to 2013. *JAMA Pediatr*. 2017;171:194-196.
7. Patrick SW, Faherty LJ, Dick AW, Scott TA, Dudley J, Stein BD. Association among county-level economic factors, clinician supply, metropolitan or rural location, and neonatal abstinence syndrome. *JAMA*. 2019;321:385-393.
8. Krans EE, Kim JY, Chen Q, et al. Outcomes associated with the use of medications for opioid use disorder during pregnancy. *Addiction*. 2021;116:3504-3514.
9. Corsi DJ, Hsu H, Fell DB, Wen SW, Walker M. Association of maternal opioid use in pregnancy with adverse perinatal outcomes in Ontario, Canada, from 2012 to 2018. *JAMA Netw Open*. 2020;3:e208256.
10. Jarlenski MP, Paul NC, Krans EE. Polysubstance use among pregnant women with opioid use disorder in the United States, 2007–2016. *Obstet Gynecol*. 2020;136:556-564.
11. Piske M, Homayra F, Min JE, et al. Opioid use disorder and perinatal outcomes. *Pediatrics*. 2021;148:e2021050279.
12. White A, Lundahl B, Bryan MA, et al. Pregnancy and the opioid crisis: heightened effects of COVID-19. *J Addict Med*. 2022;16:e2-e4.
13. Graeve R, Balalian AA, Richter M, et al. Infants' prenatal exposure to opioids and the association with birth outcomes: a systematic review and meta-analysis. *Paediatr Perinat Epidemiol*. 2022;36:125-143.
14. Ruwanpathirana R, Abdel-Latif ME, Burns L, et al. Prematurity reduces the severity and need for treatment of neonatal abstinence syndrome. *Acta Paediatr*. 2015;104:e188-e194.
15. Straub L, Huybrechts KF, Hernández-Díaz S, et al. Trajectories of prescription opioid utilization during pregnancy among prepregnancy chronic users and risk of neonatal opioid withdrawal syndrome. *Am J Epidemiol*. 2022;191:208-219.
16. Milliren CE, Melvin P, Ozonoff A. Pediatric hospital readmissions for infants with neonatal opioid withdrawal syndrome, 2016–2019. *Hosp Pediatr*. 2021;11:979-988.
17. Uebel H, Wright IM, Burns L, et al. Reasons for rehospitalization in children who had neonatal abstinence syndrome. *Pediatrics*. 2015;136:e811-e820.
18. Kocherlakota P. Pharmacological therapy for neonatal abstinence syndrome. In: Benitz W, Smith PB, Polin R, eds. *Infectious Disease and Pharmacology: Neonatology Questions and Controversies*. Philadelphia, PA: Elsevier; 2018:243-259.
19. Bianchi DW. *Neonatal Opioid Withdrawal Syndrome: The NIH Response*. Available at: https://www.wcpinst.org/wp-content/uploads/2017/09/Dr-Bianchi-Presentation-Neonatal.pdf. Accessed February 2, 2022.
20. Dave CV, Goodin A, Zhu Y, et al. Prevalence of maternal-risk factors related to neonatal abstinence syndrome in a commercial claims database: 2011–2015. *Pharmacotherapy*. 2019;39:1005-1011.
21. Kanemura A, Masamoto H, Kinjo T, et al. Evaluation of neonatal withdrawal syndrome in neonates delivered by women taking psychotropic or anticonvulsant drugs: a retrospective chart review of the effects of multiple medications and breastfeeding. *Eur J Obstet Gynecol Reprod Biol*. 2020;254:226-230.
22. Chiang KV, Okoroh EM, Kasehagen LJ, Garcia-Saavedra LF, Ko JY. Standardization of state definitions for neonatal abstinence syndrome surveillance and the opioid crisis. *Am J Public Health*. 2019;109:1193-1197.
23. Council of State and Territorial Epidemiologists. *Neonatal Abstinence Syndrome Standardized Case Definition*. Available at: https://cdn.ymaws.com/www.cste.org/resource/resmgr/ps/2019ps/19-MCH-01_NAS_updated_5.7.19.pdf. Accessed February 3, 2023.
24. Maalouf FI, Cooper WO, Stratton SM, et al. Positive predictive value of administrative data for neonatal abstinence syndrome. *Pediatrics*. 2019;143:e20174183.
25. Jilani SM, Jones HE, Grossman M, et al. Standardizing the clinical definition of opioid withdrawal in the neonate. *J Pediatr*. 2022;243:33-39.e1.
26. Finnegan LP, Connaughton Jr JF, Kron RE, Emich JP. Neonatal abstinence syndrome: assessment and management. *Addict Dis*. 1975;2:141-158.
27. Wolff K, Perez-Montesano P. Opioid neonatal abstinence syndrome. Controversies and implications for practice. *Curr Drug Abuse Rev*. 2014;7:44-58.
28. Schiff DM, Grossman MR. Beyond the Finnegan scoring system: novel assessment and diagnostic techniques for the opioid-exposed infant. *Semin Fetal* Neonatal Med. 2019;24:115-120.
29. D'Apolito KD. Assessing neonates for neonatal abstinence. Are you reliable? *J Perinat Neonat Nurs*. 2014;28:220-231.
30. Lipsitz PJ. A proposed narcotic withdrawal score for use with newborn infants. A pragmatic evaluation of its efficacy. *Clin Pediatr*. 1975;14:592-594.
31. Ostrea EM, Chavez CJ, Strauss ME. A study of factors that influence the severity of neonatal narcotic withdrawal. *J Pediatr*. 1976;88:642-645.
32. Jones HE, Seashore C, Johnson E, et al. Psychometric assessment of the neonatal abstinence scoring system and the MOTHER NAS scale. *Am J Addict*. 2016;25:370-373.
33. Gomez Pomar E, Finnegan LP, Devlin L, et al. Simplification of the Finnegan neonatal abstinence scoring system: retrospective study of two institutions in the USA. *BMJ Open*. 2017;7:e016176.

34. Chisamore B, Labana S, Blitz S, Ordean A. A comparison of morphine delivery in neonatal opioid withdrawal. *Subst Abuse*. 2016;10:49-54.
35. Wachman EM, Grossman M, Schiff DM, et al. Quality improvement initiative to improve inpatient outcomes for Neonatal Abstinence Syndrome. *J Perinatol*. 2018;38:1114-1122.
36. Grossman MR, Berkwitt AK, Osborn RR, et al. An initiative to improve the quality of care of infants with neonatal abstinence syndrome. *Pediatrics*. 2017;139:e20263360.
37. Verklan MT. Time for the Finnegan Neonatal Abstinence Syndrome Scoring Tool to be retired? *J Perinat Neonatal Nurs*. 2019;33:276-277.
38. Kocherlakota P, Qian EC, Patel VC, et al. A new scoring system for the assessment of neonatal abstinence syndrome. *Am J Perinatol*. 2020;37:333-340.
39. MacVicar S, Kelly LE. Systematic mixed study of nonpharmacological management of neonatal abstinence syndrome. *Birth*. 2019;46:428-438.
40. Ryan G, Dooley J, Gerber Finn L, Kelly L. Nonpharmacological management of neonatal abstinence syndrome: a review of the literature. *J Matern Fetal Neonatal Med*. 2019;32:1735-1740.
41. Edwards L, Brown LF. Nonpharmacological management of neonatal abstinence syndrome. An integrated review. *Neonatal Netw*. 2016;35:305-313.
42. MacMillan KDL, Rendon CP, Verma K, Riblet N, Washer DB, Holmes AV. Association of rooming-in with outcomes for neonatal abstinence syndrome: a systematic review and meta-analysis. *JAMA Pediatr*. 2018;172:345-351.
43. Holmes AV, Atwood EC, Whalen B, et al. Rooming-in to treat neonatal abstinence syndrome: improved family-centered care at lower cost. *Pediatrics*. 2016;137:e20152929.
44. Kondili E, Duryea DG. The role of mother-infant bond in neonatal abstinence syndrome (NAS) management. *Arch Psychiatr Nurs*. 2019;33:267-274.
45. Myers HA, Batten S, Brewer TL. Breastfeeding: an evidence-based intervention for neonatal abstinence syndrome. *Worldviews Evid Based Nurs*. 2021;18:350-351.
46. Clark RRS. Breastfeeding in women on opioid maintenance therapy: a review of policy and practice. *J Midwifery Womens Health*. 2019;64:545-558.
47. Chu L, McGrath JM, Qiao J, et al. A meta-analysis of breastfeeding effects for infants with neonatal abstinence syndrome. *Nurs Res*. 2022;71:54-65.
48. Mehta A, Forbes KD, Kuppala VS. Current status of the management of neonatal abstinence syndrome: results of a national survey. *J Invest Med*. 2012;60:376.
49. Shuman CJ, Wilson R, VanAntwerp K, Morgan M, Weber A. Elucidating the context for implementing nonpharmacologic care for neonatal opioid withdrawal syndrome: a qualitative study of perinatal nurses. *BMC Pediatr*. 2021;21:489.
50. MacMillan KDL, Morrison TM, Melvin P, Diop H, Gupta M, Wachman EM. Impact of Coronavirus Disease-2019 on hospital care for neonatal opioid withdrawal syndrome. *J Pediatr*. 2022;245:47-55.
51. Pahl A, Young L, Buus-Frank ME, Marcellus L, Soll R. Non-pharmacological care for opioid withdrawal in newborns. *Cochrane Database Syst Rev*. 2020;12:CD013217.
52. Lisonkova S, Richter LL, Ting J, et al. Neonatal abstinence syndrome and associated neonatal and maternal mortality and morbidity. *Pediatrics*. 2019;144:e20183664.
53. Milliren CE, Gupta M, Graham DA, Melvin P, Jorina M, Ozonoff A. Hospital variation in neonatal abstinence syndrome incidence, treatment modalities, resource use, and costs across pediatric hospitals in the United States, 2013 to 2016. *Hosp Pediatr*. 2018;8:44-48.
54. Young LW, Hu Z, Annett RD, et al. Site-level variation in the characteristics and care of infants with neonatal opioid withdrawal. *Pediatrics*. 2021;147:e2020008839.
55. Sanlorenzo LA, Cooper WO, Dudley JA, Stratton S, Maalouf FI, Patrick SW. Increased severity of neonatal abstinence syndrome associated with concomitant antenatal opioid and benzodiazepine exposure. *Hosp Pediatr*. 2019;9:569-575.
56. Patrick SW, Barfield WD, Poindexter BB. Neonatal opioid withdrawal syndrome. *Pediatrics*. 2020;146:e2020029074.
57. Hudak ML, Tan RC, American Academy of Pediatrics Committee on Drugs, Committee on Fetus and Newborn. Neonatal drug withdrawal. *Pediatrics*. 2012;29:e540-e560.
58. McPherson C. Pharmacotherapy for neonatal abstinence syndrome: choosing the right opioid or no opioid at all. *Neonatal Netw*. 2016;35:314-320.
59. Elliott MR, Cunliffe P, Demianczuk N, Robertson CMT. Frequency of newborn behaviours associated with neonatal abstinence syndrome: a hospital-based study. *J Obstet Gynaecol Can*. 2004;26:25-34.
60. Maalouf F, Cooper WO, Slaughter JC, Dudley J, Patrick SW. Outpatient pharmacotherapy for neonatal abstinence syndrome. *J Pediatr*. 2018;199:151-157.e1.
61. Finnegan L, Kaltenach K. Neonatal abstinence syndrome. In: Hoekalman R, Friedman S, Nelson N, Sidel H, eds. *Primary Pediatric Care*. St. Louis, MO: Mosby-Yearbook; 1992:1367-1378.
62. Parikh A, Gopalakrishnan M, Azeem A, Booth A, El-Metwally D. Racial association and pharmacotherapy in neonatal opioid withdrawal syndrome. *J Perinatol*. 2019;39:1370-1376.
63. Pourcyrous M, Elabiad MT, Rana D, Gaston KP, DeBaer L, Dhanireddy R. Racial differences in opioid withdrawal syndrome among neonates with intrauterine opioid exposure. *Pediatr Res*. 2021;90:459-463.
64. van Hoogdalem MW, McPhail BT, Han D, et al. Pharmacotherapy of neonatal opioid withdrawal syndrome: a review of pharmacokinetics and pharmacodynamics. *Expert Opin Drug Metab Toxicol*. 2021;17:87-103.
65. McPhail BT, Emoto C, Butler D, Fukuda T, Akinbi H, Vinks AA. Opioid treatment for neonatal opioid withdrawal syndrome: current challenges and future approaches. *J Clin Pharmacol*. 2021;61:857-870.
66. Tang F, Ng CM, Bada HS, Leggas M. Clinical pharmacology and dosing regimen optimization of neonatal opioid withdrawal syndrome treatments. *Clin Transl Sci*. 2021;14:1231-1249.
67. Chay PC, Duffy BJ, Walker JS. Pharmacokinetic-pharmacodynamic relationships of morphine in neonates. *Clin Pharmacol Ther*. 1992;51:334-342.
68. Moore JN, Gastonguay MR, Ng CM, et al. The pharmacokinetics and pharmacodynamics of buprenorphine in neonatal abstinence syndrome. *Clin Pharmacol Ther*. 2018;103:1029-1037.
69. Siu A, Robinson CA. Neonatal abstinence syndrome: essentials for the practitioner. *J Pediatr Pharmacol Ther*. 2014;19:147-155.
70. Sauberan J, Rossi S, Kim JH. Stability of dilute oral morphine solution for neonatal abstinence syndrome. *J Addict Med*. 2013;7:113-115.
71. Mikkelsen S, Feilberg VL, Christensen CB, Lundstrøm KE. Morphine pharmacokinetics in premature and mature newborn infants. *Acta Paediatr*. 1994;83:1025-1028.
72. DeAtley HN, Burton A, Fraley MD. Evaluation of the effectiveness of two morphine protocols to treat neonatal abstinence syndrome in a level II nursery in a community hospital. *Pharmacotherapy*. 2017;37:856-860.

73. Kelly LE, Knoppert D, Roukema H, Rieder MJ, Koren G. Oral morphine weaning for neonatal abstinence syndrome at home compared with in-hospital: an observational cohort study. *Paediatr Drugs*. 2015;17:151-157.
74. Mian P, Tibboel D, Wildschut ED, van den Anker JN, Allegaert K. Morphine treatment for neonatal abstinence syndrome: huge dosing variability underscores the need for a better clinical study design. *Minerva Pediatr*. 2019;71:263-286.
75. Kapur BM, Hutson JR, Chibber T, Luk A, Selby P. Methadone: a review of drug–drug and pathophysiological interactions. *Crit Rev Clin Lab Sci*. 2011;48:171-195.
76. Ward RM, Drover DR, Hammer GB, et al. The pharmacokinetics of methadone and its metabolites in neonates, infants, and children. *Paediatr Anaesth*. 2014;24:591-601.
77. Backes CH, Backes CR, Gardner D, Nankervis CA, Giannone PJ, Cordero L. Neonatal abstinence syndrome: transitioning methadone-treated infants from an inpatient to an outpatient setting. *J Perinatol*. 2012;32:425-430.
78. Napolitano A, Theophilopoulos D, Seng SK, Calhoun DA. Pharmacologic management of neonatal abstinence syndrome in a community hospital. *Clin Obstet Gynecol*. 2013;56:193-201.
79. Parikh R, Hussain T, Holder G, Bhoyar A, Ewer AK. Maternal methadone therapy increases QTc interval in newborn infants. *Arch Dis Child Fetal Neonatal Ed*. 2011;96:F141-F143.
80. Snyder K, Maurer S, Riley M, et al. Effect of methadone on QTc in infants. *Early Hum Dev*. 2021;156:105348.
81. Mangat AK, Schmölzer GM, Kraft WK. Pharmacological and nonpharmacological treatments for the neonatal abstinence syndrome (NAS). *Semin Fetal Neonatal Med*. 2019;24:133-141.
82. Walsh SL, Preston KL, Stitzer ML, Cone EJ, Bigelow GE. Clinical pharmacology of buprenorphine: ceiling effects at high doses. *Clin Pharmacol Ther*. 1994;55:569-580.
83. Bell SG. Buprenorphine: a newer drug for treating neonatal abstinence syndrome. *Neonatal Netw*. 2012;31:178-183.
84. Ng CM, Dombrowsky E, Lin H, et al. Population pharmacokinetic model of sublingual buprenorphine in neonatal abstinence syndrome. *Pharmacotherapy*. 2015;35:670-680.
85. Anagnostis EA, Sadaka RF, Sailor LA, Moody DE, Dysart KC, Kraft WK. Formulation of buprenorphine for sublingual use in neonates. *J Pediatr Pharmacol Ther*. 2011;16:281-284.
86. Moore JN, Gastonguay MR, Ng CM, et al. The pharmacokinetics and pharmacodynamics of buprenorphine in neonatal abstinence syndrome. *Clin Pharmacol Ther*. 2018;103:1029-1037.
87. Simon AE, Freund MP, Archer SW, Bremer AA. Toward the use of buprenorphine in infants for neonatal opioid withdrawal syndrome: summary of an NIH workshop. *J Perinatol*. 2021; 41:1213-1215.
88. Lainwala S, Brown ER, Weinschenk NP, Blackwell MT, Hagadorn JI. A retrospective study of length of hospital stay in infants treated for neonatal abstinence syndrome with methadone versus oral morphine preparations. *Adv Neonatal Care*. 2005;5:265-272.
89. Hall ES, Wexelblatt SL, Crowley M, et al. A multicenter cohort study of treatments and hospital outcomes in neonatal abstinence syndrome. *Pediatrics*. 2014;134:e527-e534.
90. Patrick SW, Kaplan HC, Passarella M, Davis MM, Lorch SA. Variation in treatment of neonatal abstinence syndrome in US children's hospitals, 2004–2011. *J Perinatol*. 2014;34:867-872.
91. Lee J, Hulman S, Musci Jr M, Stang E. Neonatal abstinence syndrome: influence of a combined inpatient/outpatient methadone treatment regimen on the average length of stay of a Medicaid NICU population. *Popul Health Manag*. 2015;18: 392-397.
92. Karna P. Pharmacological treatment and duration of therapy for neonatal abstinence syndrome at Michigan State Quality Collaborative. Paper presented at Pediatric Academic Societies Annual Meeting, San Diego, CA, April 25–28, 2015.
93. Young ME, Hager SJ, Spurlock D. Retrospective chart review comparing morphine and methadone in neonates treated for neonatal abstinence syndrome. *Am J Health Syst Pharm*. 2015;72: S162-S167.
94. Brown MS, Hayes MJ, Thornton LM. Methadone versus morphine for treatment of neonatal abstinence syndrome: a prospective randomized clinical trial. *J Perinatol*. 2015;35: 278-283.
95. Burke S, Beckwith AM. Morphine versus methadone treatment for neonatal withdrawal and impact on early infant development. *Glob Pediatr Health*. 2017;4:2333794X17721128.
96. Davis JM, Shenberger J, Terrin N, et al. Comparison of safety and efficacy of methadone vs. morphine for treatment of neonatal abstinence syndrome: a randomized clinical trial. *JAMA Pediatr*. 2018;172:741-748.
97. Tolia VN, Murthy K, Bennett MM, et al. Morphine vs. methadone treatment for infants with neonatal abstinence syndrome. *J Pediatr*. 2018;203:185-189.
98. Czynski AJ, Davis JM, Dansereau LM, et al. Neurodevelopmental outcomes of neonates randomized to morphine or methadone for treatment of neonatal abstinence syndrome. *J Pediatr*. 2020;219:146-151.
99. Xiao F, Yan K, Zhou W. Methadone versus morphine treatment outcomes in neonatal abstinence syndrome: a meta-analysis. *J Paediatr Child Health*. 2019;55:1177-1182.
100. Wachman EM, Werler MM. Pharmacologic treatment for neonatal abstinence syndrome: which medication is best? *JAMA Pediatr*. 2019;173:221-223.
101. Disher T, Gullickson C, Singh B, et al. Pharmacological treatments for neonatal abstinence syndrome: a systematic review and network meta-analysis. *JAMA Pediatr*. 2019;173: 234-243.
102. Slowiczek L, Hein DJ, Cochrane ZR, Gregory PJ. Morphine and methadone for neonatal abstinence syndrome: a systematic review. *Neonatal Netw*. 2018;37:365-371.
103. Zankl A, Martin J, Davey JG, Osborn DA. Opioid treatment for opioid withdrawal in newborn infants. *Cochrane Database Syst Rev*. 2021;7:CD002059.
104. Kraft WK, Gibson E, Dysart K, et al. Sublingual buprenorphine for treatment of neonatal abstinence syndrome: a randomized trial. *Pediatrics*. 2008;122:e601-e607.
105. Kraft WK, Dysart K, Greenspan JS, Gibson E, Kaltenbach K, Ehrlich ME. Revised dose schema of sublingual buprenorphine in the treatment of the neonatal opioid abstinence syndrome. *Addiction*. 2011;106:574-580.
106. Kraft WK, Adeniyi-Jones SC, Chervoneva I, et al. Buprenorphine for the treatment of the neonatal abstinence syndrome. *N Engl J Med*. 2017;376:2341-2348.
107. Hall ES, Isemann BT, Wexelblatt SL, et al. A cohort comparison of buprenorphine versus methadone treatment for neonatal abstinence syndrome. *J Pediatr*. 2016;170:39-44.
108. Hall ES, Rice WR, Folger AT, Wexelblatt SL. Comparison of neonatal abstinence syndrome treatment with sublingual buprenorphine versus conventional opioids. *Am J Perinatol*. 2018;35:405-412.
109. Taleghani AA, Isemann BT, Rice WR, Ward LP, Wedig KE, Akinbi HT. Buprenorphine pharmacotherapy for the management of neonatal abstinence syndrome in methadone-exposed neonates. *Pediatr Neonatal Pain*. 2019;1:33-38.

110. Bhandary S, Lambeth T, Holmes A, Pylipow M. Using buprenorphine to treat neonatal abstinence syndrome: a quality improvement study. *J Perinatol*. 2021;41:1480-1486.
111. Hein S, Clouser B, Tamim MM, Lockett D, Brauer K, Cooper L. Eat, Sleep, Console and adjunctive buprenorphine improved outcomes in neonatal opioid withdrawal syndrome. *Adv Neonatal Care*. 2021;21:41-48.
112. Kraft WK. Buprenorphine in neonatal abstinence syndrome. *Clin Pharmacol Ther*. 2018;103:112-119.
113. Ghazanfarpour M, Najafi MN, Roozbeh N. Therapeutic approaches for neonatal abstinence syndrome: a systemic review of randomized clinical trials. *Daru*. 2019;27:423-431.
114. Bishop BM. Buprenorphine for the treatment of neonatal abstinence syndrome. *J Pharm Technol*. 2018;34:266-272.
115. Frazier LM, Bobby LE, Gawronski KM. Emerging therapies for the treatment of neonatal abstinence syndrome. *J Matern Fetal Neonatal Med*. 2022;35:987-995.
116. Czynski AJ, Laptook AR. The time is NOW: filling the gaps in treatment of opioid-exposed infants: a prospective, pragmatic, randomized control drug trial. *R I Med J*. 2021;104:17-21.
117. Hall ES, Wexelblatt SL, Crowley M, et al. Implementation of a neonatal abstinence syndrome weaning protocol: a multicenter cohort study. *Pediatrics*. 2015;136:e803-e810.
118. Jones HE, Kaltenbach K, Heil SH, et al. Neonatal abstinence syndrome after methadone or buprenorphine exposure. *N Engl J Med*. 2010;363:2320-2331.
119. Hartgrove MJ, Meschke LI, King TL, Saunders C. Treating infants with neonatal abstinence syndrome: an examination of three protocols. *J Perinatol*. 2019;39:1377-1383.
120. Wachman EM, Minear S, Hirashima M, et al. Standard fixed-schedule methadone taper versus symptom-triggered methadone approach for treatment of neonatal opioid withdrawal syndrome. *Hosp Pediatr*. 2019;9:576-584.
121. Hall ES, Meinzen-Derr J, Wexelblatt SL. Cohort analysis of a pharmacokinetic-modeled methadone weaning optimization for neonatal abstinence syndrome. *J Pediatr*. 2015;167:1221-1225.
122. Mizuno T, McPhail BT, Kamatkar S, et al. Physiologic indirect response modeling to describe buprenorphine pharmacodynamics in newborns treated for neonatal opioid withdrawal syndrome. *Clin Pharmacokinet*. 2021;60:249-259.
123. McPhail BT, Emoto C, Fukuda T, et al. Utilizing pediatric physiologically based pharmacokinetic models to examine factors that contribute to methadone pharmacokinetic variability in neonatal abstinence syndrome patients. *J Clin Pharmacol*. 2020;60:453-465.
124. Pacifici GM. Clinical pharmacology of phenobarbital in neonates: effects, metabolism and pharmacokinetics. *Curr Pediatr Rev*. 2016;12:48-54.
125. Streetz VN, Gildon BL, Thompson DF. Role of clonidine in neonatal abstinence syndrome: a systematic review. *Ann Pharmacother*. 2016;50:301-310.
126. Löscher W, Rogawski M. How theories evolved concerning the mechanism of action of barbiturates. *Epilepsia*. 2012;53:12-25.
127. Bio LL, Siu A, Poon CY. Update on the pharmacologic management of neonatal abstinence syndrome. *J Perinatol*. 2011; 31:692-701.
128. O'Grady MJ, Hopewell J, White MJ. Management of neonatal abstinence syndrome: a national survey and review of practice. *Arch Dis Child*. 2009;94:F249-F252.
129. Farwell JR, Lee YJ, Hirtz DG, Sulzbacher SI, Ellenberg JH, Nelson KB. Phenobarbital for febrile seizures–effects on intelligence and on seizure recurrence. *N Engl J Med*. 1990;322:364-369.
130. Zankl A, Martin J, Davey JG, Osborn DA. Sedatives for opioid withdrawal in newborn infants. *Cochrane Database Syst Rev*. 2021;5:CD002053.
131. Gold MS, Redmond Jr DE, Kleber HD. Clonidine blocks acute opiate-withdrawal symptoms. *Lancet*. 1978;2:599-602.
132. Meddock RP, Bloemer D. Evaluation of the cardiovascular effects of clonidine in neonates treated for neonatal abstinence syndrome. *J Pediatr Pharmacol Ther*. 2018;23:473-478.
133. Lu D, Harmanjeet H, Wanandy T, Paine M, Peterson GM, Patel RP. Physicochemical stability of extemporaneously prepared clonidine solutions for use in neonatal abstinence syndrome. *J Clin Pharm Ther*. 2019;44:883-887.
134. Bada HS, Sithisarn T, Gibson J, et al. Morphine versus clonidine for neonatal abstinence syndrome. *Pediatrics*. 2015;135: e383-e391.
135. Coyle MG, Ferguson A, Lagasse L, Oh W, Lester B. Diluted tincture of opium (DTO) and phenobarbital versus DTO alone for neonatal opiate withdrawal in term infants. *J Pediatr*. 2002;140:561-564.
136. Agthe AH, Kim GR, Mathias KB, et al. Clonidine as an adjunct therapy to opioids for neonatal abstinence syndrome: a randomized controlled trial. *Pediatrics*. 2009;123:e849-e856.
137. Esmaeili A, Keinhorst AK, Schuster T, Beske F, Schlosser R, Bastanier C. Treatment of neonatal abstinence syndrome with clonidine and chloral hydrate. *Acta Paediatr*. 2010;99:209-214.
138. Bader MY, Zaghloul N, Repholz AA, et al. Retrospective review following the addition of clonidine to a neonatal abstinence syndrome treatment algorithm. *Front Pediatr*. 2021;9:632836.
139. Gullickson C, Kuhle S, Campbell-Yeo M. Comparison of outcomes between morphine and concomitant morphine and clonidine treatments for neonatal abstinence syndrome. *Acta Paediatr*. 2019;108:271-274.
140. Surran B, Visintainer P, Chamberlain S, Kopcza K, Shah B, Singh R. Efficacy of clonidine versus phenobarbital in reducing neonatal morphine sulfate therapy days for neonatal abstinence syndrome. A prospective randomized clinical trial. *J Perinatol*. 2013;33:954-959.
141. Devlin LA, Lau T, Radmacher PG. Decreasing total medication exposure and length of stay while completing withdrawal for neonatal abstinence syndrome during the neonatal hospital stay. *Front Pediatr*. 2017;5:216.
142. Brusseau C, Burnette T, Heidel RE. Clonidine versus phenobarbital as adjunctive therapy for neonatal abstinence syndrome. *J Perinatol*. 2020;40:1050-1055.
143. Merhar SL, Ounpraseuth S, Devlin LA, et al. Phenobarbital and clonidine as secondary medications for neonatal opioid withdrawal syndrome. *Pediatrics*. 2021;147:e2020017830.
144. Al-Muhtasib N, Sepulveda-Rodriguez A, Vicini S, Forcelli PA. Neonatal phenobarbital exposure disrupts GABAergic synaptic maturation in rat CA1 neurons. *Epilepsia*. 2018;59:333-344.

Chapter 16

Vasodilator Drugs for Pulmonary Hypertension in Bronchopulmonary Dysplasia

Rachel T. Sullivan, MD; Rachel K. Hopper, MD

Key Points

- Pulmonary hypertension (PH) is an important comorbidity associated with bronchopulmonary dysplasia that increases risk of right ventricular failure and death in premature infants.
- First-line treatment is aimed at correction of the respiratory status by optimizing lung volumes, oxygenation, and ventilation and eliminating sources of pulmonary inflammation, such as infection or aspiration.
- Depending on disease severity, PH-targeted therapies may be used in conjunction with or after respiratory optimization.
- PH-targeted therapies are directed at three main pathways regulating pulmonary vascular
- Tone: nitric oxide, endothelin, and prostacyclin.

Introduction

Infants born extremely prematurely are at risk for bronchopulmonary dysplasia (BPD), or chronic lung disease of prematurity. Based on recommendations from a 2001 National Institutes of Health workshop, BPD is defined by the presence and type of respiratory support required at 36 weeks postmenstrual age in infants born at less than 32 weeks gestation.[1] The lung parenchymal features of BPD have changed since the introduction of surfactant therapy, with "new" BPD characterized primarily by immature alveolar development and significantly less pulmonary fibrosis compared to "old" BPD, first described in 1967.[2,3] Nonetheless, the incidence of BPD has remained essentially unchanged, with approximately 40% of extremely premature infants developing BPD.[4–10] With nearly one in 10 infants born prematurely in the United States, BPD results in a significant healthcare burden.[6,11]

The development of pulmonary hypertension (PH) is an important potential consequence of BPD. PH is defined as an elevated mean pulmonary arterial pressure greater than 20 mmHg, with precapillary PH further defined by a pulmonary vascular resistance of at least 3 Wood units, indexed for body surface area ($WU \cdot m^2$).[12,13] Approximately 20% of infants with BPD develop PH, the frequency of which increases with BPD severity.[14–19] Importantly, PH imparts significant risk for mortality; a recent meta-analysis reported 16% mortality prior to discharge and 40% mortality within the first 2 years of life.[14,20,21] Despite this early mortality, most survivors have resolution of PH and are able to discontinue PH therapies by 2 years of age.[20,21] PH in infants with BPD is associated with impaired somatic growth and neurodevelopment.[22] Although treating the underlying respiratory disease and promoting lung growth are key strategies in the management of BPD-associated PH (BPD-PH), targeted PH therapy is often employed for infants with persistent or severe PH. This chapter focuses on the use of pulmonary vasodilators in infants with BPD-PH.

Pathophysiology and Risk Factors

BPD-PH pathophysiology is complex and related to a combination of both pre- and postnatal factors. Central to the development of both BPD and PH is the immature alveolar and pulmonary vascular development associated with premature birth. Preterm birth during the late canalicular to saccular stage of

TABLE 16.1 Risk Factors for Development of BPD-Associated PH

Prenatal Factors	Postnatal Factors
Maternal hypertensive vascular disease of pregnancy Anomalies of the placenta Intrauterine growth restriction and associated conditions (e.g., oligohydramnios, small for gestational age) Chorioamnionitis or other infections Fetal and/or maternal epigenic changes	Toxicity from prolonged hyperoxic exposure Toxicity from prolonged hypoxemic exposure Physical trauma from mechanical ventilation and related support Sepsis or other infections Hemodynamic alterations related to patent ductus arteriosus or congenital heart disease Retinopathy or prematurity Necrotizing enterocolitis Stenosis of one or more pulmonary veins

Reproduced with permission from Malloy KW, Austin ED. Pulmonary hypertension in the child with bronchopulmonary dysplasia. *Pediatr Pulmonol*. 2021;56(11):3546–3556.

lung development results in a reduced number of alveoli that appear architecturally simplified and are accompanied by fewer blood vessels than fully developed lungs.[2,17,23–25] Postnatal vascular injury from periods of hypoxia or hyperoxia, inflammation secondary to sepsis or aspiration, and/or hemodynamic influence of cardiac shunt lesions may promote pulmonary vasoconstriction and muscularization of the pulmonary arteries.[17,26] Ultimately, these factors together confer a risk of BPD-PH due to a significantly decreased vascular surface area, elevated pulmonary vascular tone, and pathologic vascular changes (Table 16.1).

There are a number of recognized risk factors that affect the development of BPD and BPD-PH, the most significant being lung disease severity. Generally, the risk for BPD-PH increases with more severe BPD. However, infants with no or mild BPD may develop PH, whereas some with severe BPD never develop PH, highlighting additional pre- and postnatal contributors.[14] Prenatal factors affecting lung development, including fetal growth restriction and oligohydramnios, impart increased risk for BPD and BPD-PH.[7,15,27] Early evidence of PH at 7 days of age is associated with the development of late PH at 36 weeks postmenstrual age and may reflect a reduced pulmonary vascular bed.[28] Other postnatal factors associated with BPD-PH include indices of impaired development, lung disease severity and systemic inflammation, lower gestational age, duration of mechanical ventilation, duration of hospitalization, sepsis, necrotizing enterocolitis, and retinopathy of prematurity.[14,29]

Diagnosis

Establishing the correct diagnosis is imperative in the appropriate treatment of BPD-PH. Clinical signs of PH may be vague and overlap considerably with BPD.[30] Because PH may be triggered by worsening respiratory status, symptoms may include tachypnea, respiratory distress, and hypoxia. On cardiac exam, infants with PH may have a loud second heart sound, palpable right ventricular impulse, and a systolic murmur related to tricuspid valve insufficiency. Some infants may present with signs of right ventricular failure related to BPD-PH, including tachycardia, hepatomegaly, peripheral edema, and poor growth. Hypoxia may be present in infants with right-to-left shunts from elevated pulmonary vascular resistance, manifested as either systemic hypoxia (in the case of an intracardiac shunt) or a pre- and post-ductal saturation differential (in the case of a patent ductus arteriosus). Conversely, BPD-PH may be present with no overt clinical signs. Therefore, multiple expert panels recommend echocardiographic screening for BPD-PH in at-risk infants at 36 weeks postmenstrual age (Figure 16.1).[12,31,32] However, criteria to define those most "at-risk" for BPD-PH and the most appropriate screening protocols remain controversial.[33] Serum brain natriuretic peptide is often used in combination with echocardiography as a biomarker of pulmonary hypertension and/or right heart failure in BPD-PH.[34]

Transthoracic echocardiogram is the most commonly used modality to screen for PH and identify shunt lesions. In addition to characterizing cardiac anatomy, echocardiography may estimate the right

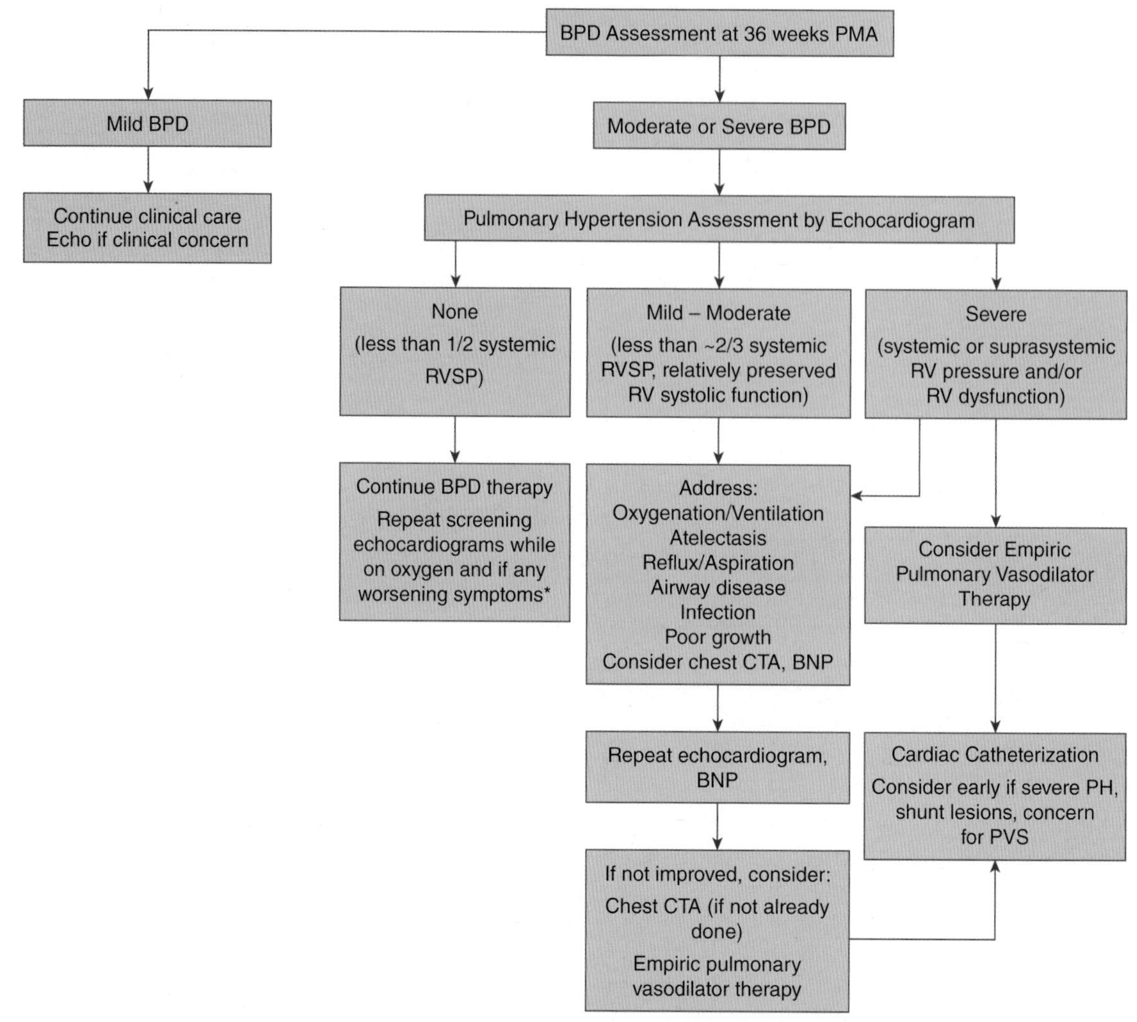

Fig. 16.1 A suggested echocardiographic screening and management protocol for bronchopulmonary dysplasia-associated pulmonary hypertension. Screening echocardiogram is recommended at 36 weeks postmenstrual age for premature infants born at less than 32 weeks postmenstrual age with moderate or severe BPD. The protocol outlines the next management steps, particularly in infants found to have PH, including additional work-up and when to consider PH-targeted pharmacotherapy. *The timing of screening echocardiograms is determined by individual patient risk factors and clinical concern. BNP, brain natriuretic peptide; BPD, bronchopulmonary dysplasia; CTA, chest computed tomography angiography; PMA, postmenstrual age; PH, pulmonary hypertension; PVS, pulmonary vein stenosis; RV, right ventricle; RVSP, right ventricle systolic pressure. (Adapted with permission from Krishnan U, Feinstein JA, Adatia I, et al. Evaluation and management of pulmonary hypertension in children with bronchopulmonary dysplasia. *J Pediatr.* 2017;188:24–34.e1.)

ventricular (RV) systolic pressure by Doppler assessment of a tricuspid regurgitation jet. Similarly, Doppler interrogation of patent ductus arteriosus flow may estimate systolic pulmonary artery pressure. When flattening of the interventricular septum at end systole is observed, it suggests that the RV pressure is at least half the systemic systolic pressure.[35] Pulmonary vein stenosis is increasingly recognized in premature infants, which may cause postcapillary PH, and should be included in PH assessment. Finally, RV hypertrophy, dilation, and systolic function reflect both PH severity and duration and are important factors when selecting pulmonary vasodilator therapy.

When PH is suggested by echocardiogram, additional imaging modalities are often used to determine if there are potential structural contributors to PH.

Chest computed tomography angiography can assess for pulmonary vascular anomalies, such as pulmonary vein stenosis or peripheral pulmonary arterial stenoses, which may contribute to RV hypertension yet not be apparent by echocardiogram. Chest computed tomography angiography also effectively characterizes the airways and lung parenchyma, highlighting airway malacia, atelectasis, or other structural abnormalities that alter clinical management.[12,31,36] Cardiac magnetic resonance imaging may have specific indications in this population (e.g., defining degree of cardiac shunt or cardiac and pulmonary vascular anatomy). However, it is less commonly used to assess lung parenchyma, and the need for anesthesia limits its clinical utility in most centers.[36,37]

Cardiac catheterization is the gold standard for the diagnosis of PH, as it provides direct hemodynamic measurements, angiographic assessment of the pulmonary vasculature, and calculation of the pulmonary vascular resistance. Catheterization also provides a means to diagnose and potentially intervene if anatomic abnormalities, such as cardiac shunts and pulmonary vein stenosis, are observed. Catheterization should be undertaken with caution and by providers experienced in the care of infants with BPD-PH, given the small patient size, potential clinical instability, and known risk for periprocedural adverse events in those with PH.[38,39] Depending on diagnostic certainty by echocardiogram, PH-targeted therapy may be initiated without catheterization if the perceived risk of the procedure outweighs the clinical benefit. Catheterization, however, should be undertaken in cases of diagnostic uncertainty, when additional anatomic and hemodynamic information may alter therapeutic decisions, when infants have an unexpected response to pulmonary vasodilator therapy, and for assessment of disease severity when considering combination PH-targeted therapies.[31,32]

Management

NON-PHARMACOLOGIC MANAGEMENT

When BPD-PH is diagnosed, optimization of the respiratory status should occur prior to initiation of pulmonary vasodilator therapy, with a focus on correcting factors that promote pulmonary vasoconstriction, such as hypoxia, hypercapnia, acidosis, inflammation, atelectasis, and alveolar hyperexpansion. In cases of hypoxia, supplemental oxygen should be used to target systemic saturations of 92% to 95% to avoid oxygen toxicity.[31] Decisions regarding respiratory support and ventilator settings are often challenging in infants with BPD due to the heterogeneity of lung disease, with atelectasis, cystic changes, and air trapping occurring concomitantly in many cases. Pulmonary vascular resistance is lowest at functional residual capacity and may be negatively impacted by both alveolar under- and overexpansion. Consequently, ventilation strategies in BPD generally target higher tidal volumes, lower respiratory rates, and longer inspiratory times.[40] Diuretics may be considered in the setting of pulmonary edema, cardiac shunt lesions, or right heart dilation. Vasoactive medications such as milrinone or dopamine may be considered in the management of PH-associated right heart failure.

Feeding evaluation should be undertaken in any infant without an identifiable cause of BPD-PH or if radiographic or clinical signs suggest aspiration. Evaluation may include assessment by a feeding therapist and fluoroscopic swallow study. An empiric trial of transpyloric feeds may be considered to assess the potential influence of aspiration on the PH, particularly when a formal swallow study cannot be undertaken or is unrevealing.

PHARMACOLOGIC MANAGEMENT

PH targeted therapies primarily promote vasodilation of the pulmonary arteries. There are three main pathways that may be targeted by pulmonary vasodilators: nitric oxide, endothelin, and prostacyclin. The mechanisms of each pathway are summarized in Figure 16.2. Medications and recommended dosing for the most commonly used pulmonary vasodilators in BPD-PH are summarized in Table 16.2.

Nitric Oxide Pathway

Nitric oxide is an endogenous pulmonary vasodilator produced by the vascular endothelium. Nitric oxide interacts with the vascular smooth muscle by stimulating soluble guanylate cyclase–mediated production of cyclic guanosine monophosphate (cGMP), which promotes smooth muscle relaxation and vasodilation.[41,42] Ultimately, the enzyme phosphodiesterase type 5 (PDE5) catabolizes cGMP breakdown. Medications targeting the nitric oxide pathway function by working toward the common endpoint of increasing cGMP, which is primarily achieved by either providing

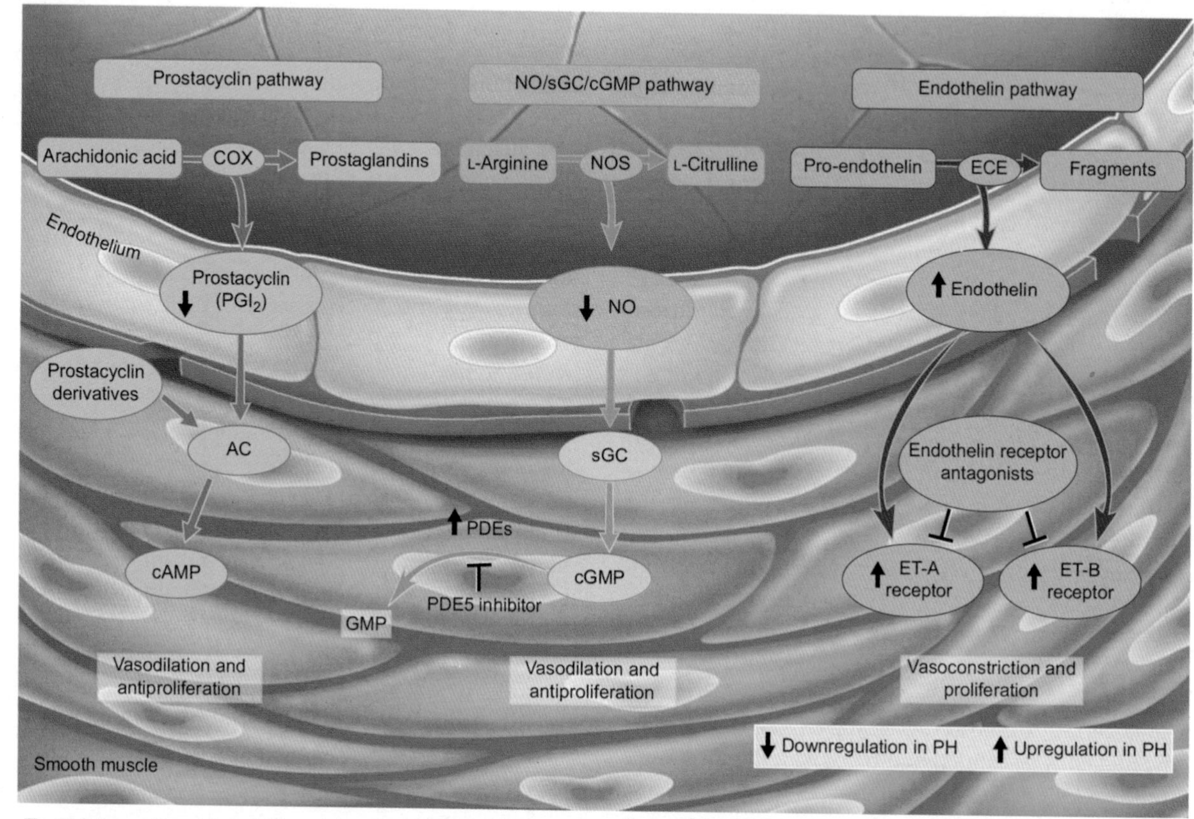

Fig. 16.2 Key pathways targeted by pulmonary vasodilator therapies, which include the prostacyclin, nitric oxide, and endothelin pathways. AC, adenylate cyclase; cAMP, cyclic adenosine monophosphate; cGMP, cyclic guanosine monophosphate; COX, cyclo-oxygenase; ECE, endothelin converting enzyme; ET, endothelin; GMP, guanosine monophosphate; NO, nitric oxide; NOS, NO synthase; PDE, phosphodiesterase; PH, pulmonary hypertension; sGC, soluble guanylate cyclase. (Ghofrani HA, Grimminger F. Modulating cGMP to treat lung diseases. *Handb Exp Pharmacol* 2009; 191: 469–483.)

exogenous nitric oxide or preventing cGMP breakdown by inhibiting PDE5.

Inhaled Nitric Oxide

Exogenous nitric oxide is a fast-acting medication delivered via inhalation that promptly diffuses into the pulmonary vasculature and acts as a selective pulmonary vasodilator. Inhaled nitric oxide (iNO) preferentially acts on ventilated portions of lung, thus improving ventilation and perfusion matching.[43] Upon entering the circulation, nitric oxide is inactivated by very rapid, high-affinity binding to oxyhemoglobin. The nitric oxide and hemoglobin in this complex are co-oxidized to produce nitrate and methemoglobin.[44] Because of its rapid inactivation, the effects of iNO are transient and limited to the pulmonary vasculature. Multiple studies, including in neonates with persistent pulmonary hypertension of the newborn (PPHN), have demonstrated no evidence of systemic hypotension to suggest systemic vasodilatory effects.[45–47] iNO is administered most dependably via invasive mechanical ventilation, although it may be delivered via non-invasive respiratory support with the understanding that dosage may have to be increased due to less efficient delivery.[48] Therapy is typically initiated at 20 parts per million, with early studies demonstrating limited additional hemodynamic benefit at higher doses.[49] Infants may develop rebound PH with the discontinuation of iNO, likely related to downregulation of endogenous nitric oxide synthase activity.[50] Risk for rebound PH may be

TABLE 16.2 Common Pulmonary Vasodilator Therapies for BPD-Associated PH

Medication/ Class	Mechanism of Action	Dose/Titration	Additional Considerations
Inhaled nitric oxide	Exogenous nitric oxide	Typically initiated at 20 ppm	$\dot{V}/\dot{Q}$ matching benefits Less dependable delivery with non-invasive respiratory support Gradual weaning required
Sildenafil	PDE5 inhibitor	Start at half dose with gradual uptitration Infants and <10 kg: 1 mg/kg TID 10–19 kg: 10 mg TID 20–39 kg: 20 mg TID 40+ kg: 20–40 mg TID	Side effects: hypotension, gastroesophageal reflux, headache, irritability, priapism
Bosentan	Endothelin receptor antagonist	Start at half dose with gradual uptitration. Infants and <10 kg: 2 mg/kg BID 10–19 kg: 31.25 mg BID 20–39 kg: 62.5 mg BID 40+ kg: 125 mg BID	Side effects: liver dysfunction/transaminitis, anemia, rhinitis, fluid retention REMS program monitoring: monthly LFTs, monthly pregnancy test in women of childbearing age
Epoprostenol	Prostacyclin	IV: start at 1 ng/kg/min, uptitrating gradually to effect Inhaled: initiate at 50 ng/kg/min	IV side effects: hypotension, gastrointestinal disturbance, flushing, nausea, diarrhea, headache; dedicated line required Inhaled side effects: potential damage to valves or filters of mechanical ventilator Short half-life (2–5 minutes) creates risk for PH crisis with infusion interruption.
Treprostinil	Prostacyclin	SQ/IV: start at 2 ng/kg/min, uptitrating gradually to initial goal of ~20–40 ng/kg/min	Side effects are similar to those of epoprostenol; with subcutaneous use, can have local catheter infusion-site pain. Longer half-life (4–5 hours) confers less risk for PH crisis with brief infusion interruption.

BID, two times daily; *IV,* intravenous; *LFTs,* liver function tests; *PDE5,* phosphodiesterase 5; *PH,* pulmonary hypertension; *ppm,* parts per million; *REMS,* risk evaluation and mitigation strategy; *TID,* three times daily; $\dot{V}/\dot{Q}$, ventilation/perfusion.

mitigated by gradual weaning, particularly with small increments at lower doses, prior to discontinuation.[51]

iNO has been most rigorously studied in the treatment of PPHN in term infants. These studies demonstrated that iNO decreased the need for extracorporeal life support but did not significantly impact mortality or hospital length of stay.[42,46,52] The use of iNO in premature infants is more controversial, and a consensus statement from the American Academy of Pediatrics did not support the use of iNO in premature infants at <34 weeks postmenstrual age based on available evidence.[53] However, this statement acknowledged rare clinical situations, including PH, for which iNO may be of benefit. The North American Pediatric Pulmonary Hypertension Network recently published recommendations for the use of iNO in premature infants with severe BPD-PH.[54] Although not currently a long-term therapeutic option in outpatients, iNO is an optimal choice in the critically ill infant with acute BPD-PH exacerbation, which may occur secondary to respiratory decompensation or infection.[55]

PDE5 Inhibitors

PDE5 inhibitors, such as sildenafil and tadalafil, are the most well-studied and commonly used class of PH-targeted therapy for the treatment of BPD-PH.[31] In preclinical rodent BPD models, sildenafil improved hyperoxia-induced alveolar simplification, pulmonary vasculogenesis, pulmonary fibrosis, and right ventricular hypertrophy.[56–59]

The first clinical use of sildenafil in the treatment of BPD-PH was published by Hon and colleagues in 2005.[60]

A majority of the experience with sildenafil in BPD-PH has been gleaned from single-center case reports and retrospective cohort studies, as there are no large randomized controlled trials of sildenafil in BPD-PH. A meta-analysis of five retrospective observational studies found hemodynamic improvement (estimated pulmonary artery pressure decreasing by ≥20%) in 69% of subjects and improvement in respiratory scores in 15%. Importantly, there were no serious adverse events and no clear effects on mortality.[61] Tan and colleagues[62] reported a decrease in systolic pulmonary arterial pressures in infants with BPD who received sildenafil, from a median of 56.5 mmHg before to 34.3 mmHg after a median of 4 weeks of treatment (Figure 16.3). Retrospective studies have demonstrated that a majority of patients are able to wean off of pulmonary vasodilator therapy due to resolution of PH, typically within 2 years of initiation.[63] None of these reports compared outcomes in untreated controls.

In published studies, sildenafil has a favorable safety profile in BPD-PH, with a minority of patients experiencing systemic hypotension or priapism due to systemic vasodilatory effects.[63–67] In a large single-center retrospective cohort of 99 infants with BPD-PH treated with sildenafil, the medication was discontinued in just 7.1% due to adverse effects.[63] An additional concern with systemically administered PH-targeted therapy is the potential for ventilation/perfusion ($\dot{V}/\dot{Q}$) mismatch and resultant hypoxemia due to the vasodilation of both ventilated and non-ventilated portions of lung. Systemic hypoxemia has been rarely encountered with sildenafil administration, and sildenafil treatment may result in an improved respiratory status in a subset of patients.[61–63,66]

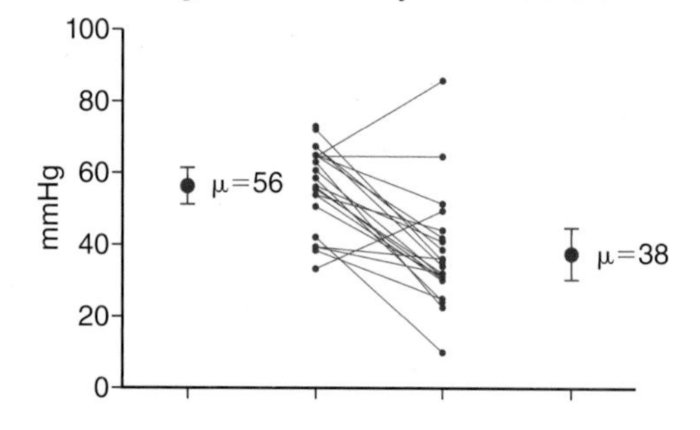

Fig. 16.3 Hemodynamic response to sildenafil therapy in patients with bronchopulmonary dysplasia-associated pulmonary hypertension. Right ventricular systolic pressure decreased from a median of 56.5 to 34.3 mmHg after a median of 4 weeks of treatment. (Reproduced with permission from Tan K, Krishnamurthy MB, O'Heney JL, Paul E, Sehgal A. Sildenafil therapy in bronchopulmonary dysplasia-associated pulmonary hypertension: a retrospective study of efficacy and safety. *Eur J Pediatr.* 2015;174(8):1109–1115.)

The safety of sildenafil in children was questioned after publication from the STARTS trial, a randomized controlled trial that evaluated the use of sildenafil monotherapy in treatment-naïve children ages 1 to 17 years with pulmonary arterial hypertension (PAH). Short-term outcome data demonstrated improvement in hemodynamics and functional class at medium to high doses and marginal efficacy in increasing peak oxygen consumption.[68] Longer term data in the STARTS-2 extension study, however, demonstrated increased 3-year mortality in the children treated with high-dose sildenafil (up to 80 mg three times daily).[69] This prompted the U.S. Food and Drug Administration (FDA) to release a drug safety communication in 2012 recommending against the use of sildenafil in pediatric patients. Experts in pediatric PH, along with the European Medicines Agency, voiced support for the use of sildenafil in pediatric PH, noting concern regarding the methodology in STARTS-2 but advising avoidance of high doses; the FDA warning was subsequently tempered and ultimately in January 2023 the FDA announced approval of sildenafil for pulmonary arterial hypertension in pediatric patients aged 1-17.[70] Importantly, the applicability of these findings to BPD-PH is unclear given that the STARTS trial did not include children with PH secondary to lung disease (such as BPD-PH) and the FDA statement only applies to pediatric children ages 1 to 17 years.

Sildenafil is often considered first-line therapy for the treatment of BPD-PH.[32,71] Sildenafil is most commonly administered enterally at a goal dose of 1 mg/kg three times daily. Sildenafil should be initiated at lower doses to monitor for potential side effects. Although titration schedules may vary institutionally, most providers start medication at a fraction of the dose and advance to full dose after a minimum of three doses, depending on tolerance. Sildenafil may also be administered intravenously, although doing so requires dosage adjustment to 0.25 to 0.5 mg/kg/dose, and it must be administered more slowly over 60 minutes given the risk of systemic hypotension.[71]

Although generally well tolerated, side effects of PDE5 inhibitors include flushing, hypotension, gastroesophageal reflux, emesis, headache, and priapism. The pediatric usage of tadalafil, a longer acting PDE5 inhibitor, is increasing given the relative ease of once daily dosing; however, pediatric studies have not evaluated its use in BPD-PH, and dosage has not been established in children <3 years of age.[12,72,73]

Soluble Guanylate Cyclase Stimulators

Riociguat, the newest medication in this pathway, is a soluble guanylate cyclase stimulator. It is approved for the treatment of adults with PAH and chronic thromboembolic pulmonary hypertension.[74] Two studies in BPD-PH animal models have demonstrated improved alveolar and pulmonary vascular development.[75,76] However, given the few published studies and minimal experience in children, riociguat is not currently widely used for treatment of BPD-PH.[77]

Endothelin Pathway

Endothelin Receptor Antagonists

Endothelin-1 is a potent vasoconstrictor produced by vascular endothelial cells that exerts its vasoconstrictive and pro-proliferative effects by binding to two receptor subtypes (types A and B) (Figure 16.2).[42] In preclinical animal models of BPD, endothelin receptor antagonism promotes vasodilation and attenuates pathologic alveolar and pulmonary vascular remodeling.[78,79] Elevated levels of both endothelin-1 and its precursor, pro-endothelin-1, have been associated with increased risk for prolonged respiratory support and development of BPD in premature infants,[80–83] making this an attractive target pathway for pharmacotherapy.

The dual endothelial receptor antagonist bosentan is approved by the FDA for the treatment of idiopathic or congenital PAH in patients 3 years and older, with studies demonstrating treatment-related improvement in hemodynamics and functional class.[84–88] Use of bosentan for the treatment of PPHN has shown varying clinical efficacy.[89–91] Furthermore, there is a paucity of data regarding the clinical efficacy of bosentan in BPD-PH. A small single-center case series showed significant hemodynamic improvement in BPD-PH in two infants treated with bosentan monotherapy and two infants treated with bosentan + sildenafil dual therapy.[92] With minimal objective data, the use of bosentan in BPD-PH is largely based on expert opinion and experience. Bosentan may be considered in the treatment of BPD-PH, frequently as adjunctive therapy to PDE5 inhibitor use.[32,71,93]

Bosentan is administered enterally, with goal dose of 2 mg/kg twice daily in children <10 kg and fixed dosing at weights above 10 kg. Potential side effects include elevated transaminases, fluid retention, rhinitis, anemia, hypotension, and teratogenicity. Transaminase elevation is less commonly seen in children but may be exacerbated during viral illness.[31] Routine lab monitoring for hepatotoxicity, anemia, and pregnancy, as applicable, is required by an FDA Risk Evaluation and Mitigation Strategy program.[12] Caregivers who may be pregnant are advised to exercise caution when handling bosentan because of potential teratogenic effects. Bosentan induces the cytochrome P450 enzyme, CYP3A4, which may impact the metabolism of multiple other drugs, including sildenafil. Co-administration of bosentan and sildenafil can result in decreased sildenafil and increased bosentan serum concentrations, although currently no specific medication dosage adjustments are recommended.[94] As with PDE5 inhibitors, there are similar theoretical concerns regarding potential risk for $\dot{V}/\dot{Q}$ mismatch with bosentan. Clinical trials are lacking in BPD-PH, but this side effect has not been reported.

Ambrisentan is a longer acting endothelin receptor antagonist specific to endothelin receptor subtype A; its pediatric usage is increasing in the treatment of PAH given the relative ease of once daily dosing and improved side-effect profile relative to bosentan. However, pediatric studies have not evaluated its use in BPD-PH, and the optimal dosage has not been established in children <5 years of age.[12,95] Similarly, macitentan is a novel dual endothelin receptor antagonist approved for treatment of PAH in adults. Although several small case series suggest benefit in children with PAH, studies of pediatric pharmacokinetics and the use of macitentan in BPD-PH are needed.[96,97]

Prostacyclin Pathway

Therapies targeting the prostacyclin pathway mimic endogenous endothelium-derived prostacyclin, or prostaglandin I_2 (PGI_2). In the pulmonary vasculature, PGI_2 binds to its receptor and stimulates cyclic adenosine monophosphate to promote pulmonary vasodilation and inhibit smooth muscle cell proliferation (Figure 16.2).[42] Several studies suggest that PGI_2 plays an important role in early pulmonary vascular tone and development. Decreased prostaglandin synthesis has been associated with both PPHN and decreased angiogenesis in a preclinical lamb model.[98] Similarly, iloprost, a prostacyclin analog, attenuated hyperoxia-induced alveolar and microvascular maldevelopment in a BPD mouse model.[99] Elevated levels of endogenous prostacyclin in tracheal aspirates of preterm infants were seemingly protective and associated with lower mean inspiratory oxygen and shorter duration of mechanical ventilation.[100]

Synthetic PGI_2 and prostacyclin analogs are used in the clinical treatment of PH, with multiple modes of administration, including intravenous, subcutaneous, inhaled, and oral routes. Prostacyclin therapies, particularly continuously administered intravenous or subcutaneous varieties, are considered the most potent class of medications used in the treatment of PAH. Prostacyclin therapy is primarily reserved for patients who have severe PH, show the presence of right heart failure, or have failed other first-line therapies. Small retrospective series have shown that inhaled epoprostenol, intravenous epoprostenol, intravenous treprostinil, and oral beraprost have efficacy in the treatment of PPHN in infants, including a subset of infants with PH related to congenital diaphragmatic hernia.[101–107] A small, single-institution series showed improvement in echocardiographic indices of PH after initiation of subcutaneous treprostinil for severe BPD-PH.[104] A retrospective cohort study of children with PH (including 43% with PH related to developmental lung disease, a category including bronchopulmonary dysplasia and congenital diaphragmatic hernia) showed that prostacyclin therapy was associated with an early and sustained improvement in echocardiographic assessment of RV performance and clinical biomarkers of PH.[108] Despite promising small studies, real-world use of prostacyclin therapy for BPD-PH is largely based on pediatric and adult PAH treatment algorithms, and these therapies are reserved for patients with high-risk features such as RV failure, disease progression, or severe hemodynamic alterations.[12,13]

The pharmacokinetics and dosing of prostacyclin therapies vary widely based on medication composition and delivery modality. Epoprostenol, or synthetic PGI_2, was the first prostacyclin therapy developed for the treatment of PH. Epoprostenol can be administered continuously intravenously or by inhalation through a ventilator. Epoprostenol has a very short half-life of 5 to 6 minutes. Although this allows for rapid escalation of dose in critical scenarios, it also conveys a risk of rebound PH crisis with abrupt medication discontinuation. Treprostinil is a more stable prostacyclin analog that may be administered continuously by an intravenous or subcutaneous route, via inhalation, or enterally. Treprostinil has a longer half-life of 4 to 5 hours, decreasing the risk of PH crisis in the event of brief infusion interruption. Iloprost is another chemically stable prostacyclin analog that may be intermittently administered every 1 to 4 hours through a ventilator or continuously.

Side effects of systemically administered prostacyclin therapy are in large part related to off-target binding to prostacyclin receptors in other organs, which include systemic hypotension, flushing, headache, extremity or jaw pain, nausea, and diarrhea.[109] A dedicated central line is required for intravenous formulations, which imparts additional risk for central-line–associated bloodstream infections. Side effects of subcutaneously administered medication include catheter site pain or superficial infection, although catheter site pain may be less severe in infants and small children compared to adolescents and adults.

As with other pulmonary vasodilators, there is potential for $\dot{V}/\dot{Q}$ mismatch secondary to systemic prostacyclin therapy. A single-center retrospective study of prostacyclin use in 36 children under 1 year of age, including 25% with BPD-PH, reported discontinuation of the drug due to desaturation in two infants with severe lung disease with high baseline oxygen requirements.[110] Conversely, in the cohort of infants with BPD-PH described by Nees and colleagues,[63] none of the 21 patients treated with systemic prostacyclin therapy but four of the 35 patients treated with inhaled iloprost discontinued medication due to desaturation. Inhaled medications may require specific ventilator modifications or trigger bronchoconstriction. Inhaled prostacyclin does not undergo rapid breakdown upon entering the bloodstream like iNO, although hypotension is rarely seen at clinically relevant doses, suggesting that vasodilation is mostly limited to the pulmonary vasculature.[111,112]

There are newer oral prostacyclin therapies—namely, oral treprostinil and the prostaglandin receptor agonist selexipag. Although there are reports of their use in older children and adolescents, the data are limited in infants and young children, with none specific to BPD-PH.

Drug Safety and Efficacy

One challenge in the treatment of BPD-PH is the lack of rigorous clinical trials and evidence-based, standardized treatment regimens. A majority of studies for all classes of pulmonary vasodilator therapies in BPD-PH are retrospective, often with small sample sizes from single institutions. As described above, all classes of systemic pulmonary vasodilators have potential side effects related to systemic vasodilation and/or off-target receptor effects. Multiple studies have demonstrated that PDE5 inhibitors, endothelin receptor antagonists, and systemic prostacyclin therapies generally have a favorable safety profile and are well tolerated in infants.[61,110,113,114] Potential for $\dot{V}/\dot{Q}$ mismatch with resultant systemic hypoxemia is of particular concern with the use of all systemic vasodilator therapies in BPD-PH, given the presence of concomitant heterogeneous lung disease. Although systemic saturations are not consistently documented in the published literature, worsening hypoxia was not reported as a significant side effect in most studies that evaluated drug safety. However, this variable may be challenging to evaluate, as it may be confounded by hypoxia related to right to left intracardiac shunting associated with severe PH. Anecdotally, clinically relevant systemic hypoxia related to $\dot{V}/\dot{Q}$ mismatch is rarely encountered in clinical practice. Regardless, because of the complex nature of disease, potential for side effects, and often tenuous status of infants with BPD-PH, the involvement of providers with expertise in the use of these therapies is recommended.

Drug Influence on Long-Term Outcomes

The recommended PH screening protocols for infants with BPD raises the question of whether the early identification and treatment of BPD-PH improve the associated mortality. Published studies show that these medications have benefit in improving short-term pulmonary vascular hemodynamics. However, there remains considerable early mortality in the BPD-PH population. The 101-patient BPD-PH cohort described by Nees and colleagues[63] showed that the use of sildenafil, treprostinil, and bosentan was not associated with a higher risk of mortality. Furthermore, despite the 33% mortality in the overall cohort, those who survived to hospital discharge did well over time with low post-discharge mortality; a majority discontinued pulmonary vasodilator therapy.[63] PH-targeted therapy has the potential to improve mortality by providing clinical stabilization so that the infant can ultimately achieve pulmonary vascular remodeling and postnatal lung growth. Conversely, one could argue that PH-targeted therapies may not improve mortality if lung growth and the associated increase in pulmonary vascular surface area are the primary mediators of survival and resolution of PH. Although the BPD-PH population has considerable respiratory and non-cardiopulmonary morbidities that may contribute to mortality, screening protocols for BPD-PH in a majority of centers are in their early phases of implementation, as the recommendations put out by the North American and European PH communities were released in 2016 and 2017.[32,71] Mehler and colleagues[115] described a single-institution experience of echocardiographic screening, although this study does not allow for assessment of this screening algorithm on mortality. By study design, the described BPD-PH cohort was one that survived to hospital discharge. There were no post-discharge deaths, and all described patients received sildenafil monotherapy, which was later discontinued in 100% of infants, making this a relatively healthy population when compared to other retrospective BPD-PH cohorts. Notably, there were three deaths in infants with BPD-PH prior to discharge, which were not further described.[115] The publication of short- and long-term outcomes after implementation of BPD-PH screening protocols will be crucial in determining the impact of PH-targeted therapy on mortality.

Prevention of Bronchopulmonary Dysplasia

An aspirational means of preventing BPD-PH would be the prevention of BPD. Despite identification of risk factors for BPD and BPD-PH, it is challenging to clinically predict which infants will be affected by either condition. Multiple peri- and postnatal interventions have been investigated for their utility in reducing the incidence of BPD. Vitamin A, caffeine, and systemic and inhaled steroids have all demonstrated some potential benefit in improving BPD incidence, although their widespread use is controversial.[116–122] The pulmonary vasodilators iNO and sildenafil have also been explored for their ability to prevent BPD. Nitric oxide use in premature infants has not been found to improve mortality or BPD incidence, and its use is currently recommended only in those with evidence of PH.[54,123,124] Empiric use of the PDE5 inhibitor sildenafil in preclinical models showed potential for the prevention of alveolar and pulmonary vascular changes in BPD models.[57–59] Unfortunately, these benefits have not been replicated in pilot clinical studies.[125,126] Stem cell therapy is rapidly emerging as a potential therapeutic tool for the prevention and treatment of BPD, with promising preclinical studies showing improvements in lung structure, inflammation, and PH in animal models. A number of phase I and II clinical trials are underway.[127]

Conclusions

In summary, PH is an important potential consequence of BPD, which imparts significant mortality risk early in life. Pulmonary vasodilator therapies provide a means to improve patient hemodynamics and clinical status. The use of pulmonary vasodilator therapies is primarily off-label usage with no definitive evidence-based treatment protocols. For this reason, the involvement of providers with expertise in pediatric PH and PH-targeted therapies is important, and all providers involved in the care of patients using these medications should have a basic understanding of the mechanism of action and potential side effects of these medications.

REFERENCES

1. Jobe AH, Bancalari E. Bronchopulmonary dysplasia. *Am J Respir Crit Care Med*. 2001;163(7):1723-1729.
2. Husain AN, Siddiqui NH, Stocker JT. Pathology of arrested acinar development in postsurfactant bronchopulmonary dysplasia. *Hum Pathol*. 1998;29(7):710-717.
3. Northway WH, Rosan RC, Porter DY. Pulmonary disease following respirator therapy of hyaline-membrane disease. *N Engl J Med*. 1967;276(7):357-368.
4. Coalson JJ. Pathology of new bronchopulmonary dysplasia. *Semin Neonatol*. 2003;8(1):73-81.
5. Day CL, Ryan RM. Bronchopulmonary dysplasia: new becomes old again! *Pediatr Res*. 2017;81(1-2):210-213.
6. Davidson L, Berkelhamer S. Bronchopulmonary dysplasia: chronic lung disease of infancy and long-term pulmonary outcomes. *J Clin Med*. 2017;6(1):1-20.
7. Berkelhamer SK, Mestan KK, Steinhorn R. An update on the diagnosis and management of bronchopulmonary dysplasia (BPD)-associated pulmonary hypertension. *Semin Perinatol*. 2018;42(7):432-443.
8. Stoll BJ, Hansen NI, Bell EF, et al. Trends in care practices, morbidity, and mortality of extremely preterm neonates, 1993–2012. *JAMA*. 2015;314(10):1039-1051.
9. Zysman-Colman Z, Tremblay GM, Bandeali S, Landry JS. Bronchopulmonary dysplasia – trends over three decades. *Paediatr Child Health*. 2013;18(2):86-90.
10. Cuevas Guaman M, Gien J, Baker C, Zhang H, Austin E, Collaco J. Point prevalence, clinical characteristics, and treatment variation for infants with severe bronchopulmonary dysplasia. *Am J Perinatol*. 2015;32(10):960-967.
11. Purisch SE, Gyamfi-Bannerman C. Epidemiology of preterm birth. *Semin Perinatol*. 2017;41(7):387-391.
12. Abman SH, Hansmann G, Archer SL, et al. Pediatric pulmonary hypertension: guidelines from the American Heart Association and American Thoracic Society. *Circulation*. 2015;132(21):2037-2099.
13. Rosenzweig EB, Abman SH, Adatia I, et al. Paediatric pulmonary arterial hypertension: updates on definition, classification, diagnostics and management. *Eur Respir J*. 2019;53(1):1-18.
14. Arjaans S, Zwart EAH, Ploegstra M, et al. Identification of gaps in the current knowledge on pulmonary hypertension in extremely preterm infants: a systematic review and meta-analysis. *Paediatr Perinat Epidemiol*. 2018;32(3):258-267.
15. Kim DH, Kim HS, Choi CW, Kim EK, Kim BI, Choi JH. Risk factors for pulmonary artery hypertension in preterm infants with moderate or severe bronchopulmonary dysplasia. *Neonatology*. 2012;101(1):40-46.
16. Bhat R, Salas AA, Foster C, Carlo WA, Ambalavanan N. Prospective analysis of pulmonary hypertension in extremely low birth weight infants. *Pediatrics*. 2012;129(3):e682-e689.
17. Mourani PM, Abman SH. Pulmonary hypertension and vascular abnormalities in bronchopulmonary dysplasia. *Clin Perinatol*. 2015;42(4):839-855.
18. Fitzgerald D, Evans N, Van Asperen P, Henderson-Smart D. Subclinical persisting pulmonary hypertension in chronic neonatal lung disease. *Arch Dis Child Fetal Neonatal Ed*. 1994;70(2):F118-F122.
19. Weismann CG, Asnes JD, Bazzy-Asaad A, Tolomeo C, Ehrenkranz RA, Bizzarro MJ. Pulmonary hypertension in preterm infants: results of a prospective screening program. *J Perinatol*. 2017;37(5):572-577.
20. Khemani E, McElhinney DB, Rhein L, et al. Pulmonary artery hypertension in formerly premature infants with bronchopulmonary dysplasia: clinical features and outcomes in the surfactant era. *Pediatrics*. 2007;120(6):1260-1269.
21. Altit G, Bhombal S, Hopper RK, Tacy TA, Feinstein J. Death or resolution: the "natural history" of pulmonary hypertension in bronchopulmonary dysplasia. *J Perinatol*. 2019;39(3):415-425.
22. Nakanishi H, Uchiyama A, Kusuda S. Impact of pulmonary hypertension on neurodevelopmental outcome in preterm infants with bronchopulmonary dysplasia: a cohort study. *J Perinatol*. 2016;36(10):890-896.

23. Baraldi E, Filippone M. Chronic lung disease after premature birth. *N Engl J Med*. 2007;357:1946-1955.
24. Thebaud B, Ladha F, Michelakis ED, et al. Vascular endothelial growth factor gene therapy increases survival, promotes lung angiogenesis, and prevents alveolar damage in hyperoxia-induced lung injury: evidence that angiogenesis participates in alveolarization. *Circulation*. 2005;112(16):2477-2486.
25. Bhatt AJ, Pryhuber GS, Huyck H, Watkins RH, Metlay LA, Maniscalco WM. Disrupted pulmonary vasculature and decreased vascular endothelial growth factor, Flt-1, and TIE-2 in human infants dying with bronchopulmonary dysplasia. *Am J Respir Crit Care Med*. 2001;164(10):1971-1980.
26. Malloy KW, Austin ED. Pulmonary hypertension in the child with bronchopulmonary dysplasia. *Pediatr Pulmonol*. 2021;56(11): 3546-3556.
27. Check J, Gotteiner N, Liu X, et al. Fetal growth restriction and pulmonary hypertension in premature infants with bronchopulmonary dysplasia. *J Perinatol*. 2013;33(7):553-557.
28. Mourani PM, Sontag MK, Younoszai A, et al. Early pulmonary vascular disease in preterm infants at risk for bronchopulmonary dysplasia. *Am J Respir Crit Care Med*. 2015;191(1):87-95.
29. Nagiub M, Kanaan U, Simon D, Guglani L. Risk factors for development of pulmonary hypertension in infants with bronchopulmonary dysplasia: systematic review and meta-analysis. *Paediatr Respir Rev*. 2017;23:27-32.
30. Varghese N, Rios D. Pulmonary hypertension associated with bronchopulmonary dysplasia: a review. *Pediatr Allergy Immunol Pulmonol*. 2019;32(4):140-148.
31. Krishnan U, Feinstein JA, Adatia I, et al. Evaluation and management of pulmonary hypertension in children with bronchopulmonary dysplasia. *J Pediatr*. 2017;9(188):24-34.
32. Hilgendorff A, Apitz C, Bonnet D, Hansmann G. Pulmonary hypertension associated with acute or chronic lung diseases in the preterm and term neonate and infant. The European Paediatric Pulmonary Vascular Disease Network, endorsed by ISHLT and DGPK. *Heart*. 2016;102(suppl 2):ii49-ii56.
33. Suresh G, King BC, Jain SK. Screening for pulmonary hypertension in preterm infants—not ready for prime time. *J Perinatol*. 2018;38(3):206-210.
34. Avitabile CM, Ansems S, Wang Y, et al. Accuracy of brain natriuretic peptide for diagnosing pulmonary hypertension in severe bronchopulmonary dysplasia. *Neonatology*. 2019;116(2): 147-153.
35. King ME, Braun H, Goldblatt A, Liberthson R, Weyman AE. Interventricular septal configuration as a predictor of right ventricular systolic hypertension in children: a cross-sectional echocardiographic study. *Circulation*. 1983;68(1):68-75.
36. Semple T, Akhtar MR, Owens CM. Imaging bronchopulmonary dysplasia—a multimodality update. *Front Med (Lausanne)*. 2017;4(88):1-7.
37. Critser PJ, Higano NS, Tkach JA, et al. Cardiac magnetic resonance imaging evaluation of neonatal bronchopulmonary dysplasia–associated pulmonary hypertension. *Am J Respir Crit Care Med*. 2020;201(1):73-82.
38. Bernier ML, Jacob AI, Collaco JM, McGrath-Morrow SA, Romer LH, Unegbu CC. Perioperative events in children with pulmonary hypertension undergoing non-cardiac procedures. *Pulm Circ*. 2018;8(1):1-10.
39. del Cerro MJ, Moledina S, Haworth SG, et al. Cardiac catheterization in children with pulmonary hypertensive vascular disease: consensus statement from the Pulmonary Vascular Research Institute, Pediatric and Congenital Heart Disease Task Forces. *Pulm Circ*. 2016;6(1):118-125.
40. Sindelar R, Shepherd EG, Ågren J, et al. Established severe BPD: is there a way out? Change of ventilatory paradigms. *Pediatr Res*. 2021;90(6):1139-1146.
41. Humbert M, Sitbon O, Simmonneau G. Treatment of pulmonary arterial hypertension. *N Engl J Med*. 2004;351:1425-1436.
42. Porta NFM, Steinhorn RH. Pulmonary vasodilator therapy in the NICU: inhaled nitric oxide, sildenafil, and other pulmonary vasodilating agents. *Clin Perinatol*. 2012;39(1):149-164.
43. Yu B, Ichinose F, Bloch DB, Zapol WM. Inhaled nitric oxide. *Br J Pharmacol*. 2019;176(2):246-255.
44. Kelm M. Nitric oxide metabolism and breakdown. *Biochim Biophys Acta*. 1999;1411(2-3):273-289.
45. Kinsella JP, Neish SR, Shaffer E, Abman SH. Low-dose inhalational nitric oxide in persistent pulmonary hypertension of the newborn. *Lancet*. 1992;340(8823):819-820.
46. Roberts J. Inhaled nitric oxide in persistent pulmonary hypertension of the newborn. *Lancet*. 1992;340(8823):818-819.
47. Frostell CG, Blomqvist H, Hedenstierna G, Lundberg J, Zapol WM. Inhalational nitric oxide selectively reverses human hypoxic pulmonary vasoconstriction without causing systemic vasodilation. *Anesthesiology*. 1993;78:427-435.
48. DiBlasi RM, Dupras D, Kearney C, Costa E, Griebel JL. Nitric oxide delivery by neonatal noninvasive respiratory support devices. *Respir Care*. 2015;60(2):219-230.
49. Tworetzky W, Bristow J, Moore P, et al. Inhaled nitric oxide in neonates with persistent pulmonary hypertension. *Lancet*. 2001;357(9250):118-120.
50. Black SM, Heidersbach RS, McMullan DM, Bekker JM, Johengen MJ, Fineman JR. Inhaled nitric oxide inhibits NOS activity in lambs: potential mechanism for rebound pulmonary hypertension. *Am J Physiol*. 1999;277(5):H1849-H1856.
51. Davidson D, Barefield ES, Kattwinkel J, et al. Safety of withdrawing inhaled nitric oxide therapy in persistent pulmonary hypertension of the newborn. *Pediatrics*. 1999;104(2):231-236.
52. Neonatal Inhaled Nitrix Oxide Study Group. Inhaled nitric oxide in full-term and nearly full-term infants with hypoxic respiratory failure. *N Engl J Med*. 1997;336:597-604.
53. Cole FS, Alleyne C, Barks JDE, et al. NIH Consensus Development Conference Statement: inhaled nitric-oxide therapy for premature infants. *Pediatrics*. 2011;127(2):363-369.
54. Kinsella JP, Steinhorn RH, Krishnan US, et al. Recommendations for the use of inhaled nitric oxide therapy in premature newborns with severe pulmonary hypertension. *J Pediatr*. 2016;170:312-314.
55. Hansmann G, Koestenberger M, Alastalo TP, et al. 2019 updated consensus statement on the diagnosis and treatment of pediatric pulmonary hypertension: the European Pediatric Pulmonary Vascular Disease Network (EPPVDN), endorsed by AEPC, ESPR and ISHLT. *J Heart Lung Transplant*. 2019;38(9): 879-901.
56. Ladha F, Bonnet S, Eaton F, Hashimoto K, Korbutt G, Thébaud B. Sildenafil improves alveolar growth and pulmonary hypertension in hyperoxia-induced lung injury. *Am J Respir Crit Care Med*. 2005;172(6):750-756.
57. de Visser YP, Walther FJ, Laghmani EH, Boersma H, van der Laarse A, Wagenaar GT. Sildenafil attenuates pulmonary inflammation and fibrin deposition, mortality and right ventricular hypertrophy in neonatal hyperoxic lung injury. *Respir Res*. 2009;10(30).
58. Park HS, Park JW, Kim HJ, et al. Sildenafil alleviates bronchopulmonary dysplasia in neonatal rats by activating the hypoxia-inducible factor signaling pathway. *Am J Respir Cell Mol Biol*. 2013;48(1):105-113.

59. Heilman RP, Lagoski MB, Lee KJ, et al. Right ventricular cyclic nucleotide signaling is decreased in hyperoxia-induced pulmonary hypertension in neonatal mice. *Am J Physiol Heart Circ Physiol*. 2015;308(12):H1575-H1582.
60. Hon KL, Cheung KL, Siu KL, et al. Oral sildenafil for treatment of severe pulmonary hypertension in an infant. *Neonatology*. 2005;88(2):109-112.
61. van der Graaf M, Rojer LA, Helbing WA, Reiss IKM, Etnel JRG, Bartelds B. Sildenafil for bronchopulmonary dysplasia and pulmonary hypertension: a meta-analysis. *Pulm Circ*. 2019;9(3):1-8.
62. Tan K, Krishnamurthy MB, O'Heney JL, Paul E, Sehgal A. Sildenafil therapy in bronchopulmonary dysplasia-associated pulmonary hypertension: a retrospective study of efficacy and safety. *Eur J Pediatr*. 2015;174(8):1109-1115.
63. Nees SN, Rosenzweig EB, Cohen JL, Valencia Villeda GA, Krishnan US. Targeted therapy for pulmonary hypertension in premature infants. *Children*. 2020;7(8):97.
64. Mourani PM, Sontag MK, Ivy DD, Abman SH. Effects of long-term sildenafil treatment for pulmonary hypertension in infants with chronic lung disease. *J Pediatr*. 2009;154(3):379-384.e2.
65. Nyp M, Sandritter T, Poppinga N, Simon C, Truog WE. Sildenafil citrate, bronchopulmonary dysplasia and disordered pulmonary gas exchange: any benefits? *J Perinatol*. 2012;32(1):64-69.
66. Trottier-Boucher MN, Lapointe A, Malo J, et al. Sildenafil for the treatment of pulmonary arterial hypertension in infants with bronchopulmonary dysplasia. *Pediatr Cardiol*. 2015;36(6):1255-1260.
67. Cohen JL, Nees SN, Valencia GA, Rosenzweig EB, Krishnan US. Sildenafil use in children with pulmonary hypertension. *J Pediatr*. 2019;205:29-34.e1.
68. Barst RJ, Ivy DD, Gaitan G, et al. A randomized, double-blind, placebo-controlled, dose-ranging study of oral sildenafil citrate in treatment-naive children with pulmonary arterial hypertension. *Circulation*. 2012;125(2):324-334.
69. Barst RJ, Beghetti M, Pulido T, et al. STARTS-2: long-term survival with oral sildenafil monotherapy in treatment-naive pediatric pulmonary arterial hypertension. *Circulation*. 2014;129(19):1914-1923.
70. Abman SH, Kinsella JP, Rosenzweig EB, et al. Implications of the U.S. Food and Drug Administration warning against the use of sildenafil for the treatment of pediatric pulmonary hypertension. *Am J Respir Crit Care Med*. 2013;187(6):572-575.
71. Krishnan U. Evaluation and management of pulmonary hypertension in children with bronchopulmonary dysplasia. *J Pediatr*. 2017;188:24-34.e1.
72. Ivy D, Bonnet D, Berger RM, Meyer GMB, Baygani S, Li B. Efficacy and safety of tadalafil in a pediatric population with pulmonary arterial hypertension: phase 3 randomized, double-blind placebo-controlled study. *Pulm Circ*. 2021;11(3):1-8.
73. Takatsuki S, Calderbank M, Ivy DD. Initial experience with tadalafil in pediatric pulmonary arterial hypertension. *Pediatr Cardiol*. 2012;33(5):683-688.
74. Klinger JR, Chakinala MM, Langleben D, Rosenkranz S, Sitbon O. Riociguat: clinical research and evolving role in therapy. *Br J Clin Pharmacol*. 2021;87(7):2645-2662.
75. Donda K, Zambrano R, Moon Y, et al. Riociguat prevents hyperoxia-induced lung injury and pulmonary hypertension in neonatal rats without effects on long bone growth. *PLoS One*. 2018;13(7):e0199927.
76. Katsuragi S, Ishida H, Suginobe H, et al. Riociguat can ameliorate bronchopulmonary dysplasia in the SU5416 induced rat experimental model. *Exp Lung Res*. 2021;47(8):382-389.
77. Spreemann T, Bertram H, Happel CM, Kozlik-Feldmann R, Hansmann G. First-in-child use of the oral soluble guanylate cyclase stimulator riociguat in pulmonary arterial hypertension. *Pulm Circ*. 2018;8(3):1-6.
78. Ambalavanan N, Bulger A, Murphy-Ullrich J, Oparil S, Chen YF. Endothelin-A receptor blockade prevents and partially reverses neonatal hypoxic pulmonary vascular remodeling. *Pediatr Res*. 2005;57(5 Part 1):631-636.
79. Gien J, Tseng N, Seedorf G, Kuhn K, Abman SH. Endothelin-1–Rho kinase interactions impair lung structure and cause pulmonary hypertension after bleomycin exposure in neonatal rat pups. *Am J Physiol Lung Cell Mol Physiol*. 2016;311(6):L1090-L1100.
80. Niu JO, Munshi UK, Siddiq MM, Parton LA. Early increase in endothelin-1 in tracheal aspirates of preterm infants: correlation with bronchopulmonary dysplasia. *J Pediatr*. 1998;132(6):965-970.
81. El Sayed M, Sherif L, Said R, El-Wakkad A, EL-Refay A, Aly H. Endothelin-1 and *L*-arginine in preterm infants with respiratory distress. *Am J Perinatol*. 2011;28(02):129-136.
82. Baumann P, Fouzas S, Pramana I, et al. Plasma proendothelin-1 as an early marker of bronchopulmonary dysplasia. *Neonatology*. 2015;108(4):293-296.
83. Gerull R, Neumann RP, Atkinson A, Bernasconi L, Schulzke SM, Wellmann S. Respiratory morbidity in preterm infants predicted by natriuretic peptide (MR-proANP) and endothelin-1 (CT-proET-1). *Pediatr Res*. 2022;91(6):1478-1484.
84. Rosenzweig EB, Ivy DD, Widlitz A, et al. Effects of long-term bosentan in children with pulmonary arterial hypertension. *J Am Coll Cardiol*. 2005;46(4):697-704.
85. Ivy DD, Rosenzweig EB, Lemarié JC, Brand M, Rosenberg D, Barst RJ. Long-term outcomes in children with pulmonary arterial hypertension treated with bosentan in real-world clinical settings. *Am J Cardiol*. 2010;106(9):1332-1338.
86. Maiya S. Response to bosentan in children with pulmonary hypertension. *Heart*. 2006;92(5):664-670.
87. Hislop AA, Moledina S, Foster H, Schulze-Neick I, Haworth SG. Long-term efficacy of bosentan in treatment of pulmonary arterial hypertension in children. *Eur Respir J*. 2011;38(1):70-77.
88. Berger RMF, Haworth SG, Bonnet D, et al. FUTURE-2: results from an open-label, long-term safety and tolerability extension study using the pediatric FormUlation of bosenTan in pUlmonary arterial hypeRtEnsion. *Int J Cardiol*. 2016;202:52-58.
89. Mohamed WA, Ismail M. A randomized, double-blind, placebo-controlled, prospective study of bosentan for the treatment of persistent pulmonary hypertension of the newborn. *J Perinatol*. 2012;32(8):608-613.
90. Steinhorn RH, Fineman J, Kusic-Pajic A, et al. Bosentan as adjunctive therapy for persistent pulmonary hypertension of the newborn: results of the randomized multicenter placebo-controlled exploratory trial. *J Pediatr*. 2016;177:90-96.e3.
91. Maneenil G, Thatrimontrichai A, Janjindamai W, Dissaneevate S. Effect of bosentan therapy in persistent pulmonary hypertension of the newborn. *Pediatr Neonatol*. 2018;59(1):58-64.
92. Krishnan U, Krishnan S, Gewitz M. Treatment of pulmonary hypertension in children with chronic lung disease with newer oral therapies. *Pediatr Cardiol*. 2008;29(6):1082-1086.
93. Hansmann G, Sallmon H, Roehr CC, et al. Pulmonary hypertension in bronchopulmonary dysplasia. *Pediatr Res*. 2021;89(3):446-455.
94. Burgess G, Hoogkamer H, Collings L, Dingemanse J. Mutual pharmacokinetic interactions between steady-state bosentan and sildenafil. *Eur J Clin Pharmacol*. 2008;64(1):43-50.

95. Takatsuki S, Rosenzweig EB, Zuckerman W, Brady D, Calderbank M, Ivy DD. Clinical safety, pharmacokinetics, and efficacy of ambrisentan therapy in children with pulmonary arterial hypertension. *Pediatr Pulmonol*. 2013;48(1):27-34.
96. Albinni S, Pavo I, Kitzmueller E, Michel-Behnke I. Macitentan in infants and children with pulmonary hypertensive vascular disease. Feasibility, tolerability and practical issues – a single-centre experience. *Pulm Circ*. 2021;11(1):1-10.
97. Schweintzger S, Koestenberger M, Schlagenhauf A, et al. Safety and efficacy of the endothelin receptor antagonist macitentan in pediatric pulmonary hypertension. *Cardiovasc Diagn Ther*. 2020;10(5):1675-1685.
98. Mahajan CN, Afolayan AJ, Eis A, Teng RJ, Konduri GG. Altered prostanoid metabolism contributes to impaired angiogenesis in persistent pulmonary hypertension in a fetal lamb model. *Pediatr Res*. 2015;77(3):455-462.
99. Olave N, Lal CV, Halloran B, Bhandari V, Ambalavanan N. Iloprost attenuates hyperoxia-mediated impairment of lung development in newborn mice. *Am J Physiol Lung Cell Mol Physiol*. 2018;315(4):L535-L544.
100. Lassus P, Viinikka L, Ylikorkala O, Pohjavuori M, Andersson S. Pulmonary prostacyclin is associated with less severe respiratory distress in preterm infants. *Early Hum Dev*. 2002;67 (1-2):11-18.
101. Kelly LK, Porta NFM, Goodman DM, Carroll CL, Steinhorn RH. Inhaled prostacyclin for term infants with persistent pulmonary hypertension refractory to inhaled nitric oxide. *J Pediatr*. 2002;141(6):830-832.
102. Berger-Caron F, Piedboeuf B, Morissette G, et al. Inhaled epoprostenol for pulmonary hypertension treatment in neonates: a 12-year experience. *Am J Perinatol*. 2019;36(11):1142-1149.
103. Ahmad KA, Banales J, Henderson CL, Ramos SE, Brandt KM, Powers GC. Intravenous epoprostenol improves oxygenation index in patients with persistent pulmonary hypertension of the newborn refractory to nitric oxide. *J Perinatol*. 2018;38(9): 1212-1219.
104. Turbenson MN, Radosevich JJ, Manuel V, Feldman J. Transitioning from intravenous to subcutaneous prostacyclin therapy in neonates with severe pulmonary hypertension. *J Pediatr Pharmacol Ther*. 2020;25(7):647-653.
105. Lawrence KM, Hedrick HL, Monk HM, et al. Treprostinil improves persistent pulmonary hypertension associated with congenital diaphragmatic hernia. *J Pediatr*. 2018;200:44-49.
106. Nakwan N, Nakwan N, Wannaro J. Persistent pulmonary hypertension of the newborn successfully treated with beraprost sodium: a retrospective chart review. *Neonatology*. 2011; 99(1):32-37.
107. Jozefkowicz M, Haag DF, Mazzucchelli MT, Salgado G, Fariña D. Neonates effects and tolerability of treprostinil in hypertension with persistent pulmonary. *Am J Perinatol*. 2020;37(9): 939-946.
108. Hopper RK, Wang Y, DeMatteo V, et al. Right ventricular function mirrors clinical improvement with use of prostacyclin analogues in pediatric pulmonary hypertension. *Pulm Circ*. 2018;8(2):1-8.
109. Lang IM, Gaine SP. Recent advances in targeting the prostacyclin pathway in pulmonary arterial hypertension. *Eur Respir Rev*. 2015;24:630-641.
110. McIntyre CM, Hanna BD, Rintoul N, Ramsey EZ. Safety of epoprostenol and treprostinil in children less than 12 months of age. *Pulm Circ*. 2013;3(4):862-869.
111. Walmrath D, Schneider T, Pilch J, Grimminger F, Seeger W. Aerosolised prostacyclin in adult respiratory distress syndrome. *Lancet*. 1993;342(8877):961-962.
112. Zwissler B, Kemming G, Habler O, et al. Inhaled prostacyclin (PGI2) versus inhaled nitric oxide in adult respiratory distress syndrome. *Am J Respir Crit Care Med*. 1996;154(6):1671-1677.
113. More K, Athalye-Jape GK, Rao SC, Patole SK. Endothelin receptor antagonists for persistent pulmonary hypertension in term and late preterm infants. *Cochrane Database Syst Rev*. 2016;(8):CD010531.
114. Levy M, Del Cerro MJ, Nadaud S, et al. Safety, efficacy and management of subcutaneous treprostinil infusions in the treatment of severe pediatric pulmonary hypertension. *Int J Cardiol*. 2018;264:153-157.
115. Mehler K, Udink Ten Cate FE, Keller T, Bangen U, Kribs A, Oberthuer A. An echocardiographic screening program helps to identify pulmonary hypertension in extremely low birthweight infants with and without bronchopulmonary dysplasia: a single-center experience. *Neonatology*. 2018;113(1):81-88.
116. Darlow BA, Graham PJ, Rojas-Reyes MX. Vitamin A supplementation to prevent mortality and short- and long-term morbidity in very low birth weight infants. *Cochrane Database Syst Rev*. 2016;2016(8):CD000501.
117. Kua KP, Lee SWH. Systematic review and meta-analysis of clinical outcomes of early caffeine therapy in preterm neonates. *Br J Clin Pharmacol*. 2017;83(1):180-191.
118. Taha D, Kirkby S, Nawab U, et al. Early caffeine therapy for prevention of bronchopulmonary dysplasia in preterm infants. *J Matern Fetal Neonatal Med*. 2014;27(16):1698-1702.
119. Doyle LW, Cheong JL, Hay S, Manley BJ, Halliday HL. Early (<7 days) systemic postnatal corticosteroids for prevention of bronchopulmonary dysplasia in preterm infants. *Cochrane Database Syst Rev*. 2021;2021(10):CD001146.
120. Doyle LW, Cheong JL, Hay S, Manley BJ, Halliday HL. Late (≥ 7 days) systemic postnatal corticosteroids for prevention of bronchopulmonary dysplasia in preterm infants. *Cochrane Database Syst Rev*. 2021;2021(11):CD001145.
121. Greenberg RG, Gayam S, Savage D, et al. Furosemide exposure and prevention of bronchopulmonary dysplasia in premature infants. *J Pediatr*. 2019;208:134-140.e2.
122. Mandell EW, Kratimenos P, Abman SH, Steinhorn RH. Drugs for the prevention and treatment of bronchopulmonary dysplasia. *Clin Perinatol*. 2019;46(2):291-310.
123. Askie LM, Ballard RA. Inhaled nitric oxide in preterm infants: an individual- patient data meta-analysis of randomized trials. *Pediatrics*. 2011;128(4):729-739.
124. Donohue PK, Gilmore MM, Cristofalo E, et al. Inhaled nitric oxide in preterm infants: a systematic review. *Pediatrics*. 2011;127(2):e414-e422.
125. König K, Barfield CP, Guy KJ, Drew SM, Andersen CC. The effect of sildenafil on evolving bronchopulmonary dysplasia in extremely preterm infants: a randomised controlled pilot study. *J Matern Fetal Neonatal Med*. 2014;27(5):439-444.
126. Abounahia FF, Abu-Jarir R, Abounahia MF, et al. Prophylactic sildenafil in preterm infants at risk of bronchopulmonary dysplasia: a pilot randomized, double-blinded, placebo-controlled trial. *Clin Drug Investig*. 2019;39(11):1093-1107.
127. Nitkin CR, Rajasingh J, Pisano C, Besner GE, Thébaud B, Sampath V. Stem cell therapy for preventing neonatal diseases in the 21st century: current understanding and challenges. *Pediatr Res*. 2020;87(2):265-276.

Chapter **17**

Drug-Associated Acute Kidney Injury in Neonates

Mina H. Hanna, MD

Key Points

- Drug-associated acute kidney injury is common in neonates and has important implications for therapeutic decisions and patient clinical outcomes.
- This chapter reviews the mechanisms of nephrotoxin-induced acute kidney injury and the various medications that are widely used in neonatal intensive care units.
- Our ability to understand the fundamental principles of management of drug-induced nephrotoxicity requires a multidisciplinary approach aimed at earlier recognition and close monitoring.

Introduction

Acute kidney injury (AKI) is defined as sudden impairment in kidney function that results in the inability to maintain adequate fluid, electrolyte, and waste product homeostasis. AKI occurs commonly in critically ill children, with varying degrees of severity, and it is associated with increased morbidity and mortality.[1] AKI can have important short-term consequences (e.g., longer duration of mechanical ventilation or ICU hospitalization) and long-term consequences (e.g., chronic kidney disease, hypertension). Critically ill newborns represent a high-risk population for developing drug-associated renal injury because of incomplete maturation of the kidney; furthermore, they are often exposed to numerous nephrotoxic medications. Drug-associated AKI may compromise the formation and development of nephrons, particularly in preterm neonates, who have incomplete nephrogenesis. There is no treatment for established AKI in this vulnerable population. Because of this, the focus has shifted to identifying modifiable risk factors that could prevent or delay the progression of AKI. In particular, nephrotoxic medications are a prevalent and potentially preventable cause of AKI in newborns. The purpose of this chapter is to briefly summarize what is known about drug-associated nephrotoxicity in neonates, highlighting the potential long-term implications of neonatal AKI.

Background

The Assessment of Worldwide Acute Kidney injury Epidemiology in Neonates (AWAKEN) study reported that AKI occurred in 30% of critically ill neonates and was associated with increased length of stay, duration of mechanical ventilation, and mortality.[2] The traditional approach to determine renal injury in neonates is based on two classical biochemical markers, serum creatinine (SCr) and blood urea nitrogen. Although these indices are valid indicators of renal function, their use in the neonatal period is associated with some limitations. Neonatal SCr initially reflects maternal values, and, rather than maintaining a steady state, these levels then decline at varying rates over days to weeks depending on gestational age, such that changes (or lack of change) in SCr may be difficult to interpret when evaluating for AKI. Rather than using arbitrary, binary AKI definitions (SCr $>$1.5 mg/dL, urine output $<$0.5 mL/kg/hr), several new neonatal studies have used modifications of the Acute Kidney Injury Network (AKIN) staging system or the risk, injury, failure, loss, and end-stage renal disease (RIFLE) classification. These standardized frameworks have allowed better comparisons across studies, have shown consistently that even

TABLE 17.1 KDIGO Classification of Neonatal AKI

Stage	SCr	Urine Output
0	No change in SCr *or* SCr rise <0.3 mg/dL	≥0.5 mL/kg/hr
1	SCr rise ≥0.3 mg/dL within 48 hr *or* SCr rise ≥1.5–1.9× reference SCr* within 7 days	<0.5 mL/kg/hr for 6–12 hr
2	SCr rise ≥2×–2.9× reference SCr*	<0.5 mL/kg/hr for ≥12 hr
3	SCr rise ≥3× reference SCr* *or* SCr ≥2.5 mg/dL** *or* Receipt of dialysis	<0.3 mL/kg/hr for ≥24 hr *or* Anuria for ≥12 hr

Differences between the proposed neonatal AKI definition and KDIGO are indicated by asterisks.
*Reference SCr is defined as the lowest previous SCr value.
**SCr value of 2.5 mg/dL represents <10 mL/min/1.73 m^2.
AKI, acute kidney injury; *KDIGO,* kidney disease improving global outcomes.

mild degrees of AKI portend poor outcomes, and have demonstrated worse outcomes with progressive AKI severity. Alternatively, Jetton and Askenazi[3] proposed a standardized neonatal AKI definition based on the Kidney Disease Improving Global Outcomes (KDIGO) definition adopted in 2012. In this modified KDIGO definition, the baseline SCr is assumed to be the lowest SCr level noted in each infant. Also, the SCr threshold for stage 3 AKI was reduced to 2.5 mg/dL rather than the usual KDIGO threshold of 4 mg/dL. The neonatal modified KDIGO definition and classification of AKI (Table 17.1) have been adopted by many researchers.

AKI epidemiologic data in neonates are sparse and mostly from single-center studies. AKI has been reported in 18% of very-low-birth-weight (VLBW) infants,[4] 30% to 50% of infants following congenital heart surgery,[5] 71% of neonates with congenital diaphragmatic hernia receiving extracorporeal membrane oxygenation,[6] and 38% of neonates with perinatal asphyxia.[7] In addition to the unique nature of neonatal renal development and physiology, several perinatal and postnatal risk factors predispose critically ill neonates to AKI. Insults such as hypoperfusion and nephrotoxic medication exposure can be classified as pre-renal or intrinsic. Hypoperfusion is a result of cardiovascular decompensation and hypotension due to a variety of reasons, such as hypoxemia, blood loss, sepsis, or patent ductus arteriosus. In these settings, healthy regulation of blood flow via dilatation of the afferent arterioles by prostaglandins and vasoconstriction of both efferent and afferent arterioles by angiotensin is often impaired, resulting in oliguria.[8] Nephrotoxic insults cause AKI by decreasing renal perfusion, causing direct tubular injury, triggering an episode of interstitial nephritis, or causing tubular obstruction. Although a few studies have evaluated drug-induced AKI epidemiology in older children, data on neonatal nephrotoxic medication–associated AKI are scarce. The most widely used nephrotoxic medications in the neonatal intensive care unit (NICU) are antibiotics, antifungals, non-steroidal anti-inflammatory drugs (NSAIDs), and diuretics. In a retrospective cohort study of 52,061 infants in 127 NICUs,[9] the median antibiotic exposure was close to one-quarter of all patient days, with a range across units from 2.4% to 97%. At all levels of care, from intermediate to units that provide the highest level of critical care, antibiotic use was independent of proven infection, necrotizing enterocolitis, surgical volume, or mortality, with a 40-fold variation in NICU antibiotic use.

AKI was independently associated with increased mortality and length of hospitalization in VLBW infants.[10] Early recognition and ongoing surveillance of modifiable risk factors that could prevent or delay progression of AKI in neonates is important. Because of the limitations of traditional definitions and biomarkers of AKI and because in most cases the etiology of AKI is multifactorial, drug-associated AKI represents the most common potentially avoidable type of AKI in neonates.

Nephrotoxin-Induced AKI

Drug-associated AKI occurs through a variety of mechanisms. The underlying neonatal susceptibility to drug toxicity plays an important role in AKI development. Additionally, the inherent nephrotoxicity of drugs and the transport and metabolism of medications by the kidneys are important factors in the progression of AKI. In hospitalized children, predisposing factors such as age, pharmacogenetics, underlying disease, dosage of the nephrotoxin, and concomitant medication determine and influence the severity of nephrotoxic insult.[11] Critically ill neonates are at higher risk for nephrotoxicity in the setting of hypotension, organ ischemia, multiple organ dysfunction, and concurrent nephrotoxic medication exposure.[12] Renal blood flow is proportionally reduced in preterm infants compared with full-term infants, making the preterm kidney more vulnerable to hypoperfusion.

A meta-analysis of risk factors for AKI in critically ill adult patients showed 53% greater odds of developing AKI with each additional nephrotoxic drug received (odds ratio, 1.53; confidence interval [CI], 1.09–2.14).[13] Moffett et al.[14] found that both the number of nephrotoxic drugs and duration of exposure were positively correlated with development of AKI in hospitalized non-critically ill children. In this cohort, age was protective, so infants were at higher risk of developing AKI. The majority of nephrotoxic medications to which patients were exposed were antimicrobial agents (52%). A pharmacoepidemiologic study of exposure to nephrotoxic medications among critically ill children in a pediatric intensive care unit (PICU) showed that furosemide (administered to 67.8% of patients), vancomycin (28.7%), and gentamicin (21.4%) were the most frequently administered. Patients who developed AKI were more likely to be exposed to at least one nephrotoxic medication, and risk increased with an increasing number of nephrotoxic medications.[15]

The potential for adverse drug events among neonates is likely greater than that among children.[16] However, neonates remain an understudied population. In the U.S. Food and Drug Administration (FDA) database for pediatric studies submitted between 1997 and 2010 involving 406 pediatric labeling changes, only 6% of the studies included new neonatal information.[17] A retrospective review of a national database collected prospectively showed that only 35% of the most commonly prescribed medications in NICUs are FDA approved for infants. In this large cohort, the 10 most commonly reported medication exposures were ampicillin, gentamicin, caffeine, vancomycin, beractant, furosemide, fentanyl, dopamine, midazolam, and calfactant. For extremely low-birth-weight (ELBW) infants, the 10 most commonly reported drug exposures were gentamicin, ampicillin, caffeine, vancomycin, furosemide, dopamine, beractant, indomethacin, fentanyl, and albuterol.[18] A single-center study of nephrotoxic medication exposure in VLBW neonates showed that 86.9% were exposed to at least one nephrotoxic medication during their hospital stay, and the neonates with the greatest cumulative exposure were at the highest risk of acquiring AKI. This study showed that VLBW infants were exposed to approximately 2 weeks of nephrotoxic medications before discharge, or on 1 of every 6 days of hospitalization. The greatest exposures occurred among the smallest and most immature infants and in those who experienced AKI.[19]

Although many medications are eliminated by the kidneys, data about renal processing of medications used in neonates are limited. Medication-induced AKI occurs through mechanisms that involve their inherent toxicity, as well as their transport and handling by the kidneys. Neonatal variability in developmental pharmacokinetics, pharmacodynamics, and pharmacogenetics, combined with heterogeneity in the underlying pathophysiology of nephrotoxicity, leads to uneven responses to medications. The two major pathways that mediate drug clearance are glomerular filtration and tubular secretion (sometimes in combination). Therefore, tubular cells and the surrounding interstitium are exposed to potentially nephrotoxic medications via apical contact and cellular uptake or by transport from the basolateral circulation through cells with subsequent apical efflux into the urine.[20] Then, as drugs are concentrated as they move from the proximal tubules into the loop of Henle and distal tubules, there is increased potential for tubulointerstitial injury. Additionally, distal nephrons can be injured secondary to precipitation of drug crystals within tubule lumens with the formation of obstructive drug-containing casts.[21] A panel of international pediatric and adult nephrologists and pharmacists developed a standardized description of the phenotype for drug-associated kidney disease in hospitalized patients. The four general categories include AKI, glomerular disorders, nephrolithiasis, and tubular dysfunction. Underlying mechanisms can be either dose dependent or dose independent (as in acute interstitial nephritis).[22] Each phenotype is based on primary and secondary criteria, and at least one primary criterion must be met for all drugs suspected of causing drug-induced kidney disease. For each phenotype definition, the following critical elements from the Bradford–Hill causation criteria must be met:

1. The drug exposure must be at least 24 hours preceding the event.
2. There should be biological plausibility for the causal drug, based on known mechanisms of drug effect, metabolism, and immunogenicity.
3. Complete data surrounding the period of drug exposure (including but not limited to comorbidities, additional nephrotoxic exposures, exposure to contrast agents, surgical procedures, blood pressure, and urine output) are required to account for concomitant risks.
4. The strength of the relationship between the attributable drug and the phenotype should be based on drug exposure duration, extent of primary and secondary criteria met, and the time course of the injury.

Nephrotoxic Medications

ACYCLOVIR

Acyclovir, used in neonates for the treatment of herpes simplex viral infections, is excreted in the urine through both filtration and secretion. It is relatively insoluble in urine. Nephrotoxicity is observed in 17% to 35% of patients,[23] typically develops within 48 hours of initiation of treatment,[24] and warrants diligent monitoring throughout treatment. Acyclovir-associated renal injury is classically attributed to tubular obstruction secondary to drug crystallization, but direct tubular toxicity from acyclovir metabolites may also contribute.[25] Additionally, acyclovir is transported by organic acid transporters shared with certain beta-lactam antibiotics (particularly ceftriaxone), which may increase the risk of nephrotoxicity. Nephrotoxicity is more likely in those with impaired renal function, concurrent nephrotoxic exposures, and reduced intravascular volume. Therefore, to mitigate the nephrotoxic potential it is recommended to adequately hydrate patients, administer the medication over 1 to 2 hours, adjust dosage in those with decreased renal function, and avoid concurrent nephrotoxic medication exposure.

AMINOGLYCOSIDES

Aminoglycosides are commonly used for the treatment of neonates with suspected sepsis or documented Gram-negative infections. A recent retrospective review of a large database showed that gentamicin was the most commonly used medication for ELBW infants in the NICU.[18] Risk factors for nephrotoxicity include low birth weight, concurrent nephrotoxic medications, prematurity, hypovolemia, sepsis, and hypoxic ischemic encephalopathy.[26] Aminoglycoside nephrotoxicity is classically non-oliguric in nature and develops later in the treatment course. As a result of their impact on tubular function, aminoglycoside-induced renal injury may be associated with electrolyte abnormalities, including hypomagnesemia, hypokalemia, hypophosphatemia, and acidosis.

Aminoglycosides are freely filtered into the urine, accumulate in the proximal tubules by endocytosis and cationic transporters, and are almost entirely excreted by the kidneys.[26] Approximately 10% to 15% of filtered aminoglycosides accumulate in the renal cortex in concentrations that may exceed measured systemic concentrations. Intracellular aminoglycoside accumulation damages proximal tubular cells by lysosomal accumulation, membrane disruption, disruption of protein production, disruption of mitochondrial adenosine triphosphate production, and oxidative stress.[27] Aminoglycoside toxicity may be also characterized by acute tubular necrosis, tubular obstruction from dead cells sloughing into the tubule, distal tubular dysfunction, polyuria, and antidiuretic hormone resistance.

The true incidence of AKI related to aminoglycoside exposure is unclear in neonates, but epidemiological studies will benefit from the use of updated neonatal AKI definitions. Estimated rates of aminoglycoside-associated nephrotoxicity in neonates vary depending on the definition used and the population studied. A recent narrative review included 10 studies of gentamicin use in neonates, where nephrotoxicity was assessed using serum creatinine.[26] Seven of these studies reported no nephrotoxicity, and the remaining three reported various rates, the maximum being 27%, highlighting the lack of standardized criteria for diagnosing aminoglycoside nephrotoxicity. A 10-day, open-label, prospective study of gentamicin in critically ill neonates during the first week of life showed that 27% of infants developed AKI (23/84), and two infants had abnormal renal function 1 week after stopping gentamicin. Mean gentamicin clearance measured after the first dose increased with gestational age.[28] A prospective trial showed that urinary excretion of the marker of renal tubular injury *N*-acetyl-β-D-glucosaminidase (178 ng/mol Cr, IQR: 104-698 vs. 32 ng/mol Cr, IQR: 9-82; $p < 0.001$) and of neutrophil gelatinase–associated lipocalin (569 ng/mol Cr, IQR: 168-1,681 vs. 222 ng/mol Cr, IQR: 90-497; $p < 0.05$), were higher in neonates treated with gentamicin compared to controls and preceded the peak of serum creatinine and decrease in urine output.[29] These studies have shown that aminoglycoside exposure results in elevation of urinary biomarkers, including those that signify proximal tubular damage, irrespective of rise in serum creatinine,[30] suggesting that damage resulting from aminoglycoside exposure may not be detected by the traditional criterion of a rise in serum creatinine.

To prevent aminoglycoside-associated renal injury, clinicians should diligently monitor drug levels and renal function while an infant is on therapy. Therapeutic drug monitoring is felt to be helpful for monitoring both efficacy and toxicity. Because of differential accumulation of aminoglycosides in the renal cortex, toxicity may occur despite therapeutic drug levels. Elevated trough levels suggest reduced renal clearance of aminoglycosides. This may reflect pre-existing renal dysfunction but is also considered to be a risk factor for developing nephrotoxicity.[31] Optimal dosing of aminoglycosides in critically ill neonates is challenging because of the pathologic alterations that accompany severe illness in this vulnerable population. To maximize therapeutic benefits and minimize toxicity, extended interval aminoglycoside dosing regimens have been adopted, based on favorable pharmacokinetics, but they have yet to be shown to impact rates of nephrotoxicity in neonates.[32]

AMPHOTERICIN B

Invasive fungal infections are an important cause of nosocomial infection in the NICU, especially in the extremely premature infants. They are associated with significant mortality and adverse neurodevelopmental outcomes. Amphotericin B is used as empiric therapy for neonatal fungal infections. Nephrotoxicity represents the most significant side effect to amphotericin B and results from renal vasoconstriction, decreased glomerular filtration rate (GFR), and distal tubular toxicity.[27] The direct toxicity and increased tubular membrane permeability account for the characteristic electrolyte abnormalities associated with amphotericin B (hypokalemia, hyponatremia, acidosis, and hypomagnesemia). The nephrotoxicity associated with amphotericin B in neonates is typically milder than in older children and is transient, but it may be associated with significant morbidity. Liposomal formulations of amphotericin B are larger and therefore less cleared by glomerular filtration, so these formulations are less nephrotoxic.[33] Nephrotoxicity while using liposomal formulations in neonates is commonly transient in nature but occurs in 0% to 20% of exposed infants.[34] Risk factors for nephrotoxicity include longer treatment duration, nephrotoxic medications, and severity of illness. The risk of nephrotoxicity can be diminished by avoiding concurrent nephrotoxic medication exposure and potentially by increasing sodium intake (>4 mEq/kg/day).[35]

RENIN–ANGIOTENSIN SYSTEM BLOCKERS

The renin–angiotensin system is critical to fetal renal development and contributes significantly to renal vascular resistance during the neonatal period through its vasoconstrictive activity. In the kidney, angiotensin acts primarily as a vasoconstrictor at the efferent arteriole (post-glomerulus) to maintain glomerular filtration. The consequences of blockade of the renin–angiotensin system using angiotensin-converting enzyme inhibitors (ACEIs), such as captopril and lisinopril, or angiotensin receptor blockers, such as olmesartan or valsartan, on the developing fetus are well described and include renal failure, oligohydramnios, death, arterial hypotension, intrauterine growth retardation, respiratory distress syndrome, pulmonary hypoplasia, hypocalvaria, limb defects, persistent patent ductus arteriosus, and cerebral complications.[36] A retrospective study performed through the Midwest Pediatric Nephrology Consortium showed that fetopathy caused by renin–angiotensin system blockers continues to be a cause of considerable morbidity, with more severe renal complications associated with exposure after the first trimester. This highlights the importance of emphasizing the risk of fetopathy whenever clinicians prescribe renin–angiotensin system blockers to women of childbearing age.[37]

Given the potential deleterious impact on postnatal renal development, it may be appropriate to avoid the use of ACEIs in neonates <32 weeks of age, in whom nephrogenesis may not be complete. In a study of captopril treatment in neonates with congenital heart disease, AKI occurred in 14% of patients and was reversible in all patients.[38] AKI induced by ACEIs is typically reversible with dose adjustment, increased renal perfusion, or medication discontinuation. Because neonatal kidneys are known to be sensitive to renin–angiotensin system blockade, ACEIs should be started at low doses and titrated slowly with diligent monitoring of electrolytes and renal function. To mitigate the risk of AKI with ACE inhibition, practitioners should closely monitor intravascular volume (particularly in infants on diuretic therapy) and be cautious about concomitant use of NSAIDs.[39]

DIURETICS

Diuretics are commonly used in the NICU to remove excess extracellular fluid secondary to various conditions such as bronchopulmonary dysplasia. Diuretics target sodium and water reabsorption in different nephron segments (e.g., loop diuretics target the loop of Henle; thiazides and spironolactone, the distal tubule). A recent survey of U.S. neonatologists involving hypothetical clinical scenarios suggests that diuretic therapy for VLBW infants in the first 28 days of life is common, despite limited evidence of benefit from randomized trials.[40] Most respondents expected sustained improvements in pulmonary mechanics, decreased days on mechanical ventilation, and decreased length of stay, despite a lack of evidence in current literature. In a review of a large national dataset from 1996 to 2005, Clark et al.[41] reported furosemide to be the seventh most commonly prescribed drug in the NICU, with 8% to 9% of all NICU patients receiving at least one dose. A later analysis of this same database (1997–2011) found that 37% of infants <32 weeks' gestation and <1500 g birth weight (39,357/107,542) were exposed to at least one diuretic; furosemide was the most commonly used (93% with ≥1 recorded dose).[42] Using the same database, Bamat et al.[43] found that almost 95% of infants <32 weeks' gestation with bronchopulmonary dysplasia were exposed to loop diuretics at least once during hospital admission, with the duration of use ranging from 7.3% to 49.4% of all hospital days.

In a multicenter retrospective study using the Pediatric Hospital Information System (PHIS) database, 76% of infants with AKI (1801/2379) received at least one dose of diuretics, whereas only 16% of those without a diagnosis of AKI (11,075/69,242) were treated with this medication class. Among infants with AKI, treatment with diuretics was associated with younger gestational age and lower birth weight. For infants receiving diuretics (and 99% of these received furosemide), the median duration was 18 days, with slightly over half of these receiving diuretics for ≥5 consecutive days. In neonates with AKI, treatment with diuretics was significantly associated with increased mortality, need for mechanical ventilation, and length of stay.[44] Diuretics may also add to the nephrotoxicity of other medications (including aminoglycosides) secondary to intravascular volume depletion and GFR reduction.[45]

Despite the lack of evidence that diuretic administration can prevent or decrease the severity of AKI, early use of furosemide has been proposed to prevent the progression of AKI. Furosemide is often administered in the setting of AKI in an attempt to ameliorate the severity of injury by increasing renal blood flow through the stimulation of prostaglandins production, decreasing renal oxygen consumption (blockade of cotransporter activity), and clearing of tubular debris by maintaining luminal salt and water and thus urine flow. Diuretics have been shown in several adult studies to be potentially detrimental or to lack clear effectiveness for improving survival or renal recovery.[46] The role of diuretics in either improving or causing renal injury in neonates remains unclear.

All neonates receiving diuretics should have regular monitoring of electrolytes, and those receiving prolonged loop diuretic treatment should be screened for nephrocalcinosis due to hypercalciuria. It is also imperative to critically monitor intravascular volume status and blood pressure when using aggressive diuresis to avoid hypovolemia.[27]

NON-STEROIDAL ANTI-INFLAMMATORY DRUGS

Neonates have high levels of circulating prostaglandins, which play an integral role in renal water clearance and in increasing renal blood flow by vasodilation of the afferent arteriole. High prostaglandin levels during the neonatal period act as a key counter-regulatory mechanism to offset the highly vasoconstrictive milieu following birth. Inhibiting prostaglandin synthesis can profoundly decrease neonatal renal blood flow and GFR, causing transient oliguria. Prenatal exposure to NSAID medications can adversely impact renal function with a range of effects from transient oliguria to oligohydramnios depending on timing and duration of exposure.[47] NSAIDs are mainly used in the NICU to decrease circulating prostaglandin in preterm infants as prophylaxis for the prevention of intraventricular hemorrhage or as pharmacologic treatment of persistent patent ductus arteriosus. NSAID-induced AKI is most frequently related to exposure to ibuprofen or indomethacin and is typically transient in nature; however, occasionally this may be complicated by oliguria, fluid overload, and electrolyte abnormalities. Nephrotoxic side effects are less severe with ibuprofen.[48] To prevent NSAID-induced AKI, clinicians should ensure adequate intravascular volume, consider using the lowest effective dose, and avoid the use of concomitant nephrotoxic medications.

RADIOCONTRAST AGENTS

There are few data on the incidence of radiocontrast-associated AKI in neonates. In children, the incidence is about 10%. Pre-existing reduced renal function is an important risk factor for AKI with radiocontrast exposures.[49] Neonates have physiologically reduced GFR to begin with; however, this likely represents a different phenomenon compared with patients who have underlying pathological chronic kidney disease. It is unclear whether the risk of contrast-induced AKI in neonates is higher or lower than in older children. Proposed interventions recommended for reno-protection before contrast administration include hydration with saline or sodium bicarbonate and the use of *N*-acetylcysteine.[49] Ensuring adequate hydration is reasonable in neonates who might be considered at risk for contrast nephropathy (e.g., preexisting or recent recovery from acute tubular necrosis or severe AKI, receiving multiple nephrotoxic drugs). However, the use of *N*-acetylcysteine cannot be recommended in neonates due to the lack of proven efficacy and experience.[27]

VANCOMYCIN

The role of vancomycin as a nephrotoxin remains controversial, particularly in the setting of monotherapy with appropriate medication levels. A retrospective observational cohort study demonstrated infrequent occurrence of AKI with single vancomycin use. However, the presence of a patent ductus arteriosus, concomitant NSAID use, ≥1 positive blood cultures, low birth weight, or higher severity of illness and risk of mortality scores were associated with an increased risk of nephrotoxicity.[50] In the past, vancomycin adverse effects were related to formulation impurities, a situation that has since been remedied. The proposed mechanism of nephrotoxicity is speculated to be related to oxidative proximal tubular damage. Retrospective studies suggest that neonates with higher vancomycin trough concentrations or those receiving concomitant nephrotoxins and/or diuretics are at higher risk for AKI.[51] Similarly, a single-center cohort study showed that patients with piperacillin–tazobactam added to vancomycin exhibited an increased incidence of nephrotoxicity, with an odds ratio of 2.48 (P = 0.032), and a steady-state vancomycin trough concentration of 15 µg/mL or greater was also associated with an increased risk.[52] Animal studies suggest that vancomycin may potentiate the nephrotoxic effects of aminoglycosides. Given the ability to monitor vancomycin levels and its potential for nephrotoxicity, vancomycin monitoring protocols should be instituted with at least daily review of nephrotoxic medications.[39]

Management of Drug-Associated AKI

There is no treatment for established AKI; therefore, prevention is the key. To decrease the incidence of nephrotoxin-associated AKI in hospitalized patients, the development of algorithms to screen, monitor, and intervene to reduce harm produced by medications could significantly improve outcomes. These programs would regularly evaluate infants who are at risk for nephrotoxic injury, develop lab monitoring processes for those at risk, and institute intervention strategies to limit the damage caused by nephrotoxic medications. One such approach relies on daily evaluations by a multidisciplinary team that includes input from nurses, physicians, residents, and pharmacists. The Nephrotoxic Injury Negated by Just-in-Time Action (NINJA) initiative is a multicenter collaborative aiming to address the issue of pediatric nephrotoxic AKI. Its mission statement is that "nephrotoxic medications should only be used for as long as they are needed." NINJA is an electronic health record–driven surveillance program whereby all non-critically ill patients are screened for exposure to three or more nephrotoxic medications or 3 or more days of aminoglycoside exposure. Those who are identified as exposed using these criteria are monitored daily for increases in SCr.

Goldstein et al.[53] showed that the use of specific criteria to trigger a SCr nephrotoxin–AKI surveillance process resulted in a 42% reduction in the number of days with AKI (AKI intensity). Additionally, these investigators also showed that implementation of daily SCr measurements as part of a hospital-wide quality initiative led to earlier and increased detection of aminoglycoside-associated AKI compared to SCr measurement every other day in a cohort of hospitalized children. Stoops et al.[54] have since extended monitoring to critically ill neonates and reported that such a program reduced nephrotoxic medications exposures and decreased AKI rates.

The following steps represent the fundamental principles of management of drug-induced nephrotoxicity:

1. Measure SCr before administration of potentially nephrotoxic drugs to establish baseline glomerular function, recognizing that even small increments in creatinine are an independent risk factor for increased morbidity and mortality.
2. Take periodic measurements of serum electrolytes and assess acid–base status, because abnormalities can develop before glomerular dysfunction is detectable.
3. Ensure adequate hydration and sodium repletion before administration of a nephrotoxic drug.
4. Avoid the simultaneous use of two or more different nephrotoxic drugs.
5. Adjust drug dosage in accordance with organ functional status, distribution volume, and drug pharmacokinetics.
6. Determine if a nephrotoxic drug has specific measures to prevent or attenuate its potential for renal damage.
7. Avoid harmful medication interactions (e.g., NSAIDs, angiotensin-converting enzymes), and use the minimal effective dose (e.g., daily vs. multiple-daily aminoglycoside doses).
8. If AKI occurs, also consider other causes of AKI that may be contributing, including ischemia, renal vein thrombosis, or the presence of undetected renal development abnormalities (which may be screened for by performing a renal ultrasound).
9. Finally, reassess the dosing of other medications in the setting of AKI.[27]

Regular monitoring of kidney function and drug levels (where applicable) should be protocolized to monitor for the development and progression of AKI.

Long-Term Effects of Drug-Associated AKI in Neonates

Although AKI is often thought of as a component of multiple organ dysfunction syndrome, it likely also exacerbates delay in recovery from that condition.[55] Animal models indicate that acute kidney injury induces a loss of renal microvessels ("vascular dropout"), resulting from endothelial phenotypic transition combined with an impaired regenerative capacity. Emerging evidence suggests that AKI may thereby increase the long-term risk of chronic kidney disease (CKD) in surviving children. Mammen et al.[56] found a substantial risk of CKD 1 to 3 years after AKI in the pediatric intensive care unit, with 10% of patients fulfilling the National Kidney Foundation's Kidney Disease Outcomes Quality Initiative (KDOQI) definition and almost 50% being identified as being at risk for developing CKD (mildly decreased GFR, hypertension, and/or hyperfiltration). In a retrospective cohort study, children who developed AKI (using pediatric RIFLE criteria) associated with nephrotoxin exposure ($\geq$3 days of aminoglycosides or $\geq$3 nephrotoxins simultaneously for 1 day) had a relative risk of 3.84 (95% CI, 1.57–9.40; $P < 0.05$) for developing one or more signs of CKD, including reduced estimated GFR, hyperfiltration, proteinuria, or hypertension, at 6 months compared to controls (nephrotoxin exposure but no AKI).[57] Newborns who sustain AKI in the neonatal period may not develop changes in their GFR (measured SCr) until they go through a growth spurt at adolescence.[58] Neonates with low birth weight, low gestational age, cardiac surgery, urologic malformations, need for mechanical ventilation, or inotropic use are especially prone to long-term sequelae after episodes of AKI.[59] Because preterm neonates are born with underdeveloped nephrons and low nephron numbers, the negative impact of nephrotoxin exposure on renal outcomes may be substantial. Nephrotoxic medication exposure during nephrogenesis could interfere with nephron generation, contributing to a particular magnitude of renal damage. Such adjunctive damage could further increase the risk of CKD in children born prematurely.[60] A meta-analysis performed by White et al.[61] reported that preterm infants (birthweight <2500 g) have nearly twice the odds of having a low GFR, microalbuminuria, end-stage renal disease, and hypertension in latter life than their term counterparts.

The duration of established AKI may impact long-term outcomes. Critically ill children who had earlier resolution or improvement of AKI severity had a lower mortality rate than those who had persistent AKI.[55] The development of improved diagnostic tools must be coupled with the development of further strategies to minimize the nephrotoxic consequences of drugs. Given the significant long-term health sequelae as described above, it is essential that children with AKI events be followed after the episode to screen for the development of CKD. KDIGO practice guidelines recommend an evaluation 3 months after the acute episode and then at least annually if no signs of renal disease are detected.[12]

REFERENCES

1. Zappitelli M. Epidemiology and diagnosis of acute kidney injury. *Semin Nephrol.* 2008;28(5):436-446.
2. Jetton JG, Boohaker LJ, Sethi SK, et al. Incidence and outcomes of neonatal acute kidney injury (AWAKEN): a multicentre, multinational, observational cohort study. *Lancet Child Adolesc Health.* 2017;1(3):184-194.
3. Jetton JG, Askenazi DJ. Update on acute kidney injury in the neonate. *Curr Opin Pediatr.* 2012;24(2):191-196.
4. Koralkar R, Ambalavanan N, Levitan EB, McGwin G, Goldstein S, Askenazi D. Acute kidney injury reduces survival in very low birth weight infants. *Pediatr Res.* 2011;69(4):354-358.
5. Blinder JJ, Goldstein SL, Lee VV, et al. Congenital heart surgery in infants: effects of acute kidney injury on outcomes. *J Thorac Cardiovasc Surg.* 2012;143(2):368-374.
6. Gadepalli SK, Selewski DT, Drongowski RA, Mychaliska GB. Acute kidney injury in congenital diaphragmatic hernia requiring extracorporeal life support: an insidious problem. *J Pediatr Surg.* 2011;46(4):630-635.
7. Selewski DT, Jordan BK, Askenazi DJ, Dechert RE, Sarkar S. Acute kidney injury in asphyxiated newborns treated with therapeutic hypothermia. *J Pediatr.* 2013;162(4):725-729.e1.
8. Stritzke A, Thomas S, Amin H, Fusch C, Lodha A. Renal consequences of preterm birth. *Mol Cell Pediatr.* 2017;4(1):2.
9. Schulman J, Dimand RJ, Lee HC, Duenas GV, Bennett MV, Gould JB. Neonatal intensive care unit antibiotic use. *Pediatrics.* 2015;135(5):826-833.
10. Carmody JB, Swanson JR, Rhone ET, Charlton JR. Recognition and reporting of AKI in very low birth weight infants. *Clin J Am Soc Nephrol.* 2014;9(12):2036-2043.
11. Patzer L. Nephrotoxicity as a cause of acute kidney injury in children. *Pediatr Nephrol.* 2008;23(12):2159-2173.
12. Nada A, Bonachea EM, Askenazi DJ. Acute kidney injury in the fetus and neonate. *Semin Fetal Neonatal Med.* 2017;22(2):90-97.
13. Cartin-Ceba R, Kashiouris M, Plataki M, Kor DJ, Gajic O, Casey ET. Risk factors for development of acute kidney injury in critically ill patients: a systematic review and meta-analysis of observational studies. *Crit Care Res Pract.* 2012;2012:691013.
14. Moffett BS, Goldstein SL. Acute kidney injury and increasing nephrotoxic-medication exposure in noncritically-ill children. *Clin J Am Soc Nephrol.* 2011;6(4):856-863.
15. Slater MB, Gruneir A, Rochon PA, Howard AW, Koren G, Parshuram CS. Identifying high-risk medications associated with acute kidney injury in critically ill patients: a pharmacoepidemiologic evaluation. *Paediatr Drugs.* 2017;19(1):59-67.
16. Moore TJ, Weiss SR, Kaplan S, Blaisdell CJ. Reported adverse drug events in infants and children under 2 years of age. *Pediatrics.* 2002;110(5):e53.
17. Laughon MM, Avant D, Tripathi N, et al. Drug labeling and exposure in neonates. *JAMA Pediatr.* 2014;168(2):130-136.
18. Hsieh EM, Hornik CP, Clark RH, et al. Medication use in the neonatal intensive care unit. *Am J Perinatol.* 2014;31(9):811-821.
19. Rhone ET, Carmody JB, Swanson JR, Charlton JR. Nephrotoxic medication exposure in very low birth weight infants. *J Matern Fetal Neonatal Med.* 2014;27(14):1485-1490.
20. Perazella MA. Renal vulnerability to drug toxicity. *Clin J Am Soc Nephrol.* 2009;4(7):1275-1283.
21. Luque Y, Louis K, Jouanneau C, et al. Vancomycin-associated cast nephropathy. *J Am Soc Nephrol.* 2017;28(6):1723-1728.
22. Mehta RL, Awdishu L, Davenport A, et al. Phenotype standardization for drug-induced kidney disease. *Kidney Int.* 2015;88(2):226-234.
23. Kimberlin DW, Lin CY, Jacobs RF, et al. Safety and efficacy of high-dose intravenous acyclovir in the management of neonatal herpes simplex virus infections. *Pediatrics.* 2001;108(2):230-238.
24. Rao S, Abzug MJ, Carosone-Link P, et al. Intravenous acyclovir and renal dysfunction in children: a matched case control study. *J Pediatr.* 2015;166(6):1462-1468.e1-e4.
25. Steinberg I, Kimberlin DW. Acyclovir dosing and acute kidney injury: deviations and direction. *J Pediatr.* 2015;166(6):1341-1344.
26. Kent A, Turner MA, Sharland M, Heath PT. Aminoglycoside toxicity in neonates: something to worry about? *Expert Rev Anti Infect Ther.* 2014;12(3):319-331.
27. Zappitelli M, Selewski DT, Askenazi DJ. Nephrotoxic medication exposure and acute kidney injury in neonates. *NeoReviews.* 2012;13(7):e420-e427.
28. Martinkova J, Pokorna P, Zahora J, et al. Tolerability and outcomes of kinetically guided therapy with gentamicin in critically ill neonates during the first week of life: an open-label, prospective study. *Clin Ther.* 2010;32(14):2400-2414.
29. Jansen D, Peters E, Heemskerk S, et al. Tubular injury biomarkers to detect gentamicin-induced acute kidney injury in the neonatal intensive care unit. *Am J Perinatol.* 2016;33(2):180-187.
30. McWilliam SJ, Antoine DJ, Sabbisetti V, et al. Mechanism-based urinary biomarkers to identify the potential for aminoglycoside-induced nephrotoxicity in premature neonates: a proof-of-concept study. *PLoS One.* 2012;7(8):e43809.

31. McWilliam SJ, Antoine DJ, Smyth RL, Pirmohamed M. Aminoglycoside-induced nephrotoxicity in children. *Pediatr Nephrol.* 2017;32(11):2015-2025.
32. Rao SC, Srinivasjois R, Moon K. One dose per day compared to multiple doses per day of gentamicin for treatment of suspected or proven sepsis in neonates. *Cochrane Database Syst Rev.* 2016;12:CD005091.
33. Turkova A, Roilides E, Sharland M. Amphotericin B in neonates: deoxycholate or lipid formulation as first-line therapy - is there a 'right' choice? *Curr Opin Infect Dis.* 2011;24(2):163-171.
34. Karadag-Oncel E, Ozsurekci Y, Yurdakok M, Kara A. Is liposomal amphotericin B really safety in neonates? *Early Hum Dev.* 2013;89(1):35-36.
35. Turcu R, Patterson MJ, Omar S. Influence of sodium intake on amphotericin B-induced nephrotoxicity among extremely premature infants. *Pediatr Nephrol.* 2009;24(3):497-505.
36. Bullo M, Tschumi S, Bucher BS, Bianchetti MG, Simonetti GD. Pregnancy outcome following exposure to angiotensin-converting enzyme inhibitors or angiotensin receptor antagonists: a systematic review. *Hypertension.* 2012;60(2):444-450.
37. Nadeem S, Hashmat S, Defreitas MJ, et al. Renin angiotensin system blocker fetopathy: a Midwest Pediatric Nephrology Consortium report. *J Pediatr.* 2015;167(4):881-885.
38. Gantenbein MH, Bauersfeld U, Baenziger O, et al. Side effects of angiotensin converting enzyme inhibitor (captopril) in newborns and young infants. *J Perinat Med.* 2008;36(5):448-452.
39. Hanna MH, Askenazi DJ, Selewski DT. Drug-induced acute kidney injury in neonates. *Curr Opin Pediatr.* 2016;28(2):180-187.
40. Hagadorn JI, Sanders MR, Staves C, Herson VC, Daigle K. Diuretics for very low birth weight infants in the first 28 days: a survey of the U.S. neonatologists. *J Perinatol.* 2011;31(10):677-681.
41. Clark RH, Bloom BT, Spitzer AR, Gerstmann DR. Reported medication use in the neonatal intensive care unit: data from a large national data set. *Pediatrics.* 2006;117(6):1979-1987.
42. Laughon MM, Chantala K, Aliaga S, et al. Diuretic exposure in premature infants from 1997 to 2011. *Am J Perinatol.* 2015;32(1):49-56.
43. Bamat NA, Nelin TD, Eichenwald EC, et al. Loop diuretics in severe bronchopulmonary dysplasia: cumulative use and associations with mortality and age at discharge. *J Pediatr.* 2021;231:43-49.e3.
44. Mohamed TH, Klamer B, Mahan JD, Spencer JD, Slaughter JL. Diuretic therapy and acute kidney injury in preterm neonates and infants. *Pediatr Nephrol.* 2020;36(12):3981-3991.
45. Ho KM, Power BM. Benefits and risks of furosemide in acute kidney injury. *Anaesthesia.* 2010;65(3):283-293.
46. Bagshaw SM, Bellomo R, Kellum JA. Oliguria, volume overload, and loop diuretics. *Crit Care Med.* 2008;36(suppl 4):S172-S178.
47. Antonucci R, Zaffanello M, Puxeddu E, et al. Use of non-steroidal anti-inflammatory drugs in pregnancy: impact on the fetus and newborn. *Curr Drug Metab.* 2012;13(4):474-490.
48. Ohlsson A, Walia R, Shah SS. Ibuprofen for the treatment of patent ductus arteriosus in preterm or low birth weight (or both) infants. *Cochrane Database Syst Rev.* 2020;2:CD003481.
49. Brasch RC. Contrast media toxicity in children. *Pediatr Radiol.* 2008;38(suppl 2):S281-S284.
50. Constance JE, Balch AH, Stockmann C, et al. A propensity-matched cohort study of vancomycin-associated nephrotoxicity in neonates. *Arch Dis Child Fetal Neonatal Ed.* 2016;101(3):F236-F243.
51. McKamy S, Hernandez E, Jahng M, Moriwaki T, Deveikis A, Le J. Incidence and risk factors influencing the development of vancomycin nephrotoxicity in children. *J Pediatr.* 2011;158(3):422-426.
52. Burgess LD, Drew RH. Comparison of the incidence of vancomycin-induced nephrotoxicity in hospitalized patients with and without concomitant piperacillin-tazobactam. *Pharmacotherapy.* 2014;34(7):670-676.
53. Goldstein SL, Kirkendall E, Nguyen H, et al. Electronic health record identification of nephrotoxin exposure and associated acute kidney injury. *Pediatrics.* 2013;132(3):e756-e767.
54. Stoops C, Stone S, Evans E, et al. Baby NINJA (nephrotoxic injury negated by just-in-time action): reduction of nephrotoxic medication-associated acute kidney injury in the neonatal intensive care unit. *J Pediatr.* 2019;215:223-228.e6.
55. Sanchez-Pinto LN, Goldstein SL, Schneider JB, Khemani RG. Association between progression and improvement of acute kidney injury and mortality in critically ill children. *Pediatr Crit Care Med.* 2015;16(8):703-710.
56. Mammen C, Al Abbas A, Skippen P, et al. Long-term risk of CKD in children surviving episodes of acute kidney injury in the intensive care unit: a prospective cohort study. *Am J Kidney Dis.* 2012;59(4):523-530.
57. Menon S, Kirkendall ES, Nguyen H, Goldstein SL. Acute kidney injury associated with high nephrotoxic medication exposure leads to chronic kidney disease after 6 months. *J Pediatr.* 2014;165(3):522-527.e2.
58. Goldstein SL. Renal recovery at different ages. *Nephron Clin Pract.* 2014;127(1-4):21-24.
59. Lee CC, Chan OW, Lai MY, et al. Incidence and outcomes of acute kidney injury in extremely-low-birth-weight infants. *PLoS One.* 2017;12(11):e0187764.
60. Zaffanello M, Bassareo PP, Cataldi L, Antonucci R, Biban P, Fanos V. Long-term effects of neonatal drugs on the kidney. *J Matern Fetal Neonatal Med.* 2010;23(suppl 3):87-89.
61. White SL, Perkovic V, Cass A, et al. Is low birth weight an antecedent of CKD in later life? A systematic review of observational studies. *Am J Kidney Dis.* 2009;54(2):248-261.

SECTION 3

Immunology

Chapter 18

Recent Advances and Controversies in Inborn Errors of Immunity Presenting in the Newborn Period

Julie J. Kim-Chang, MD; John W. Sleasman, MD

Key Points

- Inborn errors of immunity (IEI) presenting in the newborn period include immune deficiencies affecting cellular and humoral immunity, diseases of immune dysregulation, congenital defects in phagocyte function, defects in intrinsic and innate immunity, and autoinflammatory disorders.
- There are many syndromes associated with IEI that can be recognized in the newborn period through extra-immune manifestations.
- However, many newborns with IEI appear healthy until they acquire infections or develop immune dysregulation.
- Implementation of newborn screening (NBS) for severe combined immunodeficiency (SCID) in the US have facilitated early identification of T-cell immunodeficiency
- Premature birth alone can result in abnormal newborn screening for SCID. Suggested algorithm for evaluation of pre-term infants with abnormal NBS for SCID are outlined in this chapter.
- Majority of IEIs evident in the newborn period are severe conditions that require immediate definitive diagnosis and management soon after birth.
- The application of molecular genetics have significantly improved the accuracy of diagnosing specific IEIs. Precise genetic diagnosis helps guide medical management, assessment of risk for associated complications, determine prognosis, and predict long-term outcomes.
- Management of neonates with IEI vary depending on the diagnosis and include preventive therapy (preventing nosocomial and opportunistic infections and GVHD), bridge therapy (enzyme replacement therapy or biological agents), and curative therapy (hematopoietic stem cell transplantation, gene therapy, and cultured thymus tissue implantation).

Inborn Errors of Immunity Presenting in the Newborn Period

Recent advances in the diagnosis and management options for infants with inborn errors of immunity (IEIs) have resulted in improved outcomes but also created new challenges and controversies regarding the medical management of IEIs during the newborn period. Highlighted developments for this chapter include the application of newborn screening for early identification of newborns with T-cell immune deficiency, the application of molecular diagnostics allowing for rapid definitive diagnosis of IEIs, and the use of novel therapies that drastically improve outcomes. Over the past decade, the number of monogenic IEIs discovered has increased, many of which can be recognized during the newborn period. The International Union of Immunological Societies (IUIS) Expert Committee Classification system categorizes over 400 genetic defects identified in human IEIs according to distinct clinical and laboratory phenotypes.[1] These IEIs present with increased susceptibility to infections, as well as diverse clinical phenotypes, including autoimmunity, auto-inflammation, allergy, and/or malignancy. IEIs that may present in the neonatal period are listed in Table 18.1 based on IUIS classification.

IMMUNE DEFICIENCIES AFFECTING CELLULAR AND HUMORAL IMMUNITY

T-cell and combined immunodeficiency disorders commonly present in early infancy. If infants present with opportunistic infections such as *Pneumocystis*

TABLE 18.1 IUIS Classification of IEIS Seen in the Newborn Period

1. Immune deficiencies affecting cellular and humoral immunity
   a. Severe combined immune deficiency (SCID), categorized based on T, B, NK phenotype: $T^-B^-NK^-$, $T^-B^-NK^+$, $T^-B^+NK^-$, $T^-B^+NK^+$
   b. Combined immunodeficiency (CID) less profound than SCID: major histocompatibility complex (MHC) I/MHC II deficiencies, zeta-chain associated protein kinase 70 kDa (ZAP-70) deficiency, Dedicator of cytokinesis 8 (DOCK8) deficiency, DOCK2 deficiency, CDL40L/CD40 deficiency, caspase recruitment domain family member 11 (CARD11) deficiency
2. CID with associated or syndromic features
   a. CID due to thymic defects with additional congenital anomalies: DiGeorge/22q11.2 deletion syndrome, CHARGE (coloboma, heart defects, atresia of the choanae, retarded growth, genital abnormalities, and ear abnormalities) syndrome, forkhead box N1 (FOXN1) deficiency, paired box 1 (PAX1) deficiency, Jacobson syndrome
   b. Wiskott–Aldrich syndrome (WAS)
   c. Ataxia telangiectasia
   d. Cartilage hair hypoplasia (CHH)
   e. Dyskeratosis congenita
   f. Comel–Netherton syndrome
   g. NF-κB essential modulator (NEMO) deficiency syndrome
   h. CID with gastrointestinal involvement in infancy: trichohepatoenteric syndrome (TTC37, SKIV2L), immunodeficiency with multiple intestinal atresias, hepatic venoocclusive disease with immunodeficiency (VODI)
3. Predominantly antibody deficiencies
   a. Congenital agammaglobulinemia
   b. Other antibody deficiencies: hyper-IgM syndromes, transient hypogammaglobulinemia of infancy
4. Diseases of immune dysregulation
   a. Hemophagocytic lymphohistiocytosis (HLH) and Epstein–Barr virus (EBV) susceptibility: familial hemophagocytic lymphohistiocytosis syndrome, inborn errors of immunity (IEIs) associated with HLH (Chediak–Higashi syndrome, Griscelli syndrome type 2, X-linked inhibitor of apoptosis protein [XIAP] deficiency)
   b. Syndromes with autoimmunity and regulatory T-cell defects: immune dysregulation, polyendocrinophathy, enteropathy, X-linked (IPEX), IL-10R deficiency
5. Congenital defects in phagocytes
   a. Congenital neutropenia
   b. Functional defects: leukocyte adhesion deficiency (LAD), chronic granulomatous disease (CGD)
6. Defects in intrinsic and innate immunity
   a. Bacterial and parasitic infections: chronic mucocutaneous candidiasis (CMC)
   b. Mycobacterial and viral infections: Toll-like receptor 3 (TLR3) pathway defects
7. Autoinflammatory disorders
   a. Recurrent and systemic inflammation with urticarial rash: neonatal onset multi-inflammatory disease (NOMID)

jirovecii pneumonia (PJP or PCP), *Mycobacterium avium* or *tuberculosis*, invasive fungal infections (*Candida*), or disseminated viral infections, it should raise suspicion for cell-mediated immunodeficiency. These infants may also present with manifestations of graft-versus-host disease (GVHD), including erythematous rash, hepatosplenomegaly, and chronic diarrhea, during the neonatal period due to maternally derived T cells or transfusions with non-irradiated blood products.[2] Compared to B-cell and other primary immune deficiency diseases, individuals with defects in cell-mediated immunity are more likely to present with initial clinical manifestations soon after birth.[3]

Severe Combined Immune Deficiency

Severe combined immune deficiency (SCID) is a group of rare genetic disorders with an absence of T, B, and/or natural killer (NK) cells, predisposing the infant to early life-threatening infections and death within the first 2 years of life. This condition is classified based on the presence or absence of T, B, and NK cellular phenotypes: $T^-B^+NK^+$, $T^-B^+NK^-$, $T^-B^-NK^+$, or $T^-B^-NK^-$.

$T^-B^-NK^-$ SCID

Adenosine deaminase (ADA) deficiency is the most common form of this SCID phenotype, with severe lymphopenia and absent T, B, and NK cells. Reticular dysgenesis can have similar lymphocyte distribution, but all hematopoietic lineages are affected. ADA deficiency results in the intracellular accumulation of adenosine, 2′-deoxyadenosine, and ultimately deoxyadenosine triphosphate (deoxyATP), which leads to feedback inhibition of ribonucleotide reductase, resulting in impaired DNA synthesis.[4] Accumulation 2′-deoxyadenosine, a cellular toxin, causes chromosome breakage, as well.

$T^-B^-NK^+$ SCID

Defects in recombinase-activation genes (RAGs) most commonly present with this phenotype. *RAG1* and *RAG2* play a critical role in somatic rearrangement and assembly of variable, diversity, and joining gene segments of immunoglobulins and antigen receptors for T and B cells. Defects in *RAG1/2* lead to absent T and B cells with intact NK cells.[5] Defects in other proteins involved in non-homologous end joining and DNA repair, including Artemis (*DCLRE1C*), DNA ligase IV, Cernunnos, and DNA-PKcs, also lead to similar phenotype. DNA repair enzyme defects lead to radiosensitivity, malignancy, and extraimmune manifestations such as microcephaly and facial dysmorphisms.[3] Hypomorphic mutations of these genes can lead to phenotype of combined immunodeficiency (CID) with partial T and B cell function and immune dysregulation involving oligoclonal and activated T-cell expansion, with clinical presentation of early onset erythroderma, hepatosplenomegaly, and autoimmune cytopenias.[5]

$T^-B^+NK^-$ SCID

Abnormal signaling through the interleukin receptor common gamma chain (γc) or the downstream pathway results in this phenotype with absent T cells, low NK cells, and normal or increased B cells.[6] X-linked SCID is the most common form of SCID. Mutations in the common γc lead to impaired signaling of multiple cytokines that signal through this receptor, including interleukin (IL)-2, IL-4, IL-7, IL-15, and IL-21. Janus kinase 3 (JAK3) deficiency leads to an identical phenotype, but it is inherited as an autosomal recessive (AR) trait. JAK3 associates with the common γc receptor for downstream signaling.[3]

$T^-B^+NK^+$ SCID

In this subtype, T cells fail to develop, but B cells and NK cells are spared.[2,3] IL-7Rα deficiency results in intrathymic arrest in T-cell development. Mutations in antigen receptor genes including CD45 and CD3 chain (CD3δ, CD3ϵ, CD3ζ) also result in this phenotype.[7]

Combined Immune Deficiencies Less Profound Than SCID

Clinical phenotypes of CID are less profound and more variable than SCID. Hypomorphic mutations of the genes that cause SCID such as *RAG1/2* may lead to a CID phenotype with partial defects in T, B, and/or NK cell function.[1,2] Major histocompatibility complex (MHC) I or II deficiencies are characterized by isolated low CD8 or CD4 numbers presenting with failure to thrive and recurrent respiratory and/or gastrointestinal infections. Zeta-chain associated protein kinase 70 kDa (ZAP-70) deficiency with defective T-cell receptor signaling results in poor cellular proliferation to mitogens with normal CD3 and CD4 but low CD8 numbers, and it may present with immune dysregulation.

Dedicator of cytokinesis 8 (DOCK8) deficiency presents with low T, B, and NK cell numbers, early-onset severe atopic disease (eczema, food allergies), refractory viral infections (human papillomavirus, herpes simplex virus [HSV], varicella zoster virus, molluscum), eosinophilia, and elevated immunoglobulin E (IgE). DOCK2 deficiency presents with early invasive herpes viruses and bacterial infections with defective NK cell function with normal number.[1,8]

CD40 ligand deficiency (X-linked) or CD40 deficiency (AR), previously classified as hyper-IgM syndromes, present with sinopulmonary and/or gastrointestinal infections with pyogenic bacteria, opportunistic infections (*PJP* pneumonia, *Cryptosporidium* cholangitis), neutropenia with perirectal abscesses and oral ulcers, and immune phenotype showing normal to high IgM; low to absent IgG, IgA, and IgE; and defects in T-cell proliferation with normal to low T-cell numbers.[1,9] Caspase recruitment domain family member 11 (CARD11) deficiency presents with severe susceptibility to bacterial and opportunistic infections and is characterized by normal numbers of T and B lymphocytes, increased number of transitional B cells, T-cell dysfunction, and hypo- to agammaglobulinemia.

CID With Associated or Syndromic Features

Conditions that affect cellular and humoral immunity often involve other organ systems. Representative examples that may present in the newborn period are listed below. CID due to thymic defects with additional congenital anomalies includes 22q11.2 deletion syndrome (DiGeorge syndrome [DGS]); CHARGE syndrome (an acronym for coloboma, heart defects, atresia of the choanae, retarded growth, genital abnormalities, and ear abnormalities); forkhead box N1 (*FOXN1*) deficiency/haploinsufficiency; paired box 1 (*PAX1*) deficiency; embryopathy associated with infants born to diabetic mothers; and Jacobsen syndrome.

DGS (22q11.2 deletion syndrome) results from defective development of the pharyngeal pouch system. It is characterized by congenital conotruncal cardiac anomalies, facial dysmorphism, hypocalcemia due to hypoparathyroidism, and varying degrees of thymic output ranging from athymia to normal thymic function.[10] The majority of infants with DGS have heterozygous deletions in chromosome 22q11.2, but genetic deletions in chromosomes 10p13 and 17p13, as well as diabetic embryopathy, may present with similar phenotypes.[10,11] The inheritance of 22q11.2 deletion is autosomal dominant, but most cases result from de novo microdeletions. *TBX1* has been identified as a candidate gene deleted in this region possibly responsible for the clinical phenotype of DGS. The 22q11.2 deletion is relatively common, affecting 1 in 5000 births and 1 in 1000 fetuses.[12,13] Infants with DGS may present with neonatal tetany and seizures due to hypocalcemia resulting from hypoparathyroidism. Speech abnormalities due to velopharyngeal insufficiency, developmental and language delay, learning disabilities, and neuropsychiatric problems including schizophrenia are common.[10] The majority of patients with DGS have mild thymic hypoplasia (termed partial DGS), and their T-cell numbers and function improve over time, but autoimmunity is common. Approximately 0.5% to 1% of DGS cases have complete athymia with absent T cells (naïve T cells < 50 cells/μL, termed complete DGS).[14] Some develop atypical phenotype with oligoclonal T-cell expansion, rash, and lymphadenopathy resembling Omenn syndrome or autologous GVHD.

CHARGE syndrome is associated with mutations in the chromodomain helicase DNA-binding protein 7 (*CHD7*) gene on chromosome 8q12 or semaphorin-3E gene (*SEMA3E*) on chromosome 7q21.[15] Patients characteristically present with coloboma of the eyes, choanal atresia, heart anomalies, central nervous system abnormalities, developmental/growth retardation, and genital and ear malformations.[16] Infants with CHARGE syndrome may present with thymic hypoplasia or aplasia.

In *FOXN1* deficiency, loss of FOXN1 function results in thymic agenesis and premature thymic involution. This condition is inherited autosomal recessive, and patients may present at birth with alopecia totalis, nail dystrophy, and severe T-cell immunodeficiency. Infants with *FOXN1* haploinsufficiency may present with thymic hypoplasia with recurrent viral and bacterial respiratory tract infections in infancy, but T-cell lymphopenia can normalize by adulthood.[17]

PAX1 deficiency, inherited autosomal dominant (AD), results in aberrant development of thymic epithelial cells, as well as other pharyngeal pouch tissues, leading to T-cell lymphopenia and orofaciocervical syndrome characterized by facial dysmorphism (long face, narrow mandible), shoulder girdle abnormalities, hearing loss, and mild intellectual disability.[18]

Jacobsen syndrome is a rare syndrome that occurs due to partial deletion of the long arm of chromosome 11. Most common clinical features include pre- and postnatal growth retardation, characteristic facial dysmorphism, and thrombocytopenia/platelet dysfunction (Paris–Trousseau syndrome). Cognitive function may range from normal intelligence to moderate intellectual disability. Patients may present with recurrent otitis media, sinusitis, and upper and/or lower respiratory tract infections. Patients with Jacobsen syndrome may present with a combined immunodeficiency phenotype, with low memory B cells, impaired response to *S. pneumoniae* polysaccharide vaccine, and low T- and NK-cell numbers for age.[19]

Wiskott–Aldrich syndrome (WAS) is a CID with associated congenital thrombocytopenia. Inherited X-linked, classical presentation of WAS includes eczema, thrombocytopenia (small platelets with poor aggregation), and immunodeficiency, with increased risk for autoimmunity and lymphoid malignancies. The immunoglobulin profile is characteristic, with elevated IgA and IgE levels and low IgM levels. The most common complication of WAS in infancy is hemorrhage, a major cause of morbidity and mortality. There is an increased susceptibility to severe disseminated infections with herpesviruses and encapsulated bacteria.[20] Diagnosis is confirmed with genetic mutations in the *WASP* (Wiskott–Aldrich syndrome protein) gene. Hypomorphic mutations of the *WASP* gene results in a milder variant with isolated X-linked thrombocytopenia, and transactivating mutations cause X-linked neutropenia and myelodysplasia.[20] Infants with WAS may experience an accelerated phase, presenting as hemophagocytic lymphohistiocytosis.

Ataxia telangiectasia is an autosomal recessive disorder caused by mutations in the DNA repair enzyme *ATM* (ataxia telangiectasia mutated) gene. Patients with ataxia telangiectasia present with ataxia and ocular telangiectasia, with an increased risk of infections and malignancy that is rarely evident in the newborn period.[21] However, the enzyme defect can also cause thymic hypoplasia, resulting in low T-cell receptor excision circle (TREC) levels and abnormal SCID newborn screen.[22] Levels of α-fetoprotein are typically increased, as are the proportion of γδ T cells. Radiation sensitivity increases the risk for lymphoreticular malignancies.

Trichohepatoenteric syndrome is a rare condition of neonatal enteropathy characterized by intractable diarrhea, woolly hair, intrauterine growth restriction, facial dysmorphism, and short stature.[23] Infants may also present with liver cirrhosis, platelet abnormalities, and immunodeficiency. The immune phenotype is variable and may include hypogammaglobulinemia, low antibody responses, and variably low switched-memory B cells.[1] It is inherited autosomal recessive, with mutations in either *TTC37* or *SKIV2L*. Inherited AR *TTC7A* mutation is responsible for the condition. Infants present with multiple intestinal atresias and thymic structural abnormalities leading to bacterial, fungal, and viral infections.[24] It is often identified prenatally with intrauterine polyhydramnios and early demise, and some present with a SCID phenotype. Immunological phenotype is heterogeneous with normal B cells in general, accompanied by markedly decreased immunoglobulins due to intestinal losses, and normal to absent T cells with variable T cell function.[25]

Hepatic veno-occlusive disease with immunodeficiency (VODI) is characterized by primary immunodeficiency with terminal hepatic lobular vascular occlusion and hepatic fibrosis, which may present as hepatomegaly or liver failure. It is inherited autosomal recessive due to mutations/variants in the *SP110* gene, and the onset of disease occurs prior to 6 months of age. Infants are susceptible to bacterial and opportunistic infections including *PJP*, mucocutaneous candidiasis, or disseminated viral infections. Immune phenotyping shows serum IgG, IgA, and IgM levels low for age; low memory B cells; absent lymph node germinal centers; and defective T-cell memory with normal T-cell numbers and normal proliferative response to mitogens.[26]

Cartilage hair hypoplasia is a condition of immuno-osseous dysplasia that results from mutation of the RNAse mitochondrial ribonucleoprotein *(RMRP)* gene. It is characterized by short-limbed dwarfism, metaphyseal dysplasia, sparse hair, increased risk for malignancies, and bone marrow failure with varying degrees of immunodeficiency ranging from SCID to normal thymic function.[27] Cartilage hair hypoplasia presenting with SCID requires hematopoietic stem cell transplantation (HSCT), which corrects immunodeficiency and autoimmunity but not musculoskeletal or growth findings. Bowel function should be closely monitored during the first year of life, as Hirschsprung's disease is common. Other rare immune-osseous dysplasias that may present in early infancy include *MYSM1* deficiency, microcephalic osteodysplastic primordial dwarfism type 1, and immunoskeletal dysplasia with neurodevelopmental abnormalities.[1]

Dyskeratosis congenita (DC) is characterized by a triad of nail dystrophy, abnormal skin pigmentation, and oral leukoplakia. Patients with DC are predisposed to development of bone marrow failure, leukemia, and cancers. Immune phenotypes vary, but lymphopenia with low B-cell numbers and decreased T-cell function occur frequently.[28] Disease onset in infancy is associated with more severe immunologic and somatic features, especially severe enteropathy.[28] The inheritance pattern varies, and most present with mild phenotype.

The classical presentation of Comel–Netherton syndrome includes a triad of congenital ichthyosiform erythema, "bamboo hair" (*trichorrhexis invaginata*), and atopy.[29] This condition is inherited autosomal recessive due to mutations in the serine protease inhibitor of the serine protease inhibitor Kazal-type 5 gene (*SPINK5*).[30] Infants typically present in infancy with generalized scaling erythroderma, failure to thrive, and bacterial infections, and they may experience life-threatening hypernatremic dehydration from water loss through the dysfunctional skin barrier. These infants generally have elevated IgE and IgA with decreased memory B cells.

The inherited X-linked NF-κB essential modulator (NEMO) deficiency syndrome is characterized by anhidrotic ectodermal dysplasia with immunodeficiency (EDA-ID) due to abnormal development of ectodermal tissue. Hypomorphic mutations in the inhibitor of nuclear factor kappa B kinase regulatory subunit gamma (*IKBKG*) gene encoding NEMO protein lead to EDA-ID, and loss-of-function mutations of *IKBKG* lead to X-linked incontinentia pigmenti, usually lethal in male fetuses.[31] Typical presentation includes conical teeth, sparse scalp hair, frontal bossing, absence of sweat glands, and early severe and multiple bacterial infections with pyogenic bacteria (*S. aureus*, *S. pneumoniae*, or *H. influenzae*) or atypical mycobacteria.[32] Immune function varies with a range of T-, B-, and NK-cell dysfunction, but low memory B cells and impaired T-cell receptor activation is common.[31] Infants may present with eczematous dermatitis at birth, and life expectancy depends on the degree of immune deficiency.

Predominantly Antibody Deficiencies

Antibody deficiencies are characterized by bacterial sinopulmonary infections, meningitis, and sepsis, as well as persistent enteroviral infections of the gastrointestinal tract or central nervous system.[3] Antibody deficiencies are difficult to recognize in the newborn period due to passively acquired maternal IgG antibodies through the placenta and the low IgA levels that are characteristic of normal newborns. Maternal antibodies can be detected through the first 18 months of life.[33] Immunoglobulin deficiency generally becomes apparent after 6 months of age but may be detected earlier, especially in preterm infants.

Congenital X-linked agammaglobulinemia (XLA) is the most common form and results from mutations in the gene encoding B-cell–specific src-associated tyrosine kinase (Bruton's tyrosine kinase [BTK]). Without BTK, B-cell development stops in the pre-B-cell stage, leading to absent B cells in the blood, which can be detected by flow cytometry.[34,35] T-cell number and function are normal. Newborn infants with XLA may present with overwhelming enteroviral sepsis.[35] Rarely, autosomal recessive forms of congenital agammaglobulinemia may present similarly and occur due to a defect in the μ heavy chain, Igα, Igβ, BLNK, or λ5.[1]

Hyper-IgM (HIGM) syndromes are antibody deficiency disorders that involve defects in immunoglobulin class switch recombination, characterized by isolated normal or elevated levels of IgM with low or absent levels of immunoglobulin isotypes IgG, IgA, and IgE.[9] Defects in CD40L and CD40 were classified in this category, but they have recently been reclassified as combined immunodeficiency, as T-cell deficiency is also involved. Currently, genetic mutations in *AID*, *UNG*, *INO80*, and *MSH6*, which are all rare, fall under this classification.[1] Infants with HIGM suffer recurrent or severe bacterial infections and have enlarged lymph nodes and germinal centers.

Transient hypogammaglobulinemia of infancy (THI) is defined by IgG levels greater than 2 standard deviations below the age-appropriate range in infants over 6 months of age. The IgG levels are typically less than 400 mg/dL, and IgA and IgM levels may also be low. The ability of these infants to make specific antibodies is frequently near normal range, and most infants with THI are not susceptible to infection, so the question remains as to whether THI is a true immunodeficiency or an extension of the physiologic nadir that occurs as maternally transferred antibody wanes and the infant begins to produce its own antibodies.[36,37] Infants with THI may present with chronic or recurrent respiratory infections, with ear and sinus infections being the most common. Increased risk of infection in THI does not decrease with the use of intravenous immunoglobulin.[37] Most children with THI develop age-appropriate IgG levels by age 3.

DISEASES OF IMMUNE DYSREGULATION

Hemophagocytic lymphohistiocytosis (HLH) is a condition of immune dysregulation involving a hyperinflammatory response associated with aberrant activation of macrophages and lymphocytes leading to overwhelming cytokine release. Infants may present in the newborn period with persistent fever, splenomegaly, cytopenia, hypertriglyceridemia, and/or hypofibrinogenemia. Elevated ferritin, soluble IL-2Rα, granzyme B, and soluble CD163 levels and reduced NK cell function are common. Bone marrow or liver biopsy showing evidence of hemophagocytosis is diagnostic. There are primary or familial HLH and secondary forms of HLH.[38,39] Familial HLH is categorized into five subtypes that are associated with inherited gene mutations that impact T- and NK-cell functions involved in target cell cytolysis.[38,39] Identified mutations to date include mutations in *PRF1*, *UNC13D*, *STX11*, and *STXBP2*. Acutely ill HLH patients with deteriorating organ function are treated with systemic and/or intrathecal chemotherapy.[40,41] Secondary HLH may be triggered by infections (most commonly Epstein–Barr virus), autoinflammatory and autoimmune conditions, malignancy, human immunodeficiency virus infection, HSCT, immunosuppression, or metabolic diseases.

IEIs associated with HLH that can present in the newborn period include WAS, Chediak–Higashi syndrome (CHS), Gricelli syndrome 2 (GS2), and X-linked inhibitor of apoptosis protein (XIAP) deficiency. CHS is an autosomal recessive condition of impaired cytotoxicity characterized by oculocutaneous albinism (gray–silvery hair, hypopigmented eyes), recurrent bacterial infections, and peripheral neuropathy, with pathognomonic giant cytoplasmic granules in leukocytes and platelets. Identification of a pathogenic variant in the *CHS1/LYST* gene confirms the diagnosis. Early HSCT is the treatment of choice, as most individuals with CHS develop an accelerated phase consistent with HLH.[42] HSCT corrects hematologic and immunologic defects but does not prevent development of neurological deterioration.[43] GS2 presents similarly with partial albinism (silvery–gray hair), neutropenia, thrombocytopenia, and progressive neurologic deterioration. Inherited AR, GS2 results from a pathogenic variant in *RAB27A* leading to impaired cytotoxicity. Similar to CHS, infants with GS2 develop an accelerated phase with HLH phenotype. Microscopic examination of the hair shaft showing clumps of pigment can be diagnostic.[44] In contrast to CHS, giant cytoplasmic granules are not observed in GS2. XIAP deficiency is an X-linked condition that involves pathogenic variants in the *XIAP* gene and affects boys in early infancy. Infants may present with early-onset splenomegaly, HLH (often triggered by Epstein–Barr virus), and, to a lesser extent, intractable inflammatory bowel disease.[45]

Syndromes with autoimmunity that may present during the neonatal period include immune dysregulation, polyendocrinophathy, enteropathy, X-linked (IPEX) syndrome and IL-10R deficiency. IPEX syndrome occurs most commonly due to pathogenic variants in the *FOXP3* gene, encoding a protein necessary for the development of regulatory T cells that regulate immune cell functions including immunologic tolerance.[46] Infants typically present with autoimmune enteropathy (severe watery diarrhea), eczematous dermatitis, and type I diabetes during the neonatal period and may even be identified on fetal ultrasound.[47,48] Characteristic laboratory findings include elevated serum IgE, autoantibodies to pancreatic islet antigens, and thyroid antigens or small bowel mucosa, autoimmune cytopenias, eosinophilia, and decreased numbers of FOXP3-expressing T cells in the peripheral blood.[49] Treatment involves immune suppression prior to HSCT. Infants with IL-10 receptor deficiency present with very early-onset inflammatory bowel disease (VEO-IBD). Infants typically experience chronic diarrhea and bloody stools leading to anal ulcers and failure to thrive in severe cases, with folliculitis and skin rash being common extra-intestinal manifestations.[50] IL-10 plays a critical role in maintaining immune homeostasis in the gastrointestinal tract, and defects in IL-10 signaling lead to immune hyper-activation and excessive inflammatory response, causing extensive tissue damage. The immune profile is generally normal, so genetic testing for *IL-10* and/or *IL-10R* mutations should be considered in an infant with refractory diarrhea and failure to thrive.[51]

CONGENITAL DEFECTS IN PHAGOCYTE FUNCTION

Defective phagocyte function leads to frequent bacterial and fungal infections involving soft tissues and various organs. Leukocyte adhesion deficiency (LAD) occurs when leukocytes are unable to adhere to vascular endothelium and migrate to sites of infection or inflammation. Characteristic presentation includes delayed separation of umbilical cord in a newborn, impaired wound healing, omphalitis, and recurrent, severe bacterial infections localized to skin and mucosal surfaces. The hallmark features of LAD are an absence of pus formation at the site of infection and persistent leukocytosis. The most common subtype is LAD-I, which results from pathogenic variants in the *ITGB2* gene encoding CD18. Diagnosis can be made by flow cytometry showing absent or decreased CD18 expression, as well as expression of associated integrin molecules CD11a,

CD11b, and CD11c on leukocytes.[52] LAD-II and LAD-III subtypes do not present with delayed separation of umbilical cord and are extremely rare.

Chronic granulomatous disease (CGD) occurs due to defective phagocyte killing of catalase-positive organisms due to the inability of nicotinamide adenine dinucleotide phosphate (NADPH) oxidase to produce reactive oxygen species.[53] Infants with CGD may present with recurrent bacterial and fungal infections with catalase-positive organisms and inflammatory granulomas. Frequent sites of infection include lung, skin, lymph nodes, liver, and soft tissues. Microabscesses and non-caseating granuloma formation are common in the lungs, gastrointestinal, and genitourinary tracts. Diagnosis is made using flow cytometry–based respiratory burst assay. The X-linked form with mutations in the *CYBB* gene is most common, but AR forms exist with biallelic pathogenic variants in the *CYBA*, *NCF1*, *NCF2*, and *NCF4* genes. Defects in *NCF4* gene mildly impair respiratory burst activity (assay may be normal), but may present with severe VEO-IBD.[54]

DEFECTS IN INTRINSIC AND INNATE IMMUNITY

Chronic mucocutaneous candidiasis results from inborn errors in IL-17–mediated pathways or innate *Candida* sensing molecules.[55] Affected infants may present with recurrent mucosal or invasive infections of skin, oral cavity, esophagus, and other organs with *Candida* spp. with increased susceptibility to bacterial and viral infections, as well. Immune dysregulation may lead to development of autoimmune diseases and affect growth and development.

Gain of function (GOF) mutations in *STAT1* (inherited AD), which result in disruption of TH17 differentiation, are the most common cause of monogenic chronic mucocutaneous candidiasis. Diagnosis is made via genetic testing. Management consists mainly of antifungal prophylaxis. Targeted immunotherapy with Janus kinase 1/2 inhibitor is reported to be effective in controlling autoimmunity in *STAT1* GOF.[56]

Toll-like receptor (TLR) 3 pathway defects lead to susceptibility to HSV-1 encephalitis in humans.[57] TLR3 is an intracellular pattern recognition receptor within endolysosomes of immune cells and binds to the double-stranded RNA of replicating viruses. Mutations in the genes involved in the TLR3 signaling pathway, including *TLR3*, *UNC93B1*, *TRIF*, *TRAF3*, and *TBK1*, increase susceptibility to HSV encephalitis, which may present in early infancy.[58]

AUTOINFLAMMATORY DISORDER

Neonatal-onset multisystem inflammatory disorder (NOMID), the most severe form of cryopyrin-associated periodic syndromes that presents in the neonatal period, is caused by AD GOF mutations in the *NLRP3* gene that encodes protein cryopyrin within the inflammasome. Consequent aberrant formation and overproduction of active IL-1β lead to an augmented inflammatory response.[59] Infants present with characteristic facial features with frontal bossing, protruding eyes, and saddle-shaped nose, along with symptoms involving the skin, central nervous system, and joints. Clinical manifestations include fevers, migratory erythematous urticarial rash that appears within the first 6 weeks of life, chronic aseptic meningitis, cognitive disabilities, seizures, sensorineural hearing loss, and impaired growth with joint inflammation and bone deformities.[60] Severely affected infants may die prematurely. Treatment options include IL-1 receptor antagonist.

Diagnostic Approach to a Neonate with Suspected IEI

NEWBORN SCREENING FOR CONGENITAL T-CELL DEFICIENCIES

SCID is a fatal inborn error of immunity unless treated with HSCT or gene therapy early in life. A multi-center analysis of clinical outcomes in infants with SCID clearly demonstrated that survival improved if HSCT was initiated prior to 3 months of age.[61] Overall survival in early transplanted infants was >90% compared to only 50% for infants transplanted after 3.5 months. Treatment initiated after 6 months of age increases the risk for both infection and non-engraftment following HSCT. The impact of timing of HSCT on outcomes suggests that SCID should be considered a medical emergency warranting rapid diagnosis and treatment in affected infants.[62] Furthermore, early HSCT results in overall lower costs of care, primarily due to prevention of prolonged repeated hospitalizations.[63] Thus, SCID as well as other T-cell primary immune deficiencies meet the criteria for implementation of newborn screening (NBS). The criteria for implementing NBS include a high incidence of the disorder (>1/100,000 live births), serious morbidity or mortality associated with the condition, inability to diagnose at birth by routine physical exam, and early diagnosis and treatment leading to significant improvement of clinical outcomes.[64]

An inexpensive and sensitive assay to detect T-cell deficiencies utilizing the dried blood spot method has been developed that could be incorporated into existing NBS that uses the Guthrie card to detect other newborn conditions via NBS using a small volume of blood obtained via heel stick.[65] The assay capitalizes on arrested T-cell receptor (TCR) rearrangement in the thymus and low T-cell numbers associated with most forms of SCID.[6] As thymocytes undergo TCR rearrangement between variable, diversity, and joining segments, the intervening DNA between the genes forms a stable TREC that can be easily quantified within the dried blood spot using reverse transcription quantitative polymerase chain reaction (RT-qPCR). Normally, naïve T cells leaving the thymus in healthy infants have easily detectable TRECs; however, in infants with T-cell immune deficiencies, TREC levels are below the limit of detection for the assay. This methodology has proven to be sensitive and specific, and its low cost enables it to be included in routine newborn screening. In 2008, an initial pilot study examining all newborns in Wisconsin showed the feasibility and cost effectiveness of detecting T-cell deficiency as part of the standard newborn screening program using dried blood spots on the Guthrie card. Subsequently, implementation has expanded across the United States, as well as many other countries.[66] This method provides a quantitative detection of T-cell development within the thymus.[67] The test can identify multiple disorders of T-cell development.

Testing of dried blood spots is done in tandem with an internal positive control to ensure that the quality of the input DNA is adequate for PCR amplification. The positive control may vary among methods, although β actin or RNAaseP is used in general. If TREC copies are below the threshold for detection (fewer than 25 or 40 copies for most assays), then confirmatory testing is done using lymphocyte enumeration by flow cytometry to quantify the total numbers of T cells, B cells, and NK cells. Assessment of the proportion of memory and naïve T cells should be included in the lymphocyte enumeration. NBS for SCID has been conducted for over a decade across the United States, and the overall sensitivity of the assay has been excellent. The prevalence of SCID conditions requiring HSCT ranges from 1 in 46,000 to 1 in 80,000 live births, and the survival rate of those transplanted is greater than 90%.[68] Among the millions of newborns screened, the overall incidence of disorders associated with clinically significant T-cell lymphopenia has been about 1 in 20,000 live births. Abnormal NBS results were detected in less than 0.3% of all screened, with confirmatory cases reported in 0.016% to 0.03%.[68,69]

INTERPRETATION OF ABNORMAL TREC ASSAY IN PRETERM INFANTS

Implementation of NBS using the TREC assay unexpectedly led to identification of conditions other than SCID that affect T-cell development (Table 18.2). Among these conditions are congenital athymia, including complete DiGeorge and CHARGE syndromes; disorders of T-cell development, including trisomy 21, AT, CIDs, and secondary T-cell impairment, which lead to low TRECs; congenital heart disease; thymectomy associated with cardiac surgery; chylothorax; fetal hydrops; and loss of lymphocytes due to gastrointestinal tract malformations.[68] It is important to note that heparin contamination in the specimen results in inactivation of the Taq polymerase used in the RT-qPCR assay, leading to falsely low TREC levels and abnormal NBS for SCID. Although the majority of T-cell immune deficiencies are detected using the TREC NBS, some cellular immune deficiencies can result in normal TREC levels (Table 18.2). One of the most perplexing issues associated with NBS using the TREC assay has been the high proportion of otherwise normal very and extremely preterm infants with low TREC levels. In a recent 10-year outcome study, the rate of normal TREC levels in infants born before 37 weeks gestational age (GA) was 99.9%, similar to term infants, but only 81% were normal among extremely premature infants born prior to 28 weeks GA.[69] This has created a controversy regarding the optimal evaluation of preterm infants with abnormal NBS. Currently, there is no universally accepted algorithm for the assessment of abnormal TREC results, particularly in very and extremely premature infants. Practices vary across centers, with some sites waiting to repeat the TREC assay until the infant approaches

TABLE 18.2 Cellular Immune Deficiency Detection Using NBS TREC Assay

Typical SCID[a]	Primary Cellular Immune Deficiencies with abnormal TREC[b]	Secondary T-cell Deficiencies with Abnormal TREC	Cellular Immune Deficiencies With Normal TREC
$T^-B^-NK^-$	Ataxia-telangectasia[c]	Preterm infants	WAS syndrome
• ADA deficiency	Idiopathic T-cell lymphopenia	Congenital heart disease	MHC-I deficiency
• Reticular dysgenesis	Trisomy 21	Cardiac surgery	MHC-II deficiency
$T^-B^-NK^+$	Jacobsen syndrome	• Thymectomy	ZAP-70
• RAG1/2	Cartilage hair hypoplasia	Gastrointestinal malformations	VODI
• Artemis[c]	Dyskeratosis congenita		Human immunodeficiency virus
• DNA ligase IV[c]	DOCK8	Third-space loss	
• Cernunnos[c]	Thymus defects	• Chylothorax	
• DNA PKcs deficiency[c]	• 22q11.2 deletion	• Fetal hydrops	
$T^-B^+NK^+$	• CHARGE		
• IL-7Rα	• TBX1		
• CD45 deficiency	• FOXN1		
• CD3 chain (CD3δ, CD3ε, CD3ζ)	• PAX1		
$T^-B^+NK^-$			
• Common γc			
• JAK3 deficiency			

[a]Detected on NBS TREC, requires rapid diagnosis and intervention
[b]Variable detection with NBS TREC.
[c]Radiation sensitivity.

35 weeks GA and others repeating the assay with a new sample right away and obtaining confirmatory lymphocyte enumeration using flow cytometry if the repeat assay is abnormal.[70] The majority of preterm infants show an increase in T-cell numbers as they approach term gestational age.[71] Therefore, additional immune testing would add unnecessary costs. However, it is possible that preterm infants could have a congenital T-cell deficiency that could only be diagnosed with confirmatory testing by lymphocyte enumeration and genetic assessments. Figure 18.1 summarizes the algorithm for the initial steps in the evaluation of newborn infants with abnormal NBS using the TREC assay. Within the steps are assurances of the quality of the samples used for the initial assay, testing based on the infant's GA, and the types of confirmatory testing needed to verify abnormal test results.

LYMPHOCYTE ENUMERATION USING FLOW CYTOMETRY

Many cellular immune deficiencies affecting T cells, B cells, or NK cells can be quickly and accurately detected using diagnostic lymphocyte enumeration by flow cytometry. This method involves analysis of individual lymphocyte populations using a fluidics-based system with lasers to detect light deflection and the fluorescence of cells tagged with fluorochrome-conjugated monoclonal antibodies binding to cell surface proteins or intracellular proteins. Most monoclonal antibodies are directed at cluster of differentiation (CD) complexes that identify subpopulations of T cells, B cells, and NK cells.[72] Each monoclonal antibody has a unique fluorochrome that can be multiplexed to identify many different cell markers within a single specimen. Identification of lymphocytes is based on the uniform size and complexity of lymphocytes (termed *scatter*) and the expression of the leukocyte common antigen (CD45) on the surface of all nucleated hematopoietic cells. All T cells express CD3 on their surface, as well as either the αβ or γδ TCR complex. Co-expression of either CD4 or CD8 is present on all αβ TCR identifying $CD4^+$ helper or $CD8^+$ cytotoxic T cells. In contrast, γδ $CD3^+$ T cells do not express CD4 or CD8. B cells express both CD19 and CD20, either of which can be used in B-cell enumeration. NK cells do not express CD3 but can be identified by co-expression of CD56 and CD16. The sum of these three populations of T cells, B cells, and NK cells make up 100% of the lymphocyte populations termed the

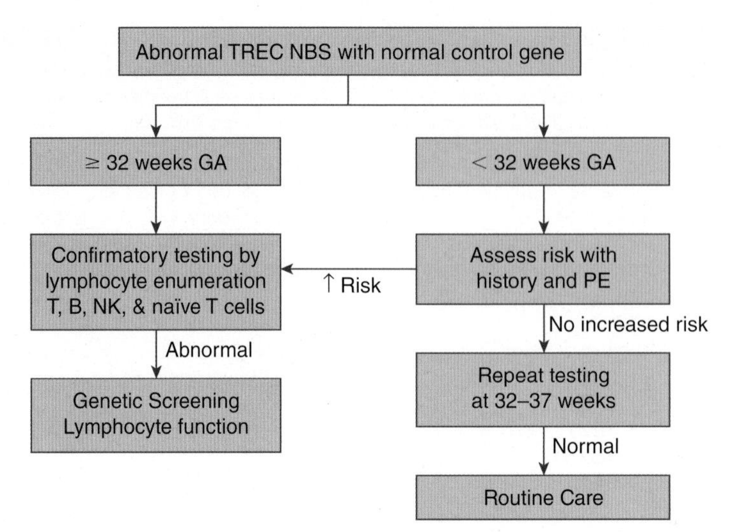

Fig. 18.1 Suggested algorithm for diagnostic approach to a newborn with an abnormal NBS for TREC. Normal control gene amplification validates the integrity of the specimen. Abnormal results in a newborn ≥ 32 weeks GA or infants < 32 weeks GA with suspicious clinical exam or history should be followed with lymphocyte enumeration by flow cytometry. If no suspicious findings, premature infants born < 32 weeks GA should have TREC assay repeated at 32 to 37 weeks. Abnormal lymphocyte enumeration should be followed by genetic studies and assessment of T-cell function.

lymphosome. The application of flow cytometry is a highly effective diagnostic tool for infants with suspected immunodeficiency. Requiring only 2 to 3 mL or less of whole blood collected in sodium heparin or ethylenediaminetetraacetic acid (EDTA), results can be obtained in a short period of time.

Although simple enumeration of T cells, B cells, and NK cells is readily available in most clinical labs, this is not adequate in the evaluation of infants with an abnormal NBS for T-cell immune deficiency. In order to accurately evaluate thymic output and T-cell development, extended lymphocyte enumeration is needed to assess the relative proportion of naïve T cells that are recent thymic emigrants, as well as memory T cells that have their own unique phenotype. Markers that identify naïve $CD3^+$ T cells are CD45RA plus an additional surface marker such as CD62L, CCR7, or CD31. Memory T cells that have encountered antigens in the germinal center and have undergone oligoclonal expansion express CD45RO. Accurate enumeration of lymphocytes requires absolute blood lymphocyte counts to be measured at the same time as flow cytometry. The percentage of each lymphocyte population is multiplied by the absolute lymphocyte count to quantify the absolute numbers of lymphocyte subsets in cells per microliter. Results must be interpreted in the context of the age of the infant, as values vary based on gestational age and continue to change throughout infancy and childhood, until they reach adult values. In term newborns, $CD3^+$ T cells make up the majority of blood lymphocytes, comprising 50 to 70% of the total lymphocyte population, percentages that are similar to those of adults but with higher absolute numbers. The normal ratio of $CD4^+$ to $CD8^+$ T cells is greater than 1.0 and generally ranges from 2:1 to 3.5:1 in term and preterm infants. Inverted CD4/CD8 ratios are abnormal, generally reflecting increased $CD8^+$ T-cell activation and expansion or a decline in $CD4^+$ T-cell numbers as in human immunodeficiency virus infection or other viral infections. B cells can make up to 20% of lymphocytes in newborns, but numbers vary greatly even in healthy infants. NK-cell percentages and numbers are higher in infants compared to adults.[73] Quantitative abnormalities may range from complete absence or pronounced deficiency or expansion in one or multiple lymphocyte populations.

LYMPHOCYTE ENUMERATION PATTERNS IN T-CELL IMMUNE DEFICIENCIES

SCID and other combined immune deficiencies associated with abnormal NBS due to low TRECs consist of multiple different clinical phenotypes reflecting the wide array of genetic conditions that lead to these disorders. However, the majority of SCID subtypes fall into four distinct patterns based on lymphocyte enumeration, highlighting the importance of flow cytometry in the evaluation of infants with abnormal NBS. Furthermore, the patterns and percentages of T, B, NK, and naïve T cells provide insight into the pathogenesis and genetic defects causing the disorders. Specific disorders were reviewed previously in this chapter. Infants with very low numbers of T cells, B cells, and NK cells ($T^-B^-NK^-$ phenotypes) will also have very low absolute lymphocyte counts. In contrast, $T^-B^-NK^+$, $T^-B^+NK^-$, or $T^-B^+NK^+$ phenotypes may have low or normal absolute lymphocyte numbers.[2,7] Taken together, lymphocyte enumeration using flow cytometry is an essential initial step in the diagnosis of cellular immune deficiencies. The results will guide the next step in confirming the diagnosis with genetic evaluation. The application of lymphocyte enumeration in the algorithm for evaluation of an infant with an abnormal TREC newborn screen is shown in Figure 18.1.

MEASUREMENT OF T-CELL FUNCTION

Assessment of lymphocyte function ex vivo is another valuable tool used in the evaluation of infants with suspected or known cellular immune deficiencies. Functional testing should be considered as an adjunct to lymphocyte enumeration, and in most cases, normal results of lymphocyte enumeration do not require further testing of cellular function, as the assays are expensive and generally require 10 mL or more of blood. The assay that has been most carefully validated and available in many clinical laboratories is the method of stimulating lymphocytes with mitogens that are plant lectins. These mitogens activate lymphocytes non-specifically to induce cellular proliferation that is quantitated by the incorporation of tritiated thymidine (^{3}H-Tdr) in cell culture. The most commonly used T-lymphocyte mitogen is phytohemagglutinin (PHA), but other plant lectins such as concanavalin A and pokeweed mitogen can also be used. Thymidine uptake by cells activated by the mitogen is compared to lymphocytes incubated in media alone. Results are expressed either as total ^{3}H-Tdr uptake or as a stimulation index that divides the maximum ^{3}H-Tdr uptake in the presence of the mitogen by the unstimulated cells without mitogen. In normal individuals, the mitogen stimulation index is 100- to 200-fold greater than the media control. Some centers use alternatives to mitogens, including stimulation with anti-CD3 monoclonal antibodies and flow cytometry–based assays using carboxyfluorescein succinimidyl ester or upregulation of CD69. However, the Primary Immunodeficiency Treatment Consortium (PIDTC) has established diagnostic criteria to use lymphocyte proliferation in response to PHA as the method of choice to assess lymphocyte function in identifying infants with typical SCID requiring expedited HSCT. Those with partial or atypical T-cell function, termed *leaky* SCID phenotypes, who are at risk for developing autoimmunity due to oligoclonal T-cell expansion, are also recommended to receive expedited HSCT, even though their T-cell dysfunction is not as severe.[74] Typical SCID is defined as mitogen proliferation that is less than 10% of the lower limit of normal for the laboratory reference standard, whereas atypical or leaky SCID is defined as proliferation that is less than 30% of the lower limit of the reference range.[74] Lymphocyte functional assays using proliferation responses to mitogens are most clinically useful in determining the likelihood of non-engraftment following HSCT or in diagnosing T-cell immune deficiencies associated with normal T-cell numbers with impaired cell signaling as is seen in ZAP-70 deficiency.

MEASUREMENTS OF ANTIBODIES

Quantitative assessments of antibody levels have limited utility in the newborn setting. Due to passively acquired maternal IgG, blood IgG levels reflect maternal transfer rather than neonatal production. Infants normally have a delayed class switch from IgM to IgA and IgG and thus have undetectable IgA at birth that continues to be substantially lower than adults throughout the first few years of life. The types of assays used in clinical laboratories to measure quantitative immunoglobulin levels pose another challenge in assessing immunoglobulins in newborns. The lower limits of detection for many standard laboratory platforms are higher than the age-appropriate ranges of IgA and IgG for term and preterm infants, limiting their utility as diagnostic tools. As a result, diagnosis of congenital antibody deficiencies is difficult during the neonatal period. Flow cytometry can be applied to detect congenital agammaglobulinemia conditions such as XLA, as these infants have no circulating $CD19^+$ or $CD20^+$ B cells. IEIs where measurement of antibody levels during the neonatal period are helpful in the diagnosis include immune dysregulation disorders that have distinct IgG, IgA, IgM, and IgE profiles such as IPEX syndrome and WAS.

TESTING PHAGOCYTIC CELL FUNCTION

Evaluation of phagocytic function begins with a complete blood count with differential, as the most common defects in neutrophil function during the newborn period are congenital neutropenias. Although rare, leukocyte adhesion deficiency can be evident in the newborn period, and diagnosis can be confirmed using flow cytometry to detect the loss of expression of CD18/11a and 11b on granulocytes, monocytes, and lymphocytes. LAD should be suspected in infants with persistently elevated white blood cell counts. Infants with CGD will have normal leukocyte counts and lymphocyte enumeration. The CGD diagnosis is made based on the neutrophil respiratory burst assay, which utilizes dihydrorhodamine (DHR) 123 and flow cytometry to measure neutrophil oxidative burst by assessing fluorescence changes in neutrophils stimulated with phorbol myristate acetate (PMA). Activation of neutrophils by PMA leads to oxidation of DHR to a fluorescent compound, rhodamine 123, which can be measured by flow cytometry. The respiratory burst assay can also detect female carriers of X-linked CGD. Although not readily available in many centers, the respiratory burst assay is a rapid and inexpensive laboratory test that can be performed in infants with suspected CGD.

DIAGNOSTIC TESTING USING MOLECULAR GENETICS

The majority of IEIs evident in the newborn period are severe conditions that require immediate definitive diagnosis and management. Furthermore, for many, definitive treatment and cure are best achieved if therapy is initiated soon after birth using HSCT, biological agents, and even gene therapy. The capacity to intervene early can dramatically alter outcomes; thus, early recognition, molecular genetic diagnosis, and proper management are critical. The application of molecular diagnostics has made a significant impact on improving the accuracy of diagnosing IEIs. Although essential for genetic counseling and assessing carrier risk, precise genetic diagnosis is also used to assess risk for associated complications, determine prognosis, and predict long-term outcomes. It is also a vital component in guiding immediate medical management of infants with IEIs, including clinical decisions involving HSCT, gene therapy, thymic implantation, and use of biological agents for definitive therapy.

Over 400 specific genes have been identified as causes of IEIs, with considerable genetic variants within those genes. Until recently, genetic diagnosis of specific genetic disorders was only available in the research setting. However, over the past 5 to 10 years, there has been an explosion in the number of clinical laboratories that are College of American Pathologists (CAP) accredited and Clinical Laboratory Improvement Amendments (CLIA) certified to perform diagnostic genetic testing. The turn-around time for most of the diagnostic gene panels is about 2 to 6 weeks, and the costs have become reasonable. Commercially available panels can be targeted for a single gene or limited number of genes associated with a specific disorder, such as SCID, or they can screen for a large number of genes associated with multiple congenital inborn errors. Gene panels utilize next-generation sequencing to identify known and unknown variants and can also detect deletions and duplications.

Although some IEIs, such as 22q11.2 deletion syndrome, can be diagnosed based on chromosomal cytogenetic studies, the majority of IEIs are associated with monogenic mutations requiring sequencing of targeted genetic regions and thus are not detected by karyotyping or microarray alone.[3,75] If initial screening does not provide a clear molecular cause for the patient's clinical phenotype, then whole exome sequencing can be performed using several available platforms. These assays involve paired-end reads and bidirectional sequencing.[76] Reads are assembled and aligned to reference gene sequences and analyzed for sequence variants. Whole exome sequencing should be done as a trio to include the index patient as well as maternal and paternal samples to identify which alleles carry the pathogenic variants. Genetic diagnosis should be moved up to an early event in the diagnostic algorithm for SCID and other conditions that should be treated early in infancy.

As genetic characterization is vital to diagnosis and management, genetic testing should be done as soon as confirmatory immune tests indicate an immune deficiency. Consultation by specialists in immunology and genetics can facilitate accurate diagnoses and the next steps in management. It should be pointed out that most children with immune deficiency lack a family history of a genetic disorder, as up to 40% of newly diagnosed cases of IEIs result from de novo mutations or compound heterozygous mutations inherited from maternal and paternal alleles. When a genetic disorder is identified, all family members at risk should be screened, as the penetrance of the gene defect may vary.[77]

Management and Treatment of Neonates with a Suspected or Known Inborn Error of Immunity

PREVENTIVE THERAPY

Preventing nosocomial and opportunistic infections as well as GVHD while maintaining clinical stability and facilitating definitive treatments is critical to the management plan.[2,3] Infants with SCID are extremely susceptible to severe, often fatal, opportunistic infections, as well as GVHD, following maternal to fetal blood transfusion or iatrogenic GVHD from transfusions with non-irradiated blood.[2] Although NBS with TREC provides early identification of infants at risk for T-cell deficiencies, it is important that plans be implemented as quickly as possible to minimize complications.[78] There are no harmonized standards for the initial management of an infant with an abnormal NBS for T-cell deficiency who has not had a confirmatory diagnosis, particularly for preterm infants younger than 32 weeks GA. In general, TREC screening results are available by the fifth to tenth day of life. Confirmatory testing using flow cytometry can provide rapid results within a few days to allow for precautions including isolation procedures, irradiated blood products, and minimizing exposure to cytomegalovirus (CMV) by holding off breastfeeding. If flow cytometry confirms T-cell immune deficiency, these precautions should continue. If the results are normal, they can be relaxed. However, management of preterm infants in which repeat TREC testing is delayed until 32 to 37 weeks can present a management challenge, particularly with respect to the potential risk for CMV acquisition from CMV-positive mothers. Most centers recommend that, for infants with confirmed SCID, CMV seropositive mothers should not breastfeed their infants.[79] Transfusion-acquired CMV poses an additional management challenge. Both infants with suspected T-cell deficiencies and premature very-low-birth-weight infants are at increased risk for disseminated CMV following transfusion of blood products from CMV-positive donors. Prevention of CMV is best achieved using CMV seronegative blood donors, although some neonatal centers use leukoreduction to minimize the risk.[80]

GVHD Prevention

GVHD can result from maternal T cells crossing the placenta during maternal-to-fetal hemorrhage, causing clinical signs of rash, hepatitis, and/or diarrhea. This condition can be confirmed by assessing for molecular chimerism in the infant's blood or skin tissue to detect infiltration of maternal T cells. GVHD can also occur when non-irradiated cellular blood products are infused into infants with T-cell deficiencies. Thus, infants with an abnormal NBS with low TRECs should receive only irradiated blood products. Infants with suspected immune deficiency associated with radiation sensitivity, such as Artemis deficiency, ligase IV deficiency, or AT should not be exposed to radiographic ionizing radiation (X-ray, computed tomography, or positron emission tomography imaging) unless they are essential and there are no reasonable alternatives (magnetic resonance imaging or ultrasonography).

Infection Prevention

Infection acquisition poses the greatest risk to morbidity and mortality among infants with SCID.[61] Interestingly, a survey carried out by the PIDTC indicated that infection rates among infants identified with SCID by NBS were higher than those known to be at risk due to family history.[79] There is not a consensus among centers with respect to the types of protective isolation and whether the isolation should take place inpatient versus outpatient for infants identified with SCID. In the inpatient setting, isolation procedures generally include universal hand hygiene and some form of personal protective equipment (gown, mask, and gloves), whereas some centers require positive-pressure isolation rooms. In the outpatient setting, most centers recommend limited visitation, immunizations for caregivers, no construction, and various requirements for siblings and pets. All PIDTC centers were harmonized with respect to antimicrobial prophylaxis given as intravenous immunoglobulin or subcutaneous immunoglobulin for immune prophylaxis and PCP prophylaxis with trimethoprim–sulfamethoxazole, generally dosed at 2.5 to 5 mg/kg/day given twice daily 3 times per week. Antifungal prophylaxis was given at most centers but fewer than half routinely used HSV prophylaxis with acyclovir.

Vaccinations with live viruses or bacillus Calmette–Guérin should not be given to infants with cellular immune deficiencies.[81] Household contacts should receive all age- and exposure-appropriate vaccines, including Severe acute respiratory syndrome coronavirus 2 (SARS-CoV-2), pertussis, and annual influenza vaccines.[82] The live attenuated measles, mumps, and rubella (MMR), varicella, and rotavirus vaccines may be administered to household contacts when indicated. MMR vaccine viruses are not transmitted to contacts, and transmission of the varicella zoster virus vaccine strain is rare.[82] If the varicella vaccine recipient develops a rash after vaccination, contact with the immune-deficient patient should be avoided until the rash resolves, although the risk of transmission is minimal unless blisters develop at the site of the vaccine administration.[82,83] The latest recommendations from the American Academy of Pediatrics and the Centers for Disease Control and Prevention for vaccinating children with immune deficiency should be followed (www.aap.org, www.cdc.gov).

CURATIVE THERAPY

Hematopoietic Stem Cell Transplantation

Early HSCT significantly improves survival and long-term outcomes for infants with many IEIs.[2,4,61] In addition to SCID and other cellular immune deficiencies, HSCT is used for other IEIs, including IPEX syndrome, CGD, primary hemophagocytic lymphohistiocytosis, WAS, congenital neutropenia, and CD40L deficiency, among others (Table 18.3).[41,84–86] The first bone marrow transplant for primary immune deficiency was done in the 1960s by Dr. Robert A. Good using a human leukocyte antigen (HLA)-matched sibling and no pre-transplant conditioning to cure a child with X-linked SCID.[87] Allogeneic HSCT from HLA-matched related donors result in the best clinical outcomes, but these donors are not always available.[61] When an HLA-matched relative is not available, stem cell sources can come from HLA-matched unrelated donors, umbilical cord stem cells, or haploidentical related donors such as a mother or father. If a haploidentical donor is used, T cells must be depleted pre-transplant to prevent

TABLE 18.3 Treatment Options for IEIS

HSCT	Enzyme Replacement/Biologics	Cultured Thymus Tissue Implant
SCID[a] (based on T, B, NK phenotype)	ADA deficiency: PEG-ADA	Congenital athymia:
CID less profound than SCID	Congenital neutropenia: GCSF	22q11.1 deletion
CID with associated features:	CGD: γ-interferon	TBX1
CHH	NOMID: IL-1 receptor antagonist (anakinra)	CHARGE
CD40L deficiency[a]		FOXN1
NEMO deficiency		PAX1
WAS[a]		Diabetic embryopathy
VODI		
Familial HLH[a]		
IEIs associated with HLH:		
CHS		
GS2		
XIAP deficiency		
Regulatory T-cell defects: IPEX[a]		
Phagocytic defects:		
Congenital neutropenia		
LAD[a]		
CGD[a]		

[a]Gene therapy as future options.

GVHD or ablated using chemotherapy post-transplant, as has been used more recently.[84] The timing, extent, and types of conditioning given to enhance stem cell engraftment vary with the molecular defect, T-cell and NK-cell function in the recipient, the donor source, existing pre-transplant complications such as GVHD or infection, and age.

The premise of the initiation of NBS using TREC is based on the assumption that early diagnosis and treatment would result in better survival following HSCT. However, in a small survey by the PIDTC, outcomes for infants with SCID identified early based on NBS or family history were similar to those for infants who were diagnosed based on clinical presentation.[88] Although these results may lead one to question the utility of universal NBS, the finding is not straightforward, as the SCID genotype, extent of immune reconstitution, and HSCT conditioning regimens all impact outcomes greatly.[89,90] Furthermore, it has been shown that long-term complications, particularly neurological outcomes, are improved in infants identified early through NBS.[91]

Gene Therapy

Gene therapy for the treatment of IEIs involves the use of autologous HSCT with the normal gene delivered to the stem cells to correct the dysfunctional gene, primarily through the use of viral vectors.[92] The modified hematopoietic stem cells are re-infused into the affected child to repopulate the bone marrow. All cells of hematopoietic origin (red blood cells, neutrophils, monocytes, and lymphocytes, including T cells, B cells, and NK cells) will then carry the normal gene. Multiple blood and immune disorders are candidates for gene therapy. Initial use of gene therapy for SCID was carried out in the 1990s. Early treatment involved the use of murine gamma-retroviral vectors. Although these early trials showed efficacy in correcting the immune dysfunction, these early vectors were associated with gene toxicity and increased risk for lymphoproliferative disease. Newer strategies have used lentiviral constructs that take advantage of the enhancer elements of the retroviral long terminal repeats and result in excellent gene delivery and safety. The autologous HSCT strategy is optimized when low-dose cytoreductive therapy is used at the time of stem cell re-infusion. Multiple clinical studies have been completed or are in progress, all supporting the efficacy and safety of gene therapy, including the successful treatment of ADA deficiency, X-linked severe combined immune deficiency, WAS, Artemis-deficient SCID, X-linked CGD, and leukocyte adhesion deficiency (Table 18.3). Gene therapy strategies are in development for primary hemophagocytic lymphohistiocytosis, X-linked lymphoproliferative disease, IPEX, and autosomal recessive CGD. Gene therapy is also being utilized for metabolic disorders involving monocytes and hemoglobinopathies, including thalassemia and sickle cell disease. As with HSCT, gene therapy does not correct the nonhematologic manifestations of these disorders.

Cultured Thymus Tissue Implantation for Congenital Athymia

Congenital athymia is considered part of the spectrum of $T^{-}B^{+}NK^{+}$ SCID that occurs due to the failure of the thymus to form in utero. Underlying genetic or syndromic conditions associated with congenital athymia include complete DiGeorge syndrome (22q11.2), CHARGE syndrome, diabetic embryopathy, severe FOXN1 deficiency, and PAX1 deficiency.[1,14,93] The lack of thymic tissue leads to a complete absence of naïve T cells, resulting in increased risk for infection, as well as autoimmunity manifested by autologous GVHD and autoimmune cytopenias. Without treatment, the condition is associated with a very high mortality rate. Cultured thymus tissue (CTT) is produced from donated human thymus tissue and surgically implanted in the recipient's body (Table 18.3). The thymus tissue used to produce CTT is obtained from infant donors who are ≤9 months and undergoing elective cardiac surgery that requires partial thymectomy.[93,94] The donated tissue is aseptically processed and cultured for 12 to 21 days to produce CTT. The manufacturing process depletes most of the donor thymocytes from the tissue but preserves the thymic epithelial cells and tissue structure. Following culture ex vivo, the thymic epithelial tissues are implanted into the quadriceps muscles of the recipient. Because infants with congenital athymia lack functional T cells, the procedure is done without HLA matching or GVHD prophylaxis. However, infants who show signs of GVHD due to oligoclonal T-cell expansion prior to CTT require T-cell ablation, generally with anti-thymocyte globulin.[95] T-cell immune reconstitution based on naïve T-cell enumeration and mitogen proliferation can be detected at approximately 6 to 12 months after the implantation, and recipients can then safely be weaned from immune and antimicrobial prophylaxis and vaccines can be administered.[93] However, post-CTT implantation T-cell counts typically remain less than the 10th percentile for age.

Treatment with Enzyme Replacement or Biological Agents

HSCT and gene therapy are considered curative treatments for many IEIs, but there are multiple biological treatment options available to use when curative therapy is not available or as a measure to bridge to the curative therapy (Table 18.3). For example, most forms of severe congenital neutropenia respond well to treatment with granulocyte colony-stimulating factor (G-CSF), and patients can be maintained on this treatment for many years. However, if the child fails to respond to the initial use of G-CSF, or if the child develops myelodysplastic syndrome or acute myeloid leukemia, then the best option would be to proceed to HSCT.[96] Enzyme replacement therapy with elapegademase, a recombinant adenosine deaminase conjugated to monomethoxypolyethylene glycol (PEG-ADA), is given by subcutaneous injection for the treatment of ADA deficiency. PEG-ADA has been used prior to definitive gene therapy or HSCT, but many patients have been successfully maintained on PEG-ADA for many years.[97,98] Similarly, patients with CGD can be treated with γ interferon, with mixed results.[99] In contrast, there is currently no definitive treatment available for NOMID, the severe phenotype of CAPS. However, these infants can be effectively treated with anti-IL-1 agents such as anakinra, the current treatment of choice for neonates, although it is not effective against joint or bone problems.[100]

REFERENCES

1. Bousfiha A, Jeddane L, Picard C, et al. Human inborn errors of immunity: 2019 update of the IUIS phenotypical classification. *J Clin Immunol.* 2020;40(1):66-81.
2. Buckley RH. Primary cellular immunodeficiencies. *J Allergy Clin Immunol.* 2002;109(5):747-757.
3. Notarangelo LD. Primary immunodeficiencies. *J Allergy Clin Immunol.* 2010;125(2 suppl 2):S182-S194.
4. Hershfield MS. Adenosine deaminase deficiency: clinical expression, molecular basis, and therapy. *Semin Hematol.* 1998;35(4):291-298.
5. Villa A, Notarangelo LD. *RAG* gene defects at the verge of immunodeficiency and immune dysregulation. *Immunol Rev.* 2019; 287(1):73-90.
6. Sleasman JW, Harville TO, White GB, George JF, Barrett DJ, Goodenow MM. Arrested rearrangement of TCR V beta genes in thymocytes from children with X-linked severe combined immunodeficiency disease. *J Immunol.* 1994;153(1):442-448.
7. Roberts JL, Lauritsen JP, Cooney M, et al. T⁻B⁺NK⁺ severe combined immunodeficiency caused by complete deficiency of the CD3zeta subunit of the T-cell antigen receptor complex. *Blood.* 2007;109(8):3198-3206.
8. Dobbs K, Dominguez Conde C, Zhang SY, et al. Inherited DOCK2 deficiency in patients with early-onset invasive infections. *N Engl J Med.* 2015;372(25):2409-2422.
9. de la Morena MT. Clinical phenotypes of hyper-IgM syndromes. *J Allergy Clin Immunol Pract.* 2016;4(6):1023-1036.
10. Sullivan KE. Chromosome 22q11.2 deletion syndrome: DiGeorge syndrome/velocardiofacial syndrome. *Immunol Allergy Clin North Am.* 2008;28(2):353-366.
11. Lindstrand A, Malmgren H, Verri A, et al. Molecular and clinical characterization of patients with overlapping 10p deletions. *Am J Med Genet A.* 2010;152A(5):1233-1243.
12. Botto LD, May K, Fernhoff PM, et al. A population-based study of the 22q11.2 deletion: phenotype, incidence, and contribution to major birth defects in the population. *Pediatrics.* 2003;112(1 Pt 1):101-107.
13. Grati FR, Molina Gomes D, Ferreira JC, et al. Prevalence of recurrent pathogenic microdeletions and microduplications in over 9500 pregnancies. *Prenat Diagn.* 2015;35(8):801-809.
14. Markert ML, Devlin BH, Alexieff MJ, et al. Review of 54 patients with complete DiGeorge anomaly enrolled in protocols for thymus transplantation: outcome of 44 consecutive transplants. *Blood.* 2007;109(10):4539-4547.
15. Jyonouchi S, McDonald-McGinn DM, Bale S, Zackai EH, Sullivan KE. CHARGE (coloboma, heart defect, atresia choanae, retarded growth and development, genital hypoplasia, ear anomalies/deafness) syndrome and chromosome 22q11.2 deletion syndrome: a comparison of immunologic and nonimmunologic phenotypic features. *Pediatrics.* 2009;123(5):e871-e877.
16. Hale CL, Niederriter AN, Green GE, Martin DM. Atypical phenotypes associated with pathogenic CHD7 variants and a proposal for broadening CHARGE syndrome clinical diagnostic criteria. *Am J Med Genet A.* 2016;170A(2):344-354.
17. Bosticardo M, Yamazaki Y, Cowan J, et al. Heterozygous *FOXN1* variants cause low TRECs and severe T cell lymphopenia, revealing a crucial role of FOXN1 in supporting early thymopoiesis. *Am J Hum Genet.* 2019;105(3):549-561.
18. Giardino G, Borzacchiello C, De Luca M, et al. T-cell immunodeficiencies with congenital alterations of thymic development: genes implicated and differential immunological and clinical features. *Front Immunol.* 2020;11:1837.
19. Dalm VA, Driessen GJ, Barendregt BH, van Hagen PM, van der Burg M. The 11q terminal deletion disorder Jacobsen syndrome is a syndromic primary immunodeficiency. *J Clin Immunol.* 2015; 35(8):761-768.
20. Ochs HD, Thrasher AJ. The Wiskott–Aldrich syndrome. *J Allergy Clin Immunol.* 2006;117(4):725-738; quiz 739.
21. Lavin MF. Ataxia-telangiectasia: from a rare disorder to a paradigm for cell signalling and cancer. *Nat Rev Mol Cell Biol.* 2008;9(10):759-769.
22. van Os NJH, Jansen AFM, van Deuren M, et al. Ataxia-telangiectasia: immunodeficiency and survival. *Clin Immunol.* 2017;178:45-55.
23. Busoni VB, Lemale J, Dubern B, et al. IBD-like features in syndromic diarrhea/trichohepatoenteric syndrome. *J Pediatr Gastroenterol Nutr.* 2017;64(1):37-41.

24. Lien R, Lin YF, Lai MW, et al. Novel mutations of the tetratricopeptide repeat domain 7A gene and phenotype/genotype comparison. *Front Immunol.* 2017;8:1066.
25. Mou W, Yang S, Guo R, et al. A novel homozygous TTC7A missense mutation results in familial multiple intestinal atresia and combined immunodeficiency. *Front Immunol.* 2021;12:759308.
26. Cliffe ST, Bloch DB, Suryani S, et al. Clinical, molecular, and cellular immunologic findings in patients with SP110-associated veno-occlusive disease with immunodeficiency syndrome. *J Allergy Clin Immunol.* 2012;130(3):735-742.e6.
27. Kostjukovits S, Klemetti P, Valta H, et al. Analysis of clinical and immunologic phenotype in a large cohort of children and adults with cartilage-hair hypoplasia. *J Allergy Clin Immunol.* 2017;140(2):612-614.e5.
28. Jyonouchi S, Forbes L, Ruchelli E, Sullivan KE. Dyskeratosis congenita: a combined immunodeficiency with broad clinical spectrum—a single-center pediatric experience. *Pediatr Allergy Immunol.* 2011;22(3):313-319.
29. Netherton EW. A unique case of trichorrhexis nodosa; bamboo hairs. *AMA Arch Derm.* 1958;78(4):483-487.
30. Chavanas S, Bodemer C, Rochat A, et al. Mutations in *SPINK5*, encoding a serine protease inhibitor, cause Netherton syndrome. *Nat Genet.* 2000;25(2):141-142.
31. Fusco F, Pescatore A, Conte MI, et al. EDA-ID and IP, two faces of the same coin: how the same *IKBKG/NEMO* mutation affecting the NF-κB pathway can cause immunodeficiency and/or inflammation. *Int Rev Immunol.* 2015;34(6):445-459.
32. Puel A, Picard C, Ku CL, Smahi A, Casanova JL. Inherited disorders of NF-κB-mediated immunity in man. *Curr Opin Immunol.* 2004;16(1):34-41.
33. Lewis DB, Wilson CB. Developmental immunology and role of host defenses in fetal and neonatal susceptibility to infection. In: Remington JS, Klein JO, Wilson CB, Baker CJ, eds. *Infectious Diseases of the Fetus and Newborn Infant*. 6th ed. Philadelphia, PA: Elsevier Saunders; 2006:87-210.
34. Cunningham-Rundles C, Ponda PP. Molecular defects in T- and B-cell primary immunodeficiency diseases. *Nat Rev Immunol.* 2005;5(11):880-892.
35. Ochs HD, Smith CI. X-linked agammaglobulinemia. A clinical and molecular analysis. *Medicine (Baltimore).* 1996;75(6):287-299.
36. Tiller Jr TL, Buckley RH. Transient hypogammaglobulinemia of infancy: review of the literature, clinical and immunologic features of 11 new cases, and long-term follow-up. *J Pediatr.* 1978; 92(3):347-353.
37. Sandberg K, Fasth A, Berger A, et al. Preterm infants with low immunoglobulin G levels have increased risk of neonatal sepsis but do not benefit from prophylactic immunoglobulin G. *J Pediatr.* 2000;137(5):623-628.
38. Verbsky JW, Grossman WJ. Hemophagocytic lymphohistiocytosis: diagnosis, pathophysiology, treatment, and future perspectives. *Ann Med.* 2006;38(1):20-31.
39. Ishii E. Hemophagocytic lymphohistiocytosis in children: pathogenesis and treatment. *Front Pediatr.* 2016;4:47.
40. Trottestam H, Horne A, Arico M, et al. Chemoimmunotherapy for hemophagocytic lymphohistiocytosis: long-term results of the HLH-94 treatment protocol. *Blood.* 2011;118(17):4577-4584.
41. Marsh RA, Haddad E. How I treat primary haemophagocytic lymphohistiocytosis. *Br J Haematol.* 2018;182(2):185-199.
42. Kaplan J, De Domenico I, Ward DM. Chediak–Higashi syndrome. *Curr Opin Hematol.* 2008;15(1):22-29.
43. Eapen M, DeLaat CA, Baker KS, et al. Hematopoietic cell transplantation for Chediak–Higashi syndrome. *Bone Marrow Transplant.* 2007;39(7):411-415.
44. Masri A, Bakri FG, Al-Hussaini M, et al. Griscelli syndrome type 2: a rare and lethal disorder. *J Child Neurol.* 2008;23(8):964-967.
45. Marsh RA, Madden L, Kitchen BJ, et al. XIAP deficiency: a unique primary immunodeficiency best classified as X-linked familial hemophagocytic lymphohistiocytosis and not as X-linked lymphoproliferative disease. *Blood.* 2010;116(7):1079-1082.
46. Bennett CL, Christie J, Ramsdell F, et al. The immune dysregulation, polyendocrinopathy, enteropathy, X-linked syndrome (IPEX) is caused by mutations of *FOXP3*. *Nat Genet.* 2001;27(1):20-21.
47. Torgerson TR, Ochs HD. Immune dysregulation, polyendocrinopathy, enteropathy, X-linked: forkhead box protein 3 mutations and lack of regulatory T cells. *J Allergy Clin Immunol.* 2007; 120(4):744-750; quiz 751-752.
48. Louie RJ, Tan QK, Gilner JB, et al. Novel pathogenic variants in *FOXP3* in fetuses with echogenic bowel and skin desquamation identified by ultrasound. *Am J Med Genet A.* 2017;173(5): 1219-1225.
49. Gambineri E, Perroni L, Passerini L, et al. Clinical and molecular profile of a new series of patients with immune dysregulation, polyendocrinopathy, enteropathy, X-linked syndrome: inconsistent correlation between forkhead box protein 3 expression and disease severity. *J Allergy Clin Immunol.* 2008;122(6):1105-1112.e1.
50. Yazdani R, Moazzami B, Madani SP, et al. Candidiasis associated with very early onset inflammatory bowel disease: first IL10RB deficient case from the National Iranian Registry and review of the literature. *Clin Immunol.* 2019;205:35-42.
51. Hutchins AP, Diez D, Miranda-Saavedra D. The IL-10/STAT3–mediated anti-inflammatory response: recent developments and future challenges. *Brief Funct Genomics.* 2013;12(6):489-498.
52. Cabanillas D, Regairaz L, Deswarte C, et al. Leukocyte adhesion deficiency type 1 (LAD1) with expressed but nonfunctional CD11/CD18. *J Clin Immunol.* 2016;36(7):627-630.
53. Holland SM. Chronic granulomatous disease. *Hematol Oncol Clin North Am.* 2013;27(1):89-99, viii.
54. van de Geer A, Nieto-Patlan A, Kuhns DB, et al. Inherited p40phox deficiency differs from classic chronic granulomatous disease. *J Clin Invest.* 2018;128(9):3957-3975.
55. Shamriz O, Tal Y, Talmon A, Nahum A. Chronic mucocutaneous candidiasis in early life: insights into immune mechanisms and novel targeted therapies. *Front Immunol.* 2020;11:593289.
56. Weinacht KG, Charbonnier LM, Alroqi F, et al. Ruxolitinib reverses dysregulated T helper cell responses and controls autoimmunity caused by a novel signal transducer and activator of transcription 1 (STAT1) gain-of-function mutation. *J Allergy Clin Immunol.* 2017;139(5):1629-1640.e2.
57. Zhang SY, Jouanguy E, Ugolini S, et al. TLR3 deficiency in patients with herpes simplex encephalitis. *Science.* 2007;317(5844): 1522-1527.
58. Lim HK, Seppanen M, Hautala T, et al. TLR3 deficiency in herpes simplex encephalitis: high allelic heterogeneity and recurrence risk. *Neurology.* 2014;83(21):1888-1897.
59. Baroja-Mazo A, Martin-Sanchez F, Gomez AI, et al. The NLRP3 inflammasome is released as a particulate danger signal that amplifies the inflammatory response. *Nat Immunol.* 2014;15(8): 738-748.
60. Finetti M, Omenetti A, Federici S, Caorsi R, Gattorno M. Chronic infantile neurological cutaneous and articular (CINCA) syndrome: a review. *Orphanet J Rare Dis.* 2016;11(1):167.
61. Pai SY, Logan BR, Griffith LM, et al. Transplantation outcomes for severe combined immunodeficiency, 2000–2009. *N Engl J Med.* 2014;371(5):434-446.
62. Puck JM, SCID Newborn Screening Working Group. Population-based newborn screening for severe combined immunodeficiency:

steps toward implementation. *J Allergy Clin Immunol.* 2007;120(4):760-768.
63. Kubiak C, Jyonouchi S, Kuo C, et al. Fiscal implications of newborn screening in the diagnosis of severe combined immunodeficiency. *J Allergy Clin Immunol Pract.* 2014;2(6):697-702.
64. American College of Medical Genetics. Newborn screening: toward a uniform screening panel and system. *Genet Med.* 2006;8(suppl 1):1S-252S.
65. Chan K, Puck JM. Development of population-based newborn screening for severe combined immunodeficiency. *J Allergy Clin Immunol.* 2005;115(2):391-398.
66. Chase NM, Verbsky JW, Routes JM. Newborn screening for T-cell deficiency. *Curr Opin Allergy Clin Immunol.* 2010;10(6):521-525.
67. Baker MW, Grossman WJ, Laessig RH, et al. Development of a routine newborn screening protocol for severe combined immunodeficiency. *J Allergy Clin Immunol.* 2009;124(3):522-527.
68. Kwan A, Abraham RS, Currier R, et al. Newborn screening for severe combined immunodeficiency in 11 screening programs in the United States. *JAMA.* 2014;312(7):729-738.
69. Hale JE, Platt CD, Bonilla FA, et al. Ten years of newborn screening for severe combined immunodeficiency (SCID) in Massachusetts. *J Allergy Clin Immunol Pract.* 2021;9(5):2060-2067.e2.
70. Knight V, Heimall JR, Wright N, et al. Follow-up for an abnormal newborn screen for severe combined immunodeficiencies (NBS SCID): a Clinical Immunology Society (CIS) survey of current practices. *Int J Neonatal Screen.* 2020;6(3):52.
71. Remaschi G, Ricci S, Cortimiglia M, et al. TREC and KREC in very preterm infants: reference values and effects of maternal and neonatal factors. *J Matern Fetal Neonatal Med.* 2021;34(23):3946-3951.
72. Brown M, Wittwer C. Flow cytometry: principles and clinical applications in hematology. *Clin Chem.* 2000;46(8 Pt 2):1221-1229.
73. Shearer WT, Rosenblatt HM, Gelman RS, et al. Lymphocyte subsets in healthy children from birth through 18 years of age: the Pediatric AIDS Clinical Trials Group P1009 study. *J Allergy Clin Immunol.* 2003;112(5):973-980.
74. Shearer WT, Dunn E, Notarangelo LD, et al. Establishing diagnostic criteria for severe combined immunodeficiency disease (SCID), leaky SCID, and Omenn syndrome: the Primary Immune Deficiency Treatment Consortium experience. *J Allergy Clin Immunol.* 2014;133(4):1092-1098.
75. Pena LDM, Jiang YH, Schoch K, et al. Looking beyond the exome: a phenotype-first approach to molecular diagnostic resolution in rare and undiagnosed diseases. *Genet Med.* 2018;20(4):464-469.
76. Green RC, Berg JS, Grody WW, et al. ACMG recommendations for reporting of incidental findings in clinical exome and genome sequencing. *Genet Med.* 2013;15(7):565-574.
77. Shashi V, McConkie-Rosell A, Schoch K, et al. Practical considerations in the clinical application of whole-exome sequencing. *Clin Genet.* 2016;89(2):173-181.
78. Michniacki TF, Seth D, Secord E. Severe combined immunodeficiency: a review for neonatal clinicians. *NeoReviews.* 2019;20(6):e326-e335.
79. Dorsey MJ, Wright NAM, Chaimowitz NS, et al. Infections in infants with SCID: isolation, infection screening, and prophylaxis in PIDTC centers. *J Clin Immunol.* 2021;41(1):38-50.
80. Harmon CM, Cooling L. Current strategies and future directions for the prevention of transfusion-transmitted cytomegalovirus. *Int J Clin Transfus Med.* 2017;5:49-59.
81. Succi RC, Farhat CK. Vaccination in special situations. *J Pediatr (Rio J).* 2006;82(suppl 3):S91-S100.
82. Medical Advisory Committee of the Immune Deficiency Foundation, Shearer WT, Fleisher TA, et al. Recommendations for live viral and bacterial vaccines in immunodeficient patients and their close contacts. *J Allergy Clin Immunol.* 2014;133(4):961-966.
83. Grossberg R, Harpaz R, Rubtcova E, Loparev V, Seward JF, Schmid DS. Secondary transmission of varicella vaccine virus in a chronic care facility for children. *J Pediatr.* 2006;148(6):842-844.
84. Slatter MA, Gennery AR. Hematopoietic cell transplantation in primary immunodeficiency - conventional and emerging indications. *Expert Rev Clin Immunol.* 2018;14(2):103-114.
85. França TT, Barreiros LA, Al-Ramadi BK, Ochs HD, Cabral-Marques O, Condino-Neto A. CD40 ligand deficiency: treatment strategies and novel therapeutic perspectives. *Expert Rev Clin Immunol.* 2019;15(5):529-540.
86. Dorsey MJ, Petrovic A, Morrow MR, Dishaw LJ, Sleasman JW. FOXP3 expression following bone marrow transplantation for IPEX syndrome after reduced-intensity conditioning. *Immunol Res.* 2009;44(1-3):179-184.
87. Meuwissen HJ, Gatti RA, Terasaki PI, Hong R, Good RA. Treatment of lymphopenic hypogammaglobulinemia and bone-marrow aplasia by transplantation of allogeneic marrow. Crucial role of histocompatiility matching. *N Engl J Med.* 1969;281(13):691-697.
88. Heimall J, Logan BR, Cowan MJ, et al. Immune reconstitution and survival of 100 SCID patients post-hematopoietic cell transplant: a PIDTC natural history study. *Blood.* 2017;130(25):2718-2727.
89. van der Burg M, Mahlaoui N, Gaspar HB, Pai SY. Universal newborn screening for severe combined immunodeficiency (SCID). *Front Pediatr.* 2019;7:373.
90. Haddad E, Logan BR, Griffith LM. SCID genotype and 6-month posttransplant CD4 count predict survival and immune recovery. *Blood.* 2018;132(17):1737-1749.
91. Dvorak CC, Puck JM, Wahlstrom JT, Dorsey M, Melton A, Cowan MJ. Neurologic event-free survival demonstrates a benefit for SCID patients diagnosed by newborn screening. *Blood Adv.* 2017;1(20):1694-1698.
92. Kohn LA, Kohn DB. Gene therapies for primary immune deficiencies. *Front Immunol.* 2021;12:648951.
93. Markert ML, Gupton SE, McCarthy EA. Experience with cultured thymus tissue in 105 children. *J Allergy Clin Immunol.* 2022;149(2):747-757.
94. Enzyvant Therapeutics. RETHYMIC (Allogeneic processed thymus tissue–agdc) [package insert]. Cambridge, MA: Enzyvant Therapeutics, Inc.; 2021.
95. Markert ML, Alexieff MJ, Li J, et al. Postnatal thymus transplantation with immunosuppression as treatment for DiGeorge syndrome. *Blood.* 2004;104(8):2574-2581.
96. Skokowa J, Dale DC, Touw IP, Zeidler C, Welte K. Severe congenital neutropenias. *Nat Rev Dis Primers.* 2017;3:17032.
97. Hershfield MS. PEG-ADA replacement therapy for adenosine deaminase deficiency: an update after 8.5 years. *Clin Immunol Immunopathol.* 1995;76(3 Pt 2):S228-S232.
98. Ferrua F, Aiuti A. Twenty-five years of gene therapy for ADA-SCID: from bubble babies to an approved drug. *Hum Gene Ther.* 2017;28(11):972-981.
99. International Chronic Granulomatous Disease Cooperative Study Group. A controlled trial of interferon gamma to prevent infection in chronic granulomatous disease. *N Engl J Med.* 1991;324(8):509-516.
100. Welzel T, Kuemmerle-Deschner JB. Diagnosis and management of the cryopyrin-associated periodic syndromes (CAPS): what do we know today? *J Clin Med.* 2021;10(1):128.

Chapter 19

Clinical and Molecular Markers to Assist Decision-Making in Neonatal Sepsis

Martin Stocker, MD, MME; Laura Fillistorf, MS; Eric Giannoni, MD

Key Points

- Early detection followed by rapid initiation of antimicrobial treatment and measures to prevent and treat organ dysfunction are key to optimizing the outcome of sepsis.
- Due to the non-specific presentation, the dynamic and heterogeneous nature of sepsis, and the difficulties in objectively defining clinical signs, there is no combination of clinical markers that offers high diagnostic accuracy.
- Molecular markers mainly assess the systemic inflammatory response, which is neither sensitive nor specific of sepsis.
- Predictive algorithms using single or multiple variables are informative for risk stratification but have a low to moderate accuracy to detect neonatal sepsis before overt clinical deterioration.
- The lack of precision and overestimation of the performance of current diagnostics lead to delays in the initiation of treatment in some patients and unnecessary exposure to antibiotics in many newborns.
- We propose a conceptual framework to assist clinicians in decision-making for suspected neonatal sepsis that takes into account the baseline incidence of sepsis, the presence of additional risk factors, a dynamic assessment of vital signs, clinical and molecular markers, microbiology, consideration of alternative diagnoses, and risk–benefit ratio of antibiotics in a given patient.

Introduction

Neonatal sepsis is characterized by non-specific signs and difficulty in distinguishing it from non-infectious conditions, but also by a rapid progression toward dysfunction of vital organs, high mortality, and a risk of lifelong disability, especially in preterm infants. Therefore, clinicians have a low threshold to initiate empirical antibiotics. In fact, suspected neonatal infection or "rule-out sepsis" is one of the most common diagnoses in neonatal units, and antibiotics are among the most frequently prescribed medications.[1–3] However, in the vast majority of cases, cultures remain negative, and sepsis is subsequently ruled out. Therefore, the current approach leads to substantial overtreatment with antibiotics, and exposes neonates to colonization with antibiotic resistant bacteria. Antibiotic treatment also induces perturbations in early-life microbiota with potentially long-lasting negative impact on the individual's health.[4] Accurate diagnostic algorithms and tools are needed to accelerate the diagnosis of neonatal sepsis while minimizing overtreatment. Currently, most published studies analyzing risk factors, clinical signs, and biomarkers/molecular markers have major limitations regarding design (observational studies), size (insufficient power to prove safety), and strategy (lack of acknowledging important factors such as baseline sepsis incidence or focusing on a single or a limited set of clinical or molecular markers).

This chapter presents the current state of knowledge on the use of clinical and molecular markers to guide the management of neonatal sepsis, based on data from high-income countries. The diagnostic value of and potential pitfalls in the interpretation of clinical and laboratory data to guide decisions to start, stop, or continue antimicrobial treatment and for risk stratification are reviewed. Moreover, we discuss how clinical and molecular markers can be integrated in a framework aiming at optimizing the decision-making process for suspected neonatal sepsis.

Decision-Making in Neonatal Sepsis

Decision-making is the backbone of clinical medicine. Despite research and guidelines, an understanding of how decisions are made in daily clinical practice remains elusive. Very large variations in the use of antibiotics among neonatal units have been described.[5–9] To some extent, they can be explained by differences in guidelines, patient populations, level of implementation of antimicrobial stewardship programs, and leadership style at each institution.[10–12] However, it is more difficult to assess the impact of seniority, interactions between junior and senior physicians, habits, and dramatic or negative experiences on decision-making by individual clinicians and teams.[13] Excessive fear of sepsis may be a key driver for antibiotic overtreatment in neonates. Whereas a high face validity exists for this assumption, literature is scarce regarding this topic. There is some evidence from qualitative studies that fear critically influences antibiotic decision-making.[14–17] A systematic review of qualitative studies regarding physician antibiotic-prescribing behavior found that complacency and fear were the most influential intrinsic factors.[18] Moreover, when faced with similar scenarios, individual clinicians may not always make the same decisions.[19] Decision-making in neonatal sepsis is affected by bias, a systematic deviation toward overtreatment, and noise, a random scatter.[20]

The decision to start antibiotics is typically based on a prediction made by the clinician that a particular patient has an ongoing bacterial infection. Some predictive judgments are verifiable, but this is rarely the case in neonatal sepsis. One can only be certain that starting antibiotics was the correct decision if the patient has an unambiguous proof of infection, documented by a positive and non-contaminated blood or cerebrospinal fluid culture. As this is rarely the case in clinical practice, many decisions regarding initiation and termination of antibiotics are made under conditions of uncertainty. The quality of unverifiable judgments can only be assessed by the quality of the thought process that produces them.[20]

Cognitive biases in the interpretation of clinical scenarios (including data from clinical and molecular markers of sepsis) contribute to inadequate antibiotic prescribing practices.[21] However, the capacity of clinicians to make predictions might be greater than expected. In a prospective study of 347 patients admitted to a neonatal and a pediatric intensive care unit, physicians were asked, based on all available information, to provide an estimate of the presence of serious infection at every ward round.[22] In cases for which empirical antibiotics were started, predictions made at initiation of antibiotics discriminated well patients who were later deemed to have culture-proven sepsis from non-infectious episodes (area under the receiver operating characteristic curve [AUROC] = 0.88). But, only 14% of antibiotic courses were administered for episodes of proven systemic bacterial infection, suggesting that accurate predictions do not always translate into appropriate clinical decisions. Clinical and molecular markers should not be considered as single measurements allowing to rule in or rule out sepsis on their own. They should be interpreted building on evidence-based data on their diagnostic value and their potential to add value to the judgment of physicians and improve patient outcomes as part of an overall structured approach to optimize antibiotic use in early life. As an example, the Agency for Healthcare Research and Quality provides a program to improve antibiotic-prescribing practices by combining adaptive change theories and evidence-based diagnostic and treatment practices.[23] Recently, an approach based on six key questions to evaluate the objective risk of bacterial infection was proposed to guide antibiotic prescriptions in critically ill children, and overcome irrational decision-making due to the fear of missing severe bacterial infections.[24]

Conceptual Framework for Decision-Making in Neonatal Sepsis

Key aspects in the decision-making process are the determination of the probability of sepsis and the evaluation of the risk–benefit ratio of starting, not starting, or stopping antibiotics for a given patient. We provide a conceptual framework to assist clinicians in decision-making for suspected neonatal sepsis (Figure 19.1). Assessment of the probability of sepsis in a given patient can be done using a structured approach, including the following steps: (1) determination of baseline incidence of sepsis, (2) evaluation of risk factors and clinical and molecular markers and consideration of alternative diagnoses to estimate the specific probability of sepsis for an individual patient, (3) evaluation of the course of clinical and molecular markers to adapt the

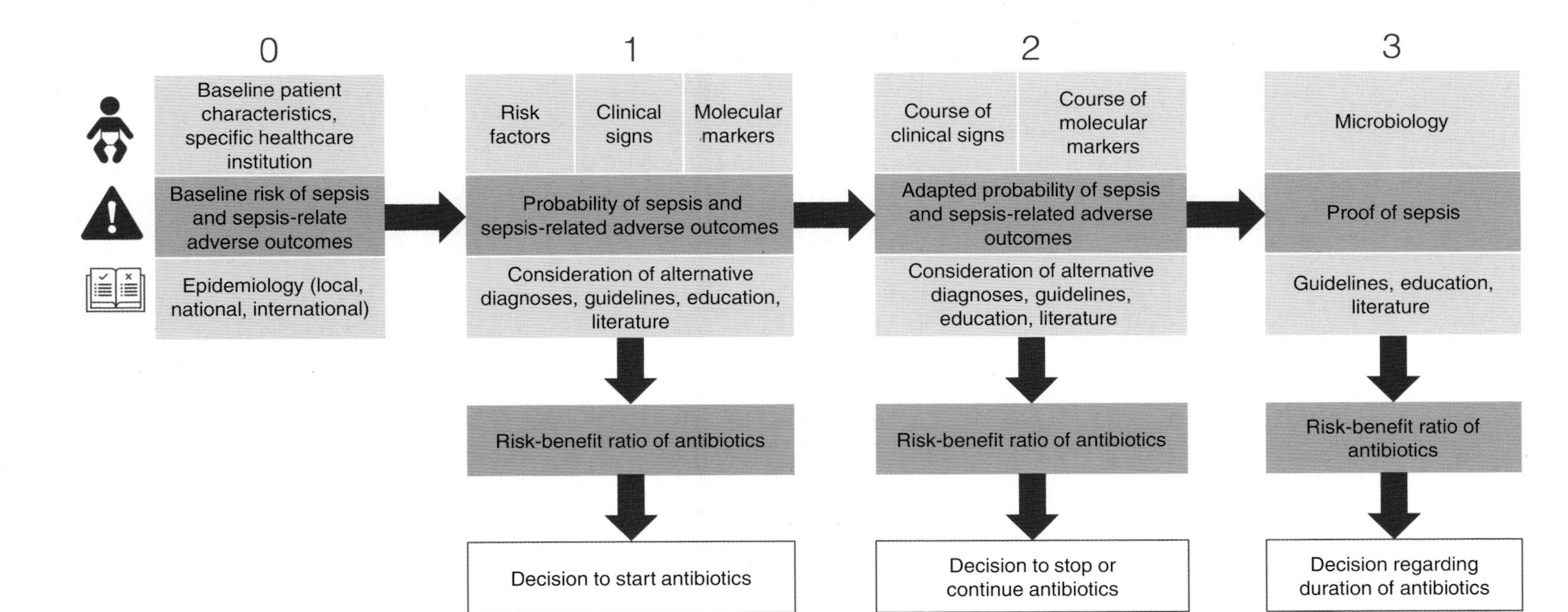

Fig. 19.1 Framework for decision-making regarding antibiotic therapy in neonates with suspected sepsis. *0,* baseline situation; *1,* before potential start of antibiotics; *2,* during antibiotic therapy with definitive diagnosis pending; and *3,* during antibiotic therapy with proof of infection.

assessment of the specific probability of sepsis, and (4) proof or definitive exclusion of sepsis with the help of microbiology results. Importantly, the course of clinical signs and serial evaluation of molecular markers will provide more information than a single assessment at the onset of symptoms. Guidelines and educational programs are key components of the decision-making framework and may assist clinicians at every step of the process.

GUIDELINES AND EDUCATION

Guidelines to standardize diagnostic workup and treatment strategies have been issued by a number of professional associations from multiple countries.[10,25–27] In general, guidelines help to reduce variability and noise in clinical care. However, wide variations in the approaches recommended in guidelines from different countries and multiple updates may contribute to a sense of uncertainty regarding the optimal approach. Reports from the United Kingdom, Germany, and The Netherlands indicate a relatively low compliance with national recommendations for neonatal sepsis.[28–30] The majority of guidelines focus mainly on early-onset sepsis (EOS), defined as sepsis that occurs within the first 72 hours after birth. Moreover, guidelines are not intended to address all clinical scenarios and are not a substitute for clinical judgment.

Education of healthcare providers is key to translating evidence from randomized control trials (RCTs) and observational studies into clinical decisions at the bedside, to the implementation of guidelines and antimicrobial stewardship programs, and to decision-making in general. Considerable knowledge gaps on sepsis have been identified among medical and nursing staff taking care of adults, resulting in 30% to 50% of patients not being triaged as urgent in the emergency department.[31,32] Conversely, improved recognition was associated with decreased mortality.[33]

DETERMINATION OF BASELINE INCIDENCE

An important, but often neglected step in risk assessment at the individual patient level is the determination of the baseline incidence of sepsis in a particular clinical scenario. Basic patient characteristics and data from epidemiologic studies, as well as local epidemiological data for the specific healthcare institution, serve as important sources of information. Neonatal sepsis presents mainly as three different scenarios, with distinct risk factors, clinical presentations, and outcomes.[34] EOS results from the transmission of pathogens from the mother in utero or at the time of birth in the context of chorioamnionitis or colonization of the birth canal by pathogens. The vast majority of neonates affected by EOS develop symptoms within 48 to 72 hours following birth. Hospital-acquired late-onset sepsis (LOS) accounts for more than 60% of all cases of neonatal sepsis and typically presents after postnatal day 3 as a nosocomial infection in premature or ill newborns treated with invasive devices. Community-acquired LOS affects predominantly term newborns discharged home after an uncomplicated birth who present to the emergency room after the first week of life. As for the majority of conditions affecting neonates, gestational age has a strong impact on incidence. Looking at both extremes, the incidence of hospital-acquired, blood culture–positive LOS ranges from 10% to 40% in extremely preterm newborns, whereas the incidence of culture-positive EOS ranges between 0.2 and 0.8 per 1000 live births in term newborns.[34–37] Incomplete knowledge or failure to take this information into account is likely to be an important contributor to the bias toward antibiotic overtreatment in neonates.

RISK–BENEFIT RATIO OF ANTIBIOTICS

Sepsis is a major cause of neonatal death and disability. The burden of neonatal sepsis is strongly influenced by gestational age, with the most premature infants being at the greatest risk of sepsis and sepsis-related adverse outcomes. Early detection of invasive infection, prompt initiation of antibiotics, and support of vital functions are key steps to reducing mortality and morbidity.[38] Antibiotics are our main response to potentially fatal bacterial diseases, and they prevent millions of deaths every year worldwide; however, there is compelling evidence that antibiotics can be harmful.[39] Antibiotic treatments are associated with increased antimicrobial resistance, risks related to drug toxicity, longer duration of hospital stay, mother–infant separation, reduced rate of breastfeeding, and higher healthcare costs.[40,41] Antibiotic exposure early in life disrupts the developing microbiome, alters host immune responses, impacts growth, and contributes to numerous diseases later in life, including asthma, obesity, and inflammatory bowel disease.[42–46] In very-low-birth-weight

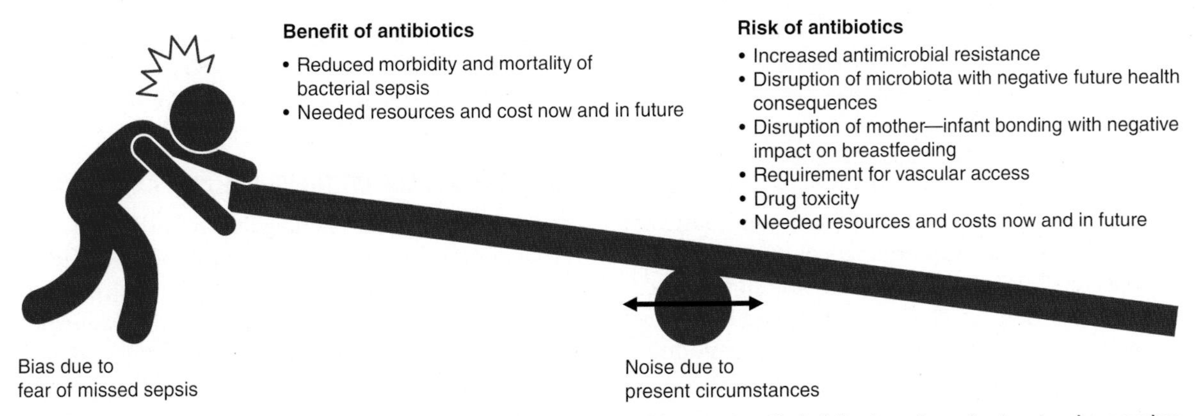

Fig. 19.2 Risk–benefit ratio of antibiotic therapy for suspected neonatal sepsis. *Bias,* a systematic deviation towards overtreatment; *noise,* a random scatter.[20]

(VLBW) preterm infants, prolonged exposure to antibiotics is associated with an increased risk of death, necrotizing enterocolitis (NEC), LOS, retinopathy of prematurity, and chronic lung disease.[47,48] Compared to adults, antibiotic treatments in newborn infants have disproportionate consequences, as the infant's microbiome and immune system are evolving and are unstable systems particularly sensitive to disruptions.[49] Therefore, balancing the trade-off between efficient sepsis care and antimicrobial stewardship is particularly challenging in neonates (Figure 19.2).[50] The problem is even more complex in preterm neonates, who are at the greatest risk of adverse outcomes of infection and are at the same time more vulnerable to the side effects of antibiotics. In summary, in neonates with suspected infection, it is key to consider not only the individual risk of sepsis and sepsis-related adverse outcomes but also the potential harms associated with antibiotics use.

ADDITIONAL RISK FACTORS

Although assessment of clinical and molecular markers is the focus of this chapter, we also briefly discuss considerations regarding additional risk factors. An in-depth discussion regarding risk factors can be found in Chapter 1. After having determined the baseline incidence of sepsis according to gestational age and clinical scenario (EOS, hospital-acquired LOS, and community-acquired LOS), the evaluation of additional risk factors is an important step for accurate estimation of the risk of developing sepsis. The main risk factors in each clinical scenario are well known from epidemiological studies. However, the impact of each individual risk factor and every possible combination of risk factors on the odds of developing sepsis may be difficult to grasp for the clinician at the bedside.[51] The Neonatal EOS Calculator is a multivariate assessment tool designed to predict the risk of EOS in late-preterm and term infants through the use of baseline incidence of EOS, objective assessment of risk factors, and clinical signs.[52] Although such an approach has an indisputable benefit to increase the capacity of physicians to assess the risk of developing EOS in individual patients, the recommendation provided by the calculator to start antibiotics at an estimated risk of EOS $\geq$3/1000 is highly controversial.[53]

Clinical Markers of Sepsis

Sepsis is a heterogeneous syndrome defined in adults as a life-threatening organ dysfunction caused by a dysregulated host response to an infection.[54] Initial manifestations are often subtle, and progression to multiorgan dysfunction, which can occur over a few hours to days, is a strong predictor of mortality.[55] In order to reduce mortality and morbidity, the optimal approach should allow clinicians to identify patients before the occurrence of significant organ dysfunction. Clinical manifestations can arise potentially from any organ and system, reflecting local and systemic invasion by pathogens, host response, and evolving organ dysfunction. This explains the diverse, unspecific, and dynamic nature of clinical signs. Due to the complex and rapid changes in organ function that occur as part of normal physiology in early life, defining cutoffs to discriminate physiology from disease and predict organ dysfunction is challenging in newborns. Moreover, many infants have abnormal physiology before the onset of sepsis due to prematurity, non-infectious complications of prematurity, or other comorbidities (such as congenital malformations). Therefore, it is particularity challenging for clinicians to diagnose neonatal sepsis at early stages and discriminate it from non-infectious conditions, as well as for researchers to study clinical manifestations of neonatal sepsis.

Clinical markers can be divided in three categories: (1) vital signs (heart rate, blood pressure, respiratory rate, oxygen saturation, and temperature), which are expressed as numerical data; (2) more complex clinical signs that depend on interpretation by healthcare professionals (e.g., apnea, retractions, poor perfusion, lethargy); and (3) treatments to support the function of vital organs (e.g., non-invasive or invasive ventilation, catecholamines), which also have a subjective component, as they depend on the decisions made by physicians.

DIAGNOSTIC VALUE OF INDIVIDUAL CLINICAL SIGNS

In a review of studies conducted from the 1950s to 1990s,[56] the most frequent clinical sign was fever (present in 50% of cases), followed by jaundice, respiratory distress, and hepatomegaly, which were observed in over 30% of cases. Recent studies show a different and heterogeneous presentation, where respiratory and cardiovascular signs are predominant, followed by neurologic and gastrointestinal manifestations and temperature changes (Table 19.1).[57–66] None of these signs has a positive predictive value (PPV) above 50%, but most of them have a negative predictive value (NPV) value of ≥70%, as invasive infection is rarely asymptomatic.

TABLE 19.1 Diagnostic Value of Clinical Signs for Culture-Positive Neonatal Sepsis

Clinical Signs	Percent of Infants with Sign	Sensitivity	Specificity	PPV	NPV	OR
Respiratory						
Apnea	30–84	40	65	14–32	73	0.5–2.7
Tachypnea	4–60	10	81	18	69	1.3–1.6
Grunting, flaring, retractions	66	—	—	—	—	—
Increased oxygen requirement	36–45	—	—	17	—	0.7–1.7
Increased respiratory support	17–64	—	—	17	—	0.6–4.3
Cardiovascular						
Tachycardia	4–82	30	81	39	74	1.1–3.1
Hypotension	5–42	19	93	8–31	—	3.5
Pallor/gray/mottled skin	23–95	—	—	—	70	1.8–2.9
Capillary refill time >2 seconds	40–63	30	81	39	74	2.8–3.3
Central-peripheral temperature difference > 2°C	71–84	79	78	45	94	16
Gastrointestinal						
Abdominal distension	5–53	20	89	43	74	0.6–1.3
Feeding intolerance	18–35	—	—	15	—	1.5–1.6
Jaundice	5	96	5	3	—	0.8
Temperature						
Hyperthermia	7–19	9–27	84–96	19–33	73–96	1.1–1.8
Hypothermia	3–18	3–36	90–97	7–44	71–96	1.9–2.6
Temperature instability	20	6–20	92–98	7–50	82–96	2.0–2.9
Neurological						
Lethargy	13–64	40	65	20–32	73	4.3
Irritability	12–14	—	—	—	—	1.0
Seizures	4	—	—	—	—	—

Data are from References 57 to 66. *OR*, odds ratio.

Apnea is a complex sign that is difficult to detect, categorize into central or peripheral, and quantify (in terms of duration and severity of associated bradycardia and desaturation) with clinical observation and monitoring devices, making data collection often imprecise. Respiratory distress manifests as tachypnea, retractions, nasal flaring, grunting, and reduced oxygen saturation (SpO_2). An increased fraction of inspired oxygen (FiO_2) and non-invasive or invasive ventilation are often considered as clinical markers of sepsis and have prognostic value for the risk of death.[34,55,67]

Peripheral vasoconstriction reduces skin perfusion and temperature of extremities, redirecting blood and heat to vital organs. Pale, gray, and/or mottled skin and increased capillary refill time are commonly used to describe poor skin perfusion during sepsis. Monitoring the central–peripheral temperature difference as a way to quantify peripheral vasoconstriction has been identified as a clinical marker of LOS in preterm newborns.[57,58] Hypotension is often a late sign of infection,[58] and its treatment with catecholamines is associated with increased risk of death.[34,55,67]

Abdominal distention, absent bowel sounds, and feeding intolerance are the manifestations of paralytic ileus, or the consequence of intra-abdominal infection. Jaundice is no longer a common sign of sepsis and has a poor diagnostic value. There is no standardized way (such as the Glasgow Coma Score) to assess the level of consciousness in neonates. Neurological manifestations of sepsis with or without central nervous system infection include lethargy, irritability, altered muscle tone, and seizures.

In a study of 127 infants with temperature symptoms in the first 3 days of life, fever, hypothermia, and temperature instability had a specificity of >90% for the diagnosis of EOS in all gestational age groups.[59] The diagnostic value of temperature seems more limited in preterm infants with suspected LOS.[60] This is not surprising, given that these patients are often cared for in incubators, which can mask temperature changes.

Published data on the diagnostic value of individual clinical signs suffer from a number of limitations. Treatments such as non-invasive or invasive ventilation, fluid therapy, caffeine, inotropes, steroids, and sedatives modify the physiology and may potentially mask signs of infection. Although some variables exist to take into account the impact of treatment on vital signs (e.g., PaO_2/FiO_2 and SpO_2/FiO_2 ratios, oxygenation index), this is not the case for many clinical signs. The diagnostic value of clinical markers of infection is influenced by gestational age, postnatal age, clinical scenario, definitions of sepsis cases, and controls. Definitions of clinical signs are often inconsistent among studies and imprecise; for example, pallor, mottling, or gray skin are often clustered into one sign. Moreover, rapid changes in clinical condition during the course of infection add complexity to the evaluation. Many studies capture single or a limited number of time points, providing low-resolution data.

ALGORITHMS BASED ON HIGH-RESOLUTION CLINICAL MARKERS OR COMBINATION OF CLINICAL MARKERS

Considering the dynamic changes that occur during sepsis, the digitalization of healthcare systems, and the strong computational capabilities that are now available, analysis of high-resolution data from continuous monitoring of vital signs is an attractive strategy to develop accurate predictive algorithms for the early detection of neonatal sepsis. In preterm newborns, reduced variability in heart rate and transient decelerations have been identified in the hours to days prior to the diagnosis of LOS. These abnormal heart rate characteristics (HRCs) were analyzed with mathematical models, leading to the development of an HRC index, which represents the fold increase in risk of sepsis during the next 48 hours.[68] HRC monitoring can be used as a non-invasive early-warning tool, alerting physicians before overt clinical deterioration. An RCT conducted in 3003 VLBW preterm infants demonstrated a reduction of mortality with continuous real-time HRC monitoring.[69] Subsequent studies showed a modest accuracy of the HRC index for the diagnosis of LOS (AUROC = 0.66 to 0.70), and a strong impact of gestational age on its performance.[70–72] A higher HRC index was associated with an increased risk of death following LOS but with low to modest diagnostic accuracy (AUROC = 0.68).[71–73]

Studies analyzing high-resolution clinical data (collected every 2 seconds) from continuous monitoring of chest impedance, electrocardiographic waveforms, and pulse oximetry in preterm infants showed a twofold increase in apnea, bradycardia, and desaturation in 43% of infants and extreme periodic breathing in

12% of infants on the day prior to diagnosis of LOS.[74,75] In a study of 1065 VLBW infants, including 123 cases of LOS and 63 cases of NEC, changes in heart rate, SpO_2, and respiratory rate were observed, and cross-correlation or co-trending of heart rate and SpO_2 had the highest diagnostic accuracy for LOS or NEC.[70] The diagnostic value of the three variables differed between the two sites where the study was conducted, highlighting the importance of external validation. Combining the three variables in a model and adding the HRC index increased diagnostic accuracy (AUROC = 0.73).

Models using multiple clinical markers achieved a greater diagnostic accuracy.[60,76,77] A machine learning–based model developed using data on five vital signs collected in electronic medical records of 715 newborns with LOS and over 2000 controls predicted LOS events 48 hours before clinical detection with an AUROC of 0.86.[76] RALIS is another algorithm based on five clinical markers (heart rate, respiratory rate, temperature, desaturation events, and bradycardia events) entered in electronic medical records at least every 3 hours, and it uses gestational age- and birthweight-specific ranges in combination with modifications from individual infants' own baselines. In a single-center retrospective study of 155 very preterm infants, RALIS predicted LOS with a sensitivity of 81%, a specificity of 80%, a PPV of 57%, and a NPV of 93% (AUROC = 0.90), and it identified LOS episodes at a mean of 43 hours earlier than standard care.[77]

Molecular Markers of Neonatal Sepsis

Over 250 biomarkers of sepsis have been studied across all age groups in more than 8000 clinical studies.[78] Numerous studies and reviews have been published regarding different molecular markers for neonatal sepsis, including white blood count (WBC); platelets; interleukin (IL)-1, IL-6, and IL-8; C-reactive protein (CRP); procalcitonin (PCT); tumor necrosis factor alpha; CD64; molecular signatures; and more.[79] Nevertheless, most studies have at least one serious limitation, including the following: (1) the study design is observational, (2) the sample size is insufficient to prove the safety of the approach, (3) the definition of sepsis is inconsistent and sepsis cases are heterogeneous, or (4) there is a lack of translation into clinical practice.[78,79] Therefore, most studies on molecular markers are not good enough to guide decision-making regarding neonatal sepsis.

Despite these limitations, molecular markers are widely used by clinicians caring for neonates with suspected or proven neonatal sepsis. Fear of missed sepsis cases and poor outcomes may be one reason for the widespread use of molecular markers. In addition, the sensitivity of the gold standard for the diagnosis of neonatal sepsis, the blood culture, is modest, and culture-negative neonatal sepsis is an ongoing debate in the medical literature.[50]

Molecular markers yield objective numbers. In the past, the description of complex situations by numbers helped to improve medical management. The Apgar score, which is nothing more than a translation of a complex situation into numbers, changed neonatal management in the first hour of life.[80] Currently, many clinicians are using molecular markers to guide their management of neonatal sepsis. The normalization of an initial increased molecular marker during antibiotic treatment may falsely induce clinicians into thinking that the neonate has culture-negative sepsis, and antibiotic treatment must be prolonged.

RCTs with a safety outcome regarding molecular markers for neonatal sepsis are scarce. Nevertheless, high-quality studies with over 1000 participants are available for CRP and PCT.[81,82] In a prospective study published more than 20 years ago, Benitz et al.[81] evaluated serial CRP levels in 1002 neonates with suspected EOS and 184 with suspected LOS. Three serial CRP levels below 10 mg/dL within 48 hours had a negative predictive value of 99.7% for EOS and 98.7% for LOS. The NeoPInS study is a RCT evaluating PCT to shorten antibiotic therapy in a cohort of over 1700 neonates suspected of neonatal sepsis.[82] With a primary classification of low, medium, and high risk for EOS, followed by PCT-guided duration of therapy, antibiotics were reduced from 65 to 55 hours in the intention-to-treat and from 64 to 52 hours in the pre-protocol analysis. The AUROC values to rule out EOS within 36 hours were 0.99 for CRP and 0.92 for PCT.[83] The main limitation of both studies is a relatively low number of culture-proven sepsis cases; therefore, the pretest probability of sepsis is low. Cantey and Bultmann pointed out in a recently published editorial that a coin flip may reach a NPV of 95% due to a low pretest probability.[84] Nevertheless, both studies showed a high NPV for CRP and PCT within 48 and 24 hours, respectively, and these results are in line with many observational studies and meta-analyses.[79]

WBC count is probably the most used biomarker in the management for neonatal sepsis, and some guidelines have incorporated it in their algorithms. In a huge retrospective cross-sectional study with more than 65,000 neonates, a WBC count below $5 \times 10^3/\mu L$ correlated with an increased risk for EOS. The time point of analysis was an important factor for accuracy, as the AUC increased from 0.52 within the first hour of life to 0.87 after 4 hours.[85] In another large observational study of EOS in 66,000 neonates, the AUC for the absolute neutrophil count and immature/total neutrophil ratio showed a similar time dependency but with an overall lower accuracy (AUROC = 0.70 to 0.87).[86] Two huge retrospective studies have confirmed the low to modest accuracy of complete blood cell count to detect EOS and LOS.[87,88] Therefore, a WBC count below $5 \times 10^3/\mu L$ may help clinicians to refine their estimate regarding the probability of infection in each patient, but it is never proof of sepsis.

No large RCTs have analyzed the PPV of molecular markers for neonatal sepsis. Small studies using CRP, PCT, IL-6, progranulin, and many more show overall poor to modest positive predictive values for neonatal sepsis.[79] Numerous non-infectious conditions influence molecular markers in neonates suspected of sepsis. In the first few days of life, perinatal factors such as vaginal versus cesarean delivery, duration of labor, maternal fever, or maternal intrapartum antibiotic prophylaxis are associated with increased CRP and IL-6. Lower gestational age, hypoxic–ischemic encephalopathy, meconium aspiration syndrome, and viral infections influence the values of CRP, PCT, and IL-6.[89] Similarly, non-infectious conditions such as maternal hypertension, preeclampsia and intrauterine growth restriction are associated with leucopenia and neutropenia in the newborn.[90] Therefore, the PPV of molecular markers is generally insufficient to support decision making for neonatal sepsis.

Researchers have tried to increase the accuracy of prediction by combining multiple molecular markers. In a prospective study analyzing CRP, PCT, sTREM-1, and pancreatic stone protein (PSP) in a group 137 neonates with suspected EOS, a panel of two molecular markers (PCT and PSP) showed the highest accuracy with an AUROC of 0.83. A panel with three or four molecular markers failed to increase accuracy.[91] A secondary analysis of the NeoPInS study, including 1678 neonates suspected of EOS and more than 10,000 biomarker measurements, showed no increase in accuracy to rule out sepsis within 36 hours with the use of a combination of CRP and PCT compared to CRP or PCT alone.[83] In a meta-analysis of 28 studies enrolling 2661 neonates with suspected sepsis that compared PCT, CRP, and presepsin alone or in combination showed similar accuracies for a combination of PCT and CRP or presepsin alone.[92] Whereas in some adult sepsis studies, panels of multiple molecular markers showed an increased accuracy,[93,94] there is a lack of evidence for this approach in neonatal sepsis.

All of the above-mentioned molecular markers are molecules produced by the host as a reaction to an infection or inflammation. This process requires time, and newer approaches using host RNA signature are one step ahead. A study of 200 infants younger than 60 days with suspected sepsis showed promising results (AUROC = 0.96).[95] A prospective observational study using a different set of RNA signatures reported a sensitivity of 95% and a specificity of 94% for bacterial infection in a randomly selected group of 279 infants out of a cohort of 1883 infants younger than 60 days with suspected sepsis.[96] These results must be confirmed in prospective trials within large cohorts of neonates, and the use of this technique is still exploratory.

As an unbalanced microbiome is a potential source of sepsis, microbiome and metabolic patterns are probably the earliest stage to look for molecular markers in the cascade of infection.[97–99] Fecal volatile organic compounds reflect microbiome patterns and host interactions.[98,99] In a multicenter cohort study of 843 preterm neonates, fecal volatile organic compounds discriminated infants with LOS from matched controls.[100] The attraction of this approach is the early stage of a signal sent even before neonatal sepsis clinically occurs.

Currently, the biggest problem may be how molecular markers are used. Several reports have shown a negative impact of the use of molecular markers. In a single-center study, initiation of antibiotic treatments was delayed in the group using molecular markers.[101] Another study reported prolonged antibiotic treatment and hospital stay with the use of repeat CRP measurements.[102] One problem is the dichotomized thinking of clinicians: If a result is not negative, then clinicians tend to see it as positive. Nature is rarely dichotomized as positive and negative but is more of a continuum, with a broad gray zone between the ends. We need to think again how to use molecular markers for neonatal sepsis. There is evidence from high-quality studies that CRP and PCT may be used to shorten antibiotic therapy in neonates started for suspected EOS. On the other hand, a WBC below $5 \times 10^3/\mu L$ is a marker signaling an increased likelihood of neonatal sepsis. But, most importantly, molecular markers must be studied and analyzed as part of an algorithm or management strategy for neonatal sepsis and not as isolated markers. We have to acknowledge that the search for molecular markers as the holy grail in the diagnosis and management of neonatal sepsis is probably futile.[78,79]

Multimodal Approaches

To overcome the limitations related to the use of clinical and molecular markers and their modest diagnostic accuracy, multimodal approaches have been applied to designing scores or algorithms to diagnose neonatal sepsis or to predict a fatal outcome (Table 19.2). The second adult sepsis definition and the 2002 pediatric consensus definition were based on systemic inflammatory response syndrome (SIRS) criteria, defined by at least two out of five abnormal variables among heart rate, respiratory rate, temperature, and leucocyte count. As in other age groups, SIRS criteria lack both sensitivity and specificity to diagnose neonatal sepsis and predict the risk of death.[80–108] Sepsis is now recognized to involve pro- and anti-inflammatory responses and major (non-immunologic) changes in the cardiovascular, neuronal, autonomic, hormonal, bioenergetic, metabolic, and coagulation systems, all of them having prognostic significance. Consequently, SIRS criteria were abandoned in the third adult sepsis definition, which uses the Sequential Organ Failure Assessment (SOFA) score to quantify organ dysfunction and predict the risk of death.[54] In neonates, dysfunction of the respiratory and cardiovascular systems plays a central role in the pathogenesis of sepsis and sepsis-related adverse outcomes.[34,55,108] A neonatal

TABLE 19.2 Diagnostic Accuracy of Prediction Models for Neonatal Sepsis

Study	Type of Data in Model	Type of Infection	Population	AUROC for Prediction of Sepsis	AUROC for Prediction of Mortality
Bekhof et al.[60]	Risk factors, clinical signs	LOS	<34 wk	0.84	—
Walker et al.[63]	Vital signs, biomarkers	LOS	All newborns	0.9	—
Fleiss et al.[67] (nSOFA)	Clinical markers, platelets	LOS	<33 wk	—	0.71–0.95
Fairchild et al.[70]	Vital signs	LOS, NEC	VLBW	0.73	—
Fairchild et al.,[70] Rio et al.,[71] Zeigler et al.[73] (HRC index)	Vital signs	LOS	All newborns/ VLBW	0.66–0.7	0.68
Song et al.[76]	Vital signs	LOS[a]	All newborns	0.86	—
Mithal et al.[77] (RALIS)	Vital signs	LOS	<32 wk	0.9	—
Joshi et al.[103]	Vital signs	LOS	<32 wk	0.84	—
Mahieu et al.[104] (NOSEP NEW-II)	Risk factors, comorbidities, clinical markers, biomarkers	LOS[a]	All newborns	0.82	—
Stocker et al.[105]	Risk factors, clinical signs, biomarkers	EOS	≥34 wk	0.83	—
Masino et al.[106]	Risk factors, clinical signs, biomarkers	LOS	All newborns	0.8	—

[a]Cases of culture-positive and culture-negative sepsis were included.

SOFA (nSOFA) score was developed to quantify the need for respiratory and hemodynamic support and thrombocytopenia.[109] A multicenter validation study of 653 preterm infants with late-onset infection showed an AUROC of 0.81 (at sepsis evaluation) to predict the risk of death.

The NOSEP score, based on dichotomized data on prolonged parenteral nutrition, presence of fever, elevated CRP, low platelets, and neutrophilia, was designed to predict nosocomial sepsis across all gestational age groups.[61] In a multicenter validation cohort including 155 episodes of culture-positive and culture-negative nosocomial sepsis, diagnostic accuracy reached an AUROC of 0.71 after several modifications of the algorithm (NOSEP New-I). Adding information on surgery, maternal hypertension, and ventilation increased diagnostic accuracy, with an AUROC of 0.82 (NOSEP New-II).[104] In a study of 53 newborns with LOS and 112 controls, a model based on sick appearance 24 hours after the start of antibiotics, elevated CRP, and increased neutrophil/lymphocyte ratio allowed identification of LOS cases with an AUROC of 0.94, suggesting a potential to assist clinicians in the decision to discontinue antibiotics.[62]

In a secondary analysis of the NeoPInS study, a machine-learning model based on 28 variables (risk factors, clinical signs, and biomarker levels) collected at the start of antibiotics achieved an AUROC of 0.83 to predict EOS in late-preterm and term infants. Interestingly, the markers with the highest predictive value were CRP and WBC count, indicating that traditional biomarkers may have a diagnostic value in multivariate models.[105] As described earlier, the Neonatal EOS Calculator is a multivariate risk assessment tool designed to predict the risk of EOS in late-preterm and term infants, using baseline incidence of EOS, objective assessment of risk factors, and clinical signs.[52] The tool provides a risk estimate and a recommendation to start empirical antibiotics when the estimated risk is ≥3/1000.[53] This approach has allowed practitioners to strongly reduce neonatal exposures to antibiotics in certain settings, but it was not designed to identify all cases of EOS.[110,111]

Overall, the performance of algorithms to detect neonatal sepsis before overt clinical deterioration is low to moderate, raising concerns regarding their potential impact on clinical decisions. However, given the limitations of current approaches, using algorithms with low to moderate diagnostic accuracy may have a positive influence on clinical outcomes, at least in certain settings. This has been demonstrated for the Neonatal EOS Calculator and the NeoPInS algorithm, which were associated with reduced exposure to antibiotics in late-preterm and term infants with suspected EOS,[82,110] and for real-time display of the HRC index, which led to a decreased mortality in very preterm newborns.[69]

Future Perspectives

It has become clear that the analysis of clinical and molecular markers requires a holistic approach rather than focusing on a single or limited set of markers. The difficulty for clinicians is to estimate the value of all available information to predict the risk of sepsis and sepsis-related adverse outcomes and to use these predictions to optimize decision-making at the bedside in a limited amount of time. Future efforts should include a consensus definition of neonatal sepsis, the development and update of guidelines and bundles, and the discovery and validation of novel clinical and molecular markers and algorithms. Evidence-based international guidelines and bundles are warranted to standardize diagnostic workup and early treatment strategies and will require the support of professional organizations to promote adherence. Although blood culture remains a gold standard, new diagnostic methods are needed to overcome the limited sensitivity and slow turn-around time of traditional microbiology. Research on molecular markers should not focus on inflammation alone but should target early signals, taking into account the heterogeneous nature of sepsis, with the goal to develop tests with high sensitivity and a rapid turn-around time. Advances in technology have led to the development of new monitoring devices. The Signal Instability Index quantifies movement based on analysis of the electrocardiographic waveform. This tool identified decreased spontaneous infant activity corresponding to lethargy hours before clinical suspicion of LOS in very preterm newborns (AUROC = 0.67).[103] Investigation of microcirculatory dysfunction using near-infrared spectroscopy or video microscopic techniques may provide a valuable contribution to early detection of sepsis and risk stratification.[112,113]

The chapter has discussed clinical and molecular markers to guide decisions regarding the start and stop of antibiotics in infants with suspected invasive infection. Clinical and molecular markers also have a potential to guide decisions regarding choice and duration of antimicrobial treatment, fluid management, catecholamines, steroids, and potentially novel adjunctive treatments during sepsis. The term "precision medicine" describes a model where medical decisions and treatments are tailored to the patient's needs using information gathered at different levels, including clinical data and omics (genomics, transcriptomics, proteomics, and metabolomics).[114]

Machine learning can analyze very large datasets on multiple clinical and molecular markers and their interactions and may find signals in combinations of variables that might be otherwise missed. A multimodal machine learning–based approach assessing patient demographics, risk factors, high-resolution clinical markers, results of common laboratory tests, and potentially novel molecular markers, as well as treatments in large cohorts of infants with well-defined phenotypes of microbiologically documented infection and accounting for the heterogeneity and the dynamic nature of sepsis, is required to identify a combination of markers with a high diagnostic accuracy. There is no doubt that, in the future, algorithms will make more accurate predictions than humans, but the performance of algorithms depends on the quality of the data used to train them.[20]

The long-term goal is to design an algorithm that considers baseline incidence, risk factors, and high-resolution clinical and molecular markers to provide a real-time and dynamic assessment of the probability of sepsis and risk of developing adverse outcomes. Such an algorithm will require robust external validation prior to evaluation of the impact of real-time displays on outcomes.

Conclusions

Current approaches based on the assessment of risk factors and clinical signs with or without the use of molecular markers lack both sensitivity and specificity, leading to delays in the initiation of treatment in some and unnecessary exposure to antibiotics in many newborns. Even if our diagnostic tools are imperfect, a structured decision-making framework integrating all available and relevant information is likely to reduce bias and noise. Machine learning–based algorithms will have an important role in guiding medical decisions in the future.

REFERENCES

1. Flannery DD, Ross RK, Mukhopadhyay S, Tribble AC, Puopolo KM, Gerber JS. Temporal trends and center variation in early antibiotic use among premature infants. *JAMA Netw Open*. 2018;1(1):e180164.
2. Schulman J, Benitz WE, Profit J, et al. Newborn antibiotic exposures and association with proven bloodstream infection. *Pediatrics*. 2019;144(5):e20191105.
3. Stark A, Smith PB, Hornik CP, et al. Medication use in the neonatal intensive care unit and changes from 2010 to 2018. *J Pediatr*. 2022;240:66-71.e4.
4. Raymond SL, Rincon JC, Wynn JL, Moldawer LL, Larson SD. Impact of early-life exposures to infections, antibiotics, and vaccines on perinatal and long-term health and disease. *Front Immunol*. 2017;8:729.
5. Schulman J, Dimand RJ, Lee HC, Duenas GV, Bennett MV, Gould JB. Neonatal intensive care unit antibiotic use. *Pediatrics*. 2015;135(5):826-833.
6. Cotten CM, Taylor S, Stoll B, et al. Prolonged duration of initial empirical antibiotic treatment is associated with increased rates of necrotizing enterocolitis and death for extremely low birth weight infants. *Pediatrics*. 2009;123(1):58-66.
7. Schulman J, Profit J, Lee HC, et al. Variations in neonatal antibiotic use. *Pediatrics*. 2018;142(3):e20180115.
8. Payton KSE, Wirtschafter D, Bennett MV, et al. Vignettes identify variation in antibiotic use for suspected early onset sepsis. *Hosp Pediatr*. 2021;11(7):770-774.
9. Giannoni E, Dimopoulou V, Klingenberg C, et al. Analysis of antibiotic exposure and early-onset neonatal sepsis in Europe, North America, and Australia. *JAMA Netw Open*. 2022;5(11):e2243691.
10. van Herk W, el Helou S, Janota J, et al. Variation in current management of term and late-preterm neonates at risk for early-onset sepsis: an international survey and review of guidelines. *Pediatr Infect Dis J*. 2016;35(5):494-500.
11. Mukhopadhyay S, Taylor JA, Von Kohorn I, et al. Variation in sepsis evaluation across a national network of nurseries. *Pediatrics*. 2017;139(3):e20162845.
12. Steinmann KE, Lehnick D, Buettcher M, et al. Impact of empowering leadership on antimicrobial stewardship: a single center study in a neonatal and pediatric intensive care unit and a literature review. *Front Pediatr*. 2018;6:294.
13. Wojcik G, Ring N, McCulloch C, Willis DS, Williams B, Kydonaki K. Understanding the complexities of antibiotic prescribing behaviour in acute hospitals: a systematic review and meta-ethnography. *Arch Public Health*. 2021;79(1):134.
14. Broom J, Broom A. Fear and hierarchy: critical influences on antibiotic decision-making in the operating theatre. *J Hosp Infect*. 2018;99(2):124-126.
15. Broom A, Broom J, Kirby E. Cultures of resistance? A Bourdieusian analysis of doctors' antibiotic prescribing. *Soc Sci Med*. 2014;110:81-88.

16. Charani E, Castro-Sanchez E, Sevdalis N, et al. Understanding the determinants of antimicrobial prescribing within hospitals: the role of "prescribing etiquette." *Clin Infect Dis*. 2013;57(2):188-196.
17. Livorsi D, Comer A, Matthias MS, Perencevich EN, Bair MJ. Factors influencing antibiotic-prescribing decisions among inpatient physicians: a qualitative investigation. *Infect Control Hosp Epidemiol*. 2015;36(9):1065-1072.
18. Teixeira Rodrigues A, Roque F, Falcão A, Figueiras A, Herdeiro MT. Understanding physician antibiotic prescribing behaviour: a systematic review of qualitative studies. *Int J Antimicrob Agents*. 2013;41(3):203-212.
19. Al-Azzawi R, Halvorsen PA, Risør T. Context and general practitioner decision-making– a scoping review of contextual influence on antibiotic prescribing. *BMC Fam Pract*. 2021;22(1):225.
20. Kahneman D, Sibony O, Sunstein CR. *Noise: A Flaw in Human Judgment*. Boston, MA: Little, Brown Spark; 2021.
21. Langford BJ, Daneman N, Leung V, Langford DJ. Cognitive bias: how understanding its impact on antibiotic prescribing decisions can help advance antimicrobial stewardship. *JAC Antimicrob Resist*. 2020;2(4):dlaa107.
22. Fischer JE, Harbarth S, Agthe AG, et al. Quantifying uncertainty: physicians' estimates of infection in critically ill neonates and children. *Clin Infect Dis*. 2004;38(10):1383-1390.
23. Tamma PD, Miller MA, Cosgrove SE. Rethinking how antibiotics are prescribed: incorporating the 4 moments of antibiotic decision making into clinical practice. *JAMA*. 2019;321(2):139-140.
24. Bruns N, Dohna-Schwake C. Antibiotics in critically ill children–a narrative review on different aspects of a rational approach. *Pediatr Res*. 2022;91(2):440-446.
25. Benitz WE, Wynn JL, Polin RA. Reappraisal of guidelines for management of neonates with suspected early-onset sepsis. *J Pediatr*. 2015;166(4):1070-1074.
26. Paul SP, Khattak H, Kini PK, Heaton PA, Goel N. NICE guideline review: neonatal infection: antibiotics for prevention and treatment (NG195). *Arch Dis Child Educ Pract Ed*. 2022;107(4):292-297.
27. Stocker M, Berger C, McDougall J, Giannoni E, Taskforce for the Swiss Society of Neonatology and the Paediatric Infectious Disease Group of Switzerland. Recommendations for term and late preterm infants at risk for perinatal bacterial infection. *Swiss Med Wkly*. 2013;143:w13873.
28. Mukherjee A, Ramalingaiah B, Kennea N, Duffy DA. Management of neonatal early onset sepsis (CG149): compliance of neonatal units in the UK with NICE recommendations. *Arch Dis Child Fetal Neonatal Ed*. 2015;100(2):F185.
29. Litz JE, Goedicke-Fritz S, Härtel C, Zemlin M, Simon A. Management of early- and late-onset sepsis: results from a survey in 80 German NICUs. *Infection*. 2019;47(4):557-564.
30. van der Weijden BM, Achten NB, Bekhof J, et al. Multicentre study found that adherence to national antibiotic recommendations for neonatal early-onset sepsis was low. *Acta Paediatr*. 2021;110(3):791-798.
31. Robson W, Beavis S, Spittle N. An audit of ward nurses' knowledge of sepsis. *Nurs Crit Care*. 2007;12(2):86-92.
32. Groenewoudt M, Roest AA, Leijten FMM, Stassen PM. Septic patients arriving with emergency medical services: a seriously ill population. *Eur J Emerg Med*. 2014;21(5):330-335.
33. Liu VX, Fielding-Singh V, Greene JD, et al. The timing of early antibiotics and hospital mortality in sepsis. *Am J Respir Crit Care Med*. 2017;196(7):856-863.
34. Giannoni E, Agyeman PKA, Stocker M, et al. Neonatal sepsis of early onset, and hospital-acquired and community-acquired late onset: a prospective population-based cohort study. *J Pediatr*. 2018;201:106-114.e4.
35. Köstlin-Gille N, Härtel C, Haug C, et al. Epidemiology of early and late onset neonatal sepsis in very low birthweight infants: data from the German Neonatal Network. *Pediatr Infect Dis J*. 2021;40(3):255-259.
36. Cailes B, Kortsalioudaki C, Buttery J, et al. Epidemiology of UK neonatal infections: the neonIN infection surveillance network. *Arch Dis Child Fetal Neonatal Ed*. 2018;103(6):F547-F553.
37. Bell EF, Hintz SR, Hansen NI, et al. Mortality, in-hospital morbidity, care practices, and 2-year outcomes for extremely preterm infants in the US, 2013–2018. *JAMA*. 2022;327(3):248-263.
38. Schmatz M, Srinivasan L, Grundmeier RW, et al. Surviving sepsis in a referral neonatal intensive care unit: association between time to antibiotic administration and in-hospital outcomes. *J Pediatr*. 2020;217:59-65.e1.
39. Cotten CM. Adverse consequences of neonatal antibiotic exposure. *Curr Opin Pediatr*. 2016;28(2):141-149.
40. Mukhopadhyay S, Lieberman ES, Puopolo KM, Riley LE, Johnson LC. Effect of early-onset sepsis evaluations on in-hospital breastfeeding practices among asymptomatic term neonates. *Hosp Pediatr*. 2015;5(4):203-210.
41. Sourour W, Sanchez V, Sourour M, et al. The association between prolonged antibiotic use in culture negative infants and length of hospital stay and total hospital costs [published online ahead of print May 11, 2021]. *Am J Perinatol*. Available at: https://doi.org/10.1055/s-0041-1729560.
42. Fjalstad JW, Esaiassen E, Juvet LK, van den Anker JN, Klingenberg C. Antibiotic therapy in neonates and impact on gut microbiota and antibiotic resistance development: a systematic review. *J Antimicrob Chemother*. 2018;73(3):569-580.
43. Wan S, Guo M, Zhang T, et al. Impact of exposure to antibiotics during pregnancy and infancy on childhood obesity: a systematic review and meta-analysis. *Obesity (Silver Spring)*. 2020;28(4):793-802.
44. Zhang Z, Wang J, Wang H, et al. Association of infant antibiotic exposure and risk of childhood asthma: a meta-analysis. *World Allergy Organ J*. 2021;14(11):100607.
45. Kamphorst K, Van Daele E, Vlieger AM, Daams JG, Knol J, van Elburg RM. Early life antibiotics and childhood gastrointestinal disorders: a systematic review. *BMJ Paediatr Open*. 2021;5(1):e001028.
46. Uzan-Yulzari A, Turta O, Belogolovski A, et al. Neonatal antibiotic exposure impairs child growth during the first six years of life by perturbing intestinal microbial colonization. *Nat Commun*. 2021;12(1):443.
47. Esaiassen E, Fjalstad JW, Juvet LK, van den Anker JN, Klingenberg C. Antibiotic exposure in neonates and early adverse outcomes: a systematic review and meta-analysis. *J Antimicrob Chemother*. 2017;72(7):1858-1870.
48. Ting JY, Synnes A, Roberts A, et al. Association between antibiotic use and neonatal mortality and morbidities in very low-birth-weight infants without culture-proven sepsis or necrotizing enterocolitis. *JAMA Pediatr*. 2016;170(12):1181-1187.
49. Gensollen T, Iyer SS, Kasper DL, Blumberg RS. How colonization by microbiota in early life shapes the immune system. *Science*. 2016;352(6285):539-544.
50. Klingenberg C, Kornelisse RF, Buonocore G, Maier RF, Stocker M. Culture-negative early-onset neonatal sepsis – at the crossroad between efficient sepsis care and antimicrobial stewardship. *Front Pediatr*. 2018;6:285.
51. Puopolo KM, Draper D, Wi S, et al. Estimating the probability of neonatal early-onset infection on the basis of maternal risk factors. *Pediatrics*. 2011;128(5):e1155-e1163.

52. Kuzniewicz MW, Puopolo KM, Fischer A, et al. A quantitative, risk-based approach to the management of neonatal early-onset sepsis. *JAMA Pediatr*. 2017;171(4):365-371.
53. Kuzniewicz MW, Walsh EM, Li S, Fischer A, Escobar GJ. Development and implementation of an early-onset sepsis calculator to guide antibiotic management in late preterm and term neonates. *Jt Comm J Qual Patient Saf*. 2016;42(5):232-239.
54. Singer M, Deutschman CS, Seymour CW, et al. The Third International Consensus Definitions for Sepsis and Septic Shock (Sepsis-3). *JAMA*. 2016;315(8):801-810.
55. Wynn JL, Kelly MS, Benjamin DK, et al. Timing of multiorgan dysfunction among hospitalized infants with fatal fulminant sepsis. *Am J Perinatol*. 2017;34(7):633-639.
56. Wilson CB, Nizet V, Maldonado YA, Remington JS, Klein JO, eds. *Remington and Klein's Infectious Diseases of the Fetus and Newborn Infant*. 8th ed. Philadelphia, PA: Saunders; 2016.
57. Ussat M, Vogtmann C, Gebauer C, Pulzer F, Thome U, Knüpfer M. The role of elevated central-peripheral temperature difference in early detection of late-onset sepsis in preterm infants. *Early Hum Dev*. 2015;91(12):677-681.
58. Leante-Castellanos JL, Martínez-Gimeno A, Cidrás-Pidré M, Martínez-Munar G, García-González A, Fuentes-Gutiérrez C. Central-peripheral temperature monitoring as a marker for diagnosing late-onset neonatal sepsis. *Pediatr Infect Dis J*. 2017;36(12):e293-e297.
59. Hofer N, Müller W, Resch B. Neonates presenting with temperature symptoms: role in the diagnosis of early onset sepsis. *Pediatr Int*. 2012;54(4):486-490.
60. Bekhof J, Reitsma JB, Kok JH, Van Straaten IHLM. Clinical signs to identify late-onset sepsis in preterm infants. *Eur J Pediatr*. 2013;172(4):501-508.
61. Mahieu LM, De Muynck AO, De Dooy JJ, Laroche SM, Van Acker KJ. Prediction of nosocomial sepsis in neonates by means of a computer-weighted bedside scoring system (NOSEP score). *Crit Care Med*. 2000;28(6):2026-2033.
62. Goldberg O, Sokolover N, Bromiker R, et al. Antibiotic discontinuation 24 h after neonatal late-onset sepsis work-up-a validated decision tree model. *Front Pediatr*. 2021;9:693882.
63. Walker SAN, Cormier M, Elligsen M, et al. Development, evaluation and validation of a screening tool for late onset bacteremia in neonates – a pilot study. *BMC Pediatr*. 2019;19(1):253.
64. Fanaroff AA, Korones SB, Wright LL, et al. Incidence, presenting features, risk factors and significance of late onset septicemia in very low birth weight infants. The National Institute of Child Health and Human Development Neonatal Research Network. *Pediatr Infect Dis J*. 1998;17(7):593-598.
65. Stoll BJ, Puopolo KM, Hansen NI, et al. Early-onset neonatal sepsis 2015 to 2017, the rise of Escherichia coli, and the need for novel prevention strategies. *JAMA Pediatr*. 2020;174(7):e200593.
66. Sullivan BA, Nagraj VP, Berry KL, et al. Clinical and vital sign changes associated with late-onset sepsis in very low birth weight infants at 3 NICUs. *J Neonatal Perinatal Med*. 2021;14(4):553-561.
67. Fleiss N, Coggins SA, Lewis AN, et al. Evaluation of the neonatal sequential organ failure assessment and mortality risk in preterm infants with late-onset infection. *JAMA Netw Open*. 2021;4(2):e2036518.
68. Griffin MP, O'Shea TM, Bissonette EA, Harrell FE, Lake DE, Moorman JR. Abnormal heart rate characteristics preceding neonatal sepsis and sepsis-like illness. *Pediatr Res*. 2003;53(6):920-926.
69. Moorman JR, Carlo WA, Kattwinkel J, et al. Mortality reduction by heart rate characteristic monitoring in very low birth weight neonates: a randomized trial. *J Pediatr*. 2011;159(6):900-906.e1.
70. Fairchild KD, Lake DE, Kattwinkel J, et al. Vital signs and their cross-correlation in sepsis and NEC: a study of 1,065 very-low-birth-weight infants in two NICUs. *Pediatr Res*. 2017;81(2):315-321.
71. Rio L, Ramelet AS, Ballabeni P, Stadelmann C, Asner S, Giannoni E. Monitoring of heart rate characteristics to detect neonatal sepsis. *Pediatr Res*. 2022;92(4):1070-1074.
72. Coggins SA, Weitkamp JH, Grunwald L, et al. Heart rate characteristic index monitoring for bloodstream infection in an NICU: a 3-year experience. *Arch Dis Child Fetal Neonatal Ed*. 2016;101(4):F329-F332.
73. Zeigler AC, Ainsworth JE, Fairchild KD, Wynn JL, Sullivan BA. Sepsis and mortality prediction in very low birth weight infants: analysis of HeRO and nSOFA [published online ahead of print May 10, 2021]. *Am J Perinatol*. Available at: https://doi.org/10.1055/s-0041-1728829.
74. Fairchild K, Mohr M, Paget-Brown A, et al. Clinical associations of immature breathing in preterm infants: part 1–central apnea. *Pediatr Res*. 2016;80(1):21-27.
75. Patel M, Mohr M, Lake D, et al. Clinical associations with immature breathing in preterm infants: part 2–periodic breathing. *Pediatr Res*. 2016;80(1):28-34.
76. Song W, Jung SY, Baek H, Choi CW, Jung YH, Yoo S. A predictive model based on machine learning for the early detection of late-onset neonatal sepsis: development and observational study. *JMIR Med Inform*. 2020;8(7):e15965.
77. Mithal LB, Yogev R, Palac HL, Kaminsky D, Gur I, Mestan KK. Vital signs analysis algorithm detects inflammatory response in premature infants with late onset sepsis and necrotizing enterocolitis. *Early Hum Dev*. 2018;117:83-89.
78. Pierrakos C, Velissaris D, Bisdorff M, Marshall JC, Vincent JL. Biomarkers of sepsis: time for a reappraisal. *Crit Care*. 2020;24(1):287.
79. Cantey JB, Lee JH. Biomarkers for the diagnosis of neonatal sepsis. *Clin Perinatol*. 2021;48(2):215-227.
80. Gawande A. *Better: A Surgeon's Notes on Performance*. Lagos, Nigeria: Metropolitan Publishers; 2007.
81. Benitz WE, Han MY, Madan A, Ramachandra P. Serial serum C-reactive protein levels in the diagnosis of neonatal infection. *Pediatrics*. 1998;102(4):E41.
82. Stocker M, van Herk W, El Helou S, et al. Procalcitonin-guided decision making for duration of antibiotic therapy in neonates with suspected early-onset sepsis: a multicentre, randomised controlled trial (NeoPIns). *Lancet*. 2017;390(10097):871-881.
83. Stocker M, van Herk W, El Helou S, et al. C-reactive protein, procalcitonin, and white blood count to rule out neonatal early-onset sepsis within 36 hours: a secondary analysis of the Neonatal Procalcitonin Intervention Study. *Clin Infect Dis*. 2021;73(2):e383-e390.
84. Cantey JB, Bultmann CR. C-reactive protein testing in late-onset neonatal sepsis: hazardous waste. *JAMA Pediatr*. 2020;174(3):235-236.
85. Newman TB, Puopolo KM, Wi S, Draper D, Escobar GJ. Interpreting complete blood counts soon after birth in newborns at risk for sepsis. *Pediatrics*. 2010;126(5):903-909.
86. Newman TB, Draper D, Puopolo KM, Wi S, Escobar GJ. Combining immature and total neutrophil counts to predict early onset sepsis in term and late preterm newborns: use of the I/T2. *Pediatr Infect Dis J*. 2014;33(8):798-802.

87. Hornik CP, Benjamin DK, Becker KC, et al. Use of the complete blood cell count in late-onset neonatal sepsis. *Pediatr Infect Dis J*. 2012;31(8):803-807.
88. Hornik CP, Benjamin DK, Becker KC, et al. Use of the complete blood cell count in early-onset neonatal sepsis. *Pediatr Infect Dis J*. 2012;31(8):799-802.
89. Tiozzo C, Mukhopadhyay S. Noninfectious influencers of early-onset sepsis biomarkers. *Pediatr Res*. 2022;91(2):425-431.
90. Del Vecchio A, Christensen RD. Neonatal neutropenia: what diagnostic evaluation is needed and when is treatment recommended? *Early Hum Dev*. 2012;88(suppl 2):S19-S24.
91. Schlapbach LJ, Graf R, Woerner A, et al. Pancreatic stone protein as a novel marker for neonatal sepsis. *Intensive Care Med*. 2013;39(4):754-763.
92. Ruan L, Chen GY, Liu Z, et al. The combination of procalcitonin and C-reactive protein or presepsin alone improves the accuracy of diagnosis of neonatal sepsis: a meta-analysis and systematic review. *Crit Care*. 2018;22(1):316.
93. Grover V, Pantelidis P, Soni N, et al. A biomarker panel (Bioscore) incorporating monocytic surface and soluble TREM-1 has high discriminative value for ventilator-associated pneumonia: a prospective observational study. *PLoS One*. 2014;9(10):e109686.
94. Kim H, Hur M, Moon HW, Yun YM, Di Somma S, GREAT Network. Multi-marker approach using procalcitonin, presepsin, galectin-3, and soluble suppression of tumorigenicity 2 for the prediction of mortality in sepsis. *Ann Intensive Care*. 2017;7(1):27.
95. Kaforou M, Herberg JA, Wright VJ, Coin LJM, Levin M. Diagnosis of bacterial infection using a 2-transcript host RNA signature in febrile infants 60 days or younger. *JAMA*. 2017;317(15): 1577-1578.
96. Mahajan P, Kuppermann N, Mejias A, et al. Association of RNA biosignatures with bacterial infections in febrile infants aged 60 days or younger. *JAMA*. 2016;316(8):846-857.
97. Graspeuntner S, Waschina S, Künzel S, et al. Gut dysbiosis with bacilli dominance and accumulation of fermentation products precedes late-onset sepsis in preterm infants. *Clin Infect Dis*. 2019;69(2):268-277.
98. Berkhout DJC, Niemarkt HJ, de Boer NKH, Benninga MA, de Meij TGJ. The potential of gut microbiota and fecal volatile organic compounds analysis as early diagnostic biomarker for necrotizing enterocolitis and sepsis in preterm infants. *Expert Rev Gastroenterol Hepatol*. 2018;12(5):457-470.
99. Niemarkt HJ, De Meij TG, van Ganzewinkel CJ, et al. Necrotizing enterocolitis, gut microbiota, and brain development: role of the brain-gut axis. *Neonatology*. 2019;115(4):423-431.
100. Berkhout DJC, van Keulen BJ, Niemarkt HJ, et al. Late-onset sepsis in preterm infants can be detected preclinically by fecal volatile organic compound analysis: a prospective, multicenter cohort study. *Clin Infect Dis*. 2019;68(1):70-77.
101. Duvoisin G, Fischer C, Maucort-Boulch D, Giannoni E. Reduction in the use of diagnostic tests in infants with risk factors for early-onset neonatal sepsis does not delay antibiotic treatment. *Swiss Med Wkly*. 2014;144:w13981.
102. Mukherjee A, Davidson L, Anguvaa L, Duffy DA, Kennea N. NICE neonatal early onset sepsis guidance: greater consistency, but more investigations, and greater length of stay. *Arch Dis Child Fetal Neonatal Ed*. 2015;100(3):F248-F249.
103. Joshi R, Kommers D, Oosterwijk L, Feijs L, van Pul C, Andriessen P. Predicting neonatal sepsis using features of heart rate variability, respiratory characteristics, and ECG-derived estimates of infant motion. *IEEE J Biomed Health Inform*. 2020; 24(3):681-692.
104. Mahieu LM, De Dooy JJ, Cossey VR, et al. Internal and external validation of the NOSEP prediction score for nosocomial sepsis in neonates. *Crit Care Med*. 2002;30(7):1459-1466.
105. Stocker M, Daunhawer I, van Herk W, et al. Machine learning used to compare the diagnostic accuracy of risk factors, clinical signs and biomarkers and to develop a new prediction model for neonatal early-onset sepsis. *Pediatr Infect Dis J*. 2022;41(3):248-254.
106. Masino AJ, Harris MC, Forsyth D, et al. Machine learning models for early sepsis recognition in the neonatal intensive care unit using readily available electronic health record data. *PLoS One*. 2019;14(2):e0212665.
107. Hofer N, Müller W, Resch B. Definitions of SIRS and sepsis in correlation with early and late onset neonatal sepsis. *J Pediatr Intensive Care*. 2012;1(1):17-23.
108. Coggins S, Harris MC, Grundmeier R, Kalb E, Nawab U, Srinivasan L. Performance of pediatric systemic inflammatory response syndrome and organ dysfunction criteria in late-onset sepsis in a quaternary neonatal intensive care unit: a case-control study. *J Pediatr*. 2020;219:133-139.e1.
109. Wynn JL, Polin RA. A neonatal sequential organ failure assessment score predicts mortality to late-onset sepsis in preterm very low birth weight infants. *Pediatr Res*. 2020;88(1): 85-90.
110. Achten NB, Klingenberg C, Benitz WE, et al. Association of use of the neonatal early-onset sepsis calculator with reduction in antibiotic therapy and safety: a systematic review and meta-analysis. *JAMA Pediatr*. 2019;173(11):1032-1040.
111. Achten NB, Plötz FB, Klingenberg C, et al. Stratification of culture-proven early-onset sepsis cases by the neonatal early-onset sepsis calculator: an individual patient data meta-analysis. *J Pediatr*. 2021;234:77-84.e8.
112. Ng NYY, Ang HHE, Tan JCL, Ho WH, Kuan WS, Chua MT. Evaluation for occult sepsis incorporating NIRS and emergency sonography. *Am J Emerg Med*. 2018;36(11):1957-1963.
113. Erdem Ö, Ince C, Tibboel D, Kuiper JW. Assessing the microcirculation with handheld vital microscopy in critically ill neonates and children: evolution of the technique and its potential for critical care. *Front Pediatr*. 2019;7:273.
114. Ng S, Strunk T, Jiang P, Muk T, Sangild PT, Currie A. Precision medicine for neonatal sepsis. *Front Mol Biosci*. 2018;5:70.

Index

Page numbers followed by "*f*" indicate figures, and "*t*" indicate tables.